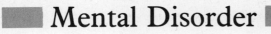 # Mental Disorder

ITS CARE AND TREATMENT

The Dyke

I have met a fortunate few
Who have never been aware that it existed;
That it stood, safely encircling their lives.
They have managed to survive, their certainties intact,
Their skies as blue as when they were first fathomed.

Taken for granted, like health and husbands,
You only notice it when the first breach appears.
The black waters enter, trickling in rivulets
And patterning the land with dark threads
Or, as the case may be, crashing across the walls,
Breaking them down and covering the fields.

When the tide ebbs, as all tides must,
The dyke will be re-built, as all dykes must
Or, as the case may be, simply patched up.
The salt mud must be made fertile.
In time, with work, or alternatively,
Without appearing to bother very much,
New grasses grow—even a few trees.

It will not happen again. The dyke is stronger,
Built to withstand further destruction.
The builder knows his apple trees will bloom;
That in the autumn fruit will appear and fall
Just as it did before, only the taste
Will have altered.
And in blossom time it will be necessary
To view the flowers from a different perspective.

Jenny Morgan

With kind permission of the publisher, MTP Press.

Mental Disorder

ITS CARE AND TREATMENT

Jack Lyttle

RMN, RGN, DN(Lond.), RNT
Senior Tutor (Psychiatry)
Inverclyde and Bute College of
Nursing and Midwifery, Greenock;
National Board for Nursing
Midwifery and Health Visiting (Scotland)

Baillière Tindall London Philadelphia Toronto
Mexico City Rio de Janeiro Sydney Tokyo Hong Kong

Baillière Tindall   1 St Anne's Road
W. B. Saunders   Eastbourne, East Sussex BN21 3UN, England

West Washington Square
Philadelphia, PA 19105, USA

1 Goldthorne Avenue
Toronto, Ontario M8Z 5T9, Canada

Apartado 26370—Cedro 512
Mexico 4, DF Mexico

Rua Evaristo da Veiga, 55, 20° andar
Rio de Janeiro—RJ, Brazil

ABP Australia Ltd, 44–50 Waterloo Road
North Ryde, NSW 2113, Australia

Ichibancho Central Building, 22–1 Ichibancho
Chiyoda-ku, Tokyo 102, Japan

10/fl, Inter-Continental Plaza, 94 Granville Road
Tsim Sha Tsui East, Kowloon, Hong Kong

First published 1986

Typeset by Phoenix Photosetting, Chatham
Printed and bound in Great Britain
by Mackays of Chatham Ltd, Kent

British Library Cataloguing in Publication Data

Lyttle, Jack
  Mental disorder: its care and treatment.
  1. Psychiatry   2. Psychiatric nursing
  I. Title
  616.89′0024613   RC484

ISBN 0–7020–1158–4

Contents

Preface

In recent years the emphasis in psychiatric care has changed very considerably. Uncritical adherence to the medical model of mental disorder has largely been replaced by broader social perspectives incorporating a skills-orientated approach to care. These changes have major implications for health care professionals as the task-orientated approach which all too often underpinned the medical model is gradually being replaced by an orientation that sees the role of the helping professions as an active and dynamic one which recognizes and responds to the individuality of clients. This changing climate is reflected in statements of educational philosophy like the training syllabus for psychiatric nurses (English and Welsh National Boards, 1982) and is also apparent at the level of practice.

To admit someone to a psychiatric hospital or unit is a major step and it is no longer defensible, on either moral or scientific grounds, to thereafter complacently subscribe to a simple regime of labelling followed by medication and sporadic involvements in recreation or industrial 'therapy' in the belief that the client's circumstances will somehow magically improve. Intervention should clearly specify problems and the psychological and psychiatric literature has long since specified a wide range of simple but effective skills which will rapidly yield positive results with a wide range of client groups. The passive and therapeutically inactive view of psychiatric nursing which was implicit in the custodial approach to care, no matter how well meaning this was, is gradually being replaced by a positive and therapeutically active approach to psychiatric nursing based on the acquisition and development of a live body of skills.

Though the focus of psychiatric care is moving steadily from hospital to community, training schemes have yet to reflect this adequately and this book is therefore largely aimed at nurses receiving hospital-based training. Some of the traditional language of medicine (e.g. 'patient', 'clinical features' and 'treatment') has been retained, largely for the purpose of expediency, though this should not be construed as an unthinking endorsement of the medical model. The book has two main aims: (1) it serves as an introduction to the principles of psychiatry, which is largely conventional in structure but which is not uncritical and which is eclectic in approach, and (2) it serves as an introduction to the principles of nursing care, which is patient-centred and which loosely adopts the format of the nursing process. I have avoided the rigid specification of desirable outcomes as to do so would deny the individuality of the client and would fail to recognize the process of continual growth and development in which our clients are involved.

The book is primarily a core text for psychiatric nurses in training, though it is hoped that it will be of value to qualified staff and to general nurses receiving psychiatric experience as well as to members of other mental health care professions (e.g. trainee social workers).

The coverage of the principles of psychiatry should obviate the need to buy an ancillary psychiatric test against which to set the skills specified.

Lastly acknowledgements are due to the many people who have provided help and inspiration throughout the gestation period of this book. Graham Smith (formerly of Baillière Tindall) provided the initial impetus and his support and enthusiasm guided me through the early conceptual period and ensured that the idea for this book became a reality. Rosemary Morris of Baillière Tindall continued the process and acted as a midwife as the book's development continued. Brian McNamee read the sections on treatment in particular and provided valuable feedback on the manuscript as a whole. Tom McClymont patiently and diligently excavated library material for me, and Mrs E. Vardy typed the manuscript (showing remarkable skill in deciphering my hieroglyphic handwriting). Lastly, many of my students, too numerous to mention, commented on drafts of the manuscript and provided useful feedback, and Judith Spence carefully studied the manuscript and produced sensitive and imaginative illustrations to accompany the text. To all of these my sincere thanks.

Jack Lyttle

I

BASIC CONCEPTS

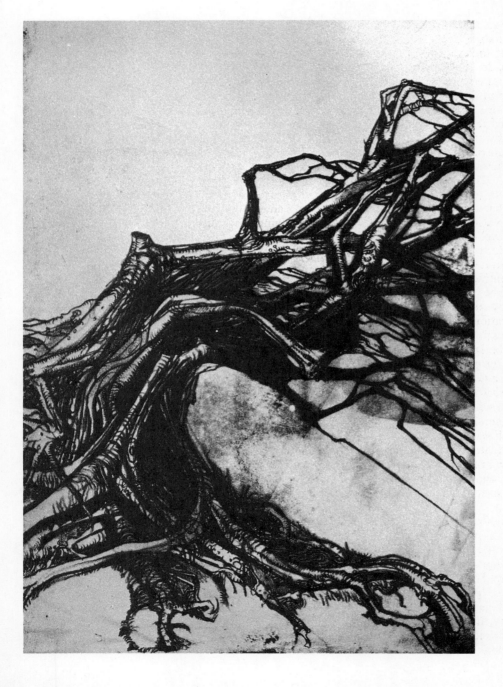

What is Mental Disorder?

> What we do about a problem is determined very largely by how we view that problem.
>
> *D. L. Davies.*

Physical Health and Illness

To most of us health and illness are familiar and important concepts. Health is that happy state of well-being which we tend to take for granted when younger and cautiously foster as we grow older.

But what is health? For most people the desirable and sought after state of health is commensurate with a smoothly functioning body, and the pursuit of health tends to involve servicing and grooming this complex and sophisticated organic machine with a fervour and energy which underlines the social importance of remaining healthy.

We wash, feed and clothe our bodies. We try to accentuate its desirable characteristics and glumly contemplate its less attractive features in the mirror. The importance and desirability of maintaining our bodies is stressed by shrill and urgent reminders from the advertising media. We must not smoke. We must eat the 'right' foods. We must eradicate our adolescent pimples and reduce our thickening waistlines. Those unspeakable spectres 'body odour' and 'bad breath' may be exorcised by having recourse to an armoury of deodorants and mouth-washes. 'Research scientists' selflessly labour in their laboratories to produce 'pH-balanced protein shampoos' and substances designed to free the human race from the ravages of dandruff. Television commercials feature young women who testify to the efficacy of these products, displaying relief and gratitude of the magnitude one would expect to be displayed to a surgeon by a patient who has been spared the prospect of an imminent and painful demise by the exercise of heroic medical skill.

When we smile we must reveal white and attractive teeth, and exercise is essential if we are to remain slim and sexually attractive. Thinning hair is frantically disguised and adverts for hair restorers and toupees abound.

Body maintenance can thus involve the expenditure of large amounts of time, energy and money and the types of activity involved vary according to the dictates of fashion.

A brief consideration of the above range of 'maintenance activities' will reveal that concepts of health transcend the purely physical. Psychological and social factors play a major part in our quest for 'health'. To be healthy is to be attractive and to be attractive is to be healthy.

We described health as a state of 'well-being' and most of us are uncomfortably aware that our psychological and social well-being is largely dependent upon the judgements of others. What others think of us may, to a greater or lesser extent, determine what we think of ourselves. If the responses of others—our social 'feedback'—indicate that we are regarded as being popular, attractive, accomplished and intelligent then we happily incorporate this gratifying information in our view of self and we can function in a relaxed and confident manner in most social settings, secure in the knowledge that we are not only accepted, and acceptable, but perhaps even admired in some ways. But if the social feedback obtained from others suggests that we are unattractive, unpopular, gauche or even stupid then this unpalatable information will be incorporated to produce a negative self-image. We may attempt to eradicate our perceived unattractiveness by improving our 'presentation of self'. We may have recourse to cosmetics and fashionable clothes and hair styles. We may learn a foreign language, take up hang-gliding, improve our vocabularies or our knowledge of music or current affairs. Attempts at improving our feeling of well-being may also include dieting, exercise or efforts to stop smoking.

Thus our sought after sense of well-being is both fragile and complex and involves dimensions other than the purely physical. The elusive nature of the concept of health is reflected in the definition offered by the World Health Organization, which suggests that health is a state of 'ideal physical, psychological

3

and social well-being and not merely the absence of disease'. Unfortunately no attempt is made to describe these ideal states.

What then of disease or illness? Surely the issues are clearer here? Illness implies loss or disturbance of function and may range from discomfort to incapacity, disability and death. We may, however, be comforted by the knowledge that doctors and nurses and other highly trained professionals—fluent in the mysteries of the body—are available to alleviate or cure illness and discomfort, backed by a formidable array of medical technology.

Thus we tend our bodies as best we can, motivated by physical, psychological and social impulses, and hopefully present any malfunctions beyond our control to the caste of professional healers.

Mental Health and Illness

But what of our minds? Our mind cannot be studied in a mirror. It cannot be groomed and maintained by recourse to cosmetics, exercise or dietary supplements. How then are we to know it and maintain it in a desirable state of well-being? How will we recognize mental disability and incapacity? and How may we deal with this if it arises?

Our everyday body awareness and maintenance activities unfortunately have no mental parallel. There is no psychological equivalent of the 'health food' shop.

Most people are only vaguely aware of the concept of mental disorder and have distorted images of this area of disability, which are coloured by fear and prejudice. People tend to avoid that which they fear, and mental illness is the disorder which most people perhaps fear more than any other, and this fear is often reflected in popular images of mental disorder.

Society has often shunned and segregated the mentally disordered, and sufferers may be treated as social lepers, as being socially 'unclean'. Sufferers may also be regarded as dangerous, alarming and unpredictably erratic. Myths and stereotypes of the 'lunatic' and 'madman' still abound and considerable stigma is still unfortunately attached to the label of mental illness. The treatment of the 'madman' in literature and the media exaggerates and perpetuates these negative stereotypes. Hollywood has made much capital from distorted and lurid accounts of madness, and has often presented the

madman as a violent and incomprehensible creature who poses a threat to the fabric of society. Ophelia floating to her watery grave bedecked with flowers and King Lear cursing the thunderstorm are familiar images of madness which capture the essentially 'alien' quality of the condition.

Small wonder that we tend to relax comfortably in our beds at night, secure in the knowledge that the mentally disordered are safely segregated in mental hospitals, cut off from the rest of society, from the mentally healthy majority.

But are the mentally ill so incomprehensibly different? If the average 'mentally healthy' person were to inspect their mind and try to become as familiar with it as they are with their body they would perhaps realize that the mentally ill are not as alien as they at first appear. We have all experienced fear, anxiety, depression, anger and suspicion and many of us have experienced life crises, or problems in living, which have disturbed our psychological and social equilibrium to a greater or lesser degree. Life may have had its 'ups and downs' and our social functioning may have been much more effective at some times than at others. The wall of complacency, from behind which we view the mentally ill, may be readily breached by stress.

In other words our social and psychological well-being is not constant but may fluctuate to a greater degree than our physical well-being. Extreme fluctuation may constitute mental disorder if it impairs our capacity to cope with the demands of everyday living.

The Difficulties of Describing Mental Health

The concept of mental health is thus difficult to reduce to a simple operational definition, and is best described cautiously. We cannot with any confidence draw a simple dividing line and insist that those characteristics falling on one side are invariably to be found only in the mentally disordered and those on the other are only to be found in the mentally healthy.

Most of us would confidently identify extreme mental disorder as 'madness', just as we would identify happiness and adjustment as evidence of 'mental health'. However, between the confusion and despair of mental illness and the peace and contentment of mental health, there stretches a wide gulf of unhappiness and maladjustment wherein we can be less sure of our perspectives. In this intermediate area the language of sociology and psychology may more usefully describe the landscape than that of medicine, despite conventional reference to 'mental illness' and 'mental health'.

This zone, intermediate between 'true madness' and 'normality', will produce many examples which may be disturbingly familiar to many people. Consider, for example, the depressed or anxious young housewife, the insomniac who cannot sleep without a tablet, the overstressed businessman who is losing control over his alcohol consumption, the truanting and 'glue-sniffing' school child, the tormented homosexual, the elderly person with failing memory and powers of concentration, the person who incessantly visits the doctor with vague aches and pains and minor complaints for which no specific cause can be found and the girl who invariably responds to stress with a 'sick headache'. Most people would agree that these individuals have a 'problem' but would shrink from describing them as 'mad' and may even hesitate to describe them as 'ill' in the conventional sense. What then has happened to these people? Are they 'ill', 'odd' or 'unhappy'?

I remember once walking along a desolate clifftop in the Hebrides. It was a cold and lonely place, scoured by strong winds blowing in from the open sea. A few trees struggled for existence in this hostile environment, warped by the forces of nature. The trees had been subject to the prevailing sea winds which reached gale force in winter and had, in consequence, grown leaning at an unnatural angle away from the sea, bowed by the gale. Others were small and stunted, undernourished by the barren and stony soil. So it may be with people. Constant stress, like the gale, may produce the response of distorted behavioural patterns as the individual leans away from stress into the defensive posture of neurosis. Poor psychological and social soil, devoid of love, affection, fulfilment and parental or environmental security may produce the stunted growths of personality disorder or maladjustment.

People, like trees, need good strong roots and a healthy climate in order to flourish. In a small percentage of mental disorders the seed itself may be faulty—there may be genetic factors—and the resultant growth may be neither vigorous nor symmetrical.

So far we have identified the fact that the mentally ill are not always incomprehensibly different from the mentally healthy, insofar as many common char-

acteristics interpenetrate both groups. Differentiation between both groups must take place if identification and treatment of mental disorder is to take place, but such differentiation should not be based on the stark assumption that mental disorder is the polar opposite of mental health and is thus remote from the comprehension of the non-sufferer.

Neurosis, the commonest form of mental disorder, often takes the form of distortions or exaggerations of 'normal' responses like anxiety or depression. There is no loss of contact with reality, although reality may be perceived in a distorted way or experienced as threatening.

In the group of major mental disorders known as the psychoses—for example, schizophrenia or manic depressive psychosis—contact with reality may be impaired or transiently lost completely. Nevertheless many of the contributory factors, and perhaps some of the causative factors, may be located within familiar areas of family dynamics and social experience. The psychoses tend to run a relapsing/remitting course; that is they tend to be characterized by relapses when the condition worsens, and remissions when the condition improves. The psychoses also show a tendency to chronicity but treatment can quickly control relapses and may prevent their reoccurrence. Treatment may maintain the sufferer from psychosis in a state of remission wherein the features of the underlying chronic disorder may be indiscernible or may only faintly colour the behaviour and responses of the individual.

Thus the belief that the mentally disordered are irretrievably estranged from the mainstream of human understanding and experience is a fiction which militates against positive understanding and treatment of their condition.

If we are to develop our understanding as a bridge between the mentally disordered and the mentally healthy, we must critically examine the language and concepts used in this area of study.

Social Dimensions of Health

Even a cursory examination will reveal that illness and health are not unmistakable categories, despite casual everyday use of the terms.

The American sociologist Eliot Freidson (1973) makes a distinction between illness as a 'biophysical state' and illness as a 'social state'. Illness as a biophysical state refers to abnormalities in biological functioning which are independent of values and judgements, for example a fractured bone exists—it is there—irrespective of people's beliefs about fractures. Biological disorders of this nature may also be described as *disease*.

By contrast, illness as a *social* state is inextricably bound up with people's beliefs, values and moral judgements. The norms of health and sickness are social and cultural norms, in the sense that in given societies, at given times, general agreement exists among its members as to what is health and what is sickness. A condition may be regarded as illness in one society and not in another. For example one South American tribe places great value on a condition regarded as a disease by Western doctors—without the brightly coloured spots on the skin, caused by dyschromic spirochaetosis, members of the tribe are regarded as unattractive and are unlikely to secure a good marriage (Dubois, 1965). Conversely, sweaty armpits, a condition regarded as a social nuisance by Westerners, often necessitates hospital treatment in Japan and is a legitimate reason for exemption from compulsory military service (Baker, 1974). Similarly an investigation of Zulu women revealed a syndrome of screaming, in which the victim might yelp for days or weeks. Fifty per cent of a large sample (616) of women were 'screamers' but were regarded as being quite normal. Thirty per cent of these women also experienced visual and auditory hallucinations; that is they had 'visions' and heard 'voices', but these hallucinations were regarded as legitimate within the context of their culture (Lee, 1961).

In medieval Europe there were many accounts of women 'hearing voices'. If the 'voices' conveyed messages from God (as in the case of Joan of Arc) or if the individual concerned experienced 'visions' of angels or celestial scenes, then they might well be regarded with awe and venerated as a saint. If the 'voices' and 'visions' were of a sexual nature then the individual concerned was liable to be regarded with alarm and revulsion and burned as a witch. The critical factor was not simply the presence of disordered perceptions; the important factor was the response of the social audience to their content. Nowadays both groups would be likely to be regarded as being ill.

The element of strong social values is particularly apparent in the consideration of mental illness and mental health. It is perhaps comforting to the majority of people to realize that the deviant who is eccentric or threatening, in comparison to the mass of his fellows, can be identified as being 'ill' and can even be 'treated' and perhaps 'cured'. In the absence or impossibility of 'cure' he can at least be safely relegated to the anonymity of the mental hospital, thus keeping those who are out of mind out of sight.

Deviance and Disease

Deviance consists of a departure from culturally accepted norms, and a deviant is one who makes such a departure and thus incurs the censure of the social 'audience'. Such departures are an integral part of many mental disorders and we have thus created the risk that eccentric, disturbing or incomprehensible behaviour may be labelled as 'illness'. Not all deviations from accepted norms are regarded as illness; some are regarded as criminality, wickedness, bad manners, heresy, sin, betrayal or madness. Sociologists have commented that there has been an increasing shift towards regarding an increased number of deviant responses as illness. In other words there has been a progressive 'medicalization' of deviance.

This trend has led the British psychiatrist Anthony Clare (1976) to suggest acidly that it seems that

The mentally healthy person is not a nuisance, does not challenge the rules, lose his temper, kick the cat, or park his car on a double yellow line. He makes no demands, passes his life quietly and productively and does not fiddle the social security, live with a mistress, or wear placards warning that the end of the world is nigh.

There is thus a risk that psychiatry may venture far from the traditions of physical medicine to colonize and control many strictly non-medical areas of social concern. The 'medicalization' and 'psychiatricization' of social problems has proceeded apace. The 'bad' may have become confused with the 'mad'.

Pearson (1975) has commented as follows:

'Crime, it is said, is an illness; youthful unrest is a maturational phase; political dissent is the result of personality quirks of "mindless militants"; a poor employment record flows from a disorder of character; poor families, or "problem" families are low on something called "interpersonal maturity".'

Many concerned observers thus feel that the 'medicalization' of deviance may create a state of affairs in which society can dispose of its dissidents by labelling them as 'mentally ill' and by suggesting that they be treated by psychiatrists and psychiatric nurses. This danger becomes particularly apparent when one considers the use of psychiatrists as a 'soft police force' in the USSR, and the resultant labelling of political deviants as 'mad'.

The deviance debate is very topical and will rapidly become familiar to any newcomer to the literature of psychiatry.

While we must temper our considerations of mental disorder with an awareness of the difficulties involved, we may also console ourselves with an awareness of the fact that there is little dispute about the plight of the mentally disordered. The torment of psychosis, the crushing weight of depression and the myriad wounds that mental disorder can inflict necessitate intervention, care and support until function returns and the individual can again cope with everyday living. The debate centres around causation and treatment and the 'grey areas' of those disorders which are not regarded as a problem by the person concerned or by a significant proportion of social observers. As a medical sociologist recently commented: 'When the so-called "hard cases" such as homosexuality are ceasing to be regarded as abnormal, one must be all the more sceptical about such "soft cases" as the personality disorders.' (Pearson, 1975)

The deviance debate certainly underlines the fact that workers in the field of mental disorder should try to avoid using their own value systems and moral beliefs to judge the actions and feelings of others.

Dimensions of Mental Health

So far we have identified the fact that the layman's concept of mental disorder may be distorted by fear and prejudice which may render understanding of the condition difficult. We have also discussed the fact that the category of 'illness' may not be as unmistakable as it at first seems, and that it may be inappropriate to many forms of mental disorder. The concept of deviance may serve to make this clearer. Many, if not most, mental 'illnesses' may be more appropriately viewed as social rather than medical disorders. Health, like illness, has many social dimensions which make its unambiguous defi-

nition difficult. This is particularly true of mental health. Nevertheless an attempt must be made to outline the suggested dimensions of mental health if any clarity of perspective is to be achieved.

Wright and Taylor (1970) list some commonly used criteria for 'normality' or mental health. These are as follows:

Happiness. Unhappiness is often the presenting feature of mental disorder and the gravity of the disorder may be assessed in terms of the degree of unhappiness it causes in the sufferer. There may be a close relationship between unhappiness and other evidence of mental disorder.

Unhappiness may be a necessary and acceptable response to the life situation of the individual—for example in grief and sympathy for others. It can, however, be regarded as evidence of disorder if it is disproportionately increased in quantity or quality—to the point of causing incapacity and enduring feelings of misery.

Efficiency. The mentally healthy person is said to display efficiency in applying his drives to fulfilling his needs satisfactorily, whether the needs are physical, psychological or social. In mental disorder, much mental energy is often directed inwardly in a way that creates internal friction and tensions at the expense of efficiency. Efficiency may be noticeably lacking in the common disorders of depression and anxiety.

Lack of anxiety. Anxiety is probably the chief component of a wide range of mental disorders, particularly the neuroses, and is often accompanied by well-marked and distressing physical symptoms. These symptoms include sweating, tension with tremors, visual disturbances, headache, 'palpitations', gastric disturbances and impairment of sleep and appetite.

Anxiety may be considered as 'fear spread thin' and, like unhappiness, may be justified—for example, examination anxiety in students or the anxiety evoked by an impending visit to the dentist.

Anxiety becomes abnormal when it permeates the inner life of the individual in a lasting and incapacitating way that cannot be explained by simple reference to external events. For example anxiety may be generated by previously unthreatening objects or situations (phobic anxiety) or when the sufferer is unaware of the reason for his anxiety (free-floating anxiety).

The mentally healthy person copes with the anxieties of everyday life without disintegration or lasting incapacity.

Lack of guilt. Guilt may reflect a need for self-punishment which may eventually become socially incapacitating if uncontrolled. Guilt is again a natural response to many situations and only becomes a problem if it becomes so pervasive as to cause incapacitating tensions with associated loss of efficiency. Equally abnormal is the individual who is incapable of guilt responses. This may be a distinguishing feature of the psychopath who lacks internal controls and is incapable of feeling guilt or remorse for his antisocial actions.

Maturity. Freud suggested that we develop from an early stage of inner disorganization in which we gratify our needs and drives without an awareness of the effects of our actions on other people. He suggested that this infantile stage was governed by the 'Pleasure Principle'. Maturity suggested movement towards the development of internal controls, of a 'conscience', as we become aware of the fact that our behaviour affects other people. We learn to forego or postpone instinctual gratification as our social awareness develops and we mature to live according to the 'Reality Principle'.

Maturity is not synonymous with the dissipation of self-seeking infantile drives but with their regulation—they linger on in the mature adult but are controlled.

The frustrated or stressed adult may revert to immature behavioural patterns, reminiscent of his childhood behaviour; that is, he may show *regression*. Excessive dependence and immaturity may be a feature of neurosis.

The sociopath (psychopath) does not seem to have developed those internal controls which give rise to behaviourally regulating feelings of guilt and remorse. His behaviour may be considered as immature insofar as he has not made an effective transition from Pleasure to Reality Principle and thus remains locked in impulsive and self-gratifying patterns of behaviour without regard for the consequences of his actions on other people.

Adjustment. Adjustment refers to the individual's capacity to adjust to the demands of society in a flexible and resilient way. This criterion implies the capacity to adjust to the demands of society in a productive and adaptable way.

Loss of adjustment and adaptability may be very apparent in the social disintegration of psychosis.

Autonomy and self-esteem. Autonomy implies independence; self-control, self-sufficiency and self-esteem imply a healthy awareness of one's positive attributes and a realistic feeling of a confidence in these attributes. The two contribute to a positive image of self.

Lack of self-sufficiency and self-esteem may be very noticeable in depression and many other mental disorders.

The ability to establish adequate emotional bonds with others. This is perhaps the cement which holds together the fabric of society and it may be noticeably lacking in the emotional impoverishment and social isolation of schizophrenia. The capacity for love and friendship is perhaps central to effective social functioning.

The psychopath is often shallow and insincere in the area of relationships and may simply 'use' others in a very manipulative way.

Contact with reality. The individual can be expected, if 'normal', to cope adequately with the realities of his group and of society and to perceive these in an undistorted way. The psychotic, however, may withdraw into an inner 'reality' in which he loses touch with the world of the observer. The boundaries of reality may become blurred and indistinct to the sufferer of psychosis and he may be unable to distinguish aspects of inner reality from external or 'true' reality; that is, 'reality testing' may be impaired.

This major symptom of mental disorder may be revealed by the disordered thought processes of the sufferer of psychosis, which indicate disordered perceptions of reality. The psychotic may express false, unshakeable beliefs which are quite unamenable to logic, these being known as *delusions*. He may, for example, express the belief that he is the victim of a conspiracy to murder him—the nurses and medical staff perhaps being considered as parties to the conspiracy—or he may believe that he is suffering from incurable illnesses, despite medical evidence to the contrary, the illnesses being imagined as punishment for imagined past misdeeds.

Thus mental health, like mental illness, has many dimensions, none of which are fixed. Our levels of happiness, adjustment, self-esteem and autonomy may fluctuate with our life circumstances, and our mental landscape is not a level plain, with health at one extreme and illness at the other. Rather it is a mountainous and sharply graduated terrain marked by the peaks of happiness and fulfilment between which lie the hollows and swamps of insecurity and unhappiness. The gulfs of mental disorder may well appear in anyone's inner landscape.

The Classification of Mental Disorder

Mental disorder is not one disorder. Rather, the term includes many categories of disorder which are divided into four major groups which we may briefly introduce at this point—neurosis, psychosis, personality disorder and mental handicap.

Neurosis (Psychoneurosis)

The neuroses constitute the commonest group of mental disorders, though the nurse is unlikely to encounter many clear-cut neurotic states amongst the in-patient population of the psychiatric hospital. Some neuroses are self-limiting and tend to resolve with changes in life circumstances, with or without the aid of the general practitioner who may prescribe drugs to reduce anxiety or alleviate depression. Others may be seen as out-patients or may attend hospital as day patients. These categories aside, there is probably a large pool of neurosis in the community in respect of which intervention is not made, as the individuals concerned cope with everyday living though fluctuations in mood and efficiency may be apparent to family and friends. The neuroses should not be regarded as trivial, however, as incapacitating levels of unhappiness and torment may well be caused by some of them.

The neuroses are essentially exaggerations of normal responses, for example depression, the psychiatric equivalent of the common cold, and anxiety, the psychiatric equivalent of headache, in terms of its prevalence. Responses like anxiety and depression should not always be regarded as evidence of illness or disorder as they may be justified by external circumstances and are usually self-limiting.

Many, if not most, of us are neurotic to a certain degree and within socially acceptable limits. We all have our idiosyncrasies and quirks of personality which may mimic neurosis on a miniature scale.

Neurosis becomes a fully blown disorder when it becomes incapacitating, as it interferes with interpersonal relationships and impairs efficiency and happiness.

There is no loss of contact with reality in neurosis—reality testing remains unimpaired and the patient retains *insight*; that is, he is aware that his functioning is impaired and may actively seek help. Personality is not disorganized, though behaviour may be greatly affected, but usually remains within socially acceptable limits despite arousing comment.

The adjective 'neurotic' has unfortunately become widely used by laymen to describe behaviour or personality characteristics of which they disapprove; the meaning of the term has thus become blurred due to its widespread use as a singularly inappropriate term of censure. Strictly speaking the term refers to recognizable and treatable responses to stress or anxiety which have affected the individual's functioning without causing disorganization of personality or loss of insight or contact with reality, though much interpersonal and social disorganization may result.

The commonest types of neurotic response are anxiety, depression, obsessive compulsive and hysteria.

Anxiety

This may be *free-floating* (with no discernible or indentifiable 'trigger' for the anxiety) or it may assume the form of a *phobia* (an exaggerated fear of a specific object or situation e.g. a phobic fear of insects or open spaces).

Depression

Depression becomes a disorder when it persists to the extent that it seems unshakeable and begins to impair efficiency.

Neurotic depression is often called *reactive* depression as it is often an unusually severe and disabling reaction to a discernible factor in the life circumstances of the patient. Precipitating factors include divorce, bereavement, chronic physical illness, unemployment and many other familiar stress factors.

Neurotic depression should not be confused with *endogenous* depression, which is a psychosis and is much more damaging in its effects on thinking and personality and has no discernible cause in external circumstances.

Obsessive compulsive neurosis

In this disorder the patient shows a blend of *obsessions* which are persistently intrusive (and often unwelcome) thoughts, and *compulsions* which are actions that the patient feels compelled to carry out. Compulsive rituals may develop, for example compulsive hand washing and elaborate checking of everyday activities. Everyday acts, like washing or dressing, may have to be carried out in a ritualistic order which may be so complex that the patient feels compelled to repeat the entire sequence to make sure they have got it right. Sequences may be repeated so many times that the day becomes a series of agonizing and time-consuming rituals.

Obsessive/compulsive states are usually responses to high anxiety levels.

Hysteria

This refers to a disorder in which the person has *unconsciously* decided to gain attention or love or escape from a difficult situation by appearing to be ill. It must not be confused with malingering, as the malingerer consciously and deliberately fakes illness and is completely aware of what he is doing.

The hysterical person may complain of blindness, deafness, paralysis or loss of memory. A man may become impotent or a woman frigid.

In hysteria, unconscious mental tensions have been converted into physical symptoms. This unconscious retreat into the 'sick role' at times of stress is probably bound up with our social ethic of caring for the sick person and feeling sorry for them.

Psychosis

The psychotic disorders form the group often regarded by lay people as being 'true' madness and form the group of disorders often requiring admission to the psychiatric hospital.

The psychoses, unlike the neuroses, are often characterized by some degree of personality deterioration or disintegration, and the psychotic may retreat into an inner world of fantasy in which there is loss of contact with reality; that is, reality testing may be impaired. To the onlooker and the family of the sufferer, the psychoses may seem much less comprehensible than the neuroses.

Insight, or awareness of disorder, may be lost or impaired and the patient may voice delusional beliefs.

The sufferer from psychosis may experience *hallucinations*, that is false perceptions which may affect one or more of the five senses (hearing, sight, smell, touch or taste). Typically he may hear 'voices' which may threaten or criticize him or may make a running commentary on his actions.

The psychoses are divided into two major groups—*organic* and *functional* psychosis.

The organic psychoses

In this group of disorders there is impairment of mental function brought about by some physical change in the brain substance. This change may be acute and temporary (for example, the cerebral poisoning brought about by acute alcohol intoxication or the delirium associated with severe systemic infection). Many of the acute forms recover within a few days or hours in the general hospital ward and psychiatric referral is unnecessary as there is no residual disorder. A smaller percentage of the acute forms may, however, leave some degree of physical change with residual chronic impairment.

Infants and the elderly are more prone to respond to the toxaemia of infection with episodes of acute brain failure of this sort, though residual impairment is unlikely in the former group.

Organic psychosis may also be of a chronic nature (for example, the permanent mental changes associated with the degeneration of brain substance occurring in some old people). Chronic brain failure of this type cannot be reversed by treatment, though the more troublesome symptoms may be considerably reduced by appropriate medical and nursing care. Chronic organic states tend to be marked by confusion and restlessness, with impaired judgement and deterioration of personality. Chronic organic psychosis will be commonly encountered by the psychiatric nurse, particularly in the psychogeriatric wards of the psychiatric hospital.

The functional psychoses

As the name suggests, these are disorders of *function* rather than structure. There are no discernible changes in the physical structure of the brain. This group includes schizophrenia, psychotic depression and manic-depressive psychosis, all of which, particularly schizophrenia, will be encountered by the psychiatric nurse.

Schizophrenia. Contrary to popular belief, this term does not refer to split personality, which is a rare hysterical disorder. In schizophrenia the mind is not split but is rather fragmented. Hallucinations and delusions are common and there is diminished awareness of reality.

Schizophrenia is a relatively common mental disorder and affects 8–10 people per 100 000 of the population. The condition accounts for approximately one half of first admissions to the psychiatric hospital and makes up an even larger percentage of long-stay patients.

Pessimistic attitudes towards schizophrenia are no longer justified however, as appropriate care often leads to early discharge, and many schizophrenics can lead productive and contented lives in the community, with or without the medications which can reduce symptoms to the point where they no longer interfere with the ability to cope with the demands of everyday living.

Psychotic depression. This major depressive reaction is also known as *endogenous* depression—the word meaning 'coming from within'. This term is used since there is usually no discernible cause in external events which could have precipitated the depression, unlike the neurosis of reactive depression which does have an identifiable cause in life circumstances.

This crippling form of depression is associated with a high suicide risk and may present with a wide range of physical symptoms such as loss of appetite, sleep disturbance, constipation and amenorrhoea. Sometimes the physical symptoms are almost as pronounced as the depressed mood and this may lead to mistaken diagnosis of physical illness.

Delusions, often of a hypochondriacal nature, may appear and thought processes may be slowed down. The overall feeling may be of guilt, worthlessness and hopeless misery and the level of mental agony experienced may be intense.

In older patients with this major depressive reaction there is often an element of associated agitation and restlessness.

Manic-depressive psychosis. This is a less common psychosis which also affects mood. In this disorder the pathological or morbid sadness of depression alternates with periods of *mania* or unreasoning exultation, which, like the depression, cannot be explained by reference to external events. The manic patient has boundless energy, both physical and psychological, in contrast to the noticeable lack of both in depression.

The patient feels elated and 'on top of the world'

and may express *grandiose delusions*; that is, he may believe himself to be someone rich and famous, or perhaps a member of the aristocracy. The manic patient has boundless energy and optimism, and experiences accelerated thought processes. The condition of mania is thus, in many ways, the opposite of depression, though the patient may plunge from the dizzying heights of mania to the depths of depression.

This alternation of mania and depression may take place on a cyclical basis which led the French to call the condition 'folie circulaire' or 'circular madness'.

Modern treatment can now interrupt this cycle and reduce the chances that mood will swing to either extreme.

Personality disorder

The third of our four categories is that of personality disorder. This group of disorders includes the sociopath (*psychopath*) who is devoid of feelings of guilt and normal human warmth. The sociopath was distastefully referred to as a 'moral defective' by the Victorians, who placed such great public value on morality. The sociopath has a disorder of character as opposed to a disorder of thought or mood. This is reflected in an inability to learn constructively from past experience and a tendency to exploit other people and persistently underrate their intelligence. The sociopath will lie, cheat, let you down again and again and come back expecting to be believed. There may be a marked intolerance of constructive advice and criticism, and above all, a total indifference to the feelings of other people.

The nurse will not encounter many clear-cut examples of this type as in-patients although she may encounter patients with sociopathic tendencies. Sociopaths are often imprisoned, as they may repeatedly break the law, or they may be treated in specialist treatment centres like the Henderson Hospital in Surrey.

Mental handicap

The term 'mentally handicapped' refers to those persons with an inborn lack of mental capacity. Their bodies develop but their minds do not, the end result being a child's mind locked in an adult's body. Intelligence fails to keep pace with physical growth but develops slowly and eventually arrests at a stage below, or well below, that of other people.

Powers of reasoning are limited, and thinking and behaviour may resemble that of a child. Such handicap may often render the person incapable of coping with simple activities of daily living and may make residential care necessary.

There may be associated physical disabilities such as deformity of cranium or tooth and jaw formation. In the well-known condition of mongolism (Down's syndrome) the eyes have a characteristic slanting appearance which is thought to bear some resemblance to the eyes of the Mongolian race.

It must be emphasized very clearly that mental handicap is a category quite distinct from mental illness and should never be confused with it. The public often confuse the two categories and this becomes apparent when terms like 'mental case' are used, or the term 'mental home' is used indiscriminately to refer to both mental hospitals and hospitals for the mentally handicapped. The media are frequently guilty of errors of this nature.

The mentally handicapped are not 'ill' in any sense of the word and, rather than treatment, they are given education and training tailored to their special needs.

It should be added that the term 'mental handicap' has replaced the older stigmatizing and derogatory terms 'mental deficiency' and 'mental subnormality'.

Mental handicap is a specialist field, quite distinct from mental illness, and, for this reason this book will discuss the condition no further but will instead refer the reader to the many excellent texts written by experts in this field.

The remainder of this text will further explore the three categories of neurosis, psychosis and personality disorder and will also discuss the problems of dependence upon alcohol or drugs.

Key Concepts

1 Illness has physical, psychological and social dimensions. In mental disorder the elements of psychological and social imbalance predominate.
2 Judgements of ideal psychological and social functioning are seldom made without reference to prevailing social, cultural and moral norms.

3 There is a risk that perceptions of mental disorder may be biased by the value system of the observer, be the observer an individual or an entire society.
4 Many mental disorders are not 'illnesses' in the accepted sense of the word, but are perhaps better viewed as responses to 'problems in living'.
5 Mental disorder is not one disorder but many.
6 Mental health cannot be simply compared to physical health as it does not have clearly demarcated boundaries.
7 The blend of characteristics referred to as mental health is not fixed but fluctuates with life circumstances.
8 Mental disorders are considered as being divided into four major categories.
9 The first of these categories is neurosis, which consists of an exaggeration of normal responses without loss of contact with reality or loss of insight. Delusions and hallucinations do not occur and hospitalization is only necessary in a small percentage of cases. This is the commonest form of mental disorder.
10 The second category discussed was psychosis, which may be organic (physical changes in the brain) or functional (no physical changes in the brain).
11 In psychosis there is often loss of contact with reality, and delusions and hallucinations are often present. Insight is lost or impaired and hospitalization is often necessary.
12 The third category mentioned was personality disorder, which is a disorder of character, and is noticeable for associated difficulties with interpersonal relationships. In psychopathy, perhaps the best known example of a disorder from this category, there is failure to learn from past experience and a tendency to exploit other people, without any associated feelings of guilt or remorse.
13 The last category mentioned was mental handicap, which is a state of incomplete or arrested mental development. The resultant lack of mental capacity often makes training and education in a residential setting necessary.
14 Mental handicap should not be confused with mental illness, the term mental illness being a collective term for neurosis, psychosis, personality disorder and related problems.

References

Baker, J. R. (1974) *Race*. Oxford: Oxford University Press.

Clare, A. (1976) *Psychiatry in Dissent*. London: Tavistock Publications.

Dubois, R. (1965). *Man Adapting*. New Haven: Yale University Press.

Freidson, E. (1973) *Profession of Medicine—A Study of the Sociology of Applied Knowledge*. New York: Dodd & Mead.

Lee, S. G. M. (1961) *Stress and Adaptation*. Leicester: Leicester University Press.

Mangen, S. P. (1982) *Sociology of Mental Health*. Edinburgh: Churchill Livingstone.

Pearson, G. (1975) *The Deviant Imagination*. London: The Macmillan Press.

Wright, D. S. & Taylor, A. (1970) *Introducing Psychology, An Experimental Approach*. Harmondsworth: Penguin Books.

2

What Causes Mental Disorder?

Who shall decide when doctors disagree?

Alexander Pope

The causes of mental disorder may be infinitely variable, and it is relatively rare to find simple cause and effect relationships which could account for its development. Exploration of this area often centres around the question as to whether heredity (nature) or environment (nurture) is more important as a determining factor—the so-called 'nature/nurture' debate. It now seems probable that the two are inseparable insofar as much mental disorder may be the result of the interaction between biological predispositions and the experiences provided by the environment. In many cases the seed of inherited predispositions may be sown into the fertile soil of a stressful environment to produce the growth of mental disorder. In some cases though, there seems little doubt that the relative influence of either genetics or environment may heavily predominate and emerge as the conspicuous aetiological factor.

Genetic Factors

There is no doubt that genetic factors are responsible for some forms of mental handicap, for example Down's syndrome, where the cells of the individual contain 47 chromosomes, and not the usual 46. Huntington's chorea, a very rare form of organic psychosis, has also been demonstrated to have a genetic mode of transmission.

Research has also suggested that the prevalence of disorders of mood (affective disorders) is significantly higher among the relatives of patients with these disorders, though concrete genetic evidence to explain this observation has not been produced. Studies of the possible aetiological factors in schizophrenia have also suggested that there may be a genetic component, though other factors (psycho-logical, social and biochemical) have also received great attention.

Many studies have been carried out on the development of schizophrenia in twins on the premise that, if there is a hereditary component, then identical twins, who develop from the same egg (monozygotic twins), will be more likely to *both* develop schizophrenia than twins who develop from different eggs (dizygotic twins). Studies indicate that the *concordance rate* (the percentage of pairs in which both twins are diagnosed as schizophrenic) is higher for monozygotic than for dizygotic twins.

Concordance rates for monzygotic twins have variously been estimated at 35–69%, while the estimation of concordance for dizygotic twins has ranged from 0 to 26% (Gottesman and Shields, 1972). The presence of schizophrenic-like traits (schizoid traits) in the relatives of schizophrenics may also be strikingly high, and it has been indicated that, if both parents are schizophrenic, the incidence of schizophrenia in the children is likely to reach 33.9%, while a further 32.2% will show schizoid traits, thus giving a total incidence of 66.1% of schizophrenia or schizoid tendencies in the children of schizophrenics, compared with an incidence of 0.8% in the general population (Heston, 1970).

While a number of studies have demonstrated high concordance rates, the concordance rates for the criteria used to make the diagnosis of schizophrenia and schizoid traits has often been regrettably low between various studies.

It has been suggested that the transmission of schizophrenia may be explained by environmental factors, insofar as the schizophrenic parent(s) may transmit the disorder to the offspring by means of faulty child-rearing practices and faulty family dynamics, rather than faulty genes. Florid schizophrenia may arise in the offspring of non-schizophrenic parents. If the disorder depended solely on heredity then one would expect a 100% concordance rate between monozygotic twins.

It seems improbable that genetic factors play a critical role in producing neurotic disorders though some personality traits, which make the individual vulnerable, may be influenced genetically.

'The Crooked Molecule that Makes Men Mad'

At the end of the nineteenth century Kraepelin detected a 'mousey odour' from the urine of schizophrenics and suggested that a chemical 'auto-intoxication' might be the cause of this most enigmatic of mental disorders (Hays, 1964). Thus began the search for the psychiatric Holy Grail, the quest for the 'crooked molecule that makes men mad' (Szasz, 1976).

The belief that a biochemical explanation might be found for schizophrenia seemed to gain support from the observation that the hallucinogenic drug lysergic acid (LSD) produced a state which transiently mimicked psychosis; that is, it was noted to be *psychotomimetic* in many of its effects. Subjects intoxicated with LSD experience vivid hallucinations, inappropriate emotions, disorders of body image and of time and space perceptions and tend to ascribe importance to otherwise unimportant stimuli. When it was pointed out that the adrenaline molecule resembled that of LSD the belief grew that schizophrenics suffered from an inborn error of metabolism and were somehow producing abnormal metabolites which were disrupting cerebral chemistry. Examination of the body fluids of schizophrenics did indeed reveal abnormal metabolites or normal metabolites present in abnormal amounts. A mood of optimism pervaded early researches only to be dampened when the mysterious substances isolated in some studies were found to be the result of chronic tea and coffee drinking or of deficiencies in institutional diets (Clare, 1976). Early optimism was succeeded by pessimism. Rodnight (1971) commented that

'Biochemists in the field (psychiatry) seem to divide their time between disproving the research of their less rigorous colleagues and adding to an increasingly long catalogue of essentially negative results; everyone regrets the failure of research in the field to contribute anything of significance to the pathology of the major mental illnesses . . . It is important to recognise the magnitude of failure.'

Research has continued with admirable tenacity, but the eagerly expected breakthrough still seems as distant as ever. It may yet happen that a chemical key will be discovered to unlock the mysteries of psychosis, but, in the meantime, it would be unfortunate if workers in the field of mental health were to regard schizophrenia as an incurable illness and thus develop blind spots in respect of the critical psychological and social dimensions of the disorder.

Environmental Factors

The individual suffering from mental disorder and his/her relatives may lay the blame on one single factor (for example, a broken love affair, overwork, study problems) thus maintaining self-esteem and shifting the responsibility from the patient and his family. This tendency to 'medicalize' life difficulties by assuming the passive 'sick role' may enable the patient to rationalize complex aetiological areas, and may result in a reluctance, on the part of both patient and family, to critically examine faulty and self-destructive approaches to living which are likely to generate more 'illness' if they remain unmodified. While simple cause and effect explanations of mental disorder are often suspect, many critical environmental variables have been examined. For example:

Stress

Coping with stress is an integral part of the natural fabric of life. From birth to death stress is the inevitable accompaniment of human existence, and, in moderate amounts, may be essential for effective functioning (Spielberger, 1979). Shakespeare commented that 'adversity maketh a strange bedfellow, but sweet'. Stress may stretch and develop our abilities and may strengthen our coping mechanisms, while almost total lack of stress may lead to boredom, inertia and inefficiency. Stress may be a potent stimulus for positive growth and development.

Individual responses to stress may vary dramatically however. Similar levels of stress may 'toughen' one individual while disabling another. The psychologist Allport wryly commented that 'The heat that hardens the egg melts the butter'.

Responses to stress may be either adaptive (reflective in an increase in coping responses) or maladaptive (reflected in neurotic responses, for example anxiety states), the latter response being more probable if levels of stress exceed capacity to cope, thus 'overwhelming' the individual.

The 'anxiety prone' individual may have been

disadvantaged by faulty parent/child relationships or childhood experiences related to withdrawal of affection or persistently negative evaluations (Perdue and Spielberger, 1966).

It is estimated that emotional stress may play a part in more than half of all medical problems, and this is reflected in the field of *psychosomatic medicine* (Gk. *psyche*—mind; *soma*—body). Hypertension, peptic ulceration, ulcerative colitis, coronary heart disease, migraine, pre-menstrual tension and some skin diseases are believed to be related to emotional stress, although an emotional factor is almost invariably part of any illness and the division between psyche and soma may be rather arbitrary.

Early learning experiences may play an important part in the development of somatic responses to stress. The child who is encouraged to stay home from school every time he has an upset stomach may be learning the visceral responses that lead to chronic dyspepsia or peptic ulceration, while the child who receives attention and concern whenever a mild allergy leads to wheezing or respiratory discomfort may progress to fully flown asthma attacks.

Major changes in life circumstances may add significantly to overall stress levels, particularly if several overlap. Thomas H. Holmes, at the University of Washington, has developed a Survey of Recent Experiences which consists of 43 different life changes that have been related to stress and scaled in life change units (LCU) in terms of the demands for adaptation they make on the individual (Table 1). You may wish to calculate your own LCU rating.

Major life changes which may raise the level of stress over the threshold of coping include bereavement, divorce, unemployment, marriage, parenthood, physical illness and retirement.

Family Variables

The psychoanalyst John Bowlby suggested that temporary or permanent separation of child from parent, particularly early separation, was a critical factor in the development of adult mental disorder. Maternal deprivation was said to lead to the development of the 'affectionless personality' characterized by a basic lack of trust in other people and an inability to develop close personal relationships in adulthood (Bowlby, 1973).

This viewpoint is no longer *uncritically* accepted. Munro (1969) has suggested that there may be a case

Table 1 Holmes' Survey of Recent Experiences.

Thomas H. Holmes and his colleagues at the University of Washington School of Medicine have developed a scale for measuring the seriousness of changes in American people's lives and related their scores to their chances of becoming ill. The Survey of Recent Experiences (SRE) consists of 43 different life changes that have been scaled in life change units (LCU) for the degree of adaptation they require.

Americans are thought to run the risk of developing a major illness in the next two years if they total more than 300 LCU points. If appropriate, calculate your own LCU rating.

Life Events	Life change units
Death of spouse	100
Divorce	73
Marital separation	65
Jail term	63
Death of close family member	63
Personal injury or illness	53
Marriage	50
Fired at work	47
Marital reconciliation	45
Retirement	45
Change in health of family member	44
Pregnancy	40
Sex difficulties	39
Gain of new family member	39
Business readjustment	39
Change in financial state	38
Death of close friend	37
Change to different line of work	36
Change in number of arguments with spouse	35
Mortgage over $10 000	31
Foreclosure of mortgage or loan	30
Change in responsibilities at work	29
Son or daughter leaving home	29
Trouble with in-laws	29
Outstanding personal achievement	28
Wife begins or stops work	26
Begin or end school	26
Change in living conditions	25
Revision of personal habits	24
Trouble with boss	23
Change in work hours or conditions	20
Change in residence	20
Change in schools	20
Change in recreation	19
Change in church activities	19
Change in social activities	18
Mortgage or loan less than $10 000	17
Change in sleeping habits	16
Change in number of family get-togethers	15
Change in eating habits	15
Vacation	13
Christmas	12
Minor violations of the law	11

for linking personality disorder, suicide and 'attempted suicide' with separation, but suggests that the evidence is unconclusive regarding neurosis, schizophrenia and even depression, where Bowlby and others had proposed a specific link in terms of a chronic 'bereavement reaction'.

Birtchnell (1970) examined the association between early parental death and psychiatric hospital admissions in Scotland and concluded that the incidence of depression was no higher in patients with a history of early parental death than for a control group of non-psychiatric patients, though *severe* depression did occur more frequently in patients with such a background, the percentage difference being small however (37% for severe depression and 24% for controls).

It does appear, however, that 'broken homes' and delinquency are related (Koller and Castanos, 1970), though the concept of the 'broken home' is in itself a crude one which requires further examination. For example it has been demonstrated that homes 'broken' by divorce or separation are much more likely to be productive of delinquency than those 'broken' by parental death (Orford, 1976). Rutter (1972) has concluded that both long and short-term effects have more to do with *distortion* of relationships before, during and after separation rather than with the fact of separation itself.

Birth order has also been examined as a possibly critical variable, and it has been suggested that neurotic disturbances may be more common in eldest children and least common in youngest, though the effect is reversed for 'antisocial' disorders (Rutter et al, 1970). There is also some evidence that alcoholism is more common amongst men who were the last born in their families (Blane and Barry, 1973).

The Family as a 'Pathogenic Institution'

Some types of family have been considered as being productive of madness—as being 'pathogenic institutions'. This viewpoint is associated with the prolific writings of Laing (1964) who has suggested that the current situation within the family is at least as important as early childhood experience. He claims that seemingly irrational and schizophrenic responses are in fact 'normal responses to an abnormal situation' (Laing and Esterson, 1964), the 'abnormal situation' here being distorted and irrational family dynamics.

In analysing the family experiences of schizophrenics, Laing made use of the concept of 'double bind', developed by Bateson and furthered by Lidz. According to this notion children in certain families are subjected to contradictory demands to which it is impossible to respond satisfactorily. Contradictory demands may come from one parent or from both. For example, a mother may hold out her arms to her child and embrace her, but register displeasure when the embrace is returned. If the child embraces the mother, the mother may again register disapproval by her posture and facial expression, but respond to the child's withdrawal by saying in a hurt tone 'Don't you love me anymore?' Verbal and nonverbal communications are contradictory—mother wishes to be loved and not loved at the same time— she simultaneously invites and rejects love.

This process of 'mystification' may be generally compounded further by the parents expecting the child to behave in one particular way while they behave in quite another. Thus parents destroy the individual by mystifying family life and surrounding the child by overwhelming social and psychological stresses, thus making 'reality' so threatening and confusing that the child gradually retreats into the sanctuary of fantasy and, eventually, psychosis. Laing comments that psychotherapists became increasingly aware that 'if their patients were *disturbed*, their families were often *very disturbing*' (Laing, 1967).

The behaviour that is called schizophrenia is, according to this argument, a strategy by means of which a person can live in an unliveable situation— can tolerate the intolerable. Laing suggests that schizophrenics are driven mad by the structure and organization of society. A crazy society increasingly drives people mad. The family is the basic unit of society and captures its craziness in microcosm.

'A child born today in the United Kingdom stands a ten times greater chance of being admitted to a mental hospital than to a University, and about one fifth of mental hospital admissions are diagnosed as schizophrenic. This can be taken as an indication that we are driving our children mad more effectively than we are genuinely educating them. Perhaps it is our very way of educating them that is driving them mad.'

Laing, 1967

Laing's work has attracted both veneration and vituperation. It has been enshrined by the broad left as encapsulating a scathing indictment of bourgeois society and it has been roundly condemned by many social scientists as being mystical, confused and unscientific.

It has been pointed out that, as no 'non-schizophrenic' families were studied for comparison, we cannot say with any certainty that 'double bind' situations are typical of schizophrenic families (Mangen, 1982).

Laing's work may be speculative but it is also intriguing and is imbued with a deeply humanistic concern for the plight of the mentally disordered.

The 'Anti-Psychiatry' Viewpoint

Laing's name is often coupled with that of Thomas Szasz, Professor of Psychiatry at New York University, the two being regarded as the leading theorists of the school of 'anti-psychiatry'. In fact, there is considerable divergence of opinion between the two and both have rejected the description of their views as being 'anit-psychiatry'.

Szasz (1982) suggests that, strictly speaking, illness can only affect the body, not the mind. 'Mental illness is not something a person *has*, but is something he *does* or *is*.' The argument is developed further by suggesting that 'Those who suffer and complain of their own behaviour are usually classified as "neurotic"; those whose behaviour makes others suffer, and about whom others complain, are usually classified as "psychotic"' (Szasz, 1982).

Szasz does not deny the concept of mental disorder but vigorously attacks the concept of 'mental illness'. He suggests that people who in actual fact have 'problems in living' are thrust into the 'sick role'. This error of category occurs as 'It is part of our social ethic, that is of the rules by which we play the game of life, that we ought to feel sorry for sick people and should try to be helpful to them' (Szasz, 1982).

The neurotic may thus voluntarily embrace the 'sick role' in order to receive help with 'problems in living', thus taking advantage of the Western social ethic. The psychotic may have the 'sick role' thrust upon him involuntarily as society uses it as a convenient way of labelling objectionable behaviour and further uses it to justify 'treatment' by incarceration. This viewpoint thus considers psychiatry as a form of social oppression which controls and suppresses deviant minorities, illicitly using the language of medicine to coerce behaviour into channels approved by society. Szasz suggests that many psychiatric judgements which seem medical are in fact juridical and do not so much maintain the health of the community as maintain its social stability.

Like Laing, Szasz has evoked responses of both admiration and animosity and his thinking has powerfully influenced the sociology of medicine and has led to much critical re-examination of conventional psychiatric theory and practice.

Civilization and Sanity

The psychoanalytic view, as developed by Freud, is that man is fundamentally antisocial. Powerful drives emanating from the unconscious reservoir of the *Id* continually seek outlet. Id impulses are primitive, infantile and self-centred, and an important part of psychological development consists of learning self-control of basic impulses; that is, learning to live according to the Reality Principle, as opposed to infantile patterns of behaviour governed by the Pleasure Principle.

Society must domesticate man, by checking his basic drives, if social stability is to be achieved. The energy attached to suppressed drives is then thought to be diverted into socially useful channels, for example science and the arts. This process of energy redirection was called *sublimation* by Freud, who further suggested that sublimated drives were the basis for human culture. The more drive suppression, the more sublimation, and consequently the more civilization.

However, Freud suggested that drive suppression not only leads to culturally valuable sublimation—it also leads to neurosis. If the amount of suppression is greater than the capacity of sublimation then the individual may become neurotic as basic drives become pent-up to create tensions. Thus—the more civilization, the more neurosis, and the less civilization, the less neurosis. In the case of societies in which drives may be relatively freely expressed, unchecked by rigid social structures, it is suggested that there will be less neurosis, but less civilization, as drives are not sublimated into cultural strivings.

Culture thus arises at the expense of freedom, and neurosis is a by-product, according to this view. This viewpoint overlaps, to a certain extent, with some others previously mentioned. Rigid and oppressive social structures eroding the autonomy of the individual have been the concern of Laing and others, and the resultant mechanisms of social control have been delineated by Szasz and others.

Medical vs. social models of mental disorder

The 'medical model' of psychiatry is a term used to loosely describe those viewpoints which emphasize the 'nature' side of the nature/nurture debate. Medical model approaches are based on the assumption that mental disorders are illnesses like any other illness. There is assumed to be a pathological lesion within the body which leads to disturbed function, the lesion being assumed to be genetic or biochemical. The medical model does not exclude the effect of social and psychological forces, but places them in a subordinate relationship to physical changes in the organism. The medical model lends itself to the view that the mentally disordered are suffering from illnesses which are, as yet, incurable and treatment therefore tends to be *palliative* (aimed at relieving the symptoms rather than being aimed at the, as yet, unidentified cause). Such treatments are often physical (psychotropic drugs, electroplexy and, occasionally, psychosurgery).

Critics of this approach suggest that psychiatrists are often 'medicalizing' deviance and further suggest that biochemical and genetic research may prove to be a fruitless 'wild goose chase' which diverts attention away from the critical social and psychological factors involved in the aetiology of mental disorder.

The 'social model' tends to emphasize the nurture side of the nature/nurture debate although it does not deny the importance of genetically transmitted predisposing factors. The medical model locates the problem firmly *inside* the patient, unlike the social model which locates the roots of mental disorder in social and family structures. Approaches to treatment arising from the social model tend to be non-physical—for example, psychotherapy and behaviour therapy—though many patients receive a blend of physical and non-physical treatments (for example, drugs plus psychotherapy). Schwartz and Schwartz (1964) suggested that 'The major division in psychiatry seems to be between those who emphasize an organic (medical model) view of mental illness and those who emphasize a psychodynamic view and focus on psychological or interpersonal measures.' In the same year, Strauss et al (1964) pointed out that nurses tend to 'adopt' the ideology expressed and practised by the doctor with whom they work.

The implications of the nature/nurture debate are thus considerable, and differences in treatment philosophy often loosely cluster around viewpoints which tend to be either medical or social. It should not be assumed, however, that viewpoints of mental disorder may always be crudely reduced to either a 'medical' or 'social' model. There is considerable interpenetration between the models and the 'common ground' is often considerable.

Key Concepts

1 The causes of mental disorder are complex and it is probable that several factors (physical, psychological and social) interact in most cases.
2 Historically there have been differences of opinion, some emphasizing physical explanations (particularly heredity) and some emphasizing the effects of the environment—the so-called *nature/nurture debate*.
3 It seems probable that most neuroses are substantially determined by the environment, while many psychotic disorders arise when an inherited *predisposition* is acted upon by environmental *precipitating factors*.
4 Note that it is the predisposition, not the disorder, that is inherited and not all predispositions will culminate in mental disorder.
5 It is often suggested that genetic factors predisposing to mental disorder express themselves *biochemically*, and much inconclusive research has been carried out into the chemistry of body fluids in mental disorder.
6 The importance of *stress* as a critical factor in the aetiology of mental disorder cannot be over-emphasized. In some cases (e.g. many neuroses), stress may act as a causative factor, while in others (e.g. many psychoses) it acts as a precipitating factor.
7 Mental disorder, of any sort, causes much psychosocial disorganization and some researchers suggest that this process of disorganization starts within the environment of the family—*pathogenic families* selecting vulnerable members as scapegoats and pushing them towards, or into, mental disorder.
8 The 'medical model' view of psychiatry emphasizes physical causes (e.g. heredity and its biochemical expressions) and treatments while the

'social model' viewpoints emphasize environmental determinants and stress psychological treatments. Overlap between the two viewpoints is variable but may be considerable.

References

Blane, H. T. & Barry, H. (1973) Birth order & alcoholism. *Quarterly Journal of Studies on Alcohol*, **34**: 837–852.

Birtchnell, J. (1970) Early parental death & mental illness. *British Journal of Psychiatry*, **116**: 281–313.

Bowlby, J. (1973) *Separation, Attachment and Loss, Vol. 2*. New York: Basic Books.

Clare, A. (1976) *Psychiatry in Dissent*. London: Tavistock Publications.

Gottesman, I. & Shields, J. (1972) *Schizophrenia & Genetics. A twin study vantage point*. New York: Academic Press.

Hays, P. (1964) *New Horizons in Psychiatry*. Harmondsworth: Pelican.

Heston, L. (1970) The genetics of schizophrenia and schizoid disease. *Science*, **167**: 249–256.

Koller, K. M. & Castanos, J. N. (1970) Family background in prison groups: a comparative study of parental deprivation. *British Journal of Psychiatry*, **117**: 371–380.

Laing, R. D. (1967) *The Politics of Experience*. New York: Pantheon Books (Published by Penguin 1970).

Laing, R. D. & Esterson, A. (1964) *Sanity, Madness & The Family*. Harmondsworth: Penguin Books.

Mangen, S. P. (1982) *Sociology and Mental Health*. Edinburgh: Churchill Livingstone.

Munro, A. (1969) Parent/child separation. *Archives of General Psychiatry*, **20**: 598–604.

Orford, J. (1976) *The Social Psychology of Mental Disorder*. Harmondsworth: Penguin Books.

Perdue, O. & Spielberger, C. (1966) Anxiety and the perception of punishment. *Mental Hygiene*, **50**: 390–397.

Rodnight, R. (1971) Editorial. Biochemical Research in Psychiatry. *Psychological Medicine*, **1**(5): 353–355.

Rutter, M. (1972) *Maternal Deprivation Reassessed*. Harmondsworth: Penguin Books.

Rutter, M., Tizard, J. & Whitmore, K. (1970) *Education, Health & Behaviour*. Harlow: Longman.

Schwartz, C. & Schwartz, C. G. (1964) *Social Approaches to Mental Patient Care*. New York: Columbia University Press.

Spielberger, C. (1979) *Understanding Stress and Anxiety*. London: Harper Row.

Strauss, A. et al (1964) *Psychiatric Ideologies and Institutions*. London: Collier Macmillan & New York: The Free Press of Glencoe.

Szasz, T. (1976) *Schizophrenia*—The sacred symbols of psychiatry. *British Journal of Psychiatry*, **129**: 308–316.

Szasz, T. S. (1982) *The Myth of Mental Illness*. London: Paladin.

3

Who is Mental Disorder Likely to Affect?

They see not us, nor any Sunday caller
among the geraniums and wicker chairs
for they are Jacks who climb the beanstalk
country

Tennessee Williams

If present trends continue it is likely that one in six girls who are now at school and one in nine boys can expect to spend some period of their lives as patients in a psychiatric hospital (Appleby, 1976). These figures merely reflect hospital admission rates and thus do not give an indication of the true level of mental disorder in the community. Many neuroses will not occasion treatment—the so-called '*subclinical*' *neuroses*—and many more will be treated by general practitioners. Studies suggest that up to 70% of patients seen by general practitioners may present with a major psychological component in the presenting illness (Sim, 1974).

Mental disorder may thus be treated by the psychiatrist (on either an in-patient or out-patient basis), by the general practitioner, or may remain untreated and largely undetected.

Statistics tend to be based on referrals made to psychiatric treatment agencies and seldom take account of the great numbers of patients seen by general practitioners and treated 'conservatively' by the prescription of *psychotropic drugs* (drugs which influence mood or emotional state). Nearly a fifth of all prescriptions are for psychotropic drugs.

We can only guess at the level of undiagnosed and untreated mental disorder in the community.

The Epidemiology of Mental Disorder

Epidemiology is the study of the distribution of disease and disability in the community, and epidemiological studies have revealed certain patterns to the distribution of mental disorder in the populations studied.

The concepts of *incidence* and *prevalence* are widely used in these studies and may be briefly defined as follows: the *prevalence* of a disorder is the total number of people at a given point in time who are suffering from that disorder; the *incidence* of the disorder is the number of new cases arising within a given period of time.

The prevalence of some mental disorders may be difficult to estimate as formal psychiatric referral may not take place, the sufferer being treated by the general practitioner for 'nerves', 'tension' or the physical manifestations of neurosis.

Incidence may also be difficult to estimate as knowledge about onset may be imprecise (for example, in some types of schizophrenia).

Despite the difficulties involved in studying the distribution of mental disorder some patterns or trends do consistently emerge.

Women and Mental Disorder

In general practice, where the majority of psychiatric disorders are treated, about twice as many female as male cases are identified as suffering from mental disorder (Miles, 1981). Mental disorder is also far more prevalent among married women than among married men; for single people the differences are minimal.

Studies also suggest that women are more susceptible to mental disorder during the puerperium (the months following childbirth), the pre-menstrual period and following hysterectomy (Miles, 1981). Three quarters of the users of psychotropic drugs are women (Balint et al, 1970).

These sex-related differences have been subject to somewhat incautious interpretations. The chauvinistic male may smugly regard the dramatic differences in prevalence as evidence of the biological inferiority of females while outraged feminists may regard the imbalance as further evidence of male oppression, particularly when the increase in incidence associated with marriage is revealed.

The reality may be less dramatic. The higher incidence of mental disorder in women may be a product of social and cultural expectations rather than of innate biological factors. 'One is not born, but rather becomes a woman. No biological, psychological or economic fate determines the figure that the human female presents in society; it is civilization as a whole that produces this creature.' (De Beauvoir, 1972). In other words any given society will have certain expectations about 'appropriate' behaviours for each sex, and readily discernible differences in behavioural patterns may be a product of cultural rather than biological forces.

Sociologists use the term *socialization* to describe the transmission of culture, the process whereby the individual learns to abide by the rules and practices of his social group. Many theorists have suggested that the socialization of women in Western societies ascribes an essentially passive and dependent role to them, this role being entirely a cultural artefact. It is often strongly impressed upon girls that certain behaviours are appropriately 'feminine' while others are (for them) inappropriately 'masculine'. This process of role differentiation is often apparent in the introductory reading books used in infant schools (books of the 'Janet and John' type) in which little boys are depicted as being active and vigorous while little girls are shown as being 'pretty' and assisting mother with domestic chores. These stereotyped images may be the product of a culture which essentially sees women as weak, passive and dependent, in contrast to the male role of tough, active decision maker.

Such a socialization process may produce men who are reluctant to openly display emotion and who attempt to maintain the 'stiff upper lip' appropriate to the masculine role. It may well be that the seemingly enormous difference in the incidence of mental disorder between the sexes is not as great as statistics suggest. Men may be reluctant to report failure to cope with the stresses of living as readily as women as they may fear that this would be an admission of unmasculine 'weakness'. Instead men may attempt, with limited success, to contain stress in different ways. This may partially explain the higher incidence of alcoholism in men, as alcohol is often used as 'self-medication' to combat the effects of stress.

Women may be less inhibited than men in discussing emotional problems and in presenting them for treatment, this being quite compatible with the feminine role of the 'weaker sex'. This factor may be coupled with the fact that men often have psychological and social rewards associated with work which are denied to the housebound mother of young children. One large study revealed that almost three quarters of the housewives interviewed felt dissatisfied and socially restricted by being tied to the home by young children (Oakley, 1974).

Married women are twice as likely to commit suicide than single women but single men are twice as likely to commit suicide than married men (Mangen, 1982). Marriage thus seems to 'protect' men while placing women at risk.

Social Class and Mental Disorder

The most commonly used measurement of *social class* is the scale used by the office of the Registrar General since 1911. This scale is based upon occupational groupings (see Table 2).

Many studies have suggested that there is a strong relationship between social class and mental disorder and indicate that the lowest social classes are more at risk of mental disorder, as they are of most illnesses and early death. One study of an American population revealed that social classes 4 and 5 accounted for over 78% of the patients while social class 1 accounted for only 1% of the patients (Hollingshead and Redlich, 1958). Schizophrenia is a notable example of a mental disorder which tends to display a higher prevalence in the lower social classes.

In most populations it is relatively easy to demonstrate a high prevalence of psychiatric disorder among the lower social classes but it is less easy to explain this seeming concentration of morbidity.

The theory of '*downward social drift*' has been used in an attempt to explain the seemingly inverse relationship between mental disorder and social class. This theory points out that social class is determined by occupation and suggests that chronic mental disorder may lead to loss of efficiency (see p. 7) and impaired relationships with others. As a result, the affected individual may drift down the occupational scale into occupations which are less

Table 2 Scale showing measurement of social class.

Social Class	Occupation (examples)
1 Professional	Doctors, dentists, lawyers, architects, university teachers
2 Intermediate	Nurses, pharmacists, members of parliament, school teachers
3 Skilled	Clerical workers, police, shop assistants, sales representatives
4 Semi-skilled	Agricultural workers, barmen/maids, telephone operators, postmen
5 Unskilled	Porters, labourers, cleaners, bus conductors, packers, messengers

demanding and may also move into lower class accommodation where neighbours may be more tolerant of eccentric behaviour. Behaviour which may well attract censure in middle class suburbia may be accepted without comment in cheap rented accommodation in an urban core.

One British study located the beginning of this 'downward drift' in the period preceding the first 'breakdown' and, by comparing the social class of patients with that of their fathers, indicated that patients did indeed tend to gravitate downwards to a lower social class than that of their families (Goldberg and Morrison, 1963). This finding has not been corroborated in some other studies and the issue remains controversial.

An associated explanation of the seemingly inverse relationship between social class and mental disorder suggests that environmental stress may be a critical variable in that urban working class environments, with associated social deprivation, may be stressful and so productive of mental disorder. Unemployment (actual or potential), poor housing and high density of population may be as productive of mental disorder as it seems to be of crime and delinquency.

A third explanation is the suggestion that the lower social classes are more likely to have stigmatizing diagnostic 'labels' affixed to them than are the upper classes. This viewpoint suggests that the psychiatrist's perceptions of his patient are coloured by an awareness of his social class and that he may show reluctance to stigmatize persons of similar social status to himself. The poorly educated and possibly less articulate member of the lower social classes may also accept the stigmatizing 'label' more passively than his upper class counterpart as he may assume a subordinate role in his transactions with his psychiatrist.

There is also some evidence to suggest that lower class patients are more likely to become in-patients and to have a longer period of stay in hospital, and are more likely to be given physical methods of treatment (drugs and electroplexy) than the upper class patient. The same study revealed that prolonged psychotherapy (especially psychoanalysis) tended to be offered almost exclusively to patients from social classes 1 and 2 (Hollingshead and Redlich, 1963).

Studies of suicide also reveal a marked class differential. Completed suicidal acts are commoner in middle and upper social classes while acts of deliberate self harm (parasuicide) are commoner in the lower social classes (MacCulloch and Philip, 1972). The highest rate of parasuicide in Oxford was found to be in disadvantaged council estates (Skrimshire, 1976), while nurses appeared to be over-represented among parasuicide statistics in Oxford (Bancroft et al, 1975).

One study suggested that mental disorder in immigrant Indian women seems to be concentrated in the higher social classes (Mangen, 1975) although overall rates of mental disorder seem to be lower among the New Commonwealth immigrant population than in the host population.

Age and Susceptibility to Mental Disorder

The early age of onset of most forms of schizophrenia was noted during the nineteenth century and led to the condition being erroneously described as dementia praecox (precocious dementia). Schizophrenia still tends to manifest itself during adolescence, and the highest rates for hospitalization for males are for men in their twenties. The high male rates of schizophrenia, alcoholism and personality disorders most frequently first appear at this age. In women the two age-related high risk periods are at 40–50 years and the late twenties in the case of married women with small children (Mangen, 1975). Women tend to be treated more frequently for neurotic conditions than do men, though the incidence of alcoholism in women is rising.

Suicide rates tend to increase with age, though for parasuicide the pattern is different, the highest rates being in the late teens and early twenties with a progressive decline in the rate of parasuicide becoming apparent with increasing years (MacCulloch and Philip, 1972).

In the years of middle life the incidence of paranoid disorders increases and depressive illnesses also increase in prevalence, being the commonest form of mental disorder among those aged 60–70 years (Trethowan and Sims, 1983).

Retirement may lead to loss of self-esteem, boredom and dissatisfaction and, while it does not seem to be a major precipitating factor in the development of mental disorder, it may constitute a period of stressful social dislocation. By the time 80 years of age is attained, the prevalence of chronic brain failure rises sharply so that about one in five is affected, at least half of them severely (Trethowan and Sims, 1983).

Transcultural Psychiatry

Transcultural psychiatry is that branch of the discipline which attempts to uncover global patterns and trends in the distribution of mental disorder by considering psychiatric morbidity in a wide range of cultural settings. Some of the findings in this area of research call into question our comfortable, and often well-worn, concepts of 'normality' and 'abnormality'. For example one researcher reported that, in Ghana, 'nobody looks twice at a lorry which announces in big letters "Enemies all about me", or "Be afraid of people"' (Field, 1980). This may be added to the findings of one British researcher who reported that West African patients in British hospitals frequently have persecutory delusions which cannot necessarily be described as psychotic in origin (Copeland, 1968).

Transcultural studies of depression include a survey in which a questionnaire was completed by psychiatrists from 30 different nations, including countries in Africa, Asia, Australia, North and South America, the Middle East and Europe. All respondents reported patients displaying a core syndrome of depression, with many symptoms in common. Symptoms such as guilt and self-depreciation tended to occur only in patients of Western Christian cultural background and were largely absent in patients from other cultures (Murphy et al, 1964).

Cosmopolitan populations, like New York City, have enabled some interesting comparisons to be made between illness patterns of different ethnic groups. Poorer control of homosexual impulses and reduced levels of sexual guilt were apparent in Italian-Americans studied, while hypochondriasis, ideas of sin and guilt and alcohol abuse were more common in Irish-Americans, as was repression of troublesome sexual ideas (Opler, 1959).

In Western societies the Jews and Italians have remarkably low rates of alcoholism. A possible explanation is that alcohol consumption is an integral part of socialization and of group rites in these cultures, rather than being individual and sporadic.

The theme emerging from many cross-cultural studies is that concepts of normality and abnormality tend to be culture-specific and tend to be related to any given society's stage of social and cultural development. In many Third World cultures, aberrant behaviour, personal distress and madness may still be seen as the effects of supernatural forces. An awareness of cultural beliefs about illness and health, normality and abnormality will prove invaluable to the psychiatric nurse caring for the immigrant patient, and this awareness should be based on acceptance of the fact that beliefs or behaviours which may seem odd or incomprehensible in the context of Western society may actually be appropriate to the norms of the patient's parent culture. Dubos has commented that

'Living things can survive and function effectively only if they adapt themselves to the peculiarities of each individual situation. For some sulphur bacteria nature is a Mexican spring with extremely acid water at a very high temperature; for the reindeer moss, it is a rock surface in the frozen atmosphere of the Arctic. Nature for fishes is ocean, lake or stream, and for the desert rat it is a place where never a drop of water is available. The word "nature" also means very different things to different men.'

Dubos, 1980

Sociologists use the word *ethnocentricity* to describe the tendency to judge the beliefs and behaviours of others against the standards of our own culture and to regard with suspicion that which seems disturbingly alien. The ethnocentric approach may lead the nurse to reject the unfamiliar, and perhaps even to 'label' it as abnormal. Ethnocentricity constitutes a formidable barrier to understanding.

Key Concepts

1 Statistics suggest that women are far more prone to mental disorder than men.
2 This may be the result of female attitudes to illness rather than the result of biological factors, and these attitudes are products of the socialization process.
3 *Social class* has been related to mental disorder and there seems to be much more psychiatric morbidity in most lower class populations studied.
4 Again this may be a product, not of biological factors, but of social ones (downward social mobility, environmental deprivation and class differences in diagnosis and treatment).
5 Studies of age as a variable suggest that psychoses appear at an early age (particularly in men) while neuroses tend to occur more

frequently in women and tend to reach peak incidence at 40–50 years and also in married women with young families.

6 Completed suicide is commoner in the older middle class male while parasuicide is commoner in the younger lower class female.

7 *Transcultural* studies reveal variations in concepts of health and disorder and suggest that beliefs and behaviour cannot always be effectively studied outwith the context of the parent culture.

References

Appleby, M. (1976) *Understanding Mental Illness*. Kent: Hodder & Stoughton.

Balint, M., Hunt, J., Joyce, D., Marinker, M. & Woodstock, J. (1970) Treatment or Diagnosis: a study of repeated prescriptions in general practice. London: Tavistock Publications.

Bancroft, J., Reynolds, F., Simken, S. & Smith, J. (1975) Self-poisoning and self-injury in the Oxford area. *British Journal of Preventive & Social Medicine*, **29**: 170–177.

Copeland, J. R. (1968) Aspects of mental illness in West African students. *Social Psychiatry*, **3**: 7–13.

De Beauvoir, S. (1972) *The Female Eunuch*. London: Paladin.

Dubos, R. (1980) The mirage of health. In Mechanic, D. (Ed.) *Readings in Medical Sociology*. New York: Free Press.

Field, M. J. (1980) In Mechanic, D. (Ed.) *Readings in Medical Sociology*. Harmondsworth: Free Press.

Goldberg, D. & Morrison, S. L. (1963) Schizophrenia and social class. *British Journal of Psychiatry*, **109**: 785–802.

Hollingshead, A. & Redlich, R. (1958) *Social Class and Mental Illness*. New York: John Wiley.

MacCulloch, J. W. & Philip, A. E. (1972) *Suicidal Behaviour*. Oxford: Pergamon Press.

Mangen, S. P. (1975) Self-poisoning and self-injury in the Oxford area. *British Journal of Preventive & Social Medicine*, **29**: 170–177.

Mangen, S. P. (1982) *Sociology and Mental Health*. Edinburgh: Churchill Livingstone.

Miles, A. (1981) *The Mentally Ill in Contemporary Society*. Oxford: Martin Robertson.

Murphy, H., Wittkower, E. & Chance, N. (1964) Cross-cultural enquiry into the symptomatology of depression. *Transcultural Psychiatric Research Review*, **1**(1): 5–18.

Oakley, A. (1974) *The Sociology of Housework*. Oxford: Martin Robertson.

Opler, M. K. (Ed.) (1959) Cultural differences in mental disorders. In *Culture and Mental Health*. London: Macmillan.

Sim, M. (1974) *Guide to Psychiatry*. Edinburgh: Churchill Livingstone.

Skrimshire, A. M. (1976) A small area analysis of self-poisoning and self-injury in the region of Oxford. *Journal of Biosocial Science*, **8**: 85–112.

Trethowan, W. & Sims, A. C. (1983) *Psychiatry, 5th edn*. London: Baillière Tindall.

4

How Does Mental Disorder Affect People?

The effects of mental disorder range from distortion or exaggeration of normal responses to serious disorganization of the personality. In the case of neurosis the behaviour and speech of the patient may not differ markedly from that of the average person, while psychosis may be marked by strange or perplexing departures from behavioural norms. Mental disorder may affect *behaviour, speech, thinking, mood* and *perception*, and the possible combinations of effects are enormous. If the nurse is to make sense of the wealth of clinical features apparent in the average ward she must learn to organize her awareness of the effects of mental disorder and should learn to systematically describe and record what she sees and hears. This, of necessity, involves learning the vocabulary of psychiatry and time spent on learning basic descriptive terms will reduce the likelihood of the nurse giving rambling and confused accounts of patient behaviour when a simple and short psychiatric term will neatly capture the essence of what is being described. It is therefore suggested that the nurse make herself thoroughly familiar with the contents of this chapter before proceeding to any consideration of the mental disorders themselves.

The language of medicine still tends to be used in describing the effects of mental disorder insofar as most textbooks speak of the *signs* and *symptoms* of mental disorder (these sometimes being referred to collectively as the *clinical features* of the mental disorder). The nurse should remember that a *symptom* is a subjective complaint reported by the patient (e.g. pain, anxiety, depression), while a *sign* is an objective change which can be noted by an outside observer (e.g. hand-wringing, pacing up and down, restlessness). While the nurse should familiarize herself with the descriptive language of psychiatry she must resist any tendency to reduce the patient to a 'parcel of signs and symptoms'. Purely descriptive language enables us to record *how* the patient behaves but tells us nothing about *why* he behaves as he does, though it may enable us to consider some possibilities while rejecting others.

The purely descriptive approach typified psychiatry in its earlier stages, when lengthy inventories of signs and symptoms were compiled with little attempt being made to explain *why* patients behaved and thought as they did.

The description of changes in the patient's behaviour or thought processes is not an end in itself, but is merely part of the first step of assessing patients in order that problems may be identified and an appropriate care plan designed to meet them.

Overenthusiastic use of descriptive terms simply denies the individuality of the patient; the nurse should try to see the person behind the symptoms. The 'standard' depressed, anxious or schizophrenic patient does not exist—*patients are people and people are individuals*.

The clinical features of mental disorder may be grouped into the following four major categories: disorders of thought, disorders of perception, disorders of mood and disorders of behaviour.

Disorders of Thought (Table 3)

In mental disorder, various abnormal ideas or beliefs may preoccupy the patient. The most characteristic of these is the *delusion*.

A delusion may be defined as 'a false belief which is out of keeping with the patient's background and which is unamenable to logic'.

Delusions are held with an overwhelming sense of conviction and cannot be corrected by an appeal to reason. Delusions do *not* occur in neurosis, but are a hallmark of psychotic disorders.

Delusions may be of many types, including the following:

Persecutory delusions (paranoid delusions)

The patient believes himself to be the victim of a plot or conspiracy and often believes that this 'plot' to harm him is the work of some powerful organization

Table 3 Disturbances of thought (and associated disorders of content of speech).

Delusions
   persecution
   guilt
   hypochondriasis
   somatic
   nihilistic
   religiose
   influence
	occur in psychosis, *never* neurosis, and may be primary or secondary, systematized or unsystematized

Ideas of reference: often accompany persecutory delusions

Concrete thinking

Flight of ideas

Clang association

Pressure of speech

Poverty of thought

Thought blocking

Knight's move thinking

Word salad

Verbigeration (perseveration)

Circumstantiality

Neologisms

Obsessions

Overvalued ideas

Phobias

Amnesia

Hypermnesia

such as the police, the Catholic Church or the Communist Party. Sometimes the persecutory delusions centre around neighbours or workmates and the patient may claim that attempts are being made to poison, gas or electrocute him. These feelings may co-exist with *ideas of reference*; that is, the belief that casual remarks or actions of people he meets are intended to have some special significance for him. For example, the patient may notice someone wearing a red tie and this may be interpreted as a 'sign' that he is being followed by Communist agents. A retired nurse who had developed a paranoid psychosis entertained the delusional belief that she was to be torn to pieces by wild animals. When she turned on her television set and saw a natural history programme about lions this was interpreted as a further 'warning' to her. Even passers-by walking their dogs was regarded as another 'sign' that she was to be dismembered by animals.

Persecutory delusions (usually accompanied by ideas of reference) occur in a variety of psychotic disorders, namely schizophrenia, paranoid states, organic psychoses and affective psychoses (psychoses of mood—notably endogenous depression). In endogenous depression the persecutory delusions may be part of an overall picture of guilt and self-blame. Persecutory delusions tend to arise in middle-aged or elderly persons and are the commonest type of delusion. The patient experiencing these delusions will often be extremely tormented by them and there may be a high suicide risk in this case.

Delusions of grandeur

These are delusions of exalted status and the patient may believe himself to be a member of the aristocracy or the Royal Family or perhaps even God or Jesus Christ. Delusions of this type lead the patient to believe that he has unlimited wealth, power and influence, and he may unfortunately start to behave accordingly.

Delusions of grandeur are commonest in acute manic states, but may also be seen in some schizophrenic and organic disorders.

Delusions of guilt

These consist of false beliefs to the effect that the patient is guilty of horrendous misdeeds in his/her past life. The patient may bleakly describe himself as 'evil' or 'sinful' and may cite trivial misdeeds as evidence of this. These beliefs of wickedness are often coupled with the belief that the patient is to be punished by God as retribution for past 'sins'—the 'retribution' is often to take the form of lingering and painful incurable illnesses.

Hypochondriacal delusions

These must be distinguished from the feelings of hypochondriasis which are common in many neurotic disorders. The patient entertaining hypochondriacal delusions has delusions of bodily disease which are rigidly maintained despite medical evidence to the contrary. The patient may believe that he has cancer, venereal disease or bowel obstructions and may interpret these imagined illnesses as retribution for past 'sins'.

Hypochondriacal delusions may occur in endogenous depression and in some schizophrenic disorders.

Somatic delusions

These are false beliefs that the patient's body has undergone, or is undergoing, some strange anatomical transformation.

A teenage schizophrenic girl believed that her flesh was slowly changing into plastic and she would study herself in the mirror for hours, feeling her face cautiously. Somatic delusions may be less extreme and the patient may insist that his nose is enormously large or that his body is slowly shrinking.

These delusions may arise in schizophrenia.

Nihilistic delusions

The word 'nihilistic' is derived from the Latin 'nihil' meaning 'nothing' so that the phrase literally means 'delusions of nothingness'. The patient may state that he or the world has ceased to exist, that he is dead or that parts of his body (usually bowels or brain) have died or putrefied.

These delusions may arise in endogenous depression or, less commonly, in schizophrenia or organic psychosis.

Religiose delusions

These differ from religious beliefs in that they are distorted and rigidly held beliefs which would be rejected by others of the same religious persuasion, though they have their initial origin in orthodox religious beliefs. The patient may announce that he is the recipient of divine messages or revelations and that he is to save the world, perhaps describing himself as the new Messiah. The road to salvation may unfortunately be paved by rather odd practices. One patient announced that pepper contained the 'divine essence' and would 'concentrate the Christ beam' wherever it was distributed. He paraded up and down a busy city street during the rush hour, bringing traffic to a standstill, and throwing handfuls of pepper into the air as he delivered a rambling and disjointed harangue, until he was eventually arrested by two explosively sneezing constables.

These delusions are commonest in schizophrenics.

Delusions of influence (feelings of passivity)

The patient believes his thoughts and actions to be under external, alien control and may also complain that thoughts are inserted into his head (*thought insertion*) or that thoughts are being removed or 'stolen' by some strange external force (*thought withdrawal*) or may suggest that his thoughts are apparent to everyone in the room (*thought broadcasting*).

Delusions may be built up into a logical and complex system (*systematized delusions*) or may be fleeting, jumbled and disorganized (*unsystematized delusions*).

Delusions may also be primary or secondary.

Primary delusions

These arise when an everyday event suddenly assumes a special significance for the patient though this significance may be quite incomprehensible to others.

Fish (1967) describes how such a strange idea suddenly 'surfaced' in a patient's consciousness. A young Irishman was at breakfast with two fellow lodgers when one pushed the salt cellar towards him. He immediately realized that he must return home to greet the Pope who was visiting his family to reward them.

A young girl identified the onset of her schizophrenic disorder by describing how, on entering a cinema, she suddenly realized that it was 'a place for prostitutes . . . and the people were all there to judge me . . . it seemed as if I had suddenly woken up with the meaning of life' (Mayer-Gross et al, 1977).

An Englishman, on being given a biscuit by his brother-in-law, immediately *realized* that his brother-in-law was accusing him of being a homosexual and was organizing a gang to spy on him (Fish, 1967).

Primary delusions are regarded as being diagnostic of schizophrenia.

Secondary delusions

These do not 'fall from a clear blue sky' like primary delusions, but arise from an attempt by the patient to *explain* already disordered thoughts or feelings. For example, the patient who believes that he is the victim of a conspiracy to do him harm may notice the milkman smiling at him and 'realize' that the milkman is one of the conspirators and that he has placed poison in his milk.

The depressed patient may 'explain' his psychotic depression by deciding that he must be guilty of some terrible crime, and the pathologically elated patient may 'explain' his mania by deciding that he must be rich and famous.

In conclusion it is important to realize the overwhelming conviction with which delusional beliefs are held. Clare (1975) has commented that

'there appears to be no form of persuasion so effective, no method of reasoning so persuasive, that it can convince psychotic patients of the absurdity of their beliefs; no indoctrination, however brutal, ruthless or destructive, can manipulate a psychotic person into acknowledging that his beliefs *might* be in error. Psychotic persons chose to burn at the Inquisatorial stake rather than renounce delusional convictions. Mentally ill patients over the past two centuries have been exposed to the most extraordinary physical and mental humiliations, to bleedings, purgings, beatings, freezings, boilings, neglect, torture and death itself, yet their stubborn adherence to the content of their clearly delusional beliefs was not affected.'

After this eloquent and horrifying statement it is perhaps unnecessary to add that the nurse should not attempt to persuade patients of the falseness of delusional beliefs. Such attempts will not weaken the strength of delusional beliefs, but may actually increase it.

Other disorders of thought include acceleration of the thought processes (*flight of ideas*), where ideas crowd in with incredible speed colliding with and displacing one another (rather like billiard balls colliding and careering around the table). Flight of ideas may be accompanied by *clang association* in which rhymes or puns form the associating link between ideas. This is demonstrated in the following responses made by a patient in response to an enquiry by her doctor about her health during the preceding year.

'Yes, I was dumb and numb then but not deaf, I know Mrs. Ida Teff, she is dead, probably an appendicitis; I don't know whether she lost her sight, sightless Hesse, His Highness of Hesse, Sister Louise, His Highness of Baden.'

(*Jaspers, 1959*).

Flight of ideas and clang association occur in mania, in which the mental acceleration is accompanied by physical overactivity. It may also occur in schizophrenic disorders. In both instances the underlying flight of ideas may be reflected in *pressure of speech* (accelerated and disjointed speech, with or without clang association).

In severe depression the opposite effect may occur and the patient may complain of inability to gather or express thoughts (*poverty of thought*), while schizophrenics often display *thought blocking*—a sudden interruption of the stream of thought which is apparent when the patient pauses and then continues (often on a different topic). Patients often seem aware of the lengthy pauses occurring in their speech as a result of thought blocking, even though the casual observer may not notice the pauses or attach any significance to them.

Normal individuals may experience a mild degree of thought blocking in stressful situations (oral examination or job interviews).

In schizophrenia the normal logical sequence of ideas may be lost; this is apparent when the patient jumps from one idea to another without any apparent connection between the two. This is referred to as *knight's move thinking* (the knight is the only chess piece to move erratically by jumping over intervening pieces).

In some schizophrenic disorders speech content may become completely garbled so that a stream of completely disconnected and unrelated words is poured out (*word salad*) or the same word or phrase may be repeated over and over again (*verbigeration* or *perseveration*).

Concrete thinking is an inability to think conceptually, or in the abstract, and is not uncommon in schizophrenia. A person with concrete thinking will reveal it if asked to give the general meaning of a proverb (for example, 'People who live in glass houses shouldn't throw stones' may produce the explanation 'they would break the glass').

Another speech disturbance (also reflecting underlying thought disorder) is *circumstantiality* in which the patient rambles on endlessly, dragging in a multitude of irrelevant and tedious details, perhaps pausing at intervals to say 'Oh yes, where *was* I?' Circumstantiality may be apparent in the mentally handicapped and in organic psychosis but may also be readily observed in many normal people, especially those of limited intelligence or advanced years. Most people have met the 'party bore' who will drone on endlessly about the most trivial of events, driving the unfortunate victim to the point of desperation.

The schizophrenic patient may sometimes create completely new words (*neologisms*) which have meaning to the patient, but may perplex the listener. One patient spoke of the process of 'oversolarest' by which men were arousing sexual feelings in her from many miles away (Maddison and Kellehear, 1982), while a Student Nurse in the early stages of schizophrenia complained to her doctor that she was being 'sprockeled by an enema with a green band on it' (Henderson and Batchelor, 1962).

Obsessions are persistently intrusive and recurring thoughts which the patient feels unable to banish. This is a neurotic symptom and the patient recognizes the ideas to be abnormal and may be acutely distressed by troublesome obsessive thoughts. The young mother may be troubled by persistently intrusive thoughts of killing her baby or the religious person may find an obscene or blasphemous phrase continually forcing its way into consciousness no matter how hard he tries to prevent it.

Overvalued ideas fall between the two extremes of normal and delusional beliefs and consist of preoccupations with some aspect of the person's life, appearance or personality. They can assume gigantic proportions—to the point of excluding competing ideas.

Overvalued ideas may eventually develop into delusions, as in the case of the young woman who was preoccupied by her feet, insisting that they were abnormally big (overvalued idea) and who eventually 'realized' that she had a 'divine mission' to walk the length and breadth of Britain in order to announce that she was to give birth to the Son of God (delusion).

A *phobia* is an exaggerated fear of an object or situation which the individual realizes is not a true source of danger. It is a neurotic symptom as the person concerned recognizes the fear as irrational but feels powerless to control it.

Memory may be affected in mental disorder and the patient may experience *amnesia* (loss of memory) or *hypermnesia* (abnormally and indiscriminately increased memory)—the former occurring in a wide range of mental disorders (anxiety, depression, organic disorders) and the latter occurring in mania.

Disorders of Perception (Table 4)

Perception may be defined as 'the mental awareness of things through the medium of the senses' (Johnston, 1971) and consists of two steps: (a) receiving a stimulus via one of our senses, and (b) interpreting the stimulus mentally to ascribe meaning to it.

In mental disorder the process of perception may be grossly disturbed; these disturbances take the form of hallucinations and illusions.

Table 4 Disturbances of perception.

Hallucinations
  auditory
  visual
  tactile
  gustatory
  olfactory
	only occur in psychosis, *never* in neurosis

Illusions
  may occur in neurosis, psychosis, drug or alcohol
  withdrawal and in 'normals'	

Hallucinations

A hallucination may be defined as 'a false perception occurring in the absence of an external sensory stimulus'. Hallucinations may affect any of the five senses. In other words the patient may hear, see, smell, touch or taste that which does not exist. Like delusions, hallucinations indicate a break with normal external reality and may be terrifyingly real to the patient.

The definition described hallucinations as 'false perceptions' made in the absence of an 'external stimulus'. The word 'external' is a key part of the definition as there is a possibility that hallucinations may occur in response to *internal* chemical stimuli arising from disorders of brain chemistry. This viewpoint will be discussed further in the chapter on schizophrenia.

Normal persons may experience hallucinations in the course of a febrile illness or in extreme states of debilitation or fatigue, but persistent hallucinations arising in a state of clear consciousness are indicative of psychosis. Like delusions, hallucinations do *not* occur in neurosis.

Auditory hallucinations (hallucinations of hearing)

The patient may describe these as 'the voices' which may issue commands, make suggestions or give a running commentary on the patient's actions. The 'voices' may be friendly or threatening and may consist of clear and intelligible statements or garbled fragments. Hallucinations of hearing are the commonest type of hallucination and may arise in any psychotic disorder, though they are commonest in schizophrenia.

Visual hallucinations (hallucinations of sight)

The patient sees 'visions' which may be pleasant or unpleasant and may be of clearly defined people or objects or simply flashes of light, often arranged into geometrical symbols or patterns. Particularly frightening visual hallucinations occur in acute alcoholic psychosis (delirium tremens); these have led alcoholics to christen this state as 'the horrors'.

Olfactory and gustatory hallucinations

These are hallucinations of smell and taste respectively and often occur together in the same patient. The smells and tastes are often unpleasant ones and may lead the patient to deduce that his food has been poisoned (gustatory hallucination) or that he is being exposed to poisonous gas (olfactory hallucination). These hallucinations may arise in temporal lobe epilepsy, but are otherwise almost diagnostic of a schizophrenic disorder.

Tactile hallucinations

These are hallucinations of touch and may affect any part of the body surface, although they commonly centre around the genitals, causing patients to complain that they have been sexually molested during their sleep. This type of disordered perception is commonest in schizophrenia but may occur in drug withdrawal. Cocaine withdrawal can cause particularly unpleasant tactile hallucinations which the patient describes as being like insects crawling under the skin (the 'cocaine bug').

Fleeting hallucinatory experiences may occur in normal people in the twilight state between sleeping and waking (*hypnogogic hallucinations*) and a peculiar type of hallucination in which the patient or surrounding objects seems to have dwindled in size has been described by some migraine sufferers (*Lilliputian hallucinations*).

Illusions

The word 'illusion' is derived from the Latin verb 'illudere' which means 'to mock', and refers to *misinterpretations* of sensory stimuli. Under the right conditions our senses are readily deceived. The apprehensive person entering a darkened room may be startled by a coat hanging up, having momentarily misinterpreted it as a sinister figure lurking in the darkness. Similarly the apprehensive person walking alone down a dark country lane at night may misinterpret the sound of leaves rustling in the wind as footsteps following behind and may break into a run.

A tactile illusion may be readily demonstrated by crossing the fingers of the left hand and then gently resting a pen on the notch made by the tips of the crossed fingers. Close your eyes, and gently and lightly move the pen up and down. The resultant blurred perception feels like *two* pens as two separate sensory nerves, which are not usually close together, are registering touch.

Illusions are thus not abnormal and may occur more frequently in normal persons affected by fatigue or stress. In states of drug or alcohol withdrawal, illusions increase in frequency and intensity, and may shade off into true hallucinations. The alcoholic in delirium tremens may be startled by the pattern on the wallpaper as it resembles snakes to his fevered eye (illusion)—the snakes may then proceed to slide down the wall and climb up the counterpane (hallucination).

Disorders of Mood (Table 5)

Mood, or *affect*, may be defined as a state of emotional tone or feeling, and may vary from elation to depression. Mood is often affected by mental disorders, particularly in the group of disorders known as the affective disorders (disorders of mood), and such disturbance is very common. The following are some of the commoner mood disturbances which may form part of the overall clinical picture in mental disorder:

Table 5 Disturbances of mood.

Depression
Anxiety
Elation
euphoria
hypomania
mania
Incongruity and blunting of affect
'La belle indifference'
Lability of mood
Hostility
Apathy
Depersonalization and derealization

Depression

This is a state of pathological sadness in which mood is lowered to the point of distress. It may occur in 'normal' people, in neurosis and in psychosis and is discussed fully in Chapter 12.

Elation

This is the opposite of depression and refers to elevation of mood. It may be regarded as abnormal when it reaches a level unjustified by external events or becomes uncontrollable. Elation may reach the level of *hypomania*, in which elevated mood is accompanied by accelerated physical and mental activity. The extreme of mood elevation is *mania* in which psychomotor acceleration becomes almost uncontrollable and mood reaches dizzying heights of exaltation, quite unjustified by external events.

Euphoria

This is the term given to minor mood elevation accompanied by feelings of well-being, confidence and enthusiasm. Feelings of euphoria are quite normal if justified by external events and constructively expressed, but become symptomatic of mental disorder when they are inappropriate to events or inappropriately expressed. Thus the continuum of degrees of elation ranges through euphoria to hypomania to mania.

Anxiety

This is the blend of fear and uncertainty produced in response to threat, be the threat real or imagined. It is only abnormal if there is no identifiable cause (free-floating anxiety) or if the anxiety is disproportionate and produced in response to a threat which the patient realizes not to be a genuine danger (phobic anxiety).

Incongruity of affect

This is a schizophrenic symptom in which emotions expressed are inappropriate to the circumstances. A patient may respond to news of a bereavement with indifference, or indeed with levity, while news of fortunate events may produce a response of sadness. A teenage schizophrenic girl began to giggle uncontrollably during her mother's funeral and seemed to be very amused by the entire event, despite the fact that she had had a close relationship with her mother. *Blunting of affect* refers to the curious emotional shallowness shown by many schizophrenics. Emotional responses are flat and shallow and the normal range of emotional responses is absent. Before describing emotional responses as 'shallow' or 'blunted' the nurse should remember that institutionalization may also lead to emotional blunting. Incongruity of affect should not be confused with '*la belle indifference*' which is a bland lack of concern shown in the presence of distressing symptoms by patients suffering from hysteria.

Lability of mood

Mood is said to be *labile* when there are quick changes from one mood to another, often for no apparent reason or for very trivial reasons. The patient may literally be laughing one moment and crying the next. Lability of mood is common in the organic mental disorders of old age.

Hostility

This may only be regarded as abnormal when it is the prevailing mood, regardless of circumstances, and when it starts to bring about deterioration in interpersonal relationships. Hostility may be openly displayed or may find more subtle expression in stubbornness or lack of cooperation. The nurse must always be aware of the fact that hostility is often a response to hospitalization and that the causes may often be quickly identified and reduced.

Apathy

This refers to the loss of interest and drive shown by many psychiatric patients. Schizophrenia may produce apathy at an early stage of its development, and parents often complain that schizophrenic offspring are 'listless' and 'dreamy'.

Institutionalization also rapidly produces apathy and, in this case, the cause is the hospital regime, not mental disorder. Schizophrenics are particularly at risk of institutionalization and, as they may already show a tendency to apathy, must be carefully monitored in this respect.

Depersonalization

This is a state wherein the patient feels himself to be unreal. This may be described by the patient as the experience of looking at himself as a spectator or outsider, as though in a dream. There is a strange sense of loss of identity coupled with the feelings of unreality.

Derealization

This refers to the experience of things or events *outside* of the person seeming unreal. Familiar objects or persons may suddenly seem strange or unreal. Depersonalization and derealization usually occur together and may arise in almost any mental disorder, but are perhaps commonest in schizophrenia, depression and hysteria. Normal persons may experience depersonalization or derealization if fatigued or stressed, and both responses have been described by survivors of major accidents, the recently bereaved, and by persons who were inmates of Nazi concentration camps (Mayer-Gross et al, 1977).

Depersonalization may be associated with emotional blunting, and the overall effect may be distinctly unpleasant.

A classical monograph on the subject vividly describes the experiences of depersonalization and derealization:

'To the depersonalized individual the world appears strange, peculiar, foreign, dream like. Objects appear at times strangely diminished in size, at times flat. Sound appears to come from a distance . . . Patients characterize their imagery as pale and colourless, and some complain that they have altogether lost the power of imagination.

Their emotions likewise undergo marked alteration. Patients complain that they are capable of experiencing neither pain nor pleasure; love and hate have perished with them'.

(Schilder, 1982)

Disorders of behaviour (Table 6)

The term 'behaviour' refers to 'those activities of an organism *which can be observed*'. Behaviour is therefore visible and can be directly measured by the onlooker, unlike private, invisible thoughts, feelings and emotions.

This heading includes the areas of sleep, appetite and general activity level.

Table 6 Disturbances of behaviour.

Insomnia
  early insomnia (initial insomnia)
  early morning waking

Anorexia
Bulimia
Appetite suppression
Food refusal

Overactivity
Underactivity
Stupor

Flexibilitas cerea

Echopraxia
Echolalia

Negativism

Stereotypy

Compulsions

Sleep

This is disturbed in many mental disorders. There may be *initial insomnia* also known as *early insomnia* which consists of difficulty in getting to sleep. The patient may dread bedtime as he associates night-time with lying awake, tossing and turning, as the night slowly passes. *Early morning waking* refers to the tendency, shown by many severely depressed patients, to wake around or before dawn and be unable to get back to sleep again. In mental disorder, notably anxiety and depression, sleep is often restless, fitful and punctuated by nightmares.

Appetite

This may be reduced or lost (depression or anxiety), rigidly suppressed (anorexia nervosa) or dramatically increased (mania). Anorexia nervosa may also be punctuated by episodes of *bulimia*, or compulsive over-eating, and the depressed person may also have bulimic 'binges' on occasion.

The delusional patient may refuse food, believing it to be poisoned or contaminated, or may embark upon a fast—prompted by religious delusions or the belief that he is dead or that his bowels have rotted.

As general mental state improves with treatment, appetite tends to stabilize and observation of food intake can thus provide a useful indicator of progress.

General activity and behaviour

The patient may show marked overactivity (mania and schizophrenic excitement) or underactivity (depression and catatonic schizophrenia). In catatonic schizophrenia the patient may assume the rare state of *flexibilitas cerea* (waxy flexibility) in which his limbs may be arranged in any anatomically feasible position like those of a wax model. Once so arranged, the patient will maintain the resultant posture for a lengthy period of time. When moving the patient's limbs, a peculiar slight resistance is felt; like that experienced when bending soft wax.

Echopraxia

This is another schizophrenic sympton whereby the patient copies the gestures, mannerisms and gait of those around him. It may be coupled with *echolalia*, or the tendency to repeat or echo anything said to the patient.

The opposite of echopraxia is *negativism*, or the tendency to do the opposite of what is asked, and it occurs in schizophrenia. The patient showing this sign will stand up if asked to sit down or close his mouth if asked to open it.

Bizarre mannerisms and gestures are common in schizophrenia and these may have some mystic significance to the patient. An example of this is *stereotypy*, wherein the patient endlessly repeats an action or group of words, or monotonously paces up and down, carefully following a set pattern. Bizarre grimaces and facial expressions may also be shown by the schizophrenic patient.

Compulsions

These are acts which the patient feels compelled to carry out and which often assume a ritualistic significance. Compulsions are often combined with obsessions as the salient features of an obsessive/compulsive neurosis or may be apparent in schizophrenia.

Compulsions usually assume the form of compulsive washing or tidying, or repeatedly checking to ensure that simple actions have been properly carried out (for example, closing a door, turning off a tap, adjusting the position of a piece of furniture).

Stupor

This is the opposite of overactivity and refers to the slowing down of activity to the point of immobility. In such a state the patient is completely unresponsive to stimuli. Stupor is rare, but may very occasionally occur in catatonic schizophrenia or severe psychotic depressions. The nurse should beware of confusing the psychiatric use of the word stupor with the general medical use of the word. In general medicine, stupor refers to the state between full consciousness and coma, in which the patient *does* respond to painful stimuli.

Confusion and disorientation

The term *confusion* refers to a state of disordered consciousness in which facial expression, speech and behaviour usually clearly register perplexity and bewilderment. The patient has difficulty in grasping what is going on around him and may display high levels of agitation or inappropriate behaviour.

Confusion commonly reflects disturbance of brain function which may be temporary (as in toxic confusional states associated with infection or drug or alcohol withdrawal) or permanent (as in degenerative disorders of the brain).

Confusion is often associated with *disorientation*, a term used to indicate that a patient has 'lost his bearings' insofar as he is suffering from impaired ability to identify who he is, where he is, and to whom he is talking and is also experiencing difficulty in identifying the time of day, day of the week, month of the year or the year itself. If all of these difficulties are present, the patient is said to be disorientated for *time, place* and *person*.

This account of psychiatric symptomatology should enable the nurse to clearly and concisely describe the clinical features of mental disorder and should help her to relate these to the major groups of mental disorder. The nurse must beware of overenthusiastic or indiscriminate use of these terms however. They are very sticky 'labels' and may be difficult to remove once carelessly applied. In conclusion it is also important to reiterate that the nurse must try to see the patient as a person—not as a group of symptoms. Description is a beginning—not an end.

Key Concepts

1 Accurate description is essential in psychiatric nursing as mental disorder often has a complex range of effects on the individual which must be accurately and scientifically summarized.
2 Some patients will appear to be little affected by mental disorder while others will show gross disorganization of personality.
3 Mental disorder may cause disturbance of thought, perception, mood and behaviour.
4 Disturbance of thought is often reflected in distorted content of speech.
5 The commonest thought disturbance is the *delusion* (can you define this and give examples?).
6 The commonest perceptual disturbance is the *hallucination* (definition? example?).
7 Mood (*affect*) is subject to a wide range of disturbances, ranging from mania to depression, and including anxiety and the strange phenomena of depersonalization and derealization (definitions of these five disturbances?).
8 General behaviour and activity are also subject to a variety of disturbances (examples?).
9 In conclusion, the nurse must remember to try and see the person behind the symptoms. *Patients are people and people are individuals.*

References

Clare, A. (1975) *Psychiatry in Dissent*. London: Tavistock Publications.

Fish, F. J. (1967) *Clinical Psychopathology*. Bristol: Wright.

Henderson, D. K. & Batchelor, I. (1962) *Henderson & Gillespie's Textbook of Psychiatry*. Oxford: Oxford University Press.

Jaspers, K. (1959) *General Psychopathology, 7th edn*. Manchester: Manchester University Press.

Johnston, M. (1971) *Mental Health & Mental Illness*. Philadelphia: J. B. Lippincott.

Maddison, D. & Kellehear, K. J. (1982) *Psychiatric Nursing, 5th edn*. Edinburgh: Churchill Livingstone.

Mayer-Gross, W., Slater, E. & Roth, M. (1977) *Clinical Psychiatry, 3rd edn*. London: Baillière Tindall.

Sainsbury, M. J. (1980) *Key to Psychiatry, 3rd edn*. Australia: Australia & New Zealand Book Company.

Schilder, P. (1982) *Introduction to Psychoanalytic Psychiatry*. US: Human Science Publishers.

5

Personality: Its Structure and Development

> In the psychological field there is no 'generalised mind' to be controlled. There are only single, concrete minds, each one of which presents problems peculiar to itself.
>
> *Gordon W. Allport*

The word *'personality'* is derived from the Latin word 'persona', which described the mask worn during theatrical dramas, and refers to those relatively stable and enduring aspects of the individual which distinguish him from other people. The concept of uniqueness is central to the understanding of personality as each person displays an individual combination of characteristics which endows that individual with a unique identity. Personalities are as different as fingerprints.

It is helpful for the nurse to consider the concept of personality carefully as it will help her to achieve a greater understanding, not only of her patients, but of herself.

In ordinary conversation the word personality is often used imprecisely. It is common for someone to remark that an individual has a 'pleasant' or a 'poor' personality or that someone has 'lots of personality' while another may be described as not having much 'personality'. Such statements bear no relationship to the psychologist's use of the term. Used scientifically the term refers to those unique personal characteristics which shape the individual's interaction with his environment and affect his ability to get along with other people and himself.

Personality is a major factor affecting the way in which the individual copes with stress, pain, illness and crisis. It also influences the way in which the nurse perceives her patients and responds to them, as the nurse brings her own unique blend of personal characteristics into every nurse/patient interaction. Personality may determine areas of success and failure in nursing and may influence areas of ability and areas of difficulty. Our likes and dislikes, our hobbies and interests, the kind of work we enjoy, the ability to adapt to different situations and to make friends, our attitudes and beliefs; all are powerfully influenced by personality. How we behave in any given context is always a reflection of personality.

Personality does not only influence our perceptions of others: it also influences perceptions of self. Personal adjustment, self-image and, in particular, self-esteem are all influenced by the pervasive forces of personality.

Personality development is a complex and dynamic process involving constant movement and evolution, though personality always retains a certain identifiable consistency. This fact makes it possible for persons of all ages to profit and learn from positive experiences and to modify behaviour in adaptive directions. This is the rationale underlying all therapeutic endeavours on the behalf of patients.

Personality is expressed through *behaviour*, that is the visible activities of the person as opposed to the inner, private realm of thoughts, feelings and emotions which shape behaviour by focussing it through the lens of the personality. Some behaviours are valuable or useful to the individual as they help us to adapt successfully to the demands of a constantly changing environment (*adaptive behaviours*). Others are disadvantageous to the individual as they hamper successful adjustment or adaptation (*maladaptive behaviours*).

Persistent behavioural traits often reflect deeply rooted personality factors, and the nurse should resist the temptation to 'explain' behaviour simply by naming it or giving it a 'label'. For example a nurse observing an unfamiliar patient behaving irritably at breakfast may ask a colleague, who has worked on the ward longer, what is wrong with him. The colleague may say 'That's Peter; he's a poor mixer'. 'Oh,' the first nurse may say, 'that explains it'. Of course labels like 'poor mixer' do not explain anything. The nurse has fallen into the error called the *'nominal fallacy'* by psychologists (the belief that naming or labelling behaviour somehow explains it). Why is Peter a 'poor mixer'? Labels may help predict behaviour but they do not explain it.

An understanding of personality factors, including those that promote and those that hamper adjustment, will help the nurse towards greater understanding of behaviour and will reduce the tendency to 'explain' behaviour by labelling it. Understanding the complexities of behaviour and the many problems of adjustment which may beset the individual depends to a large extent on understanding the processes by which personality develops. It is therefore important to recognize the relationship between the early experiences that most human beings undergo and the development of personality.

Much of the information we have today about the development of the personality is not based upon scientific research but is derived from the psychological theories of early influential workers in this field.

Sigmund Freud (1856–1939)

The pioneering work of Freud established a general theory of the mind which has had a profound and lasting effect on twentieth century society. His theories had an explosive impact upon the psychological thinking of his times and developed the foundational theories of personality development.

In his approach to the study of the mind Freud adopted an uncompromising *determinism*; that is, he believed that mental happenings were never 'accidental' but were always determined, or caused, by forces and processes which could be scientifically described rather than discussed in the vague philosophical fashion current in his day. He also developed the concept of the *unconscious mind* and suggested that it played an active and dynamic part in determining behaviour rather than serving as a repository of ideas and memories which had fallen below the threshold of awareness because they were relatively unimportant. Freud also suggested that behaviour was always *goal-directed*, and suggested that not all of the causes of our behaviour are known to us, as many are unavailable to consciousness. Much of our motivation remains unconscious and most persons have but limited insight into the powerful hidden forces shaping behaviour.

Freud also suggested that human development followed a logical, sequential pattern and that the critical tasks of each developmental stage must be successfully completed in order to move on smoothly to the next stage. Failure to successfully

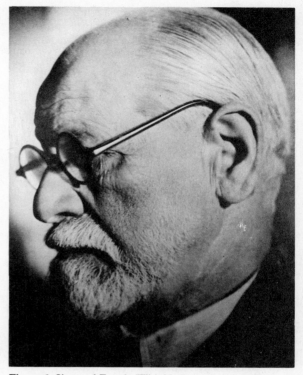

Figure 1 Sigmund Freud. (With kind permission of the Bettman Archive.)

complete the developmental tasks associated with any particular stage may lead to maladaptive behaviour as the individual shows signs of fixation at that stage. This *developmental approach* to the study of personality stresses the crucial importance of early childhood experiences in the development of human personality and suggests that many of the emotional problems of adult life may be related to negative influences occurring during the early years.

The geography of the mind

Anatomists had described the structure of the brain and Freud embarked upon a systematic attempt to chart the structure of the mind.

Freud considered the mind as consisting of three 'territories': the *conscious*, the *pre-conscious* and the *unconscious* mind. The conscious part of the mind is aware of the here and now and only functions when the individual is awake, directing the individual as he behaves in a rational, thoughtful way. Below the level of consciousness is the layer of the pre-conscious mind in which ideas and feelings are *par-*

tially forgotten, but can still be brought into consciousness if the individual concentrates on recall. Most people have had the experience of attempting to recall a forgotten piece of information (a name, date or address for example) and of being aware that the piece of information is not 'too far away'. 'It's on the tip of my tongue' people often say as they delve for the forgotten material which is close to consciousness, and whose presence can often be 'felt'. Later psychologists referred to this state as a T.O.T. state (tip of the tongue), and it usually ends as the desired piece of information is triumphantly retrieved. The pre-conscious mind serves a useful function as it is not economical to burden the conscious mind with a multitude of facts that are infrequently used and not in current demand. The pre-conscious mind also serves as a 'watchdog' as it prevents unacceptable, disturbing unconscious memories from gravitating upwards into consciousness and disturbing emotional equilibrium.

Below the level of pre-consciousness lies the vast dark territory of the unconscious mind. Medieval cartographers often marked their maps with the warning inscription 'Here there be dragons' and the same might be said of this part of our Freudian map of the mind. The territory of the unconscious is by far the biggest area of the mind and can be compared to the main hidden part of an iceberg that floats beneath the water. Above the surface, in the sunlight, lies the visible and reassuringly solid tip of the iceberg—the conscious mind. Just below the surface the outline of our iceberg would be visible for some distance as we looked down, but not immediately accessible—the pre-conscious mind. If we continued to look down from the surface to trace the contours of the iceberg, as it became invisible in the depths, our clarity of vision and perspective would be distorted and refracted by the water until we became unable to discern the shape of the ice at all. This invisible mass may be compared to the unconscious mind—submerged deep below the level of consciousness.

The unconscious is a vast storehouse for all the memories, feelings and ideas experienced by the individual during his entire lifetime. There is a continuous downward drift of material into unconsciousness, a steady silent sedimentation of discarded and unused material slowly disappearing into the depths of the unconscious. Sometimes painful or troublesome thoughts and feelings are hastily jettisoned into the depths of unconsciousness, weighted by the motivation to forget them, as to

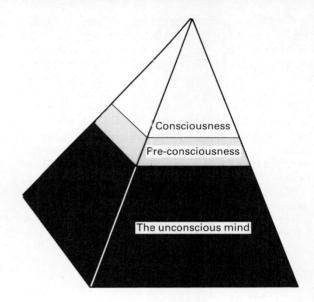

Figure 2 The three 'territories' of the mind.

contemplate them in the full light of consciousness would be too stressful.

Material consigned to the depths of unconsciousness does not cease to play a part in the mental life of the individual but creates powerful currents of psychological energy which influence behaviour because the feelings attached to the 'submerged' material continue to act as dynamic motivating forces. Material (thoughts, feelings and ideas) which has separated from consciousness, because its continued presence there would be too troublesome, is said to have been *repressed*. Excessive repression may create powerful psychological tensions in the unconscious which give rise to neurosis.

The individual is rarely aware of the unconscious mind but it reveals its presence through dreams, slips of the tongue or pen and unaccountable lapses of memory. According to this view the personality is most clearly revealed when the intellect is exercising least control. The individual's behaviour when under the influence of alcohol (in vino veritas), the content of his dreams, his occasionally 'irrational' behaviours (which he, and others, find difficult to explain as they are so 'out of character')—all of these tell us more about him than his socially controlled behaviour. The 'mask' created by social pressures and awareness of cultural expectations has slipped under these circumstances.

Thus the individual may be unaware of repressed thoughts, feelings and wishes but will display emotional and behavioural responses which are an expression of unconscious material of which he is not aware. As negative unconscious memories cannot be expressed normally, their emotional energy, or *affect*, is 'dammed up' or strangulated.

The Id, Ego and Super-Ego

Freud suggested that the newly born child is a seething mass of impulses or instinctual drives, completely devoid of any directing or guiding consciousness. This raw mass of powerful and insistent psychological energies was called the *Id* by Freud. Id simply means 'it' in Latin and this term may have been used to emphasize the impersonal nature of this part of the mind, insofar as it is detached from our conscious and rational nature. The operations of the Id are entirely unconscious and its forces provide the energy for all psychic processes.

The Id is immoral—it recognizes no codes of morality or control—and its drives are *primitive*, *infantile* and *pleasure-seeking*. The powerful forces of the Id are continually seeking outlets and are intolerant of frustration. This is apparent in consideration of the emotional and behavioural responses of the baby to frustration. The newly born baby is helpless and is completely dependent on his mother who provides food, warmth and relief from discomfort. Sometimes mother does not satisfy his needs immediately and his response is often one of violent, undiluted anger expressed in screaming, facial contortion, clenched fists and kicking legs. The baby has yet to learn that needs cannot always be satisfied immediately and that it is often necessary to delay or postpone need-gratification until the circumstances are appropriate.

Babies and small infants live according to what Freud called the *Pleasure Principle*, that is the tendency to seek avoidance of pain and to seek the gratification of primitive, instinctual needs (*primary wishes*) in a selfish and impulsive way. That is to say, the Id avoids pain at all costs and seeks to maintain pleasure. Pleasure, in this sense, means the release of tensions, and pain refers to the presence of unwelcome tensions (hunger, cold, fear and anxiety).

The primary wish fulfilment impulses, which reflect the crude pleasure-seeking strivings of the Id, cannot continue to be freely expressed if the developing individual is to adjust satisfactorily to the environment. The individual learns to gradually tolerate delays of satisfaction, and this process commences when the baby realizes that the breast or bottle is part of the environment rather than part of his own body. As awareness of external reality develops, the restraining impulses of the *Reality Principle* become apparent.

The Reality Principle accepts that primitive pleasure-seeking patterns of behaviour are not always appropriate, that the individual is *not* the 'centre of the universe', and that the environment is populated by many others who may respond negatively to his unrestrained expression of Id impulses. In other words the baby realizes that there exists an external world to which he must adapt by renouncing immediate and selfish gratification of primitive needs.

The development of the *Ego* begins as awareness of external reality unfolds. The main method used by the Ego is *reality testing*, which enables the individual to master impulses, operate independently of parental figures and control the environment. The word ego means 'self'. This reflects the view that this part of the mind strives to integrate the total personality into a smoothly functioning integrated whole, capable of balancing the need for instinctual gratification against the realities of the environment. In the mature adult it is the distinctive pattern of ego adjustments that represents the self to others and distinguishes him from other human beings.

An unfavourable early environment, for example one which lacks a stable mother or mother-substitute, means that the developing infant lacks guidance in the difficult task of adapting to the world about him, and that ego development may be incomplete or poorly organized. The resultant adult may be more prone to neurosis as his inadequately developed ego structures break down under stress. Conscious perceptions of reality belong to the Ego, but the repression of Id impulses takes place unconsciously. To this extent the Ego has its roots in the unconscious but extends upwards into consciousness.

At a still later stage the *Super-Ego* arises to operate as that part of the mind which may be loosely equated with the 'conscience', though the concept of the Super-Ego is more than the word 'conscience' implies. The Super-Ego incorporates the standards of behaviour of people whose approval is valued by the child, and represents the development of *internal* controls as parental values and attitudes are internalized. These internalized values come to assume the same attitude towards the rest of the mind as the parents previously did towards the child, and are only partly conscious, hence the fact that the individual may sometimes feel uneasy or guilty after carrying out an action which his reason tells him is not immoral.

The Super-Ego incorporates values, standards, taboos, prohibitions and ideals, all derived at an early age from the parents or from parental figures. This internalized parental authority is blindly rigid, strictly moralistic and is as unrelenting and ruthless as the Id. Violation of these primitive and rigid codes of right and wrong will lead to the Super-Ego punishing the individual using the powerful weapons of guilt, shame or remorse. The Super-Ego will also reward behaviour compatible with its ideals by generating feelings of euphoria, satisfaction and well-being when behaviour emulates those standards believed by the Super-Ego to be desirable.

In neurosis the Super-Ego may become hypertrophied, or enlarged, and may then viciously and unrealistically punish the individual by generating crucifying feelings of guilt, worthlessness and shame as the individual fails to meet its grossly unrealistic ideals and thus experiences everyday life as an anxiety-evoking series of demands and tests to which he feels unequal. No-one could be equal to the demands of a hypertrophied Super-Ego, as it has become a ruthless and implacable tyrant.

Failure to develop adequate ego strength creates the risk of the Super-Ego rampaging through the self-esteem of the individual, as the Ego does not only deal with unruly Id impulses but must also balance these against the ideals of the Super-Ego. Thus the Ego must weigh Id impulses against the dictates of social reality, which are external, and against the internal prohibitions of the Super-Ego. In other words the Ego performs a delicate 'juggling act' between *desire* (the Id) and *duty* (the Super-Ego).

Psychosexual development

Freud suggested that human development followed a pattern of logical, sequential stages during which the basic instinctual sexual energy (*libido*) finds progressively more sophisticated targets. Libido is sexual energy but Freud used the term 'sexual' in a very broad way which included any pleasurable bodily sensation as well as the everyday meaning of the word. Libido drives emanate from the Id and may find direct expression or be rechannelled into feelings such as tenderness, friendship and pleasure in work.

The newly born baby is a seething mass of Id energies and seeks immediate gratification of these impulses as it has yet to learn to rechannel these energies into substitute activities—the Pleasure Principle still reigns supreme.

Libidinal energy (the energy of the libido) is initially focused on the mouth, as suckling is the first source of pleasurable sensation and tension relief. The newly born child cannot focus its eyes or coordinate its muscular movements, and the world is simply a 'booming, buzzing confusion' as the baby cannot discriminate between sounds. The mouth is the only reliable source of pleasurable sensory input. Freud therefore called this initial stage the *Oral Stage*, as the mouth is the primary organ of pleasure.

Pleasure may be derived from passively suckling (oral erotic phase) or, later, from aggressively biting (oral sadistic phase). Residues of the Oral Stage tend to persist into adult life. Because food and love are given simultaneously during the Oral Stage, oral needs may become synonymous with security and protective love. Adults may show oral behaviours at time of stress (cigarette smoking, chewing gum, compensatory over-eating, drinking alcohol).

The second stage is the *Anal Stage*, in which awareness of the other end of the alimentary tract develops during the second year of life. Initially the child derives pleasure from aggressively expelling faeces (anal sadistic phase) and, later, from withholding faeces (anal erotic phase). In so doing the child begins to learn control of biological functions and takes the first steps towards independence.

Toilet training means that the child experiences the first frustrating restriction of Id impulses but

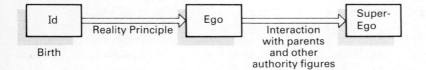

Figure 3 The relationship between the Id, Ego and Super-Ego.

also learns that he may challenge parental authority by rebellion against toilet training routines—withholding faeces or excreting in the wrong place may have a dramatic effect on parents.

The excretory function is closely bound up with social ideas of order, cleanliness and disgust, and Freud believed that over-emphasis on cleanliness during this period may produce an adult with compulsive tendencies towards cleanliness and orderliness, who would also show anxiety in response to any form of disorder (the *anal* or *anankastic personality*).

The anal stage is succeeded at age 3 or 4 by the *Phallic Stage* in which awareness of the genital area as a seat of pleasurable sensation develops. 'Phallus' means penis but Freud used the adjective 'phallic' to describe this stage in infants of both sexes.

Around this age children begin to identify with the parent of the same sex, and Freud suggested that the child unconsciously wishes to replace that parent in the family group. This resentment of the parent of the same sex is coupled with attraction for the parent of the opposite sex and is termed the *Oedipus Complex* in boys and the *Electra Complex* in girls.

Freud suggested that the Oedipus Complex was a normal development which resolved to produce the beginnings of the Super-Ego. Competitive feelings towards the father arouse unconscious fears of pun-ishment in the male child which give rise to what Freud called *castration anxiety*, and this anxiety ultimately brings about the resolution of the Oedipus Complex. The female child was thought by Freud to experience *penis envy* around this time as she becomes uncomfortably aware that she lacks this symbol of male privilege and power. While castration anxiety *resolves* the boy's attraction towards mother and resentment towards father, penis envy was thought to *bring about* attraction for father but rejection of mother by the girl as she unconsciously feels hostility towards mother for bringing her into the world 'in this shape'.

The Phallic Stage, with its associated complexes directed against the parents, is succeeded by the *Latency Stage* when the sex drive seems to disappear. Latency commences around six years of age and continues until puberty. Sexuality has *not* disappeared at this stage but simply 'goes underground'; that is, it remains latent. Infantile amnesia takes place so that people can later deny their earliest sexual feelings and experiences. During latency the child is not devoid of sexual energy but there is no qualitative development of the libido, which seems to lie dormant for this stage.

Freud saw adolescence as the final stage of personality development, characterized by reactivation of libidinal energy during the *Genital Stage*, during

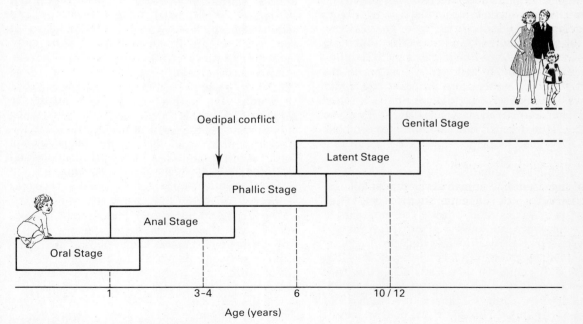

Figure 4 Psychosexual development (Freud).

which physical capacity for sex emerges. This final stage lasts for the remainder of the person's life though its most intense drives aim at satisfactory heterosexual union and beginning the life cycle anew by establishing a family.

The child in us never completely dies however, as repressed residues of oral, anal and phallic stages persist in unconsciousness. Some of the apparent unreason of adults may reflect the far-off reasoning processes of the small child within them, and the less 'serious' and less inhibited things that adults do (play, dreams, humour) are symbols of the child's legacy to the adult.

Difficulty in passing any particular psychosexual stage may be reflected in adult behaviour. For example, incompletely resolved Oedipal conflicts may produce an adult who has difficulty with authority figures and has a poor sense of sexual identity. Such an adult may be attracted to women who already have a relationship with another male, thus recreating the scenario of the Oedipus Complex. Women who have failed to resolve conflicts associated with the Electra Complex may be attracted to 'father figures' with whom they are liable to experience sexual difficulties (after all, they are symbolically committing incest).

The anal (anankastic) personality type briefly mentioned may show traits of stubbornness, independence and possessiveness derived from strong residues of retentive anal pleasures. Faeces are unconsciously associated with possessions, particularly money. As faeces were once stubbornly retained, so money may be retained by the adult— consider phrases like 'filthy rich', 'rolling in the stuff', 'throwing money down the drain' and 'stinking rich', or consider describing oneself as 'cleaned out' when no more money is available. Have you ever considered your stamp collection as symbolic faeces? Or your liking for 'good food' as an oral residue?

Freud thus saw human development as consisting of movement through a series of psychosexual stages during which control of Id impulses is learned (Ego formation), values and ideals are internalized (Super-Ego formation) and conflict with parents is resolved. The Reality Principle replaces the Pleasure Principle, though the latter never dies but remains as the child within the adult, together with repressed residues of the early psychosexual stages.

The healthy adult sublimates (rechannels) Id energies, particularly libido drives, and Freud saw civilization as the result of the renunciation of instinctual drives via the mechanism of sublimation. Art and Science are the products of sublimated libidinal energies according to Freud, though conflict may exceed the capacity of the individual to sublimate—leading to neurosis.

Civilized man is sublimated man, and the cost of civilization is neurosis according to this view. The more sublimation, the more civilization and the more neurosis. The less sublimation, the less civilization and the less neurosis.

Erik Erikson (b. 1902)

Erikson was a later psychoanalyst whose theories build upon and include Freudian concepts, but modify them to emphasize *social* rather than psychosexual development.

Erikson proposes a series of eight *psychosocial stages*, each of which is characterized by special developmental problems or 'crises', of a social nature, to be confronted (Table 7). Like Freud, Erikson believed that success, or the lack of it, in adapting to the demands of each stage influenced the individual's ability to master the critical tasks of the next period.

For Erikson the critical aspect of development is the task of facing a progressively wider range of human relationships in a way that increases the ego strength of the individual, so that he feels not only comfortable with his own identity but is sensitive to the needs of others. In other words the outcome of successful psychosocial development is a well-adjusted *social* animal.

A *sensory* phase lasts from birth to approximately 18 months and the psychosocial crisis associated with this first stage is the task of developing a sense of basic *trust*. As the needs of the vulnerable infant are consistently met, he begins to develop feelings of trust, security and self-confidence. Failure to achieve this task may produce an adult who is basically mistrustful of others and who is plagued by feelings of insecurity.

The second stage lasts from around 18 months until 3 years of age and is the muscular or toddler stage during which *autonomy* develops as the infant acquires self-control and self-government.

The third stage is the *locomotor stage* (age 3–5 years) and the critical task is now to develop initiative and assertiveness. Erikson agrees with Freud that children of this age desire to exclusively possess the parent of the opposite sex and suggests that

Table 7 Psychosocial development (Erikson).

Stages	Psychosocial crises	Significant social relations	Favourable outcome
First year of life	Trust versus mistrust	Mother or mother-substitute	Trust and optimism
Second year	Autonomy versus doubt	Parents	Sense of self-control and adequacy
Third to fifth years	Initiative versus guilt	Basic family	Purpose and direction; ability to initiate one's own activities
Sixth year to puberty	Industry versus inferiority	Neighbourhood; school	Competence in intellectual, social and physical skills
Adolescence	Identity versus confusion	Peer groups and outgroups; models of leadership	An integrated image of oneself as a unique person
Early adulthood	Intimacy versus isolation	Partners in friendship; sex, competition, cooperation	Ability to form close and lasting relationships; to make career commitments
Middle adulthood	Generativity versus self-absorption	Divided labour and shared household	Concern for family, society and future generations
The ageing years	Integrity versus despair	'Mankind'; 'My Kind'	A sense of fulfilment and satisfaction with one's life; willingness to face death

parental punitiveness and withdrawal of approval at this stage will leave a residue of guilt which will persist into adulthood.

Fourthly the *latency stage* is arrived at, during which critical school experiences develop competence in intellectual, social and physical skills. The critical task here is to develop an orientation towards *industry* versus inferiority, and feelings of self-esteem should become relatively well-organized. Failure to negotiate this stage successfully may produce lasting feelings of inferiority and rebelliousness. The rebellious child may act defiantly against others – a protective response against feelings of lack of self-worth. The latency stage extends from the sixth year until puberty.

The next stage is *adolescence* (age 12–20 years) and the critical task confronting the child is that of developing a sense of *identity*. This is the transitional stage between childhood and adulthood and is characterized by physical, psychological and social turmoil. The peer group (the person's equals) assumes great importance as emancipation from parents proceeds in preparation for social independence. Unsuccessful mastery of this stage results in a fragmented sense of self in a person who uncomfortably shifts between an adult and a child orientation.

Early adulthood (late adolescence) follows (20–25 years) and the critical task of this stage is to conquer social isolation and awkwardness to achieve social *intimacy* by developing intimate relationships with others (partners in friendship, sex, competition and cooperation). The successful completion of this stage produces the ability to form close and lasting relationships and to make effective career commitments.

Middle adulthood (25–45 years) is a stage during which the task of moving from self-absorption to *generativity*, or positive and creative social interest, are expressed in concern for family and society. Failure to complete the tasks of this period leads to stagnation and lack of goals and self-fulfilment.

The ageing years (45 years onwards) offer the task of achieving ego integrity, as opposed to despair, as the individual develops a sense of fulfilment and satisfaction with life and accepts the inevitability of death.

Erikson's model thus emphasizes the widening sphere of social relationships which confront the developing individual (mother – parents – family – school – peer group – partners – society as a whole) and identifies the 'tasks' which must be accomplished during each psychosocial stage if development is to proceed smoothly.

Jean Piaget (1896–1980)

Piaget, a Swiss psychologist, described personality development as a sequential progression, as did Freud and Erikson. Freud emphasized the psychosexual aspects of development, Erikson the psychosocial, but Piaget described *cognitive* development (Table 8); that is, he described the acquisition of cognitive structures (rules that are used for thinking and solving problems—for understanding and dealing with the world).

Like the other theorists discussed, Piaget viewed development as a series of stages. Once a stage has been successfully completed the child moves on to a more complex one until cognitive development is complete at the stage of abstract logical thinking (Table 9).

Table 8 Cognitive development (Piaget).

Stage	Approximate ages	Characterization
Sensorimotor	Birth to 2 years	Infant differentiates him or herself from objects, learns that objects continue to exist even though no longer visible (object permanence).
Preoperational	2–7 years	Uses language and can represent objects by images and words, is still egocentric and has difficulty taking the viewpoint of others. Towards the end of this stage begins to use numbers and develop conservation concepts.
Concrete operational	7–12 years	Becomes capable of logical thought, achieves conservation concepts. Develops ability to classify objects.
Formal operational	12 years and up	Can think in abstract terms, follow logical propositions, and reason by hypothesis.

Table 9 A comparison of development.

Stage	Age period	Major features	Cognitive stage (Piaget)	Psychosexual stage (Freud)	Psychosocial crisis (Erikson)
		BIRTH			
Infancy	Birth at full term to about 18 months	Locomotion established; rudimentary language; social attachment	Sensorimotor	Oral; anal	Trust vs. mistrust
Early childhood	About 18 months to about 6 years	Language well established; sex typing; group play; ends with 'readiness' for schooling	Pre-operational	Phallic; oedipal	Autonomy vs. doubt; initiative vs. guilt
Late childhood	About 6 to about 13 years	Many cognitive processes become adult except in speed of operation team play	Concrete operational	Latency (libido goes 'underground')	Industry vs. inferiority
Adolescence	About 13 to about 20 years	Begins with puberty, ends at maturity; attainment of highest level of cognition; independence from parents; sexual relationships	Formal operational	Genital	Identity vs. role diffusion
Young adulthood	About 20 to about 45 years	Career and family development			Intimacy vs. isolation
Middle age	About 45 to about 65 years	Career reaches highest level; self-assessment; 'empty nest' crisis; retirement			Generativity vs. self-absorption
Old age	About 65 years to death	Enjoy family achievements; dependency; widowhood; poor health			Integrity vs. despair
		DEATH			

Piaget divides cognitive development into four stages. The first is the *sensorimotor* period which lasts from birth until 2 years of age. The infant learns to differentiate himself from objects, seeks stimulation and learns to manipulate objects. The infant becomes aware that an object seen from a different angle has not changed its identity but remains the same object, and learns that an object which has been hidden has not disappeared but can be found again. At 4–6 months the infant will not search for an object which has been hidden. For example, if a toy is covered with a cloth as the infant watches, all interest is lost in it—out of sight out of mind. At 6–12 months the infant will lift the cloth to uncover objects hidden in this way—out of sight is no longer out of mind. At 15–18 months the infant begins to think and gain appreciation of time and space. Language (several dozen words) appears by the end of this period.

Piaget's second period of cognitive development, the *preoperational period*, lasts from approximately age 2 to 7 years and is characterized by rapid development of language ability. For the first part of this stage (age 2–4 years) the child is still egocentric (he believes that his viewpoint is the only one) and is quite unable to take the viewpoint of others. For example if a parent says 'Don't do that—you wouldn't like it if someone did that to you', the child does not understand as he is unable to place himself in the viewpoint of another.

During the later part of the preoperational period (age 4–7 years), *conservation* develops; that is, the child realizes that an object retains (conserves) the same characteristics (mass, number, volume) no matter how it is rearranged. Before conservation develops the child will be easily misled by seeming changes in object characteristics. For example, if the child watches as a volume of water is poured into a taller and narrower container it will indicate its belief that more water is now present in the second container—conservation of volume is as yet undeveloped.

If the child is shown two rows of five coins, one spaced further apart than the other, the child will report that the longer row contains more coins—number is not yet conserved. Similarly the child allowed to watch while a ball of plasticine is rolled out into a sausage shape will report that the longer piece is heavier, indicating that conservation of mass has not yet developed.

During the latter part of the preoperational period the child also develops the ability to think in terms of *classes*; that is, he is able to conceive of objects 'belonging' together on the basis of shared common characteristics. The ability to discriminate is developing.

In the period of *concrete operations* (age 7–11 years) *logic* and objectivity appear, and the period of *formal operations* (age 11–15 years) involves the final steps towards abstract thinking and conceptualization. Adult problem-solving strategies are now evolving, and teaching and imitation are especially important for learning these skills.

Not everyone reaches this stage of cognitive development; in fact, one investigation revealed that some minimally educated adults do not conserve volume (Graves, 1972).

Describing personality

Personality is a multi-dimensional phenomenon which represents a shorthand biography of the individual concerned. Attempts to describe personality, as opposed to describing those developmental factors which shape it, are essential if the scientific study of personality is to be made possible. The difficulties of effectively describing such a rich and complex phenomenon are immense. Approaches to the description of personality have the difficult task of identifying enduring groups of characteristics which occur frequently enough to make comparisons between individuals possible, yet they must try to do so in a way which is not crudely reductive of individuals into arbitrary groups which deny the uniqueness of each individual being studied.

Any given personality can be described according to its enduring *traits* (its enduring characteristics) or may be conceived of as one of a number of *types* of personality.

Allport and Odbert (1936) listed 17 953 English words used to distinguish the behaviour of one person from another—an indication of the formidable nature of the task facing researchers who would effectively describe personality. Cattel (1946) condensed this list by eliminating overlaps of meaning in an attempt to arrive at a list of universal traits, the relative presence or absence of which could be used to describe any given personality.

Cattel's research resulted in a questionnaire-type personality test (the 16PF) designed to measure the relative balances of 16 *source traits* which are present, in variable degree, in all individuals.

The *type* approach to personality description is based on the assumption that classification into types (or 'kinds') is the beginning of most sciences. If there are kinds of plants, kinds of animals, kinds of rocks, it seems logical to assume that there must be kinds (or types) of personality.

Eysenck and Eysenck (1963) proposed that personality can be understood in terms of combinations of two dimensions—stable/unstable (sometimes called 'normal'/neurotic) and introverted/extroverted.

If one bisects one dimension with the other, the result is four quadrants (see Figure 5), each descriptive of a particular personality type.

The four types of personality are:

1 Stable extrovert
2 Unstable extrovert
3 Stable introvert
4 Unstable introvert

The terms introversion and extroversion (literally 'turning inwards' and 'turning outwards') refer to the tendencies to direct mental energies inwardly and be content with one's own company (introvert) or to direct one's mental energies outwardly and to thrive in the company of others (extrovert).

The typical introvert is quiet, retiring, fond of books rather than people, reserved, cautious, serious and tends to 'look before he leaps'. The typical extrovert is sociable, likes parties, has many friends, needs people to talk to, craves excitement, is fond of practical jokes, is impulsive and does not like reading or studying by himself. The introvert tends to be reliable and is seldom aggressive, while the extrovert tends to be aggressive and is not always reliable (Eysenck and Rachman, 1965).

The other dimension—stability/instability—simply means that, at the stable end, are people whose emotions are controlled and not easily aroused, whereas the unstable end is represented by those with poor emotional control, who tend to be moody and touchy.

The problems of unstable introverts tend to be personal, while unstable extroverts are more likely to indulge in delinquent behaviour and thus get into trouble.

Extremes of each of the four types may only be dimly aware of how they are perceived by persons with very different characteristics. The stable intro-

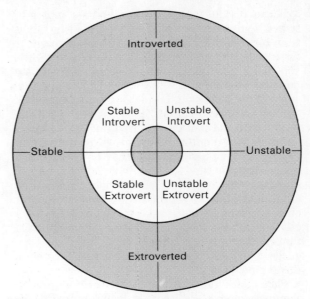

Figure 5 Type classification of personality. (From Eysenck and Eysenck with kind permission of the authors.)

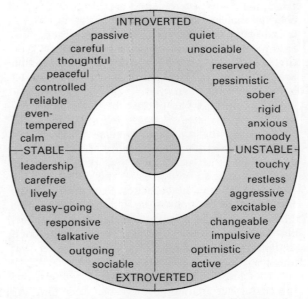

Figure 6 Dimensions of the personality. (From Eysenck and Eysenck with kind permission of the authors.)

vert may see himself as suitably prudent, sober and cautious, while the unstable extrovert may regard him as dull, miserly and boring. The unstable extrovert may see himself as 'zany', interesting and adventurous, while the stable introvert may see him as being horrifyingly erratic, undisciplined and unpredictable.

Type classifications of this sort are appealing because of their simplicity, but there is a danger that they may lend themselves to creating stereotypes, thus reducing the richness and complexity of personality to simple 'labels' which may be carelessly affixed, denying the uniqueness of each individual.

The psychoanalytical approach, derived from the theories of Freud, does not operate in terms of either 'traits' or 'types' but considers the dynamic relationships between the forces operating within any given personality (Id, Ego and Super-Ego). This approach also considers evidence of fixation at early stages of psychosexual development and emphasizes intrapsychic structures which influence personality in indirect ways.

Learning Theory is a body of knowledge which is critical of all the previously mentioned theories and instead emphasizes the context within which behaviour occurs and the ways in which it is learned. This approach suggests that behaviour is not the product of consistent *inner* tendencies but is rather the product of the interplay between the individual and the environment, insofar as behaviour is initiated and maintained by *environmental factors* such as reward or punishment. This approach suggests that behaviour is simply learned by processes of conditioning and that the organism enters the world as a 'tabula rasa' (blank tablet) to be written upon by the experiences provided by the environment. There is no place in this scheme for developmental viewpoints, which suggest the critical importance of early experiences in determining the dynamics of personality. The learning theorist sees the organism as being primarily malleable, while the theorists previously mentioned emphasize inner structures which mediate behaviour.

B. F. Skinner is an American psychologist who endorses the learning theory viewpoint. In Skinner's view we behave as we do because in past situations some behaviours have been reinforced (rewarded and thus made stronger) and others have been punished or have produced negative consequences. This viewpoint sees personality traits as *behavioural tendencies* produced by the person's history of reinforcement.

Skinner rejects the concept of internal mechanisms as being irrelevant to the scientific study of behaviour; for him *behaviour is determined by its consequences* (behaviour which is rewarded will increase in frequency and behaviour which is punished, or lacks rewarding consequences, will decrease in frequency). Thus the industrious and diligent child behaves in this way, not as the result of inner psychological forces, but because the child has been *reinforced* repeatedly for behaving in this way.

This viewpoint (sometimes called the *behaviourist* viewpoint) has been very influential in shaping our perceptions of behaviour and will be discussed more fully in Chapter 10.

The Humanistic Approach To Personality

The term *humanistic psychology* applies to a variety of approaches to the study of personality and behaviour, all of which share a belief in the importance of *holism*. The holistic perspective emphasizes the importance of studying the entire person, without reducing him to fragments (traits, types, behaviours) which may be conveniently studied by psychologists. Advocates of the humanistic viewpoint argue that psychological experiments are artificial and unnatural, and, in consequence yield results which are artificial and unnatural at worst, or trivial at best.

Humanistic psychologists disagree with the frequent use of average scores in experimental psychology. No-one is 'average'; each person is a unique individual and should be studied as such, if the complexity of the individual is not to be eradicated by 'scientific rigour'.

This viewpoint has been productive of warm, insightful therapeutic attitudes and has provided a counterbalance for some of the mechanistic and dehumanizing approaches generated by excesses of behaviourist zeal. Humanistic psychology has not, as yet, produced major contributions to our theoretical understanding of personality but has generated productive and positive therapeutic philosophies.

The Assessment of Personality

Personality is assessed *informally* all the time. When the nurse enters training she will quickly assess her classmates and select the company of those she finds congenial. To commence duty on a new ward is to be presented with the task of rapid multiple assessment—of patients and workmates.

Informal assessment of this kind is subject to many forms of error. The observer may produce a *halo effect* by noting some characteristic that she strongly likes or dislikes and then assigning this characteristic to the remaining features of the person's behaviour in a quite unwarranted way. *Stereotypes* may be used which reveal biased assumptions about the group to which the person belongs (Scots are mean, Italians are unstable, ward sisters are authoritarian, psychiatric patients are untrustworthy).

The psychologist uses *formal* methods of assessment and may measure personality by administering *personality tests* which may be designed to reveal clusters of traits (e.g. the Cattel 16PF) or to assign personality to one of a series of types (e.g. the Eysenck personality inventory – the EPI).

Most of these personality 'tests' consist of a series of statements with which the individual being tested is invited to agree or disagree. Examples of items from such a questionnaire might include the following:

I often daydream
I always tell the truth
Sometimes I worry about the future
I often doubt my own abilities
I enjoy mixing with strangers

Scoring of the answers enables the tester to assign the subject to a particular category on the basis of the association of traits revealed or the tendency towards a particular type.

Most personality tests are designed to be used with 'normals', though pathological traits might be revealed. The *Minnesota multiphasic personality inventory* is an example of a self-rating instrument designed to reveal pathological trends within the personality through comparison of the test taker's responses with those of persons having known kinds of personality disorder.

Projective personality tests are much less structured and consist of vague or ambiguous presentations which enable the subject to 'project' his own fantasies and unconscious tendencies into them. For example, the *thematic apperception test* consists of a series of pictures about which the subject is invited to tell stories. As the subject interprets each scene he says things about the characters which really apply to himself, that is he 'projects' himself into each scenario.

The *Rorschach inkblot test* is another projective test in which the individual is invited to identify his or her interpretations of a series of cards, each displaying a rather complex inkblot, thus revealing unconscious aspects of self. The Rorschach test is

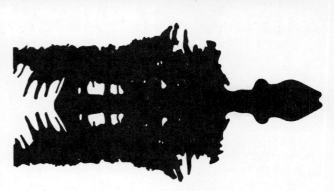

Figure 7 An inkblot similar to those used in the Rorschach test.

thought to sometimes reveal indications of incipient psychosis, though much scepticism has been expressed about the reliability of the test as there is often wide divergence between the interpretations offered by different examiners.

The field of personality study is a complex one and the student approaching this area for the first time might be forgiven for concluding that theorists are hopelessly divided in their opinions. Actually there is less disagreement than at first seems to be the case. Freud, Erikson and Piaget produced developmental theories with very different emphases, and the differences are more than simply differences of approach. Nevertheless each produced useful perspectives which together shed much light on the process of human development. Behaviourists do not totally deny the existence of internal psychological structures but rather suggest that research should concentrate on that which is observable (behaviour) rather than that which is invisible and difficult to measure with scientific precision (thoughts, feelings and emotions).

Research continues into those aspects of personality which may be inherited. For example some researchers consider the tendencies towards introversion or extroversion to be hereditary, though opinion is divided on this point.

Study of personality emphasizes the critical importance of social experiences in strengthening or weakening the structure of personality. We cannot untangle genes but the nurse can help ensure that hospitalization produces those social experiences which help promote personal growth and help to produce adaptive approaches to life difficulties.

Key Concepts

1 The term '*personality*' refers to those relatively stable and enduring aspects of the individual which distinguish him from other people.

2 Personalities are unique; no two are absolutely identical.

3 Early life experiences play a critical part in shaping personality, and personality may be thought of as a shorthand biography of the individual.

4 Personality is expressed through *behaviour* (the visible activities of the organism).

5 Behaviour may usefully promote adaptation to the environment (*adaptive* behaviour) or may interfere with successful adaptation (*maladaptive* behaviour).

6 The belief that behaviour is somehow explained by simply labelling it (the *nominal fallacy*) militates against true understanding of behaviour.

7 All individuals pass through a lifelong sequence of *stages* in personality development.

8 Much of our present knowledge about the development of personality was provided by the theories of Freud, Erikson and Piaget.

9 Freud's approach emphasized the progressive shifting of libidinal energy to various areas of the body; this is called the *psychosexual* theory of development.

10 Psychosexual theory suggests that the *libido* focusses on Oral, Anal, Phallic, Latent and Genital Stages in succession, and that residues of previous developmental stages tend to linger on in the adult.

11 Freud suggested that the mind operates on three levels—the *conscious, pre-conscious* and *unconscious* levels.

12 The unconscious mind contains the *Id*—a powerful reservoir of primitive *instincts* and *drives* which are continually seeking outlets.

13 The Id is infantile, immoral and resentful of any delay of gratification; control of its impulses is established as the *Ego* develops.

14 The *Ego* is partially conscious and *censors* impractical urges towards satisfaction of Id impulses, though it too is immoral.

15 The Ego mediates awareness of, and interaction with, external reality.

16 The *Super-Ego* develops as the values of parental figures are internalized.

17 The Super-Ego is highly *moral*, often in an irrational way, and punishes violation of its *ideals* by producing feelings of guilt, shame and remorse.

18 In psychosis, Ego boundaries are weakened (producing impaired reality testing) and in neurosis, the Super-Ego has often hypertrophied (producing crippling feelings of guilt and anxiety).

19 Erikson builds on Freud's theories by identifying eight developmental stages, each of which offers the task of developing *social* adjustment.

20 Piaget also produced a developmental model which is sequential in structure and describes four stages in *cognitive* development.

21 Personality may be described in terms of *traits* (e.g. Cattel), *types* (e.g. Eysenck), *behavioural tendencies* (e.g. Skinner) or in *psychoanalytical* terms (e.g. Freud).

22 The *humanistic* approach to personality deprecates scientific reductionism and instead adopts a *holistic* approach; that is, it emphasizes the importance of studying the *whole* person as a unique individual.

23 Assessment of personality may hinge upon theories of traits, types, behavioural patterns or psychoanalytical assessment.

24 Formal personality assessment often involves the use of *questionnaires* and may involve the use of *projective* tests.

25 Some researchers suggest that personality may be partially shaped by heredity, but the study of personality has revealed the critical importance of social experience for the individual and many therapeutic interventions aim to re-shape areas of difficulty by providing helpful and positive social experiences.

References

Allport, G. W. & Odbert, H. S. (1936) Trait names: a psycholexical study. *Psychological Monograph*, **47**(211): 402.

Cattel, R. B. (1946) *Description and Measurement of Personality*. New York: World Books.

Eysenck, H. & Eysenck, S. (1963) *The Eysenck Personality Inventory*. London: University of London Press.

Eysenck, H. & Rachman, S. (1965) *The Causes and Cures of Neurosis*. San Diego: Knapp.

Graves, A. (1972) Attainment of conservation of mass, weight and volume in minimally educated adults. *Developmental Psychology*, **7**: 233.

Hilgard, E., Atkinson, R. & Atkinson, R. (1979) *Introduction to Psychology*, 7th edn. New York: Harcourt, Brace, Jovanovich Inc.

6

How is Mental Disorder Treated?

Canst thou not minister to a mind diseas'd;
Pluck from the memory a rooted sorrow;
Raze out the written troubles of the brain;

Shakespeare: Macbeth Act V Scene III

Historical Background

An examination of the history of psychiatric treatment reveals a complex fabric in which inhumanity, compassion, superstition and scientific innovation are closely interwoven. Ancient records reveal that mental disorder has been recognized and treated for thousands of years. Egyptian medical papyri of around 1500 BC say of senility that 'The heart grows heavy and remembers not yesterday' (Henderson and Batchelor, 1962), and dream interpretation was practised in Ancient Egypt as long ago as 2900 BC (Jones, 1983).

The Old Testament records Saul's depression and attempt to commit suicide (Samuel 1:5–10) and the Ancient Greeks formally recognized mental disorder in their writings. Plato (Republic Bk XI c. 13) instructed 'If anyone is insane let him not be seen openly in the city, but let the relatives of such a person watch over him at home in the best manner they know of, and if they are negligent let them pay a fine'.

During the time of Hippocrates the mentally disordered visited the Temple of Aesculapius—the god of healing—where prayers were offered and sleeping overnight in the Temple brought relief.

The second century AD saw the emergence of chains, flogging, incarceration and starvation—often in the belief that the mentally disordered were possessed. Medieval Europe left the treatment of mental disorder to priests, and superstitious beliefs in witchcraft were used to justify the segregation and brutal ill-treatment of those persons who aroused concern or alarm as a result of disordered behaviour or beliefs. [Szasz (1973) has suggested that 'the con-

cept of mental illness serves the same social function in the modern world as did the concept of witchcraft in the late Middle Ages'.] Holy wells and springs were the subject of pilgrimages in medieval times in the hope of effecting relief of mental disorder. One such was St Fillan's Well in Scotland, mentioned by Sir Walter Scott:

Thence to St Fillan's blessed well
Whose spring can frenzied dreams dispel
And the crazed brain restore.

Marmion, Canto i, 29

Similar healing wells and springs were used in France, Finland, Belgium, Germany and England and, in modern times, the bathing of the sick at Lourdes remains an important adjunct to the spiritual exercises.

Many mentally handicapped and psychotic persons were abandoned to live as outcasts: 'When civilization grew in the Western world it grew behind walls—in castles and monasteries and small crowded cities; and the outcasts lived in the forests—madmen and idiots, lepers and escaped slaves, outlaws and felons' (Jones and Fowles, 1984).

In 1377 the Bethlehem Hospital in London was used to house mental patients, giving rise to the terms 'Bedlam' and 'Tom O'Bedlam', the latter term being used to describe the mentally handicapped or psychotic.

The country gives me proof and precedent
Of Bedlam beggars who with roaring voices . . .
Enforce their charity.

Shakespeare: King Lear, Acts III & IV

The sixteenth century saw mass burnings of witches and heretics, the Attorney General of Lorraine (who burned 900 'witches') explaining that 'Whatever is not normal is due to the Devil', though one courageous doctor protested about current theological doctrines asking 'Do figments like these move us to the torturing of harmless women?' (Szasz, 1973).

By the seventeenth century many European cities

had institutions for 'the debauched, spendthrift fathers, prodigal sons, blasphemers, men who seek to undo themselves, libertines' (Szasz, 1973). Bedlam, the Narrenturm in Vienna, the hôpital general in Paris, all incarcerated the mentally disordered under conditions of great barbarity. A visitor to Bedlam in 1753 said 'I saw a hundred spectators making sport of the miserable inhabitants, provoking them into furies of rage' (Seymer, 1956), such a visit being vividly portrayed in the Hogarth engraving 'The Rake in Bedlam' (1735).

This lack of respect for the mentally disordered was even extended to royal personages. When George III suffered attacks of maniacal excitement no hesitation was evinced in knocking him down, and one attendant boasted that he knocked him 'flat as a flounder' (Henderson and Batchelor, 1962). 'Treatment' largely consisted of restraint, bleeding, purging and beating, though attempts to use 'medication' were sporadically employed. Sydenham treated mania by prescribing a concoction which would have aroused the envy of any witch doctor—it contained the flesh and blood of vipers, wine, honey and sixty one other ingredients (Henderson and Batchelor, 1962). Many herbs were believed to be efficacious in the treatment of melancholia and other disturbances, and the substances used included chrysanthemum, saffron, rosewater, marigolds, carnations, moonwort, hellebore, lavender, gentian, opium and cannabis.

The latter part of the eighteenth century saw the emergence of an era of humane reform. Pinel in France and Tuke in England pioneered extensive reforms—removing chains and initiating coherent attempts at treatments—though historians have often over-idealized both the men and their approaches. Even Pinel believed in the efficacy of 'short sharp shocks' and the regime at the Salpetriere included the 'douche ascendante' which was a stream of cold water directed on to the anus of the naked, seated, unsuspecting patient (Jones, 1983). Pinel also observed that 'If (the madman) is met by a force convincingly superior he submits without opposition or violence. This is a great and invaluable secret in the management of well regulated hospitals' (Szasz, 1973). It has also been suggested that Pinel struck off the chains of his patients, not in response to humanitarian instincts, but because the revolutionary National Assembly wished patients to be freed as a political gesture. 'Man is born free but everywhere he is in chains' wrote Rousseau, and Pinel may have hastily endorsed the revolutionary

spirit by freeing his patients. His hospital was certainly visited twice in 1793 by Couthon, the hostile and powerful president of the Paris commune. Michel Foucault (1967) sees Pinel not as a philanthropist but as a prudent survivor.

In 1796 William Tuke opened the Retreat at York, a Quaker community, which used 'soft and mild persuasion' to treat the mentally disordered and explicitly rejected coercion and intimidation. The Retreat foreshadowed many therapeutic community principles as self-restraint and control were encouraged by an atmosphere in which the esteem of others was something to be concerned about. Despite this innovative approach the Retreat primarily offered 'moral management'; that is, the emphasis was on promoting an awareness of good and evil, of right and wrong, though it was thought that the emotions were best controlled rather than expressed or discussed.

Despite these humanitarian developments, fear and restraint played a major part in 'treatment' well into the nineteenth century. Patients were restrained in immobilizing chairs, spun to the point of collapse in revolving chairs, purged, starved and beaten. Boats and bridges were constructed which would break up and force patients to swim to the shore, and ducking chairs and cages were used to plunge pinioned patients into icy water.

The nineteenth century saw the introduction of drugs into the network of fast developing mental hospitals. Potassium bromide was widely used as a sedative, hypnotic and anticonvulsant, though excess led to bromism—a state of toxic confusion. Around the same time (the 1830s) chloral hydrate (still occasionally used today) was introduced as a sedative and hypnotic, and paraldehyde (another sedative still occasionally used) was introduced in the 1880s. It will be noted that the drugs mentioned all have a sedative effect and excessive reliance on preparations like these may simply 'place the bars of Bedlam and the locked doors *inside* the patient' (Laing, 1964). The first barbiturate (Veronal—another sedative) was introduced in 1903 and reliance on sedatives continued until the 1950s when the first *neuroleptic* drugs (i.e. the phenothiazines) were introduced.

In 1933 Sakel introduced *insulin therapy* in the belief that the hypoglycaemia associated with carefully induced insulin coma would somehow interrupt abnormal neural connections in the brain. Insulin therapy brought about improvements but it was increasingly suspected that these improvements were the results of the increased staff/patient inter-actions in the insulin unit rather than of any bioche-mical adjustments. As research cast greater suspi-cion on the rationale of insulin therapy it went into decline and disappeared in the late 1950s.

In 1935 Moniz introduced *psychosurgery* (prefron-tal leucotomy) for the management of crippling fears, obsessions and anxiety, and was awarded the Nobel Prize for Medicine in 1955 (he was shot in the spine by a leucotomized patient rendering him para-plegic). In 1938 Cerletti and Bini introduced elec-troplexy (electroconvulsive therapy or ECT)—still a major treatment for some types of mood disorder.

The fifties saw an expansion of the range of psy-chotropic drugs available, and chemotherapy became more sophisticated, many of the drugs introduced then still being in frequent use (e.g. the phenothiazines).

Treatments mentioned so far aim at bringing about some change in the physical functioning of the patient and are therefore referred to collectively as *physical methods of treatment* (e.g. chemotherapy, electroplexy and psychosurgery). Many other treatments aim to restore functioning without physi-cal intervention; that is, they treat mental disorder by mental means, and treatments of this nature (psy-chotherapy and behaviour therapy) are collectively described as *non-physical methods of treatment*.

Non-physical approaches date back to the dream interpretations of the Ancient Egyptians and the 'temple sleep' of Ancient Greece but psycho-therapy, as we know it, was first associated with Antoine Mesmer (1734–1815) who coined rather bizarre theories of 'animal magnetism' and saw all illnesses (physical and mental) as a result of disturb-ances in the flow of 'magnetic fluid'. 'Mesmerism' was soon discredited but the fact remains that many of his patients improved dramatically, not as a result of animal magnetism, but because Mesmer was giving (albeit inadvertently) effective psycho-therapy. He was a tall, charismatic individual with piercing eyes, and he made a practice of speaking commandingly to his overawed patients and sug-gesting that symptoms would disappear—as they often obligingly did. Long after 'animal magnetism' had been forgotten, the memory of the power of sug-gestion lingered on.

In 1843 an Edinburgh dentist, James Braid, coined the term '*hypnotism*', leaning heavily on some of Mesmer's techniques, and Charcot and Janet later used the technique of hypnosis in the study and treatment of hysteria.

In 1882 *Freud* began to use hypnosis to gain access to troublesome thoughts and wishes which had been repressed by his patients but was soon to abandon hypnosis as the techniques of psychoanalysis were fully worked out by him. The aim of psychoanalysis is the uncovering of unconscious conflicts and repressed experiences and Freud soon began to use three major techniques. The first technique is *free association* by the patient (the patient is encouraged to verbalize his stream of consciousness, to speak aloud any thoughts entering his mind, no matter how trivial, irrelevant, stupid or obscene they seem to him). The second technique is the formation and analysis of *transference relationships*; that is, critical early experiences are re-enacted as the patient 'transfers' emotions associated with them on to the psychoanalyst. Transference relationships may be positive or negative as the patient transfers love or hate felt for parents or significant others on to the therapist. The therapist may respond with *counter-transference* when he responds to feelings of resentment with hostility or responds to progress with feelings of pleasure. Psychoanalysts work with the transference relationship as an aid to under-standing the patient's feelings and as a method of gaining awareness of repressed conflicts. The third technique used in psychoanalysis is *interpretation* by the therapist who may interpret dreams and 'slips of the tongue', and in particular will emphasize the relationship between present feelings and past experiences. Sometimes patients will recall past experiences with a considerable discharge of pre-viously buried emotions. This discharge of emotions is often of an intensity which is surprising and dis-turbing to the patient; the discharge is called a *cath-arsis*. Cathartic experiences are often experienced as therapeutic by the patient as they may 'purge' the unconscious of troublesome repressed material and provide an increase in insight. Some of Freud's early followers broke away to establish variants of ortho-dox psychoanalysis and this group of dissenters is often collectively referred to as the *Neo-Freudians*.

Alfred Adler (1870–1937) rejected Freud's view of sexuality as the prime mover of human behaviour and established the school of *individual psychology* which emphasizes consideration of the individual's 'lifestyle' and uses re-education to establish healthier patterns and goals. Adler introduced the term 'inferiority complex' and suggested that feel-ings of inferiority were a creative force since they led to striving for superiority.

C. J. Jung (1875–1961) also disagreed with

Freud's view of sexuality and developed his own system of *analytical psychology* which emphasizes *individuation*—an innate striving for self-realization. Jung described libido as natural energy which first and foremost serves the purposes of life and which flows between the opposing poles, 'the opposites'. Many opposites can be described, for example introversion and extroversion, thinking and feeling, consciousness and unconsciousness. The natural movement of the libido (or life energy) is backwards and forwards—a movement of psychic tides. Jung called forward movement (which satisfies the demands of the conscious) *progression*, and backward movements (which satisfy the demands of the unconscious) *regression*. Progression is concerned with the active adaptation to one's environment and regression with the satisfaction of one's inner needs. Regression may be a restorative phase, as in a return to a dreamy state after a concentrated period of directed mental activity. Regression is therefore not always 'a bad thing' but is in many ways as natural a counterpart to progression as sleeping is to waking.

Jung's view of the unconscious was that it is more than a mere repository of primitive and infantile urges. The unconscious is the matrix of consciousness and in it are to be found the germs of new possibilities—the seeds of new ways of being. Jung also introduced the concept of the *collective unconscious*, a deeper stratum of the unconscious than the individual or personal unconscious, the unknown material from which our consciousness emerges. Jung suggested that the collective unconscious is shaped and influenced by the remote and distant experiences of mankind. Intellectually we are in some ways like a group of savages huddled round the comforting light and heat of the fire of conscious reason, but beyond the flickering shadows of the unconscious lies the dark (but rich) forest of the collective unconscious. This tendency to experience and apprehend life in a manner conditioned by the past history of mankind Jung called *archetypal*, and recurring symbols or motifs in art and literature (archetypes) are expressions of the primordial collective unconscious. The threatening devouring mother figure is an example. This archetype occurs throughout the history of mankind, from cave paintings to the ancient goddesses Ishtar and Isis, Kali, the Oedipus myth, the witch figure of the Middle Ages and children's fairy tales. Archetypes indicate the presence of primordial hopes, fears, wishes and instincts, and myths, in particular, are a direct expression of the collective unconscious.

Jungian therapy never loses sight of the constructive elements which can always be found in mental disorder and sees every neurosis as having an aim—an attempt to compensate for a one-sided approach to life and a voice proclaiming the existence of a side of the personality which has been neglected or repressed. Every neurosis thus has its secret strengths and the belief in the regulatory functions of the 'opposites' emphasizes that the mentally disordered are not irretrievably stranded on some alien psychic shore but are still involved in a process of psychic travel or movement. Regressive movement always has the potential to become progressive movement, and negative movement will inevitably be followed by positive movement, as light follows dark. Effective care facilitates this movement and the therapist may act as a guide on the journey.

Jung's writings are sometimes dismissed as being obscure, mystical and irrelevant to modern psychotherapy; this is, to say the least, unfortunate, as Jung's writings contain core ideas which have heavily influenced many other schools of thought. Above all Jung offers a view of psychic functioning which is positive and optimistic, and provides a

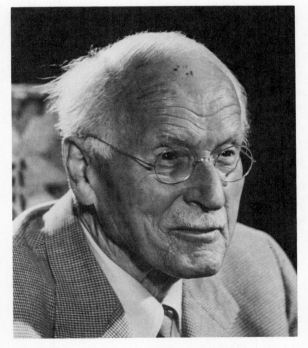

Figure 8 Carl Gustav Jung. (With kind permission of The Bettman Archive.)

much needed counterbalance to some rigid 'medical model' views of mental disorder which tend to reduce the individual to a sterile list of 'medical' symptoms, and offer little more than sedation, hospitalization and crippling loss of self-esteem. Description is a necessary first step in all sciences but in some approaches to psychiatry it has become an end in itself. Jung encourages us not only to say 'how' in describing behaviour and feelings but to ask 'why'. The warmly humanistic Jungian approach with its recognition of each individual's capacity for positive personal growth incorporates attitudes which will be an asset to any health care professional.

Otto Rank (1884–1939), also seceded from the ranks of the 'orthodox' Freudians (in 1929), examined separation anxiety and experimented with short-term therapy (orthodox Freudian or Jungian analysis usually takes some years). He introduced the concept of 'birth trauma' as the precursor of all later anxiety and this theory has a modern counterpart in Janov's theory of neurosis as a symbolization of primal pain due to the denial of primal needs.

Wilhelm Reich (1897–1957) developed 'character analysis' exploring the relationship between bodily tensions and posture, 'character armour' and psychological defences. Reich had a somewhat chequered career (he was expelled from the International Psychoanalytical Association because he was a Communist and was then expelled from the Communist Party because he was a psychoanalyst), though Reichian therapy continues in a modified form as 'bio-energetics'.

Erich Fromm (1900–1983) emphasized the interaction between the individual and society and the outcomes of stress and loneliness in industrial society, and *Karen Horney* (1885–1952) stressed the individual's need for security and also emphasized cultural and situational determinants of neurosis.

Harry Stack Sullivan (1892–1948) developed a system of psychotherapy which explored the interpersonal relationships of his patients, and *Fritz Perls* (1894–1970) devised *Gestalt therapy* in which the patient is asked to personify the warring parts of his body and mind and invent a dialogue in which they could come to agreement, completing the gestalt (or wholeness).

Perls used an approach which diverged from the techniques of psychoanalysis and his approach is an example of what became a rapidly expanding alternative school of thought—the *Humanistic* approach to psychotherapy—which emphasizes the uniqueness of the individual and adopts a person-centred approach to life's difficulties.

The humanistic approach acquired new impetus when *Carl Rogers* introduced *client-centred therapy* which became a major influence in the 1950s. This approach does not emphasize insight and does not use transference relationships. Diagnosis, interpretation and direction are avoided and the 'client's' capacity for personal growth and self-regulation is recognized and encouraged. Rogers prefers the term 'client' to 'patient' as he does not believe that persons in therapy are 'sick' or 'ill' and the term 'client-centred' is used as therapy centres around the client's perceptions, and not those of the therapist, who does not interpret or direct as would a psychoanalytically orientated therapist. Many humanistic therapists are critical of 'insight-directed' therapies, emphasizing that there is a risk that the 'patient' may be said to develop 'insight' when he agrees with the therapist's interpretation of his problems.

The humanistic approach to psychotherapy was broadened in the 1960s when *Eric Berne* introduced *transactional analysis*, which focusses on the interpersonal 'transactions' of the client. The humanistic approach 'demedicalized' psychotherapy as many humanistic approaches do not consider a qualification in medicine to be necessary (or indeed relevant) to the practice of psychotherapy. Rogers has even stated that a training in psychology may be a disadvantage as it may produce a tendency to see persons as objects to be dissected or experimentally manipulated (Rogers, 1954). The important prerequisite for effective therapy is seen to consist of the personal philosophy of the therapist which outweighs 'theory' and 'technique'. Attitudes of *warmth, empathy, acceptance* and a belief in the client's capacity for *personal growth* are seen as the critical dimensions of the therapist.

Client-centred therapy (sometimes described as Rogerian therapy) also brought psychotherapy from the consulting room into the community at large. Lay counsellors trained in the Rogerian approach are using it effectively in schools, colleges and in industry. In Britain, the National Marriage Guidance Council (founded in 1948) has relied largely on the Rogerian approach while accepting recently the Masters and Johnson programme for brief sexual therapy (Parry-Jones, 1983).

A third non-physical approach to treatment consists of *behavioural psychotherapy*, which uses techniques derived from classical (Pavlovian) and operant (Skinnerian) conditioning. This approach rejects consideration of unconscious conflicts and instead focusses on behaviour—those activities which can be *observed*. The emphasis is thus not on the private inner world of thoughts, feelings and emotions (though these are not denied) but on the public, observable and measurable realm of behaviour. This approach considers mental disorder as maladaptive patterns of learned behaviour which can be 'unlearned' by a process of 'counter-conditioning'. Learned behaviour is any behaviour present in the mature organism which was not present at birth. We are not born neurotic but learn to be neurotic (largely by processes of conditioning) and can learn to respond with adaptive behaviour to previously troublesome conditioned stimuli (see Chapters 2).

Techniques used include *systematic desensitization* which constitutes an effective treatment for phobic anxiety. The rationale is that the patient has become 'sensitized' to certain stimuli (insects, heights, public places) just as the asthmatic may have become sensitized to foreign proteins. As the asthmatic may be desensitized by giving graduated doses of the troublesome substance, so may the phobic be desensitized by gradual exposure to the troublesome environmental stimulus, thus overcoming 'social allergies'. Thus the person with a phobic fear of spiders would first be taught relaxation techniques (see Appendix 1) and would then be desensitized by approaching anxiety-evoking situations arranged in a hierarchical order (from least anxiety-evoking to most anxiety-evoking). For example, the patient may commence by looking at photographs of spiders and may then progress to models of spiders (looking and then handling)—dead spider sealed in jar—dead spider in open jar—live spider in sealed jar—live spider in open jar—entering a dusty basement where spider webs are in evidence. The patient would not move on to the next step in the hierarchy until anxiety associated with the previous step had been reduced.

The technique of *flooding* (implosion) confronts the patient with the most anxiety-evoking stimulus without a graduated approach. These techniques create a situation whereby the patient who has become conditioned to associate troublesome stimuli with responses of anxiety now associates these stimuli with responses of relaxation (counter-conditioning).

Other techniques include operant conditioning, whereby the frequency of adaptive behaviour is increased and the behaviour strengthened (reinforced) by arranging desirable consequences for these behaviours while maladaptive behaviours are decreased in frequency and strength by ensuring that no rewarding consequences follow them (for example, simple behaviour modification programmes and token economy programmes (see Chapter 10).

The range of behaviour therapy techniques is very diverse and most are successful in rapidly reducing or extinguishing certain types of troublesome responses (notably anxiety responses), though in practice techniques may be only loosely related to learning theory (Parry-Jones, 1983).

Group therapies offer psychotherapeutic intervention to a small group of individuals and aim to create a group climate of mutual support and understanding in which the individual feels free to offer his/her difficulties to the group for discussion. Listening to others reduces feelings of isolation and alienation and promotes willingness to actively consider faulty approaches to living. Problems are shared, troublesome feelings are worked through in a climate of support and encouragement and new solutions are formulated. The success of the group approach is underlined by its use in groups like Alcoholics Anonymous, Phobics Anonymous, self-help groups for depressed housewives, persons with drug problems and the use of group techniques in management and educational settings.

The *encounter group* invites the participant to 'encounter self' and began as a sensitivity-training technique for 'normals'. The emphasis is on the 'here and now' aspects of human feelings and the aim is to increase awareness. The peer group dominates the proceedings rather than the authority of the group conductor, and participants are not allowed to conceal feelings behind the convenient social façades of etiquette, privacy or 'good manners'. Stark emotional confrontations may occur and openness and emotional honesty are regarded as essential. The desired outcome is increased personal growth. The often ruthless exploration of previously 'taboo' intimate areas may be experienced as very disturbing by some participants, and the result may be a distinctly 'bad experience' (an 'encounter group neurosis' has been described). Prospective participants are advised to consider this course of action carefully; participation involves some personal risk and the experience may be very rewarding but simultaneously very punishing.

Encounter groups aiming at an increase in

'human potential' by confrontational emotional techniques have drawn upon the techniques of sensitivity training, gestalt therapy, transactional analysis and, above all, the philosophy and approach of Rogers.

Extensions of this approach have included the 'marathon group' and the 'body awareness group', and a popular American variant is the 'nude marathon group' which is based on the hopeful assumption that social pretensions and facades are discarded with clothing. (A colleague attended such a group in California and reported that he left the group with an increased awareness, not so much of his own potential, but with an increased awareness of the need for more widespread use of deodorants.)

Encounter groups are often regarded with attraction by mental health care professionals and can indeed heighten self-awareness and enable the participant to approach life difficulties (personal or those of others) with increased awareness and confidence. Prospective members should, however, ask the following questions carefully:

1 Have I carefully considered why I want to join?
2 Are my expectations of this group realistic?
3 Am I prepared to fully embrace the intimate climate of such a group?
4 Is the group I am considering joining being conducted for bona fide reasons and by a suitably experienced/qualified person?

If the answers to all four questions are 'yes' then the result may be a rewarding and enriching experience; if not, careful consideration is suggested.

Consideration of the plethora of psychotherapeutic interventions available may tend to induce little else other than confusion in the student's mind. This is unnecessary. The similarities between approaches are more marked than the differences. Total embrace of any one school of thought may be injudicious for the student but all have something to offer. For example, Freud suggests that we are not always conscious of the reasons for our behaviour and consideration of underlying forces may be fruitful. The nurse should also be able to recognize transference relationships when these (inevitably) develop between her and her patients. Cathartic experiences should not be nervously suppressed—they are usually very therapeutic.

Adler suggests that inferiority complexes may serve a positive function as they may generate positive attempts to compensate. Jung supplies the view that psychic functioning is never static—we must not complacently categorize our patients as 'with-

drawn' or 'aggressive' or 'self-defeating'—psychic movement is continual and no-one is 'frozen' in a negative state. Rank emphasizes that short-term therapy may be effective and Reich underlines the importance of the relationship between physical tensions and posture and emotional state. Fromm highlights the importance of the social background and sees man as a figure in an increasingly critical urban landscape. Gestalt therapy (Perls) emphasizes the importance of attempting to unify thinking, feeling and being, while Rogers (client-centred therapy) indicates that the would-be therapist need not recoil from offering psychotherapy on the grounds of lack of theory/qualifications but should consider his/her view of other persons as the most appropriate starting point.

The behavioural approach reveals that the reasons for many troublesome problems are not particularly complex and that relatively brief interventions may produce satisfactory results. The group approach reveals the fact that the means of resolving common difficulties is available in any ward or out-patient department and that intervention need not be either prolonged or interpretative.

The beginner is often tempted to opt for one 'school' or the other (to the exclusion of alternative viewpoints). This would be unfortunate as the approach adopted by many effective therapists is *eclectic* (drawing upon more than one school of thought). The 'purist' may achieve intellectual vigour at the expense of practical efficacy and is at risk of developing a rigid frame of reference which will help some of the clients some of the time, but will be of little help to most of the clients for most of the time. The risks of the 'purist' stance are perhaps best described by Ogden Nash:

'I give you now Professor Quist,
A conscientious scientist,
Trustees exclaimed—he never bungles
And sent him off to distant jungles,
Camped by a tropic riverside,
One day he missed his blushing bride,
She had, a guide informed him later
Been eaten by an alligator.
Professor Quist could not but smile,
You mean, he said, a crocodile.'

Many mental health care professionals profess to have open minds whereas the aforesaid area is only slightly ajar; this is unfortunate as awareness of the range of psychotherapeutic interventions available will greatly enrich perspectives on mental disorder.

Analytical or interpretative approaches should only be used once the appropriate post-basic training has been undertaken and the novice should resist the temptation to offer sweeping interpretations. Despite this proviso, an awareness of the interpretative models contributes greater understanding of human behaviour and emotions, and the student should not regard interpretative writings as a 'taboo' area but should try to enhance his/her understanding by considering each of the major perspectives.

The nurse should, for example, be able to recognize transference relationships and cathartic experiences and should be able to approach nurse/patient relationships with a broad awareness of psychodynamics, and increased sensitivity to the emotional responses of self and others. Non-directive approaches are eminently suitable for use by nursing staff, as are some variants of the humanistic approach, and these will be discussed in more detail later in this chapter.

Current Approaches To Physical Treatment

These broadly consist of:
1 Chemotherapy (use of psychotropic drugs)
2 Electroplexy
3 Psychosurgery

Chemotherapy

Most drugs used in psychiatry fall into one of three broad categories:
1 Antipsychotic (neuroleptic) drugs—formerly known as 'major tranquillizers'
2 Antidepressant (and other *mood*-stabilizing) drugs
3 Anxiolytic (anti-anxiety) drugs—formerly known as 'minor tranquillizers'

Antipsychotic (neuroleptic) drugs

These have a calming effect without dulling consciousness and many are thought to specifically reduce some troublesome symptoms of psychosis (delusions and hallucinations). The effect is thus not simply to 'tranquillize' and the introduction of these drugs (in the fifties) revolutionized psychiatry as they enabled staff to unlock wards and improve ward atmosphere and made many patients amenable to psychological and social therapies.

The antipsychotics fall into three broad groups of drugs:

(a) *The phenothiazines*. This group consists of those which are given orally and those which are given as depot (sustained release) injections, enabling many patients to be returned to the community without undue anxieties about possible failures to comply with oral medication regimes. The oral phenothiazines include chlorpromazine (Largactil), thioridazine (Melleril) and perphenazine (Fentazin), and long-acting *oral* forms include penfluridol (Semap) and pimozide (Orap), taken weekly and four days per week respectively. Depot injections include fluphenazine decanoate (Modecate); one injection of such a preparation will exert an antipsychotic effect for 2–4 weeks.

(b) *Thioxanthes*. This group includes the widely used depot preparation flupenthixol decanoate (Depixol), thought to be less likely to induce depression than fluphenazine (Modecate). The oral drug flupenthixol (Fluanxol) is actually thought to have some antidepressant properties.

(c) *Butyrophenones*. This group includes haloperidol (Serenace, Haldol) and these preparations not only have an antipsychotic effect but are also used in the treatment of manic elevation of mood. Haloperidol decanoate may be administered as a depot injection; one injection produces effects lasting for four weeks.

Antidepressant drugs

These restore mood to 'normal' levels in depression and are thought to act by correcting imbalances in cerebral chemistry. This is a very large group of drugs and includes (a) polycyclic antidepressants (b) monoamine oxidase inhibitors and (c) lithium salts.

Polycyclic antidepressants. The 'standard group of antidepressants are known as the tricyclic groups and are so-called because these compounds possess three prominent 'rings' in their chemical formula. Bicyclic ('two-ringed') and tetracyclic ('four-ringed') antidepressants have also been introduced. *Tricyclics* include imipramine (Tofranil), amitryptyline (Tryptizol) and clomipramine (Anafranil), the latter also proving useful in the treatment of obsessive/compulsive and phobic states. This group is relatively cardiotoxic and takes up to three weeks to lift mood. Some *tetracyclics* [e.g. maprotilene (Ludiomil)] are claimed to lift mood more quickly, and some bicyclics [e.g. viloxazine (Vivalan)] are claimed to have fewer adverse side-effects.

Monoamine oxidase inhibitors MAOIs. These inhibit production of the enzyme (monoamine oxidase) which 'mops up' excess of naturally occurring stimulant compounds (noradrenaline and serotonin) so that mood is gradually lifted 'naturally'. Food stuffs containing the enzyme tyramine react with these drugs to cause hypertensive crises which may be fatal, thus obliging the patient to observe a range of dietary restrictions. Largely for this reason use of MAOIs has declined, though some [e.g. phenelzine (Nardil) or tranylcypromine (Parnate)] are occasionally used in resistant depression.

Lithium salts. These occur in a wide range of natural minerals (Greek 'lithos'—stone) and are used in the treatment of disorders of mood (affective disorders). Lithium salts (introduced in 1949) exert a prophylactic effect insofar as they stabilize chronic mood disorders preventing further swings into mania or depression. It is often claimed that lithium is effective in the treatment of depressive phases of bipolar affective disorders (manic depressive psychosis), though this has not been clearly established), and it has been demonstrated to reduce the frequency and severity of both depressive and manic phases of bipolar disorders (Roth, 1983) as well as serving a useful prophylactic (or preventative) function in mood disorders.

The margin between the therapeutic and toxic doses of lithium is very small so patients should have serum lithium levels monitored, weekly for the first few weeks and at monthly intervals thereafter, to ensure that the patient has been stabilized on the drug and is not accumulating toxic levels of lithium. At least 12 hours must have elapsed between the last dose of lithium and the taking of blood for the estimation of serum lithium levels, and the nurse should ensure that the patient's medication is stopped at the appropriate time. Elderly patients may require more frequent monitoring due to decreased renal functioning associated with ageing. Lithium is marketed as lithium carbonate (Priadel, Camcolit, Phasal) though other salts of lithium are occasionally used.

The drugs introduced in this section are discussed in greater detail later in this text in relation to the disorders for which they are usually prescribed. The nurse should know the maximal dose of each drug and should also be familiar with the usual therapeutic dosage range. Side-effects and complications of drugs in use should also be familiar to the nurse as many psychotropic drugs (e.g. lithium and MOAIs) may have serious side-effects which develop insidiously and escalate rapidly. Over-sedation should also be reported immediately. A sound working knowledge of widely used drugs is essential if the nurse is to help ensure that treatment is effective and if the patient's well-being is to be effectively protected. The nurse who has not familiarized herself with the side-effects of potent psychotropic drugs is placing her patients at risk. The range of psychotropic drugs is large and continually expanding and it may happen that a patient is prescribed a drug with which the nurse is not familiar. In this case the pharmacy department should be contacted and the necessary information obtained.

Electroplexy

Electroplexy is a treatment whereby a small electrical current is briefly passed between two electrodes placed on the temples of the anaesthetized patient. The current is usually 80 volts and is administered for 0.1–0.3 second. This treatment was formerly known as *electroconvulsive therapy* (ECT), now an inappropriate term as major convulsions do *not* ensue because the patient is administered a muscle relaxant so that only a 'modified convulsion' ensues. [Before the widespread use of muscle relaxants (introduced 25 years ago) major convulsions did ensue.]

In practice there are mild tonic/clonic movements of the facial muscles and of the muscles of the hand and feet lasting for approximately 30 seconds. The term 'electroconvulsive' is not only inaccurate and misleading but will needlessly alarm patients and relatives. The treatment is safe and quick and can dramatically reduce severe depressions of a psychotic nature and may indeed be life-saving, as in the case of the suicidally depressed patient.

The use of electricity in the treatment of some types of intractable mood disorder dates back to the eighteenth century though the procedure as we now know it was introduced by Cerletti in 1938. It is not known precisely how elextroplexy alleviates mood disorders though it has been suggested that it may correct imbalances in cerebral amine neurotransmitters.

Indications for electroplexy

The use of electroplexy in certain types of depressive disorder may bring dramatic relief from crippling and tormenting symptoms.

Clinical features associated with a good response are
1 family history of depression
2 a pyknic body build (short rotund physique with a round head and short arms and legs)
3 early morning waking
4 history of weight loss
5 sudden onset of disorder
6 pronounced retardation
7 self reproach
8 duration of disorder of less than one year
9 obsessional traits
10 good insight

Unfavourable features include:
1 hypochondriasis
2 emotional lability
3 neurotic traits (in childhood or in adult life)
4 hysterical overlay to disorder
5 above average intelligence
6 fluctuating course since onset
7 depersonalization

If patients are selected carefully, the proportion showing a good response to electroplexy is 70–80% (Clare, 1976). In the main, electroplexy is used in the treatment of endogenous depressions exhibiting the indications described though it may be used to reduce manic excitement. Electroplexy has little effect on reactive depressions and Sargant and Slater (1972) have advocated its use as a diagnostic tool (no response = reactive depression). Electroplexy (like chemotherapy) is not curative but palliative (reduces or controls troublesome symptoms).

Physical contraindications

These include raised intracranial pressure, cerebral aneurysm or tumour, recent myocardial infarct or cerebrovascular accident and cardiac arrhythmias.

Bilateral and unilateral electroplexy

In bilateral electroplexy two electrodes are used, one being placed on either side of the patient's head in the temporal fossa 4 cm above the mid-point of a line drawn from the lateral angle of the eye to the external auditory meatus, so that each electrode lies over one of the temporal lobes.

The unilateral approach also uses two electrodes but in this case both electrodes are placed on the same side, one electrode often being placed in the temporal position, the other on the parietal area. In some unilateral approaches the electrodes are placed on the dominant side of the head (the left side of the head in right-handed people and most left-handed people; in two-thirds of left-handed people the left hemisphere is also dominant).

Dominant unilateral electroplexy was introduced in 1942 but is thought to cause greater than average memory disturbance after treatment. In 1957 non-dominant unilateral electroplexy was introduced whereby both electrodes are placed on the non-dominant side of the head; this is claimed to produce much less post-treatment disorientation and memory impairment than either dominant uni-lateral or bilateral approaches.

After-effects of electroplexy

Other than the therapeutic lifting of mood, some undesired after-effects may occur. Two main types of memory impairment are seen: *anterograde amnesia* (i.e. difficulty in remembering information acquired *after* treatment) and *retrograde amnesia* (e.g. difficulty in remembering information acquired *before* treatment) though these are usually short-term side-effects. The duration of memory impairment may be fairly variable and one study found that 48% of the patients studied developed detectable memory impairment after the fifth treatment and that this lasted on average for 20.1 days (Summers et al, 1979), while another study found that little memory impairment could be detected at four months and none at six months. The latter study also found that the mean recovery time to pre-treatment levels of functioning was 72 days with a range of 7–270 days (Weeks et al, 1980). Other short-term side-effects reported include confusion, headache, vomiting, impaired learning and cardiac arrhythmias (Berrios, 1983).

Non-dominant unilateral electroplexy is claimed to reduce the post-treatment incidence of memory impairment, confusion and headache though the bilateral approach is still most widely used, especially if the patient's 'handedness' is in doubt.

Number and frequency of treatments

A 'course' of treatments usually consists of four to eight treatments, two treatments per week usually being given, though both number and frequency may be varied considerably depending on the patient's response.

An approach called 'multiple monitored electroconvulsive therapy', (MMECT) whereby four to eight treatments are administered at 2-minute intervals during a single session, is finding more widespread use in the USA but has had little clinical impact in the UK (Blachly and Gowing, 1966). MMECT has attracted considerable criticism as it is feared by many critics that the risks of this approach outweigh any therapeutic gains (two MMECT deaths were reported in 1976) (Blachly, 1976). The mortality rate associated with standard approaches is very low—one death in 2594 courses of treatment (Royal College of Psychiatrists, 1981).

Stages of treatment

Treatment may be considered in three stages:
1 Physical and psychological preparation of the patient
2 Care of the patient during treatment
3 Care of the patient following treatment

Preparation of the patient

The doctor must obtain written consent from the patient, having explained the treatment and what is involved. Should the patient withdraw consent at any point the medical staff should be informed at once and treatment withheld meantime. The Mental Health Acts (England and Wales, 1983 and Scotland, 1984) (Appendix 4) contain safeguards which ensure that patients who are compulsorily detained in hospital are not given certain treatments lightly. Either consent or a second opinion are required before electroplexy can be administered. Consent warrants only one series of treatments.

The nurse may have to augment the doctor's explanation should the patient request more information. Technical discussions are rarely requested and the nurse usually has to simply underline that treatment is brief and completely painless and that a light general anaesthetic will be given to briefly put the patient 'to sleep'. It should be emphasized that the patient will not 'feel a thing' and that the only part of treatment of which the patient will be conscious will consist of two injections, one half an hour before leaving the ward (which will make the mouth feel a little dry), and the anaesthetic injection, usually administered into a small vein on the back of the hand by the anaesthe-

tist. It should also be emphasized that the patient will be accompanied to treatment by a nurse from the ward who will also be there when he/she 'wakens' from the anaesthetic. The presence of a familiar nurse is usually experienced as very reassuring by the patient. The patient should also be told that he/she will probably feel light-headed or 'fuzzy' after treatment and will remember little or nothing about it. It should be explained that this is quite normal and that the nurse will ensure that nothing important is forgotten by the patient as a note of any outstanding matters to which the patient wishes to attend that day will be taken before treatment.

The patient who is to go for treatment for the first time may be particularly apprehensive on the preceding evening and may be reassured by a little extra nursing time and the provision of the opportunity to have a chat with a patient who has benefited from electroplexy. Relatives may also need a little extra reassurance on the preceding evening. Remember that patients (and relatives) may be reluctant to verbalize anxieties about treatment as they may fear that this may make them appear weak or foolish in the eyes of others. Patients should be encouraged to talk about any anxieties experienced and the nurse should be alert to non-verbal expressions of tension.

The patient must be fasted for 6–8 hours before treatment and if treatment is given in the morning the patient will have nil by mouth from midnight preceding treatment. Should a patient be given anything to eat or drink by mistake this should be reported and treatment will usually be postponed. Half an hour before leaving the ward the patient is given a premedication of *atropine* (0.6 mg by intramuscular injection) which not only dries up salivary and bronchial secretions but also prevents bradycardia during treatment by partially blocking vagal innervation of the heart. Should the atropine be omitted for any reason, the nurse should inform the anaesthetist who will then give the atropine intravenously. Patients should be observed carefully after the atropine has been given as many may attempt to drink to relieve the dryness of the mouth caused by the drug.

Final preparations include the removal of any tight clothing, and any make-up or nail varnish which may mask cyanosis should be removed. Valuables are placed in safe keeping and the patient's wedding ring taped over if it has become loose fitting due to weight loss. Any metal objects (earrings, hairgrips) which may deflect the current are removed and the patient is asked to empty the bladder (and bowels if possible) immediately before leaving the ward. The nurse who is to accompany the patient should ensure that she has the relevant documents to take with her (consent form, electroplexy treatment record card, medication prescription and recording sheets, TPR and BP charts, and sometimes, the patient's case notes). The patient is then taken to the waiting area which should be completely separate from the treatment and recovery areas.

Care during treatment

The patient's dentures and spectacles are removed and safely stored in clearly labelled containers and the patient is asked to remove his/her shoes before lying down on the trolley. The anaesthetist must be informed of any dental crowns, bridge work and loose or carious teeth as a dislodged tooth or dental crown could obstruct the patient's airway. Preparation for the administration of the anaesthetic should be relaxed, calm and unhurried and the nurse should continue to provide reassurance. The anaesthetist gives the anaesthetic by intravenous injection (usually methohexitone which has fewer cardiac side-effects than thiopentone, the other anaesthetic occasionally chosen). The anaesthetic is followed by the muscle relaxant (usually suxamethonium which will relax all muscle groups and cause apnoea lasting approximately 2 minutes). The patient's lungs are then ventilated with 100% oxygen. Pre-treatment ventilation is necessary because of the apnoea induced by the muscle relaxant, and preventing hypoxaemia also seems to reduce the intensity of post-treatment memory deficit (there is hippocampal susceptibility to reduced oxygen tension) (Berrios, 1983).

The psychiatrist then places the electrodes (padded and soaked with electrolyte solution) on the patient's head, a rubber mouth gag is inserted (sometimes a combination mouth gag and airway is used) and the nursing staff gently restrain the patient's limbs by rolling the sheets to the side of the patient's body and bearing down on them. Direct pressure on major joints must be avoided. The current is switched on and the patient is again ventilated with oxygen once twitching has ceased. Once the anaesthetist is satisfied that the patient is breathing independently again, a Guedel-type airway is inserted, ventilation ceases and the patient is turned on to his/her side and taken to the recovery room to regain consciousness.

Care after treatment

During the immediate post-treatment period it is essential that the patient is not left unobserved. Cyanosis or abnormalities of pulse or respirations should be reported to the anaesthetist immediately. A trained nurse will be in charge of the recovery area and will be fully versed in recovery procedures. The airway should not be removed until consciousness is returning. Wait until the patient either begins to expel the airway or attempts to remove it manually. As consciousness returns the patient often becomes restless and may attempt to get out of bed while still confused. The nurse should speak to the patient in a gentle and soothing tone of voice and reassurance usually leads to discontinuation of attempts to get out of bed. The nurse should use her own name (and that of any other nurse present) as the patient may not remember these. The patient will not realize that treatment is over and should be reminded of this.

As soon as is practical the patient should be given a cup of tea while the nurse remains with him/her giving gentle reminders to reorientation. Careful observation will be necessary until post-treatment confusion has subsided, and any complaints of severe headache should be reported so that an analgesic may be prescribed and given. Mood and behaviour should be monitored and recorded throughout the course of treatment and for some weeks afterwards. It is important that nursing staff maximize the therapeutic opportunities afforded by the stabilization of mood brought about by electroplexy and the patient may now be involved in group and social activities. Mood may lag behind psychomotor retardation after the first few treatments and agitation may become apparent. Until mood lifts this agitated period is often associated with an increased risk of suicidal behaviour, and increased observation is called for.

Out-patient electroplexy

Preparation is the same as for in-patients and the patient should not leave hospital unaccompanied afterwards. If for some reason this is not possible the recovery nurse should ensure that the patient is fully recovered before he/she leaves hospital. A taxi should be ordered for the patient since patients should not be allowed to drive themselves home.

Electroplexy—the research findings

The research studies of electroplexy have tended to be patchy and poorly designed. Clare (1976) comments that of more than 200 studies carried out between 1955 and 1960, 'only ten met the most minimal requirements of a scientifically valid and reliable research effort'. Some later research studies compared anaesthetized control groups with patients given electroplexy; that is, a group of patients given an anaesthetic, muscle relaxant and electroplexy were compared with a group of similar patients who were given a muscle relaxant and an anaesthetic *only*, no current being passed. One study found that electroplexy was no more effective than an anaesthetic alone (Brill et al, 1959), a finding contradicted by later studies (Clare, 1976). A Medical Research Council study in 1965 (which did not use a control group) concluded that electroplexy was the quickest and most effective treatment for depression. Research has confirmed that the previously widespread practice of using electroplexy to treat schizophrenia is no longer justifiable. A recent survey of the research concludes that 'there is no convincing evidence that it has any effect on the more common forms of the illness' (Clare, 1976) though electroplexy will stabilize marked schizophrenic excitement or stupor.

Some research has explored the premise that much of the therapeutic gain associated with electroplexy may be associated with increased levels of staff/patient interaction (especially nurse/patient interaction) associated with treatment, though the findings are at present inconclusive.

Does electroplexy have long-term harmful effects?

This is currently a very controversial area and opinions differ sharply. Critics of electroplexy suggest that it causes brain damage, that it is often administered to unwilling patients and that we simply don't know how it works. The suggestion that electroplexy should be abandoned as no-one is quite sure how it works is perhaps the least tenable of these objections; many drugs used (without objection) in general medicine would have to be abandoned on the same grounds. The objection that electroplexy is (or was) used overenthusiastically may have some substance. Jones (1983) has commented that 'a few enthusiasts misused it (electroplexy) intensively and desperately . . . the results were disappointing and in some cases fatal' and

Clare (1976) comments that 'nothing has done the course of ECT more harm than its indiscriminate use by overenthusiastic and uncritical clinicians'.

Indiscriminate use of electroplexy is now largely a thing of the past and it is important to remember that electroplexy used to treat carefully selected patients may be life-saving. Avery and Winokur (1976) found that electroplexy-treated patients had a lower mortality rate than those treated with tricyclic antidepressants or those who remain untreated.

A major area of controversy centres around the accusation that electroplexy causes brain damage. The idea of passing electricity through a living human brain may cause intuitive feelings of apprehension in many people and the arguments advanced against electroplexy may be rooted in almost archetypal fears rather than in convincing research results. Suspicion of the unscrupulous or reckless physician may be rooted in folk memories of the eighteenth century anatomists who paid unsavoury characters to provide subjects for dissection, these usually being obtained by plundering graveyards or, in some cases, by murdering people in the teeming 'rookeries' of urban slums. Mary Shelley's novel 'Frankenstein' introduced a theme which was to be endlessly developed—the unscrupulous doctor using electricity to reanimate a cadaver assembled in an anatomical variant of the paint-by-numbers kit. In the countless cinema variations on this theme the 'monster' demonstrates his new found vitality by pursuing a succession of shrieking maidens through mist-shrouded forests, and the unscrupulous doctor is besieged in his laboratory by an incensed mob of peasants wielding burning torches. These powerful images of the unscrupulous and reckless doctor using electricity in dangerous and unethical experiments are familiar to most people. The contemporary equivalent of the torch-wielding mob seems to consist largely of irate members of voluntary organizations though some criticism has emanated from health care professionals. Many critics of electroplexy point out that exponents of the treatment attempt to justify it on the basis of flimsy anecdotal accounts of success ('Miss X, an 18-year-old typist, was much improved after one course of electroplexy and thereafter made a good recovery'). The fact remains that many attacks on electroplexy assume a similar form ('Miss Y, a 36-year-old actress, has complained that her memory has become poor following a course of electroplexy 10 years ago').

Polemical and highly emotive attacks on electroplexy have frequently assumed a similar stereotyped form. For example, Cerletti 'got the idea' for electroplexy in a slaughterhouse where he observed hogs being stunned by an electrical current before slaughter; the first patient experimented on was a tramp found wandering in a railway station and who (conveniently) had no next of kin; Metrazol (Cardiazol) treatment is then discussed in detail (Metrazol treatment consisted of inducing seizures by intravenous injection of a cerebral irritant; the treatment was hazardous, terrifying to patients and has long since been abandoned). Descriptions of electroplexy emphasizing 'flailing limbs', 'drooling mouths' and bodies 'arched in convulsions' then often follow (these bear no relationship to the actual responses during electroplexy after the administration of a muscle relaxant). One could write a similarly lurid account of any common minor surgical procedure. Imagine appendicectomy described in this journalistic style: 'the glittering scalpel slicing through the shrinking flesh', 'gloved hands groping among the tender viscera', 'the patient moaning in pain for days afterwards'.

Objectivity is often sadly lacking in criticisms of this nature. The very term 'brain damage' is vague and emotive and tends to conjure up images of wrecked personalities, of individuals reduced to 'vegetable' status. In fact the neurological side-effects being criticized specifically involve memory defects, *not* global deterioration of the mind.

There is evidence that some early approaches were hazardous and did indeed result in long-term memory defects. In some approaches patients were given as many as 60 treatments over a four to eight week period, the developers of one such method stating of the patient: 'there is complete amnesia for all events of his life' (Cameron, 1960) and the introducers of a similar approach commenting that after treatment 'their minds are like clean slates on which we can write' (Kennedy and Anchel, 1948). The names given to these earlier approaches often reflect the expected outcome of treatment: 'annihilation therapy', 'blitz electric shock therapy', 'regressive electric shock therapy', though the only current approach involving multiple treatments is multiple monitored electroconvulsive therapy, an American approach which is arousing some concern and which is being closely monitored.

Berrios (1983) summarizes the neurological findings (based on uncontrolled post-mortem reports and animal findings) as follows: glial, neuronal and blood vessel changes, petechial haemorrhages and palatal myoclonus (spasmodic contractions) secondary to pons bleeding.

There are, however, no consistent research findings to indicate that moderate use of electroplexy in carefully selected patients produces lasting ill-effects which would militate against its use as a treatment method. The adverse findings criticize multiple treatment approaches and their possible long-term effects. It is important to balance criticisms against an awareness of the gains made possible by electroplexy. Jones (1983) comments that

'No longer were groups of silent, miserable patients to be seen in admission wards. The Suicidal Caution Card on which each nurse had to sign that he or she knew that the patient needed constant observation 24 hours per day became a thing of the past, and tube feeding of the resistive self starving patient was no longer necessary . . . (electroplexy) produced rapid improvement and rendered the patient susceptible to proper nursing care'.

Controversy tends to centre around not so much the *use* of electroplexy but occasional instances of what is perceived as *abuse* of electroplexy. Clare (1976) comments that

'ECT is a much abused and over-used method of treatment. Psychiatrists who persist in abusing it have only themselves to blame if the public . . . concludes that the treatment is a fraud and an anachronism and demands its abolition'.

Psychosurgery

The term 'psychosurgery' refers to a variety of techniques aimed at the destruction or removal of normal brain tissue (or apparently normal tissue) for the purpose of altering certain behaviour and should not be confused with neurosurgery aimed at removing recognizable pathological lesions (e.g. tumours, cysts or scars). This approach has its origins in 1875 when the British neurologist, Sir David Ferrier, removed a large portion of the frontal lobes of the brain in monkeys producing 'a remarkable change in the animals' characters and dispositions'. In 1888 Buckhardt isolated the frontal lobes in a violent patient by severing their connecting tracts, obtaining poor results and engendering much fierce opposition from colleagues. In 1912 three patients in Russia were the subjects of similar attempts to surgically isolate 'overactive' areas of the brain and the results were again described as 'miserable'.

Nothing more happened in the surgical treatment of mental disorder until the 1930s when the Portuguese neuropsychiatrist, Egas Moniz, fired by a promising series of results from recent animal experiments, introduced psychosurgical techniques which were to be widely adopted. Moniz initially used alcohol injections to coagulate frontal tracts but rapidly turned to the use of a steel cutter (a 'leucotome') to sever tracts leading to the frontal lobes claiming that the operation reduced aggressive behaviour in chronic schizophrenia. The procedure became known as *leucotomy* (from the Greek words for cutting and white) as the white tracts leading to the frontal lobes were reached via burr holes in the skull and were cut using a surgical cutter.

In the USA the procedure was adopted by W. Freeman and J. Watts (who used the term *lobotomy* for the operation). By 1950 Freeman and Watts had operated on over 1000 patients using the approach which was by then described as 'standard prefrontal leucotomy' (or lobotomy). The estimated world figure for such procedures has been given as over 20000 (Clare, 1976).

The early days of the Freeman–Watts era were characterized by an alarmingly uncritical adoption of the new approach. Schurr (1973) says of surgeons carrying out leucotomies: 'these included any surgeon of whatever experience who was willing to undertake them' and Clare (1976) speaks of the 'knife-happy' tendency of some surgeons. The Freeman–Watts partnership ended in 1954 when Freeman approached the undersurface of the frontal lobe by pushing an ice pick through the frontal sinus at the root of the nose while the patient was rendered unconscious by ECT. This seemingly blithe disregard for the principles of both surgery and anaesthesia seems to have proved too much for Watts. Short-term results for leucotomy had seemed promising but post-operative evaluation was often superficial and haphazard.

As the first flush of pioneer enthusiasm abated, more sober assessment of the long-term results revealed some alarming dimensions. Robins (1958), at Runwell Hospital, assessed the clinical outcome in 198 patients treated with leucotomy (using a control group). He found that leucotomy did not appear to improve the chances of discharge from hospital, accelerate discharge, reduce the possibility of readmission, delay readmission, reduce the number of admissions or improve hospital behaviour as judged at ward level. Undesirable side-effects were also now being reported (loss of creativity, loss of initiative, memory impairment, epilepsy, incontinence) as were dangerous complications (infection and haemorrhage). The advocates of psychosurgery insisted that these undesirable side-effects only affected a minority of patients but the critics protested vehemently that psychosurgery was dangerous, largely ineffective and unethical. Breggin (1972) has bluntly said 'To the extent that psychosurgery "blunts" the individual, I personally feel that it partially kills the individual . . . it should be against the law to take *part* of a person's life even with his consent'.

The number of psychosurgical operations carried out began to decline as controversy mounted; between 1942 and 1954 more than 10000 patients were operated on in Great Britain; between 1974 and 1976 431 psychosurgical operations were carried out in Britain and the number is steadily declining (Evans, 1983). The majority of the criticisms arise out of studies of patients who had the Freeman–Watts standard prefrontal leucotomy: an alarmingly unsophisticated surgical technique in which a burr hole was made in each side of the head and a leucotome introduced and blindly swept in an arc, hopefully dividing as much white matter as possible. Two-thirds of the early operations were also carried out on persons suffering from schizophrenia, a group now known to yield the least satisfactory results. Advocates of psychosurgery point out that selection is now more informed and that psychosurgical techniques in current use are far more sophisticated than the crude lacerations produced by the Freeman–Watts technique.

Stereotactic methods have now replaced free-hand techniques; that is, lesion sites are located by calculating their coordinates in relation to vertical, horizontal and parasagittal planes to a three-dimensional accuracy of 1 mm. There is minimal destruction of surrounding tissue and it is claimed that there are fewer side-effects. Surgical interventions now mostly aim to produce lesions in or around the limbic system, a collection of mid-brain structures (consisting of hypothalamus, the anterior thalamic nuclei, the angulate gyrus and the hippocampus) which influence the elaboration and expression of emotional and affective tone. The hypothalamus also plays a crucial role in the integration of appetite, sleep, sexual drive and hormonal function.

Some of the psychosurgical techniques in current use include *stereotactic limbic leucotomy* where lesions are placed into anterior limbic sites using a cryogenic probe or radiofrequency coagulation. The skull is immobilized during surgery using a Leksell stereotactic frame and the lesions are placed with great accuracy. *Stereotactic subcaudate tractotomy*—ceramic rods containing seeds of the radioactive isotope yttrium—are inserted in two lines of three into the anterior subcaudate tracts. The seeds have a half-life of about 62 hours and gradually produce a lesion about 25 mm long. *Multifocal leucocoagulation* involves stereotactic implantation into the frontal lobes of gold wire electrodes which are activated selectively and repetitively over about six months to produce lesions of a gradually increasing size, according to clinical response. *Stereotactic anterior cingulotomy* (cingulumotomy, cingulotractotomy) produces cingular lesions, sometimes using yttrium implants. *Bimedial leucotomy* is an open procedure, carried out under direct vision, which uses a metal sucker to induce lesions extending into the ventromedial segment of each frontal lobe. This procedure has been carried out on a large number of patients at the Maudsley Hospital and elsewhere (Evans, 1983). Coagulation of the amygdala (*amygdalotomy*) and of parts of the hypothalamus (*hypothalotomy*) have also been carried out, the latter being used in the treatment of individuals with a history of sexual violence.

Some critics continue to insist that even if such procedures were effective they would not be acceptable on ethical grounds. A major refrain in criticisms of psychosurgery is that these procedures are often carried out to induce social conformity rather than medical stability.

Freeman (1971) published a paper in which he reiterated his advocacy of psychosurgery, illustrating his case with anecdotal accounts of the benefits of psychosurgery (after surgery one patient, a physician, 'established a ten man medical clinic and flies his own plane'; another, a psychiatrist, 'established an after-care clinic and went into private practice'). Cynics may feel that increased aeronautical ability or business acumen are rather strange outcomes to be approvingly offered as criteria of success. Clare (1976) comments of this paper: 'Freeman's paper is somewhat more interesting with regard to the insight (unwittingly provided?) which he gives his readers into his conception of illness and health than for what it has to say about a formidable, irreversible method of treatment'.

An Indian neurosurgeon, Balasubramaniam, used psychosurgery to treat 'hyperactivity in 115 patients of whom three were under five and another 36 under eleven', approvingly recording that 'remarkable improvements' occurred. One patient is described as becoming 'quiet, bashful and . . . a model of good behaviour' (Balasubramaniam et al, 1970). Two Japanese surgeons used amygdalotomy on 27 children aged from 5 to 13 years suffering from 'poor concentration' and 'unsteadiness', and reported that surgery produced a degree of 'satisfactory obedience' (Narabayashi et al, 1966).

The controversy continues and psychosurgery continues to have its advocates as well as its critics. Sargant and Slater (1972) are perhaps the best known advocates of psychosurgery and they ascribe the decline in psychosurgery in the USA to 'ideological' attacks and claim that 'The damage done (sic) even to a mature and differentiated personality, as a rule, is so slight as to be beyond detection by clinical methods'. These authors continue to advocate psychosurgery in schizophrenia but do not cite any research findings (other than 30-year-old studies) to support this view.

Evans (1983) summarizes the current indications for psychosurgery as follows:

1 Severe, persistent, treatment-resistant depression
2 Anxiety or obsessive/compulsive neurosis
3 Pathological aggression
4 Intractable or debilitating pain

Patients should be able to give informed consent, have failed to respond to *all other treatments* for *several years*, and not be compulsorily detained. Unfavourable prognostic signs include sociopathy, 'antisocial premorbid personality' and drug or alcohol dependence.

Evans (1983) suggests that many patients have received 'considerable benefit' from psychosurgery, describes the evidence as 'flawed' and 'far from satisfactory from a methodological viewpoint', warns against 'inappropriate emotional reactions' to the issue and concedes that 'the ethical controversy continues'.

Mental health care professionals often become involved in acrimonious debates about psychosurgery and electroplexy and there have been widely publicized examples of nurses being dismissed or disciplined for refusing to participate in physical methods of treatment. Unfortunately, these debates often centre around examples of what is perceived as abuse of a physical method of treatment, and the merits of controlled *use* are often consequently forced into the background.

Emotive attitudes, no matter how admirable the

motives from which they spring, are no substitute for informed judgements. The nurse who is experiencing cognitive dissonance in respect of her own involvement is advised to avoid polemic arguments (for or against) in favour of research findings. For a comprehensive summary of research findings the reader may wish to read Chapters 6 and 7 of Psychiatry in Dissent (Clare, 1976).

Non-physical methods of treatment

These approaches fall into the three broad categories of analytical, humanistic and behavioural therapies. Analytical approaches should only be adopted by nurses who have undertaken an appropriate post-basic course though awareness of the analytical model will provide the nurse with broader insights into human functioning. The humanistic therapies have, however, provided a variety of approaches which may be actively adopted from an early stage in training in 'pure' or in modified form.

An awareness of psychotherapy will prove to be an invaluable asset to the essential psychiatric nursing activities of *listening*, *understanding* and *clarifying* and will enable communication with the mentally disordered to be both structured and helpful to nurse and patient alike.

Approaches which emphasize the 'here and now' may be usefully employed and can have considerable problem-solving capacity with the added benefit that they also encourage greater self-awareness and increased personal growth. Some of these approaches (e.g. transactional analysis, Gestalt therapy and client-centred therapy) provide a person-centred philosophy as well as a range of therapeutic interventions and will encourage the student to embark upon the necessary task of examining his/her own attitudes, beliefs and values. The attitudes brought by the nurse to every interaction with patients play a critical part in determining what happens thereafter. The practice of self-examination should both precede and accompany interactions with clients—how many 'difficulties' with patients arise out of *your* attitudes and beliefs—rather than the patient's behaviour?

Transactional analysis

Transactional analysis is a system of social psychology originated by Eric Berne which can be used to understand, predict and change human behaviour. It is both a communication tool and a treatment method and will help the nurse to profitably consider her own responses as well as those of her patients.

Ego states

Each of us has three ways of experiencing ourselves and of relating to others which are called *ego states*. Berne labels these as *Parent*, *Adult* and *Child*, as each ego state is marked by distinctive ways of feeling, thinking and behaving characteristic of the parent, adult or child in us.

The Parent ego state is that aspect of self which has incorporated what we perceived our own parenting figures to be, say and do. The parent ego state may be nurturing (*Nurturing Parent*) or critical and judgemental (*Critical Parent*). Adoption of a parental ego state is revealed by behaviours (pat on the back, pointing, accusing or threatening finger, punitive or encouraging tone of voice, scowls, frowns, disapproving looks) and language (words and phrases like: 'should if I were you', 'don't worry', 'come on now', etc).

The *Adult* ego state or aspect of self is our computer—it solves and analyses problems in an objective way and draws upon past experience. This ego state helps the person to appraise his/her environment and to calculate possibilities and probabilities. Adoption of the adult ego state is reflected in a confident, calm voice, thoughtful expression, alertness, explaining, asking or giving information.

The *Child* ego state feels, wants and needs as we did when a child of 2–5 years old. The small child inside all of us surfaces when this ego state is used and need not do so in a negative way. 'The Child is in many ways the most valuable part of the personality and can contribute to the individual's life exactly what an actual child can contribute to family life: charm, pleasure and creativity' (Berne, 1964). However, the child may also take over with negative and disconcerting results. 'If the child in the individual is confused and unhealthy then the (interpersonal) consequences may be unfortunate' (Berne, 1964). In transactional analysis there is no such thing as an 'immature' person. There are only people in whom the Child takes over inappropriately or unproductively, but 'all such people have a complete, well-structured Adult which only needs to be uncovered or activated' (Berne, 1964). The child ego state may surface in one of two forms. The

Adapted Child modifies his behaviour under parental influences—by complying or withdrawing. The *Natural Child* spontaneously expresses rebellion, creativity or enjoyment.

The presence of the Child ego state is revealed by playfulness, flirtatiousness, giggling, swearing, sulking, nail biting, curling up, obscene gestures, excitement and helplessness. Anything that happens between two people involves their ego states and it is helpful to be able to recognize which ego state is active in each person. The three aspects of the personality should co-exist in healthy and productive balance and it is only when one or other of them disturbs this healthy balance that therapy is called for; 'otherwise each of them, Parent, Adult and Child, is entitled to equal respect and has its legitimate place in a full and productive life' (Berne, 1964).

Strokes

Strokes are the fundamental units of social interaction and stroking denotes *any* act which recognizes another's presence. These units of recognition may be *non-verbal* (a smile, a frown, a hug, a slap in the face) or *verbal* (a greeting, a compliment, an insult, a question). Strokes may be *positive* or *negative* although negative strokes are often more predictable than positive ones and the patient who is experiencing '*stroke deprivation*' may indulge in hostile or destructive behaviours as these readily guarantee situations which will satisfy stroke hunger.

Research has shown that mammals, including humans, need stroking to survive adequately (Spitz and Wolf, 1946) and long-term hospitalization may be associated with high levels of stroke deprivation. If nursing provides positive strokes (approval, warmth, affection, encouragement, praise) the tendency to seek negative strokes will be dramatically reduced. Strokes felt in the Child ego state have the greatest impact and we are better able to remain in the Adult ego state when our Child need for strokes is satisfied. The nurse should try to increase awareness of the needs of the Child in both herself and her patients.

Babcock (1978) comments that 'some nurses are taught to be efficient (Adult) and to care for others (Parent) but not to pay attention to their own needs (Child)—this leads to stroke hunger and tempts us to get strokes in crooked, painful ways'. The stroke-hungry nurse may unconsciously elicit strokes at the expense of both her patients and her colleagues by adopting authoritarian, hostile or uncooperative attitudes which lead to confrontations. Communi-

cations can be improved by adopting a policy of positive stroking (smiles, hugs, arm pats and friendly, accepting or encouraging statements).

Transactions

An exchange of strokes constitutes a *transaction* which is the unit of social intercourse. A transaction consists of a stimulus stroke and a response stroke and these strokes may emanate from any one of three available ego states. A part of me—Parent, Adult or Child—offers you a stimulus and a part of you responds to that stimulus. For example, my Child ego state says 'I'm bored!' Your Child ego state responds 'Me too!'. Your response is also the stimulus to our next transaction.

Transactions are said to be *complementary* when the ego state addressed is the one that responds. For example, one may consider two nurses studying in the college library—one sighs heavily at intervals and looks away from her books (Child), the other eventually looks up and says 'What's wrong? You seem to have something on your mind' (Adult). Complementary transactions may occur between similar or different ego states so long as the stimulus evokes a response from the 'target' ego state. If a transaction is complementary, communications will proceed smoothly.

Sometimes transactions may be *crossed*; that is, a stimulus evokes a response from an ego state other than the one addressed. The nurse sighing over her studies (Child) may have evoked a response like 'For goodness' sake, be quiet and get on with your studying' (Critical Parent). The crossed transaction involves the activation of an inappropriate ego state and the result often is that people feel misunderstood, surprised, hurt or angry. Crossed transactions are not compatible with effective communication as the persons involved are likely to withdraw from each other, change the subject or turn away.

The three available ego states may be represented diagrammatically as follows:

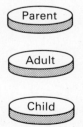

Thus when two persons (A and B) are speaking, the ego states available for use in the transaction are:

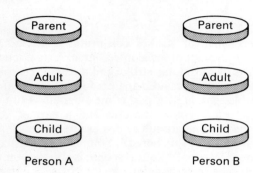

and transactions may be simply shown using these diagrams.

Consider the following exchange: Ward Sister A: 'Student nurses nowadays don't know what it means to work hard'; Ward Sister B: 'Yes, a little hard work wouldn't do most of them any harm'. This could be shown as:

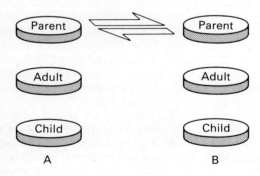

Consider another example: Patient (Person A): 'My mouth is awfully dry today. Could that be a side-effect of my tablets?' Nurse (Person B): 'Come now, Mr Smith, I think you can trust us to monitor your treatment adequately.' This could be shown as:

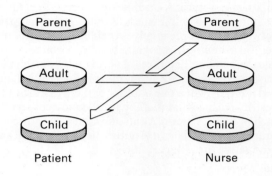

Recognizing and describing interactions in terms of the ego states involved is called transactional analysis. Ego states may change rapidly during even a short transaction. Consider a nurse chatting to one of her patients about a mutual interest, each accepting the other as an equal and both enjoying the exchange of views and information:

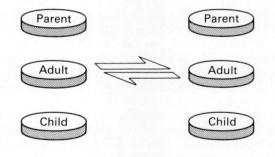

Staff Nurse appears and crossly says 'Come along, Nurse Smith, there *is* work to be done'.

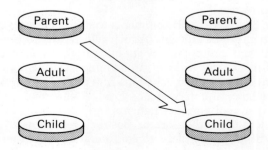

Staff Nurse leaves and the patient (sympathetic and conscious of Nurse Smith's 'loss of face') says 'What a dragon—never liked the woman myself.'

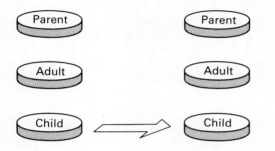

Nurse Smith says (sotto voce) 'If you ask me she's a real neurotic.'

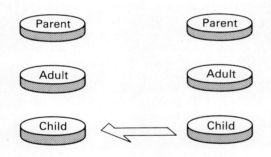

Nurse Smith's future interactions with Staff Nurse could be distorted if she now proceeds to accept the role of untrustworthy child and behaves accordingly.

For example (the next day) Staff Nurse: 'Nurse Smith, would you mind checking this drug with me?'

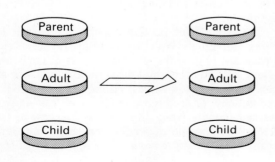

Nurse Smith: 'For goodness' sake why does something always have to be done when my meal break is due!'

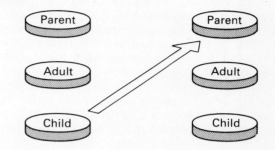

It would be more constructive for Nurse Smith to attempt to restore complementary transactions by taking advantage of a quiet moment to say to Staff Nurse: 'You know I really felt put down when you told me off yesterday and, to be honest, I'm starting to feel a little apprehensive at the prospect of working with you and I feel that this may adversely affect our working relationship if we don't discuss this now.'

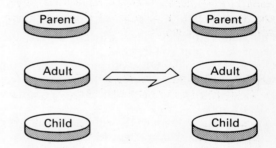

Ulterior transactions

More than two ego states are involved in this case. Under a socially acceptable transaction another message is hidden, aimed at another ego state—a hidden agenda. Often the hidden part is communicated non-verbally by facial expression, tone of voice, posture, gestures or clothes. For example, the student who always hands in his messy assignments too late may be inviting his teacher to give him a parental reprimand. Ulterior transactions take place on two levels at once—an overt level which is usually Adult to Adult and a covert level which involves the Child ego state. For example: 'Nurse Smith, I notice that Mr Jones has not been weighed this week.' (lazy—can't trust you to do anything) 'As a matter of fact he has and I have recorded his weight on the chart.' (stupid, can't you read!)

Ulterior or hidden transactions, like crossed transactions, make effective communication difficult.

Positions

Our concept of self, our position and attitudes about life are reflected in the psychological *position* assumed in interactions. Self-concept is to a great extent based on experience and on the feedback obtained from significant others. What other people think of us determines to a greater or lesser extent what we think of ourselves.

Depending on the sort of messages and experiences involved, the person sorts these out to develop a view of self or others in terms of 'being OK' or 'not being OK'. A neglected or constantly criticized child is likely to develop a negative self-concept (or self-image)—'I'm not OK' and the concept of others could very well become 'They're not OK'. Sometimes people feel OK about certain parts of themselves but not OK about others. Sometimes the concepts are connected with certain categories of people only; for example, 'Men are OK, women are not OK'.

The result may be any one of four psychological positions:

1 I'm OK, you're OK—basically accepting yourself and others.

2 I'm OK, you're *not* OK—reflected in suspicious or querulous attitudes—feeling that others are 'after you' or out to 'put you down'.

3 I'm *not* OK, you're OK—others are seen as being more successful and powerful. This can lead to feelings of inferiority and helplessness—to withdrawal or depression.

4 I'm *not* OK, you're *not* OK—life can then be perceived as meaningless and worthless.

In summary:

Position and attitudes about life (Harris, 1973)

A person in this position	feels this way about life
'I'm OK—you're OK'	'life is worth living, let's get on with it'
'I'm OK—you're not OK'	'get out of my way—who needs you?'
'I'm not OK—you're OK'	'my life is not worth much compared with you'
'I'm not OK—you're not OK'	'life is not worth anything at all—there is no point—nothing works'

Once a position is adopted people tend to collect feelings that are consistent with it; they embark upon a process of accumulating a sort of 'psychological stamp collection'. Psychological position can be changed. A person can understand how he/she got into the position of not feeling OK about self and can decide to do something about it; for example, he/she can decide to emphasize existing OK feelings, look at messages in a different way, start a different 'stamp collection'.

Games

A '*game*' in transactional analysis terms is 'an ongoing series of complementary ulterior transactions progressing to a well-defined predictable outcome' (Berne, 1964). The 'game' tends to be repetitively played and will continue to be so for as long as the outcome, the '*pay-off*', ensues. By playing 'games' the person's favourite psychological 'stamps' are collected. Psychological games are not played for fun; usually someone gets 'put down' or even hurt. Specific elements of a game are:

1 There is ostensibly a series of complementary transactions on a social level.

2 There is an ulterior transaction, that is, the underlying message of the game.

3 There is a pay-off which concludes the game and which is the real reason for playing the game.

People who are playing a game very seldom know that they are doing so. They don't play consciously and they don't recognize what is happening. Games can be played over long periods of time so long as the players observe the rules by responding in the appropriate way. Games can be played from any one of the three ego states: from the *Parent*, if the Parent's games are imitated; from the *Adult*, if they are consciously calculated even though the person may not be fully aware of the needs which the game satisfies; from the *Child*, if they are based on early life experiences and the position the child decided to adopt.

The pay-off for playing a game is different for every individual. Games can be used to avoid solving problems, to provoke attention, to reinforce beliefs about self and others and to avoid people. There are three basic roles in games: *victim*—people who feel continually discredited, helpless or 'put down'; *rescuer*—people who, disguised as helpers, in fact keep other people dependent on them and don't really help them; *persecutor*—people who impose unnecessarily strict rules on behaviour, criticize, enforce rules, make others suffer and remind them of their mistakes. These three roles can be recognized in all sorts of games, and sometimes people switch roles. The victim becomes a persecutor, the rescuer a victim.

A good example of this is the situation in which one person feels helpless and doesn't know what to do (victim) and another offers lots of advice (rescuer) only to become frustrated and resentful when the helpless person continually rejects or criticizes the advice. The victim may switch roles (becomes persecutor: 'Why don't you give me better advice? You just don't understand.') The rescuer may then become victim: ('I was only trying to help you and now you treat me like this . . .')

Berne has described many categories of game. For example, *life games*, a category including games like 'Alcoholic' in which the problem drinker plays a victim role and the spouse may alternately play the roles of persecutor and rescuer. Berne (1964) recounts the example of the female problem drinker who protested when fellow patients said nice things about her during a group therapy session. 'That's not what I want. I want to know what you really think.' She made it clear that she was seeking derogatory comments, went home and told her husband that he must promise to divorce her or have her admitted to hospital if she ever took another drink. He promised to do this and that evening she became intoxicated and was admitted to hospital where staff and patients refused to play the persecutory roles she assigned to them. She returned home where she was assured of someone who was willing to play the role she demanded.

The category of *marital games* includes games like 'Frigid Woman' in which the wife repels her husband's advances and reprimands him (you only want me for sex—you don't really love me—men are all the same). The woman may then become 'forgetful' and walk through the room half-dressed or 'forget' to take a towel into the bathroom so that her husband has to bring it to her. She may become flirtatious with other men at parties and eventually her emboldened spouse will try again, only to be rejected more indignantly; the resultant 'uproar' is the pay-off of the game as both partners may derive a perverse satisfaction from it and sexual intimacy may now be out of the question. The husband, despite his protestations, may be just as afraid of sexual intimacy as his wife and may have carefully chosen his partner to minimize the danger of

overtaxing his fragile sexual boundaries—he can now blame all on his wife.

Consulting room games include 'I'm only trying to help you' in which a mental health care professional has advice rejected and feels bewildered; after all, he followed the 'correct procedure'. Failure is ascribed wholly to the client ('after all I was only trying to help'), and bewilderment at the 'ingratitude' and 'insightlessness' of clients is the pay-off; it prevents feelings of personal inadequacy. Berne (1964) suggests that this game 'is found most commonly and in its most florid form among social workers with a certain type of training'.

Another consulting room game is 'Wooden Leg'. A victim game in which a real or imaginary handicap is used as an excuse to rationalize failure. Some people use their past as an excuse, others their sex (. . . 'I'm a woman' . . .), their age, their education and so on. The game is used to manipulate others into the role of rescuer; to make others feel guilty (the pay-off).

'Psychiatry' is a consulting room game in which mental health workers adopt the stance 'I am a healer—and I have a diploma to prove it' and 'If you don't get better it's your fault'. Patients may reciprocate by absorbing the language of psychiatry and triumphantly demonstrating that they cannot be helped. This usually involves using the Child ego state ('You will never cure me but you will teach me to be a better neurotic' i.e. play a better game of Psychiatry). Berne (1964) points out that people who play 'Psychiatry' 'can do a great deal of good providing they are professionally trained', providing that the petulant Parental ego state ('I know what is best for you—I've been trained in this sort of treatment') is replaced by an Adult position ('I will apply what therapeutic procedures I have learned in the hope that they will be of some benefit').

A variant of 'Psychiatry' is 'Archeology' in which the patient ruminates continually over childhood happenings (prompted by the therapist) thus becoming ineffective in the 'here and now' as all energies are used to consider the 'there and then'. The pay-off here can be that the patient and the therapist do not have to make any attempt to deal constructively with current difficulties.

Another category consists of *good games*, a 'good game' being one whose positive social contribution outweighs the complexity of its motivations and thus contributes both to the well-being of the other players and to the unfolding of the principal player. Examples include 'Cavalier' in which a male takes every opportunity to compliment suitable females on their good qualities, the aim being to create a climate of mutual admiration. Another 'good game' is 'Happy To Help' in which the player is consistently helpful to other people, with some ulterior motive (perhaps penance for past misdeeds or a desire to make friends in order to exploit them later, or simply a quest for prestige).

Terminating games are games in which the person who gives up a game has to learn how to obtain positive strokes and in the beginning that must be a deliberate and planned activity. Giving positive strokes to others, learning to deal realistically with the here and now, being open and honest, all these are ways of being and feeling about yourself that have to be learned. They are all incompatible with playing games. The Adult ego state is needed to break up games by analysing positions and roles and identifying the game that's being played. Adoption of roles (victim, persecutor, rescuer) can lead to persons writing a *life script* for themselves which condemns them to repeat the same series of self-defeating behaviours. *Scripts can be changed* and an effective tool for changing the faulty life script is a *contract*—a contract for change. This involves:
A decision to work on a specific problem
A statement of the precise goal
The possibility of the goal being fulfilled

The Adult ego state is the most appropriate in making a contract; the adult knows what needs to be done and how to get there. Often discomfort or dissatisfaction is the motive for wanting to change. Uncomfortable awareness of recurring problems or areas of lack of fulfilment identify the fact that a problem must be tackled, and that can involve:
Behavioural change (e.g. bad temper, problem drinking)
Attitudinal change (e.g. attitude towards self. It's not enough to concentrate on getting on with other people, you should be able to get on with yourself—enhanced belief in yourself and your potential)

The following factors are important in making a contract for change:
1 Clear statement of a goal (What do I want?)
2 A plan of action (How may I get there? and What will I want or be prepared to do to get there?)
3 A plan for evaluation (How will I know when I have reached the goal?)
4 Awareness of games (What do I do to sabotage myself?)

Some people never manage to solve a problem, never change because they don't take the problem and their own powers seriously enough. Some people spend their time *wishing* for a change, *wanting* to do something but in the meantime waiting for the arrival of the Rescuer (waiting for Sir Galahad or Santa Claus to solve things). Such an attitude will only lead to greater inertia and unhappiness. Change cannot be achieved by outsiders, however well-intentioned; change and personal growth commence within self and others can only act as midwife.

Gestalt therapy—losing our minds and coming to our senses

Gestalt is a German word meaning the 'whole', the entity formed by the particular order of its various parts. Gestalt therapy should not be confused with the gestalt theory of perception which, in essence, states that the whole (perception) is more than equal to the sum of its parts. Gestalt psychological theory predates gestalt therapy by some time and is a separate theoretical area altogether.

Gestalt therapy emphasizes self-awareness and the process of attaining insight through catharsis and was introduced by Fritz and Laura Perls in 1947. Gestalt therapy is particularly effective in helping clients who intellectualize their problems, talking about the problem without attaining any emotional contact with it. The therapist points out any intellectualization, forcing clients to confront their conflicts more directly and bringing them in touch with their emotions. Gestalt therapy has two major aims: assisting the individual to become (a) more self-aware and (b) more self-responsible.

Self-awareness means knowing yourself, becoming familiar with your own emotional patterns and tendencies. With increased self-awareness people can recognize their natural, healthy, spontaneous tendencies, all too often repressed. They can better distinguish between needs and wants, what feels good or bad, what old attitudes and habits are inappropriate or self-defeating and what new learning needs to take place.

Self-responsibility simply means recognizing what you do and whom you are. An increase in self-responsibility leads to people taking responsibility for their lives, considering a wider range of alternatives and learning to make choices that lead to personal growth rather than stagnation or defeat. Blaming other people or the situation or fate are ways in which people do not take responsibility for their lives. Gestalt therapy encourages a process whereby people learn to mobilize their own resources rather than manipulate others to achieve or ensure their well-being.

Important principles include *finishing a gestalt*: a gestalt is a figure that stands out from some background. Our psychosocial background is a complex and ever-changing whirl of experiences, events, feelings, thoughts, emotions and sense perceptions which compete for our attention and our interest. Out of this constant flow of energy some gestalt, some experience that is the combination of many individual elements, forms a pattern and captures our interest. Interest persists until some action brings this emerging gestalt to a finish, allowing it to merge into the background and leaving the foreground free for the next relevant gestalt.

Unfinished gestalts linger on to vie for our attention and much energy has to be used to suppress them if efficiency has to be maintained.

Consider a student nurse studying in the library. Her concentration is suddenly impaired as she remembers that she has to phone a friend; two gestalts are now competing for her interest. A man may be angry and mistrustful of women because he never expressed and finished his feelings of anger towards his mother. A woman may feel perpetually anxious because she never confronted the real source of her fear, perhaps a childhood belief that she is unlovable.

Resolving these situations means *finishing unfinished business*, a major aim of gestalt therapy. The person troubled by an unfinished gestalt will not cope effectively with the here and now and must be assisted to confront and finish the troublesome gestalt. Gestalt therapy thus promotes a process of self-discovery with the aim of correcting imbalances and releasing tensions; imbalance is always experienced somewhere within the organism as tension.

Direct experience

Fritz Perls liked to say that gestalt therapy was a way of 'losing your mind and coming to your senses', of dropping stultifying intellectualizations and making emotional contact with self in the here and now. We live in the present. If I am unhappy I am unhappy right now. If I want to be happy I have to develop awareness of how I am maintaining my unhappiness here and now, and then recognize and select the alternatives that will make me feel happier.

Direct experience encourages perception of self as a holistic being. There is no arbitrary separation of body and mind. The mind *is* the body and the body *is* the mind. The totality of the person is emphasized; as much importance is placed on bodily responses as on emotional ones. The troubled individual may have lost contact with his/her feelings—both physical and emotional—and is thus unable to express these feelings. Techniques like role-play and ventilation, usually taking place in a group of eight to ten members, encourage increased sensory and emotional awareness.

One of the most frequent questions a gestalt therapist asks of the person paying attention to himself or herself is 'What are you feeling now?' Feelings are facts and thoughts can be fictions. Although it is acknowledged that there are multiple causative factors that combine to produce the individual's current responses, the understanding of these factors is not believed to alleviate the present problems and they are therefore not explored.

Discharging emotion

When people repress their emotions for all of their lives, their bodies build up tension and take on the physical structure of the emotions they are not allowing themselves to feel or express. People who are angry and don't express it look angry all the time. The same is true for fear, sadness or guilt. Repressed emotion stays in the person's system influencing health, well-being and their relationships with other people. Unfinished business stays unfinished. Gestalt therapy encourages the person to 'unlock' repressed emotions by use of techniques like the 'empty chair' technique wherein the person is invited to imagine a person crucial to the unfinished gestalt in the empty chair and to embark upon an open and honest discussion of feelings towards that person. (Imagine your mother/father/husband/wife/son/daughter in the chair—tell him/her how you feel.)

The person may also be asked to invent a dialogue which personifies the warring parts of his body or mind and to try to bring about agreement between them, completing the gestalt (or wholeness). Dreams are not analysed in gestalt therapy but are rather experienced by acting them out, the individual playing all the parts in the dream. The person repressing troublesome emotions is encouraged to release them and experience them (*be* that feeling).

Double messages

Gestalt therapy encourages increased attention to actions as clues to awareness. Small gestures and non-verbal 'leakage' will often reveal feelings that the individual may not be aware of. People may make affirmative statements while shaking their heads, may verbalize affection while clenching their fists, may profess to feel close to someone but turn away from that person when seated next to him/her.

The medical model approach to psychiatry often does not encourage free emotional expression. Laing (1976) commented that

> 'I've often been asked by residents in hospital to give a patient an injection when there might be some sort of life starting up in him, perhaps a crying or whimpering or yelling or screaming' and 'drugs used in psychiatry are stoppers, not starters'.

Gestalt underlines that emotional expression is often progressive rather than regressive and emotional displays by patients should not simply be suppressed but should be worked with. The opportunities of increased self-awareness following a cathartic experience may be enormous.

Altschul (1980) acknowledges that 'the nurse's role in these newer forms of psychotherapy (gestalt and encounter groups) needs to be investigated'.

Client-centred therapy

Client-centred (non-directive) therapy was introduced by Carl Rogers in the 1950s (it is sometimes referred to as Rogerian therapy). Client-centred therapy is so called by Rogers as he sees a person in therapy not as a 'patient', and the term 'client' 'avoids the connotation that he is sick or the subject of an experiment' (Rogers, 1951). The term 'non-directive' is used to emphasize that the therapist adopts an approach which does not attempt to influence the client directly by giving directions or advice or by using direct questioning. According to Rogers people develop of their own accord, they have their own sources of growth and direction, and can become who they can be if the right conditions are provided, as a tree will grow tall and straight given the appropriate soil and climate. Therapy should provide three enabling conditions which will permit personal growth. These are that the therapist (a) is *genuine* (not authoritarian, defensive or 'professional'), (b) is carefully and accurately *emphatic* (able to enter into the client's frame or reference and understand his/her feelings) and (c) can give *unconditional positive regard* (is warm and accepting of the person, though not either approving or disapproving, i.e. does not impose conditions on her regard and acceptance).

When the client perceives these three characteristics then therapy occurs. According to Rogers these three characteristics are both necessary and sufficient for therapy of any kind. For Rogers (1961) psychotherapy means 'a relationship in which at least one of the parties has the intent of promoting the growth, development, maturity, improved functioning, improved coping with life of the other'.

According to Rogers neurosis arises out of coercive pressures placed on the individual during the socialization process. Parents feel that they know what is best for their children and may (often with the best of intentions) stifle initiative, independence and personal growth. Love and approval may be conditional on the child behaving in a way which accords with the parents' value system, the result being that the child ceases acting in a natural and spontaneous way and instead constructs a false social self to meet parental demands and expectations. Conflict (or incongruence) between what a person is actually feeling but hides, and what he/she feels they ought to do leads to chronic tension, self-doubt, anxiety and despair.

Though accepting that troublesome socialization experiences may produce an inhibited and emotionally stunted adult, this approach emphasizes the here and now.

> 'While it is true that past experience has certainly served to modify the meaning which will be perceived in present experiences, yet there is no behaviour except to meet a present need' and 'Behaviour is not "caused" by something which happened in the past. Present tensions and present needs are the only ones which the organism attempts to reduce or satisfy'.
>
> (*Rogers, 1951*)

The client-centred approach rejects interpretation, direction and 'technique'; 'No approach which relies upon knowledge, upon training, upon the acceptance of something that is *taught* is of any use' (Rogers, 1961). Instead the attitudes and orientation of the therapist are stressed. The therapist should respect the client's right to *self-direction*, should recognize his worth and dignity and should be willing for him to choose his own values. It will be apparent that this approach is heavily *person-centred* and that it completely rejects approaches based on the assumption (implicit or explicit) that clients would be better off if they let the therapist select values, standards and goals.

Rogers (1951) suggests that this approach is adopted most comfortably and effectively by 'individuals who are already striving towards an orientation which stresses the significance and worth of each person' and that it may be difficult for persons who tend to manipulate, dominate or subtly devalue others, though these needs to control and dominate—an obstacle to any form of therapeutic relationship—may be restructured by sensitivity training exercises. Training exercises using video feedback and group discussions of role-plays will do much to increase the student's self-awareness and interpersonal sensitivity.

Though rigid adherence to 'technique' is rejected, it is possible to identify some basic skills which facilitate client-centred interactions. These include *accepting* the client as he is *at this moment* and avoiding any tendency to moralize or make judgemental statements. Would *you* talk freely and confidently to someone who criticized and interrupted with value judgements? Challenging the client will simply make him defensive and resentful and implies the rather improbable belief that the therapist's value system and view of life is superior to anyone else's and could therefore be profitably adopted by clients. *Respect* and *trust* are important components of the therapeutic climate and cannot be demanded. They must be earned. It will be helpful if the therapist trusts not only the client's capacity for self-direction and personal growth but her own capacity to facilitate this growth. Client-centred therapists approach therapy with the deep conviction that this client *can* be aided to bring about positive personal change and *can* be trusted to take responsibility for his/her own life. Without basic respect for the client as a person, this climate of trust will not develop and therapy is likely to become just another consulting room game.

Empathy is the ability to see life through another person's eyes and is probably the most important factor in any therapeutic situation. Rogers writes of empathy 'It is about me as I try to perceive his experience and the meaning and the feeling and the taste and the flavour that it has for him' (Rogers, 1961). The empathic approach involves an attempt to adopt the client's frame of reference, to 'get inside his head'. Empathy does not mean that objectivity is abandoned and it should not be confused with sympathy which simply recognizes distress but makes no attempt to constructively deal with it.

Tschudin (1982) invites the reader to imagine the person who has fallen into a (psychological) ditch:

'The *sympathetic* helper goes and lies in the ditch with him and bewails the situation with him. The *unsympathetic* helper stands on the bank and shouts to the victim "come on, get yourself out of that ditch". The *emphatic* helper climbs down to the victim but keeps one foot on the bank thus being able to help the victim out of the trouble on to firm ground again.'

Ellis (1962) has emphasized the importance of objectivity: 'To provide constructive help to others is very different from becoming terribly upset for them or over them, and thereby hoping that this will magically improve matters'. Empathy means involvement but a careful, alert, calm and collected involvement.

Silence may be difficult for the budding therapist to handle. Many nurses feel that they should 'keep things going' or 'keep things moving along'. Clients need, and should be permitted, periods of silence. A reflective silence may be more productive of self-awareness than an artificially sustained dialogue. Clients need time to gather their thoughts; self-disclosure can be emotionally exhausting. Inability to handle silences is a common problem for the beginner and many students are astonished by their tendency to 'force things along' as evidenced by video feedback. The student role-playing the client will often confirm that the therapist who feels obliged to set a remorseless pace (often unconsciously) creates feelings of tension and does not permit the essential periods of reflection. Sometimes holding a hand or putting an arm around a shoulder can be a more effective message than the most elaborate verbalization.

Clarifying means helping the client to get his thoughts and feelings into focus. Often a jumbled mixture of images and ideas will be expressed and it is then helpful for the therapist to gently interject, perhaps saying something like 'Are you telling me that . . .' or 'I get the impression that you feel that you should . . .'. Vague statements should be clarified (for the benefit of both therapist and client) by saying 'Can you be more specific about that?' or 'I'm not quite sure that I know what you mean by that'.

Reflecting is one of the most basic skills of client-centred therapy and occurs when the therapist acts as a mirror to reflect back important attitudes and feelings, thus enabling the client to see himself more clearly.

'The counsellor is not telling the person what to do. He is not injecting his own words or opinions or feelings into the interview. He is picking up the other person's words and feelings and is using them to help the troubled person explore and express his feelings further'

(*Burton, 1979*)

The client may have reduced awareness of the intensity with which certain areas are discussed by him. Reflection can develop awareness of this: 'You seem angry when you talk about your son' or 'You seem sad when you mention your father' or 'I notice that you clench your fists when you talk about your husband'. Reflection involves picking up both verbal and non-verbal communications and offering these back to the client for further consideration. 'You tell me that you loved your mother yet you smile when you talk about her death', 'You seem to mention your father a lot, could we talk about him further?' 'I notice that you seem to tense up when you talk about your fiancé, would you like to discuss your feelings for him?' Significant words or phrases can be reflected: 'You say that "in a way" you were sorry to lose your job', 'You say that "for the most part" you loved your mother?'

Questions may also be reflected back to the client. For example, Client: 'Am I any better since I came into hospital?' Nurse: 'Do you feel any better since you came into hospital?' Or, Client: 'Why doesn't my father love me?' Nurse: 'Why do you feel that your father doesn't love you?' Or, Client: 'How will treatment help me?' Nurse: 'How would you like treatment to help you?'

Giving direct answers to questions of this sort blunts the movement towards personal growth, and question reflection will encourage the client to actively consider his difficulties and to consider ways of dealing with them. Remember that clients will often expect you to have 'all the answers' and often want simple 'cut and dried' solutions, which do not exist. There may be a great temptation to offer directions and advice but to do so fosters dependent transference and may result in the nurses playing a rescuer role.

Active listening is essential if clarifying and reflection are to take place and is a skill which must be practised. The active listener is not simply listening attentively but is inwardly sorting out themes, noting verbal (and non-verbal) expressions of feeling, seeking clarifications, noting incongruence and identifying material for reflection.

Useful exercises include the following: (a) pair yourself with a fellow student (A) and ask him/her to talk for 3–4 minutes and then summarize what has been said, asking (A) to point out areas of omission or key statements which he/she feels you failed to respond to. Then change places and repeat the exercise; (b) in pairs, take turns in assuming the roles of client and therapist in a simulated interaction (*co-counselling*). This will sharpen up sensitivity, awareness and listening skills. Give one another feedback. Tell your partner how their approach made you feel. Did you feel relaxed? Cautious? Trusting and trusted? Apprehensive? Angry? Accepted? Rejected? Would you feel like continuing a discussion like this? If so, why? If not, why not? What made you feel comfortable? Did anything make you feel uncomfortable? Learn from one another and learn to improvise and adapt until you arrive at a style which is comfortable for you and is perceived as congruent by the 'client'; (c) once you have revised your style, seek feedback from a larger group of your fellow students by repeating a role-play in front of them; (d) use video feedback to study your responses. Are your verbal responses congruent with your non-verbal responses? Or do they contradict them? Do you adopt a relaxed and non-threatening posture? Do you use non-verbal cues effectively to prompt and reinforce? (nods, smiles, grunts) Do you permit silences and changes of direction?

Remember that active listening does not just note what is *said*. 'The reality of the other person is not in what he reveals to you. Therefore if you would understand him, listen not to what he says but rather to what he does not say.' (Gibran, 1954)

The psyche contains many compartments or rooms. The doors to some are left open as the contents are not threatening to self and can therefore be inspected by anyone. Other doors are closed and the client cannot or will not open them because to reveal the contents would produce feelings of threat, shame, fear or vulnerability. Client-centred therapy does not attempt to break down these doors by direct questioning nor does it try to pick their locks by manipulation or interpretation. Rather it aims to produce a climate in which the client develops increased awareness of these locked areas and feels free, or able, to open them of his or her own free will.

The process of therapy

Rogers (1961) describes seven stages in the process of therapy:

First stage. Unwillingness to communicate; self-communication is about externals. Feelings, personal meanings and problems are neither recognized nor owned. There is no desire to change ('I am *not* an alcoholic', 'I could give up drugs any time if I really wanted', 'there is nothing wrong with me').

Second stage. Expression begins to flow in regard to non-self topics. Problems are perceived external to self and there is no sense of personal responsibility. Feelings are described as unowned or as past objects.

Third stage. Freer expression of feelings about self. Self seen as primarily existing in others ('I have my father's bad temper', 'my wife makes me angry', 'I wish I had more of my mother's characteristics').

Fourth stage. The 'loosening' stage; feelings are described as objects in the present though there is little open acceptance of feelings. ('I feel rather hopeless', 'I feel stupid/angry/bitter/frightened.') There is now some tendency to approach disturbing feelings.

Fifth stage. Feelings are expressed *freely* as in the present and are now very close to being fully experienced. Emotional discharges may occur but there is surprise and fright, rarely pleasure, at the feelings which 'bubble through'. There is increasing ownership of self-feelings.

Sixth stage. Feelings are experienced with full immediacy and flow to their full results. Feelings are now experienced with richness and acceptance and physiological loosening accompanies the psychological loosening (sadness is accompanied by tears, happiness by laughter). In this stage there are no longer 'problems', external or internal. The client is living subjectively a phase of his problem; it is not an object external to self and divorced from feelings.

Seventh stage. There is now a basic trust in the process of change. Personal constructs are tentatively reformulated, to be validated against further experience. Communication with self is now clear and occurs effectively. There is now an awareness of new ways of being. The client has changed but, more significantly, he has become 'an integrated process of changingness'. (Rogers, 1961).

Psychodrama

Psychodrama was introduced by Moreno in 1921 and is a form of unscripted role-play in which the patient is invited to enact his/her difficulties before an audience of fellow patients who provide commentary and suggest alternative interpretations. The actor patient (the protagonist) may recruit fellow patients to act as auxiliary egos, significant persons from the protagonist's life, and the therapist acts as director. Psychodrama encourages awareness through dramatization; in action people can become aware of unsuspected aspects of self. Catharsis and revelation may occur during the psychodrama and this approach can be particularly effective for clients who have difficulty in verbalizing feelings or who have become adept at over-intellectualizing their problems or who have become prone to introspective ruminations which reduce efficiency and stunt personal growth.

Group therapy

Psychotherapy may be effectively offered to a small group of people and indeed the group setting has certain distinct advantages of its own. The group provides feedback and support, and new-found ways of interacting and behaving may be tentatively tried in the group setting. The group offers the challenges of self-revelation but also provides an atmosphere of safety fostered by the support of other group members and the fact that any individual member is not 'in the spotlight' for all of the time. The inhibited and unassertive may learn by simply observing and listening to other members before gathering the confidence to become personally involved: 'I felt able to express what I felt for people in my group more fully than in almost any other situation I've been in' (Lieberman et al, 1973).

Benefits of groups

Groups may bring about positive change in the following areas:
   Self-esteem
   Behaviour
   Perceptions of others
   Self-awareness
   Social skills
   Motivation to tackle problems

Common outcomes also include greater confidence and an increased openness to others. Coping strategies also tend to become active rather than passive; the group experience can make participants more autonomous and self-accepting and studies reveal a growth in warmth and understanding (Pfister, 1975).

Group orientation. This usually reflects the orientation of the group conductor. Varying treatment philosophies have been translated into group practice, including psychoanalysis and other interpretive approaches, transactional analysis, gestalt therapy, client-centred therapy and behavioural approaches.

Group dynamics. Group dynamics (the processes occurring within groups) can be measured using sociometric techniques.

A useful aid to studying group processes is the *sociogram,* a simple diagram which records interactions. The group members may be represented by their initials, and arrows record the direction of interaction. For example:

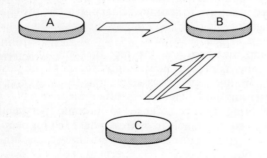

(A has spoken to B who has not replied but has engaged C in conversation. A and C have not interacted verbally at all.)

Sociograms reveal that every group has its *star* (willing or unwilling) who becomes the focus of the group. The group tends to consult the star on important issues and expects him/her to act as referee and adjudicator in disputes. For example:

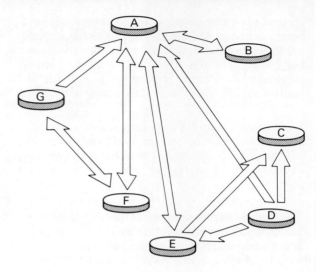

(In this example all but one of the group members have involved A.)

Any group may have its *isolate* who does not participate (C in the example above) or its *reject* who is rejected by the other group members (D in the example above).

Cliques may develop i.e. a small number of members (usually 3 or 4) who do not involve themselves in the main proceedings of the group but chat to one another, becoming a group within a group. Cliques may occasionally launch a concerted attack on another member of the group. The *mutual pair* consists of two group members who ignore the rest of the group but chat cosily to one another. Sociograms may also be used to study interactions within ward populations and to chart changes in these populations brought about by alterations in nursing approach.

Selection of group members. Bloch (1979) suggests that the following common problems can be tackled effectively in a group setting:

Self-image—lack of clear identity, low self-esteem, lack of purpose and direction

Symptomatic—anxiety, depression, poor work or study performance, ineffective coping with stress, disturbed sexual functioning

Emotional—low awareness of feelings, inability to express feelings, poor control over emotions, obsessional traits

Interpersonal functioning—inability to achieve intimacy, discomfort in group situations, specific interpersonal conflicts e.g. marital, parent/child, lack of trust, overly dependent, overly assertive, histrionic

The patient should be motivated to change and be prepared to work voluntarily on the process of change. Patients should not be coerced into joining groups as they will not benefit and may prove to be a disruptive influence. Patients who do poorly in groups include the severely depressed, the acutely disturbed schizophrenic, the paranoid personality and the very hypochondriacal.

Group contracts. A written contract may be signed by each group member to establish the framework within which the group will operate. Contracts usually include the following points:

Consumption of alcohol or unprescribed drugs before meetings is forbidden

Destructive attacks on fellow members are forbidden, though constructive criticism is permitted

No late-coming to meetings

Any absences to be covered by a medical certificate

Group proceedings to be absolutely confidential

Composition. Groups may be *homogeneous*, i.e. consist of patients with similar problems and are relatively easy to form as they have basically similar goals for all their members. *Heterogeneous* groups consist of patients with a mixture of problems.

Number. Sociometric studies suggest that ideally the group should have 7 or 8 members with a conductor and perhaps one co-conductor. If the number drops to 5 or less, the group climate becomes too intimate and searching and awkward silences become frequent. Groups consisting of more than eight members may prevent individuals obtaining sufficient time to work on their problems. Success has been claimed for very large groups (20–30) but these numbers involve the risk of the group degenerating into a disorderly public meeting.

Potential problems. These include the emergence of a reject or an isolate. Remember that anything happening in a group can be used as a learning experience if the issue is reflected back to the group for consideration and discussion: 'I notice that everyone seems to be ignoring John today, can we talk about this?' In the case of the isolate there is no substitute for simply asking the person concerned why they are not participating; try not to make this sound like a reprimand—invite discussion. In the case of the timid or hesitant group member, reinforce any verbal contributions made: 'John made a good point there', or 'can we discuss John's point a little further?'

Don't worry unduly about group members who say little but follow group proceedings closely. Positive change is often associated with the degree of emotional response made rather than the frequency of verbalizations. Group members may learn by observing others' experiences. Bandura (1973) demonstrated that subjects seeing a person rewarded for being aggressive are more liable to behave aggressively in similar situations themselves, while those seeing aggression attracting negative consequences were less likely to behave aggressively. Carlson (1984) points out that people have a strong tendency to acquire conditioned responses themselves by observing them being elicited in other people by the conditional stimulus. The seemingly uninvolved member may thus be undergoing powerful learning experiences.

Sensitivity to non-verbal cues is essential in the group leader and may be used to gently involve members: 'You seem amused/cynical/angry/disturbed/happy about that, John?' The 'star' is not always a problem. 'Can we talk about why everyone seems to expect John to provide answers for them?' 'Why do you think you tend to turn to John for answers?' 'Can you think of any characteristics attracting you to John?' 'Does John remind you of someone you once knew?' 'John, how do you feel about all this?'

Cliques and mutual pairs should be re-seated at a distance and reminded, gently, of the common objectives of the group. The group may focus resentment or hostility on a scapegoat and again the conductor should point out any blatant transference or displacement and invite discussion of this.

Don't be afraid of emotional discharges—groups often facilitate cathartic experiences. It is important that the group member is protected during the cathartic experience and that he/she learns from it afterwards.

Evaluating outcomes. Reduction of troublesome interpersonal problems may occur quite quickly, self-esteem may increase and interpersonal functioning may become smoother and more confident.

The group may vote to terminate as members feel that they have achieved their personal goals and want to try out new skills in the wider social setting. Try not to define expected outcomes too narrowly. Whitaker (1975) says of group evaluation: 'One always hopes to work at what is the frontier for each person, facilitating what is for him the next possible step . . . one's goals, or better, expectations, may continually change as the frontier changes'.

Music therapy. Music may facilitate emotional release and studies have demonstrated that the music of Tchaikovsky, Schubert and Chopin were effective in this respect (Mitchell and Zanker, 1984). Music may also have an antidepressant effect and one study (of 74 people) claimed that Mozart, Wagner, Bach and Beethoven were most effective in this respect. Of the 33 people receiving antidepressants, 27 claimed that music was more effective (O'Donnell, 1974). Music may be used as part of group therapy or, with art therapy, may constitute a medium enabling patients to project or focus their feelings and thoughts.

Behaviour therapy. This consists of a battery of approaches directed at the modification of troublesome behaviours. Symptoms are regarded as the problem rather than underlying psychic disturbances, and behaviour therapy involves setting specific treatment goals and evaluation of outcomes in objective terms. The range of interventions includes many which may usefully be adopted by the nurse. The behavioural approach is discussed in the next chapter.

Psychotherapy and the nurse

In 1956 the Expert Committee on Psychiatric Nursing of the World Health Organization emphasized that hospitalization should provide 'experiences in living' for the patient 'which will enable him to establish relationships that are less anxiety evoking and more comfortable, thereby making the prospect of further relationships less forbidding' (World Health Organization, 1956). This committee saw the nurse as playing a central role in the provision of 'therapeutic experiences' and three aspects of the nurse's role were isolated: the technical, social and interpersonal, the latter being described as 'the essential part of her task'.

In 1968 Clark reported that 'the psychotherapeutic value of the psychiatric nurse is not fully recognized at present and in future nursing staff will be required to play a more active part in therapy and should be prepared accordingly'. In 1975 Towell wrote of 'increasing emphasis on the personal relationships aspect of the nurse's role' though there was little evidence of changing treatment philosophies having any impact on nurse training curricula.

The contrasting American situation was described by Peplau in 1972:

'Clinical expertness (in psychiatric nursing) revolves around the field's unique aspect or emphasis, in this case the role of counsellor or psychotherapist . . . I wish to pinpoint why other aspects of the work in a psychiatric unit are not the central focus of psychiatric nursing . . . depth counselling such as might be employed by a psychiatric nurse specialist is seen to be the focal task of the nurse.'

Acceptance of the psychotherapeutic role of the nurse has been less widespread in the UK where curricula have tended to centre around traditional 'medical models' of care, stifling the emergent role of the psychiatric nurse.

Altschul (1972) commented that nurse/patient relationships might become more therapeutic 'if nurses felt free to discuss their relationships with patients without feeling they were contravening regulations or exposing themselves to condemnation'. She adds that 'not all psychiatrists may include a belief that nurse–patient relationships are relevant to treatment'. Some psychiatrists may see the nurse who attempts to adopt a psychotherapeutic approach as an 'amateur psychiatrist' rather than as a professional maximizing on the unique opportunities for sustained interactions with patients provided by her role. Laing (1985) can, alarmingly, still recount a conversation he had with a charge nurse (in 1984) in which the charge nurse commented: 'We don't hold much with talking to patients in this ward. Our main objective is to break the cycle of madness and get them out.' Laing himself, when working for his first university appointment, was warned by his professor not to get 'too close' to his patients and a later audience of senior psychiatric staff asked him in disbelief: 'Dr Laing, I am told that you allow your schizophrenic patients to talk to you.' (Laing, 1985) Rigid interpretations of the medical model may reduce the status of patients to that of 'things' to be controlled by a custodial nursing staff.

Despite these constraints, therapeutic development of the nurse's role continues. Quinn (1985) describes the trend towards psychotherapeutic development of the nurse's role as being 'too far gone to be reversible', adds that 'the trend towards nurses practising psychotherapy can no longer be ignored', and describes nurses as 'the new psychotherapists'.

Though therapeutic interventions by the nurse should focus on the 'here and now' rather than the 'there and then' of analytical approaches, an increasing number of nurses are undertaking post-registration courses which will enable them to interpret effectively. The patient may often wish to discuss the 'there and then' and the nurse should work with any material offered by the patient. She should simply avoid actively excavating for the 'there and then' until the appropriate specialist post-registration course has been taken.

Peplau uses the terms 'counselling' and 'psychotherapy' interchangeably, as do many writers on this area. Rogers (1942) writes that

> 'these terms (counselling and psychotherapy) will be used interchangeably because they refer to the same basic method—a series of direct contacts with the individual which aims to offer him assistance in changing his attitudes and behaviour', while Perez (1965) concludes that 'A sampling of definitions found in the relevant literature would seem to indicate that counselling and psychotherapy are pretty much the same process.'

Though all interactions aimed at bringing about change or resolving problems have obvious factors in common there are equally obvious areas of difference between approaches. The term counselling is perhaps best reserved for interventions which focus on rational conscious factors, while psychotherapy best describes interventions aimed at affective or unconscious factors, a viewpoint adopted by Bordin (1955) and Mowrer (1951).

In practice psychotherapeutic interventions may be subdivided into supportive (here and now) and interpretive (there and then) approaches, though there may be some overlap between counselling and psychotherapy and 'here and now' and 'there and then' as the focus of any interaction changes.

The 'cut-off' line A indicates the limit which should not be passed by the nurse without appropriate specialist training, and the shaded area B indicates material from the 'there and then' which may emerge during a supportive interaction. Though the impulse to analyse or interpret such material should be resisted by the novice, the nurse should not suppress discussion of it; such discussion may lead to cathartic experiences and/or increased self-awareness. Traditional reliance on chemotherapy shows signs of faltering; concern is being expressed about the addictive nature of widely used anxiolytics and there is concern about the long-term effects on the central nervous system of phenothiazines.

The need for a critical re-evaluation of the psychotherapeutic role of the nurse has never been greater.

Key Concepts

1 Psychiatric treatment acquired a scientific direction with Freud's introduction of psychoanalysis, with its emphasis on *free association* and working with *transference relationships*.
2 Psychoanalysis is an example of an *interpretive* approach.
3 Adler founded the school of *individual psychology* which emphasizes attempts to bring about healthy changes in lifestyle
4 Jung introduced *analytical psychology* which emphasizes striving for *individuation*.
5 These early non-physical (psychotherapeutic) approaches were accompanied by advances in physical methods of treatment (electroplexy and chemotherapy).
6 Perls introduced gestalt therapy which emphasizes 'here and now' realities and sensory awareness, and identifies 'unfinished gestalts'.
7 Rogers introduced *client-centred* (non-directive) therapy which takes the client's view of the world as the starting point and aims to promote personal growth.

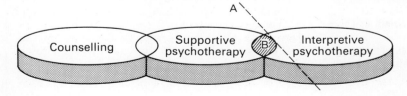

8 Berne introduced *transactional analysis* which focusses on events between people rather than events within them.
9 Transactional analysis uses the concepts of *ego-states, transactions, psychological position* and *games*.
10 These approaches may be used in either individual or group settings.

References

Altschul, A. (1972) Patient–nurse interaction. *University of Edinburgh Dept of Nursing Studies. Monograph No. 3.*

Altschul, A. (1980) Hints of maintaining patient–nurse interaction. *Nursing Times*, **76**(15): 650–652.

Avery, D. & Winokur, G. (1976) Mortality in depressed patients treated with ECT and antidepressants. *Archives of General Psychiatry*, **33**: 1029.

Babcock, D. (1978) Transactional analysis. In Backer, B. A. et al (Eds) *Psychiatric/Mental Health Nursing Contemporary Readings*. Berks: Van Nostrand Reinhold.

Balasubramaniam, V., Kanaka, T. S. & Ramamurthi, B. (1970) Surgical treatment of hyperkinetic and Behaviour Disorders. *International Surgery*, **54**: 18–23.

Bandura, A. (1973) *Aggression: A Social Learning Analysis*. Herts: Prentice-Hall.

Berne, E. (1964) *Games People Play*. Harmondsworth: Penguin Books.

Berrios, G. (1983) The convulsive therapies. In Berrios, G. E. & Dowson, J. H. (Eds). *Treatment and Management in Adult Psychiatry*. London: Baillière Tindall.

Blachly, P. (1976) MMECT. *Convulsive Therapy Bulletin*. July: p. 25.

Blachly, P. & Gowing, D. (1966) Multiple monitored electro-convulsive treatment. *Comprehensive Psychiatry*, **7**: 100–109.

Bloch, S. (1979) Group Psychotherapy. In Bloch, S. (Ed) *An Introduction to the Psychotherapies*. Oxford: Oxford University Press.

Bordin, E. (1955) Psychological Counselling. New York: Appleton-Century-Crofts.

Breggin, P. (1972) The return of lobotomy and psychosurgery. *Congressional Record*, **118**: E 1603–E 1612 (February 24).

Brill, N. Q. et al (1959) Relative effectiveness of various components of electro-convulsive therapy. *Archives of Neurological Psychiatry*, **81**: 627–635.

Burton, G. (1979) *Interpersonal Relations*. London: Tavistock Publications.

Cameron, D. (1960) Production of differential amnesia as a factor in the treatment of schizophrenia. *Comprehensive Psychiatry*, **1**: 26–34.

Carlson, N. (1984) *Psychology*. London: Allyn & Bacon.

Clare, A. (1976) *Psychiatry in Dissent*. London: Tavistock Publications.

Central Health Services Council (1968) Joint subcommittee of the standing mental health and the standing nursing advisory committees. *Psychiatric Nursing Today and Tomorrow*. London: HMSO.

Clark, (1968) *Psychiatric Nursing Today and Tomorrow*. London: HMSO.

Ellis, A. (1962) *Reason and Emotion in Psychotherapy*. New Jersey: Lyle & Stuart.

Evans, H. (1983) Psychosurgery. In Berrios, G. & Dowson, J. H. (Eds) *Treatment and Management in Adult Psychiatry*. London: Baillière Tindall.

Foucault, M. (1967) *Madness and Civilisation*. London: Tavistock Publications.

Freeman, W. (1971) Frontal lobotomy in early schizophrenia: long follow up in 415 cases. *British Journal of Psychiatry*, **114**: 1223–1246.

Gibran, K. (1954) *Sand and Foam*. London: William Heinemann.

Harris (1973) *I'm OK—You're OK*. London: Pan Books.

Henderson, D. & Batchelor, I. (1962) *Henderson and Gillespie's Textbook of Psychiatry*, 9th edn. Oxford: Oxford University Press.

Jones, W. (1983) *Ministering to Minds Diseased—A History of Psychiatric Treatment*. London: William Heinemann.

Jones, K. & Fowles, A. (1984) *Ideas on Institutions—Analysing the Literature on Long-Term Care and Custody*. London: Routledge & Kegan Paul.

Kennedy, C. & Anchel, D. (1948) Regressive electric-shock in schizophrenics refractory to other shock therapies. *Psychiatric Quarterly*, **22**: 317–320.

Laing, R. (1964) *The Divided Self*. Harmondsworth: Pelican.

Laing, R. (1976) *The Facts of Life*. Harmondsworth: Penguin Books.

Laing, R. (1985) *Wisdom, Madness and Folly—The Making of a Psychiatrist*. London: Macmillan.

Lieberman, M., Yalom, I. & Miles, M. (1973) *Encounter Groups: First Facts*. New York: Basic Books.

Medical Research Council (1965) Report by clinical psychiatry committee. *British Medical Journal*, **1**: 881.

Mitchell, S. & Zanker, A. (1984) The use of music in group therapy. *Journal of Mental Science*, **94**: 737.

Mowrer, O. (1951) Concepts and Programs of Counselling. Minnesota: University of Minnesota Press.

Narabayashi et al (1966) Long range results of stereotaxic amygdalotomy for Behaviour Disorders. *Confinia Neurologia*, **27**: 168–171.

O'Donnell, M. (1974) Editorial. An era of tranquillity. *World Medicine*, **9**: 5.

Parry-Jones, W. (1983) The development of the psychotherapies. In Weller, M. (Ed) *The Scientific Basis of Psychiatry*. London: Baillière Tindall.

Peplau, H. (1972) Interpersonal techniques—the crux of

psychiatric nursing. *American Journal of Nursing*, **62**: 50–54.

Perez, J. (1965) Counselling. Theory and Practice. Massachusetts: Addison-Wesley.

Pfister, G. (1975) Outcome of laboratory training for police officers. *Journal of Social Issues*, **31**: 115–121.

Quinn, P. (1985) The new psychotherapists. *Nursing Times*, **81**(24): 28–30. (June 12).

Robins, A. (1958) A retrospective controlled study of leucotomy in schizophrenia and affective disorders. *Journal of Mental Science*, **104**: 1025–1037.

Rogers, C. (1942) Counselling and Psychotherapy. Boston: Houghton Mifflin.

Rogers, C. (1951) *Client-Centred Therapy—Its Current Practice, Implications and Theory*. London: Constable.

Rogers, C. (1961) *On Becoming a Person—A Therapist's View of Psychotherapy*. London: Constable.

Roth, M. (1983) Management of depression and mania in clinical practice. In Berrios, G. & Dowson, J. H. (Eds) *Treatment and Management in Adult Psychiatry*. London: Baillière Tindall.

Royal College of Psychiatrists (1981) ECT—report.

Sargant, W. & Slater, E. (1972) *An Introduction to Physical Methods of Treatment in Psychiatry, 5th edn*. Edinburgh: Churchill Livingstone.

Schurr, P. (1973) Psychosurgery. *British Journal of Hospital Medicine*, **10**(1): 53–60.

Seymer, L. (1956) *A General History of Nursing*. New Zealand: Faber.

Spitz, R. & Wolf, K. (1946) Anaclitic depression. In *Psychoanalytic Study of the Child*. New York: International Universities Press.

Summers, W. K., Robins, E. & Reich, T. (1979) The natural history of acute organic mental syndrome after bilateral ECT. *Biological Psychiatry*, **14**(6): 905–912.

Szasz, T. (1973) *The Manufacture of Madness*. London: Paladin.

Towell, D. (1975) *Understanding Psychiatric Nursing*. London: Royal College of Nursing.

Tschudin, V. (1982) *Counselling Skills for Nurses*. London: Bailliére Tindall.

Weeks, D., Freeman, C. P. & Kendell, R. E. (1980) ECT—enduring cognitive deficits? *British Journal of Psychiatry*, **137**: 26–37.

Whitaker, D. (1975) Group psychotherapy. In Bannister, D. (Ed) *Issues and Approaches in the Psychological Therapies*. Chichester: John Wiley & Sons.

World Health Organization (1956) *Report of the Expert Committee on Psychiatric Nursing*.

II

THE NURSING ENVIRONMENT

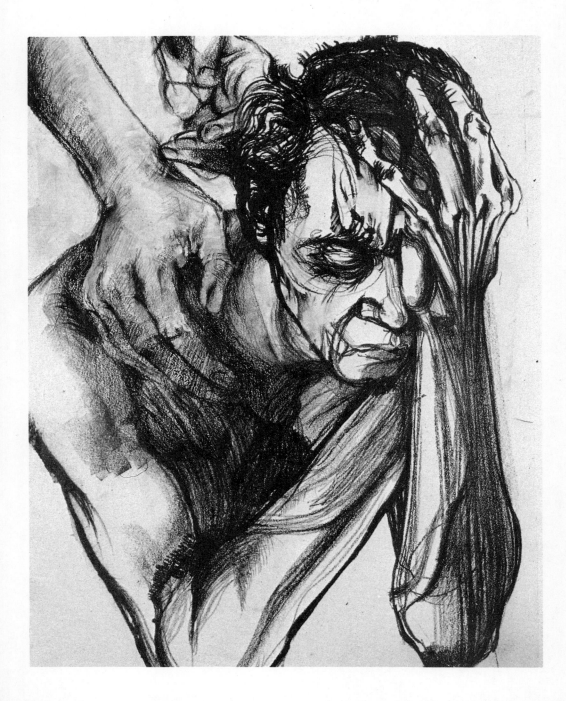

7

The Hospital Environment

> The main function of the hospital is that it should do the patient no harm.
>
> *Florence Nightingale.*

Hospitals are a regular feature of our urban landscapes. Islands of antiseptic calm and efficiency in an otherwise clamorous landscape which are often uncritically viewed as citadels of therapeutic wisdom, to the garrisons of whom we gratefully yield our pain-racked or malfunctioning bodies in order that the assaults of illness may be combated, and well-being restored.

The experience of physical illness requires certain accommodations of the patient. The white-uniformed hospital staff know what is best and autonomy must be surrendered to a great extent for the duration of hospitalization. The clinical judgements of the staff prevail and much adjustment in habits and activities of daily living may be required for the duration of hospitalization, and sometimes afterwards. These life adjustments tend to be accepted relatively uncritically as the recipients of care and treatment tend to behave as the title of their new role suggests—patients tend to be remarkably patient.

For most people hospitalization is a relatively short and positive experience—suffering has been reduced or function restored. On return to the community the ex-patient may usually resume former roles and activities and may enjoy recounting little anecdotes about the period of hospitalization to a family relieved at the return of a now stronger family member.

Psychiatric hospitals, and the patient experience offered by them, tend to differ radically from the world of the general hospital, though not necessarily in a negative way (Table 10).

Table 10 Psychiatric and general hospitalization contrasted.

	General hospital	Psychiatric hospital
Hospitalization	Of relatively short duration	Tends to be longer
Patient's attitude to hospitalization	Tends to be positive	May be negative or mixed
Staff attitudes towards patients	Patients are psychosocially equal	Patients may be socially 'distanced' from staff
Emphasis of nursing care and subculture	Physical—absent or impermanent	Psychological and social—may be fixed and highly organized
Patient's awareness of disorder and treatment	Relatively good	Relatively poor
Treatment	Usually curative	Usually palliative
Contact with community	Usually well maintained	May be atrophied or absent
Self-esteem	Usually little affected	Usually negatively affected
Stigma	Usually little or none (social identity 'unspoiled')	Almost invariably present (social identity 'spoiled')
Nature of nursing interventions	Restitutive	May be covertly or overtly retributive
Adjustment required of patient	Usually temporary and usually positively accepted	May be total (long-stay patients) and negatively received—'secondary deviance' probable 'secondary' adjustment necessary'

The buildings often differ dramatically from the modern general hospital, which now tends to be a concrete and glass tower placed in an urban core. Large psychiatric hospitals tend to be situated in the countryside, as our forefathers pursued a policy of segregating the mentally disordered from the general population, though many towns and cities have now sprawled outwards to enclose their mental hospitals, extruding concrete pseudopodia to engulf Victorian anachronisms in an embrace of motorways and high-rise flats.

Most of our large mental hospitals were built during the latter half of the nineteenth century, and they were built to last.

'There they stand', said Enoch Powell when he was Minister of Health, 'isolated, majestic, imperious, brooded over by the gigantic water-tower and chimney combined, rising unmistakeable and daunting out of the countryside—the asylums which our forefathers built with such immense solidity to express the notions of their day.'

The Victorians produced a morality as severe and uncompromising as much of their architecture. The mentally disordered were housed in asylums—places of safety—in which the philosophy was one of 'moral management'. Patients were encouraged to develop awareness of good and evil, of right and wrong behaviour, supervised by a sternly paternalistic staff who discouraged excesses of any sort and urged patients onto the path of social righteousness. The regime was one of work, plain food and conformity, in the apparent hope that healthy bodies would produce healthy minds. Physical, psychological and social restraint was freely employed and the staff always had a comforting awareness that the 'unimproved' patient was at least safely segregated in a setting where he could not offend the sensibilities of society.

The inmates of Victorian asylums were largely poor people who were expected to display suitable gratitude for the care and shelter provided. Social distance between staff and patients was great and a faint aroma of moral censure hung like a pall over the attitudes of the staff.

To be 'put away' in such an asylum carried strong overtones of moral condemnation and the likelihood of anyone re-emerging to resume his or her former place in society with an intact social identity was remote.

Thus the public view of the mental hospital and its inmates received a negative bias, which is far from dead today. Many people still unfortunately attach considerable stigma to the concept of mental disorder and entertain vague suspicions that the experience of mental disorder implies social and moral weakness which is liable to endure. Nervous jokes about the 'loony-bin' are still current and beliefs about the psychiatric hospital are still haunted by the spectres of fear and irrational prejudice.

The media have enthusiastically capitalized on public fear, credulity and superstition and have contributed in no small way to a negative 'mythology of madness' which has perpetuated destructive and absurd stereotypes about mental disorder.

Cinema coverage has no doubt implanted the lingering suspicion in many people that anyone with a history of mental disorder is at heart a mother-fixated homicidal maniac with a propensity for disturbing the ablutions of guests, armed with a carving knife.

Media documentary coverage in the seventies and eighties has, in the main, been more responsible and it is to be hoped that generations nurtured on more factual accounts of mental disorder will discard the prejudices of the parental generation.

The modern psychiatric hospital has evolved dramatically from its Victorian ancestors. Scientific psychiatry has long since succeeded moral management, and public awareness of the realities of mental disorder is now much higher, though public education still has a long way to go.

The person with mental disorder may be treated in a variety of settings. The general practitioner now treats the majority of mental disorders as the range of effective psychotropic drugs increases steadily. Out-patient clinics and community organizations offer a wide range of therapeutic facilities and the growth of support organizations in the community mushrooms encouragingly. Most general hospitals have a department of psychiatry which offers a wide range of in-patient and out-patient facilities, and psychiatric clinics offering a range of services for specific problems abound (drug or alcohol abuse, psychosexual disorders, child and family psychiatry, post-natal depression, phobias, etc.).

There is still a need for the provision of continuing care facilities for psychiatric in-patients and this facility tends to be offered within the large Victorian hospitals referred to, though the number of in-patients receiving treatment in such a setting has decreased steadily over the last decade. The avowed intention of successive governments of running down the large institutions in favour of a policy of community care has proceeded slowly and erratically. Mental health still tends to be the Cinderella of the health services.

This lack of progress is concerning for two reasons: (a) there is a 'better way of doing it' than institutional care and (b) institutional living has long been recognized to have deleterious effects on the inmate, whether the institution is a hospital, convent, prison or orphanage.

Long-term institutional care may lead to apathy, dehumanization and passive dependence on the institution which, in cumulation, renders the patient unable to resume his former place in society and may thus be considerably more damaging than the disorder leading to hospitalization in the first place. This phenomenon has been noted with alarm by a succession of observers who have recorded their concern in a body of literature which is now considerable.

Mental Bed Sores

Myerson (1939) claimed that institutional living produced a 'prison stupor' in schizophrenic patients, an assertion which was indignantly refuted by many psychiatrists who claimed that the state of passive, incurious apathy described was the end result of the schizophrenia—the patients were simply 'burnt-out schizophrenics'.

As more concerned observers entered the fray it was pointed out that this picture of dehumanization was also apparent in long-term prisoners who could hardly be described as 'burnt-out schizophrenics'.

Bettelheim and Sylvester (1948) used the term 'psychological institutionalism' to describe a similar picture in emotionally disturbed children cared for in an institution, and Martin (1955) used the term 'institutionalization' to describe the loss of volition and individuality apparent in many long-term psychiatric patients.

Russell Barton, an English psychiatrist, produced the important book *Institutional Neurosis* (1959) in which he used this term to describe the constellation of adverse effects of protracted institutional living. These effects he summarized as 'mental bed sores' and he firmly ascribed them to the effects of the institutional regime, commenting that 'It seems unlikely that mental disorders, regardless of their type, produce an end state similar to institutional neurosis. (Barton, 1976)

In 1961 the American sociologist Erving Goffman produced his book *Asylums* in which he dissects the structure of the institution to reveal those forces which may strip the inmate of individuality and lead to social atrophy.

Barton unfortunately attempted to 'medicalize' a social phenomenon as he referred to institutional neurosis' as a 'disease', thus unnaturally forcing the phenomenon into the rigid confines of the 'medical model' rather than handing the problem to social scientists for broader examination (though he does acknowledge Goffman's 'brilliant work' in the preface to the second edition of his book).

In 1962 Peter Townsend produced his book *The Last Refuge* which surveyed homes and residential institutions for the elderly. His description of the conditions he found is worth quoting:

'The day rooms were bleak and uninviting. In one of them sat forty men in high backed Windsor chairs, staring straight ahead, or down at the floor . . . the sun was shining outside but no-one was looking that way . . . Watery eyed and feeble, they looked suspiciously at our troupe of observers, and then returned to their self-imposed contemplation. They wore shapeless tweed suits and carpet slippers or boots. Life seemed to have been drained from them, all but the dregs. Their stoic resignation seemed not only attributable to infirmity and old age. They were like people who had taken so much punishment that they had become inured to pain, and robbed of all initiative.'

(*Townsend, 1962*).

Note that, as Barton does not ascribe similar states in mental hospitals to schizophrenia, Townsend does not attribute the 'loss of life' he observed to old age alone. The apathy he described '. . . seemed not only attributable to infirmity and old age'.

In 1962 Gruenberg writes of the condition, calling it 'social breakdown syndrome' and Vail (1966) summarizes the end result of rigid institutional regimes as 'dehumanization'.

It is not essential that the student learns this plethora of names for the condition produced by protracted institutional living. They are reproduced as they help convey the gist of the condition and chart the increasing concern expressed about the undesired effects of the institution. The term 'institutionalization' will be used from this point as it is less cumbersome than many others, is widely used and does not medicalize a social phenomenon.

The Total Institution

This is a term introduced by Goffman (1961) as part of his attempt to identify those institutional forces and practices which combine to erode individuality and self-esteem.

He defines the 'total institution' as 'a place of residence and work where a large number of like-situated individuals, cut off from the wider society for an appreciable period of time, together lead an enclosed, formally administered round of life' (Goffman, 1961).

Goffman uses the term *total* institution as establishments of this nature *totally* organize the life of their inmates. Those of us living in the community *work, rest* and *play* in different settings and observe different social rules and practices in each setting. Behaviour appropriate to the role of the nurse on a hospital ward may seem highly inappropriate in the pub or at home, and behaviours appropriate to the pub or home may be grossly inappropriate to the ward. The rules are different in each setting and we respond to this by wearing different social 'masks' in each setting.

In the total institution the three life activities of work, rest and play take place under the same roof and are subject to the same rules. The total institution is 'formally administered'; that is, it has many rules and regulations governing the life of the inmates, who play no part in making the rules and have little recourse to changing them.

Consideration of the characteristics of the total institution so far introduced will reveal that a variety of establishments may be so designated (psychiatric hospitals, prisons, orphanages, convents, monasteries, epileptic 'colonies', hospitals and homes for the elderly and the mentally handicapped, tuberculosis sanatoria and hospitals for the young chronic sick).

Goffman suggests that the total institution has four main characteristics. The first is '*batch living*'; that is, a 'large number of like situated individuals' sleep, work, and play under the same roof, and are subject to the same rules.

The second characteristic is '*binary management*'; that is, the existence of a system of psychological and social apartheid:

'there is a basic split between a large managed group, conveniently called inmates, and a small supervisory staff . . . each grouping tends to conceive of the other in terms of narrow, hostile stereotypes, staff often seeing inmates as secretive and untrustworthy, while inmates often see staff as condescending, high-handed and mean . . . social mobility between the two strata is grossly restricted; social distance is great and may be formally prescribed'

(*Goffman, 1961*).

The third characteristic is the '*inmate role*'; that is, the role of 'inmate' supersedes all other roles the individual has been accustomed to play. '*Role dispossession*' strips the inmate of individuality and reduces him to a number, a cypher or a diagnostic 'label'. Before admission a person may have been, for example, married, with young children, may have worked as an electrician and may have gone fishing in his spare time. After admission he no longer lives with his wife, brings up his children, works as an electrician or goes fishing. His roles of husband, father, electrician and angler (to give but a few examples) have gone to be replaced with one all-embracing role—the 'inmate' or 'patient' role.

Our social roles are the salient features of social reality for us. Social reality perishes with them to be replaced with the realities of institutional life.

The fourth characteristic of the total institution is the '*institutional culture*' to which the inmate must adapt as he embarks upon his new 'career' as an inmate or patient. Adaptation tends to take the form of '*secondary adjustments*' which are 'practices which do not directly challenge staff but allow inmates to obtain forbidden satisfactions or to obtain permitted ones by forbidden means' (Goffman, 1961).

There are four types of 'secondary adjustment': (1) the inmate may withdraw, from the painful realities of his new environment (and may then be described as 'regressed' by the staff), (2) he may become rebellious and 'fight the system' (and then be described as 'insightless' or 'uncooperative' by the staff), (3) he may become 'colonized'; that is, he may temporarily pay lip service to the system as he awaits the day of deliverance and independence, and (4) he may become 'converted', accepting the staff's

Table 11 The features of the total institution (Goffman).

Batch living
Binary management
The 'inmate role'
The 'institutional culture'

view of himself and accepting the institutional culture as valid (he may then be described as having gained 'insight' or be approvingly described as that most desirable phenomenon—the 'clean, quiet and cooperative' patient). 'The patient must "insightfully" come to take, or affect to take, the hospital's view of himself.' (Goffman, 1961)

Conventional wisdom has it that if a person goes to prison he will learn a lot of bad habits and suffer great loss of self-esteem. This viewpoint has been developed by Lemert (1967) with his introduction of the concept of *secondary deviance*. Primary deviance consists of the initial act or behaviour which incurs a negative social response (assuming the role of the 'alcoholic', 'junkie' or 'delinquent'). Secondary deviance is the *added* deviant behaviour which is incorporated in the unwritten 'job description' of the person's new role as a deviant. It is a 'means of defence, attack or adaptation to the problems created by the societal reaction to primary deviation' (Lemert, 1967) and involves a major reorganization of concepts about self. Jean Genet (1967), in *The Thief's Journal* said 'I owned to being the coward, traitor, thief and fairy they saw in me'.

The 'patient' (or 'sick') role is, in this sense, a secondary role. It carries low social status, as the person performing it is evaluated as being weak, helpless, dependent and irresponsible or untrustworthy. What other people think of us may, to a large extent, determine what we think of ourselves, and the inmate role may induce the patient to see himself as a social incompetent, and to act accordingly.

Goffman saw psychiatric nurses as the main upholders of the system. They were the key 'culture carriers' of the hospital as they were the principal teachers of the 'patient role'. The nursing staff presided over institutional ceremonies, like the 'stripping' procedures of hospitalization, and actively re-shaped the patient's concept of self (Goffman, 1961), the desired end product being the quiet and docile patient who submissively adheres to hospital routine and does not create 'difficulties' for staff or fellow patients—the easily 'managed' patient.

The world of the patient

In 1973 the psychologist Rosenhan published the memorably entitled paper *On Being Sane in Insane Places*, which recounts the experiences of a group of fake patients ('pseudopatients') admitted to a variety of American psychiatric hospitals. All of the *pseudopatients* were admitted on the basis of allegedly hearing 'voices' and all, save one, were diagnosed as schizophrenic. After admission the 'pseudopatients' ceased to simulate any abnormalities and each was instructed to behave as he 'normally' behaved. Despite their public show of sanity the 'pseudopatients' were never discovered—to the contrary, much of their behaviour was viewed suspiciously by the staff. 'Once a person is designated abnormal, all of his other behaviours and characteristics are coloured by that label. Indeed the label is so powerful that many of the pseudopatients' normal behaviours were overlooked entirely or profoundly misinterpreted.' (Rosenhan, 1973)

Rosenhan gives examples. One pseudopatient asked his physician what kind of medication he was receiving and began to write down the response. 'You needn't write it', he was told gently. 'If you have trouble remembering, just ask me again.' One kindly nurse found a pseudopatient pacing the long hospital corridors. 'Nervous, Mr X?' she asked. 'No, bored', he said. Even writing was seen as pathological. 'Patient engages in writing behaviour' was the daily nursing comment on one of the pseudopatients, who was never questioned about his writing.

Encounters with the medical staff often revealed their reluctance to embark upon any dialogue with the pseudopatients: 'Pardon me Dr X, could you tell me when I am eligible for grounds privileges?' 'Good Morning Dave. How are you today?' (moves off without waiting for a response). Nursing staff rarely enquired into the causes of patients' behaviour but tended to assume that it derived from the patient's pathology: 'never were the staff found to assume that one of themselves or the structure of the hospital had anything to do with a patient's behaviour'.

Ironically the pseudopatients were frequently detected by the patients but never by the staff: 'You're not crazy. You're a journalist, or a professor. You're checking up on the hospital'.

Rosenhan's belief that the bias towards detection of pathology distorted staff perceptions was tested in a follow-up experiment. A research and teaching hospital agreed to take part in a simple sequel, having heard of the earlier findings, but doubted that such an error could occur in their hospital. The staff were informed that during the next three months one or more pseudopatients would attempt to be admitted into the psychiatric hospital. Judgements were obtained on 193 patients who were admitted for psychiatric treatment. Forty one patients were confidently alleged to be pseudopatients by at least one member of staff. Twenty three were considered suspect by at least one psychiatrist. Nineteen were suspected by one psychiatrist *and* one other staff member. No genuine pseudopatients were admitted at all during this period.

Rosenhan comments that 'The fact that the patients often recognised normality when staff did not raises important questions'. He concludes that physicians are more likely to call a healthy person sick than a sick person healthy, as it is 'better to err on the side of caution'.

The teaching of psychiatric nurses may be responsible for imparting a similar bias. Great emphasis is often placed on the negative aspects of behaviour and lengthy lists of signs and symptoms are memorized, to be hopefully applied to patients at the first available opportunity. This bias is often revealed in nursing records where rule-breaking or deviant behaviour is carefully recorded at the expense of records of adaptive behaviour. 'Verbally abusive today'. 'Refused medication this a.m.'. 'Withdrawn and uncooperative'. 'Returned late from pass under the influence of alcohol'. If the psychiatrist functions as judge, jury and social executioner in the custodial institution, the nursing staff often act as a social police force. The importance of maintaining the institutional status quo may produce dangerous blind spots in respect of the patient's individuality and social reality, and may militate against constructive review of hospital policy.

Stanford County Prison

Three psychologists (Haney, Banks and Zimbardo, 1973) from Stanford University constructed a fake prison which yielded more evidence of the effects of institutional life on the individual.

The 'prison' was constructed in a basement corridor and consisted of three small cells, in each of which three volunteer 'prisoners' were detained. The 'prisoners' and the twelve 'guards' were selected from student volunteers, carefully chosen after a battery of tests designed to reveal the most stable and mature subjects.

The findings were that the 'guards' began to act aggressively and insultingly after a few days and some 'went far beyond their roles to engage in creative cruelty and harassment' (Haney et al, 1973)—some even remained on duty for extra hours without pay.

The experiment was terminated early, after six days, because of the 'prisoners'' reactions. Five 'prisoners' had to be released early, four because they suffered from 'extreme emotional depression, crying, rage and acute anxiety', and one because he had developed a psychosomatic rash. The remaining prisoners were delighted when the experiment was ended, though the 'guards' did not want the experiment to end, and were 'reluctant to give it up'.

The experimenters came to the conclusion that 'the extremely pathological reactions which emerged in both groups of subjects testify to the power of the social forces operating'. Gostin (1977) surveys this experiment and concludes that

'Something in the character of a secure institution itself impedes the process of rehabilitation. The typical inmate becomes passive, dependent, depressed, helpless and self deprecatory . . . The Haney study . . . clearly illustrates that it is the secure institution itself, and not the professional staff, which causes many of the problems.'

It is easy to dismiss the Rosenhan and Haney studies as 'contrived' or 'untypical' or simply 'not representative of clinical realities', and many irate critics did. Each study has a sobering postscript however—a study of long-stay 'schizophrenics' in a Wisconsin hospital revealed that a third had no past or present symptoms of the condition (Wing and Brown, 1970), and Milgram's study of obedience to authority involved an experiment in which volunteers continued to press buttons in the belief that they were administering painful and possibly fatal electric shocks to strangers when ordered to do so by an 'authority figure' (Milgram, 1965).

The total institution, and the authority relationships it incorporates, seems to engulf indiscriminately and regurgitate reluctantly, and life in the belly of the institutional 'whale' may be a pallid and dehumanizing one.

Recognizing the institutionalized patient

This is not difficult. Barton wrote of apathy, lack of initiative, loss of interest—especially in things of an impersonal nature, submissiveness, apparent inability to make plans for the future, lack of individuality, and sometimes a characteristically stooped posture and shuffling gait (Barton, 1976). He adds that there is 'a resigned acceptance that things will go on as they are—unchangingly, inevitably and indefinitely'.

The loss of interest applies to events that do not

directly affect the patient. The world outside the institution has lost reality, and even memories of past life in it may be distorted by the fractured self-esteem of the inmate role.

Changes in ward routine may elicit interest or concern, though there is often a singular lack of expressed resentment at unfair staff attitudes or behaviour—submissiveness may become deeply engrained.

In some cases there may be a stooped posture or shuffling gait associated with lack of exercise and prolonged sitting in chairs. One patient said to Barton: 'I'm terrified of being sent where the women walk about with their hands under their aprons with no signs of life in them' (Barton, 1976).

Table 12 The features of institutionalization (after Barton).

Apathy
Lack of initiative
Loss of interest—especially in things of an impersonal nature
Submissiveness
Inability to plan for the future
Lack of individuality
Stooped posture and shuffling gait (minority of cases)
Passive dependence on staff
'Institutional behaviours' ('secondary adjustments')

The patient has handed over the reins of life to hands deemed more capable, and may appear unable to make the simplest decisions—individuality and initiative have been stifled and died. Childlike dependence may be complete.

Factors in the hospital environment productive of institutionalization

The features of the total institution have already been described and many will be found to be present in long-stay wards if the yardstick provided by Goffman is used. Jones and Fowles (1984) say of Goffman: 'What he describes as a "total institution" will probably not fit any real life institution exactly. It is . . . an ideal type against which the practices of real life institutions may be measured'.

Barton carefully delineates those 'practices' which may be examined in an attempt to uncover factors in the hospital environment which may be productive of institutionalization.

The following causative factors are discussed by Barton: (a) *loss of contact with the outside world*, and (b) *enforced idleness*—the patient's day is totally organized for him. He does not decide when to get up in the morning. He does not prepare or cook his breakfast, or decide at what time it will be eaten. Routine governs his every activity. Medication follows breakfast and 'therapy' follows medication; 'therapy' may consist of dull, menial tasks or the sorting out of nuts and bolts etc., sometimes referred to as 'industrial therapy'. Lunch follows at the same time every day and, again, the patient does not select his menu, his eating companions or the place in which he eats. Afternoon 'therapy' may follow, though not all patients will be sent to a therapy department; some are simply abandoned to their own devices between meals, and the evening meal is followed by more medication. The evenings are often spent sitting in an overcrowded 'day room', contemplating a flickering television set through a haze of cigarette smoke before bed time, and the time of retiring may be dictated by the staff.

In such an environment mopping floors or cleaning out lavatories may be referred to as 'therapy', and the weeks, months, seasons and years may slip past unnoticed. Life has become devoid of landmarks and the texture afforded by the right to plan one's own day.

Barton also lists brutality, browbeating and teasing as causative factors in the aetiology of institutionalization. Overt brutality is now uncommon, though investigations into conditions at a few large psychiatric hospitals have revealed horrific instances of abuse. Fortunately such hospitals seem to be in a small, but widely publicized, minority, and overcrowding and understaffing are almost invariably associated with scenarios in which the staff may find themselves at their wits' ends.

Browbeating and teasing may still be relatively common and often do not arise from a calculated desire to humiliate or degrade. The 'social distance' between staff and patients in some long-term units, and the low status of the 'patient role', may create a scenario in which the staff loudly and abruptly criticize and control the behaviour of their charges, using language to which they themselves would take marked exception were they to have it directed against them. Patients whose delusions have an 'amusing' content may be prompted to repeat them by bored staff and may even be rewarded for so doing by being given a cigarette. Staff who believe that it is their legitimate remit to control and regulate their patients in their every activity may soon come to unthinkingly adopt social practices which deny the humanity of their patients.

Authoritarian attitudes are also listed by Barton as an aetiological factor, and staff attitudes of this nature may be rooted in anxieties arising from situations in which a small staff feel almost totally responsible for a large number of patients. Firmness may become confused with harshness and any displays of initiative by patients may be quickly stifled by an excessively paternalistic routine.

Loss of personal possessions and personal events are also listed, and the key word in this catalogue of losses is 'personal'. Goffman comments that:

> The individual ordinarily expects to exert some control over the guise in which he appears before others. For this he needs cosmetic and clothing supplies, tools for applying, arranging and repairing them, and an accessible secure place to store these supplies and tools—in short the individual will need an 'identity kit' for the management of his personal front.'
>
> *(Goffman, 1961).*

Loss of the personal 'identity kit' may be associated with the stripping rituals of hospitalization. Personal clothing may be replaced with hospital issue, haircuts may be provided by a hospital barber, whose goal is often speed rather than the aesthetic standard of the end product. Personal possessions may be discouraged by staff as they may lead to administrative difficulties (they may be lost, stolen or sold), and drab institutional anonymity may soon prevail.

Loss of personal friends often rapidly ensues. Ennals (1973) spent some time as a 'pseudopatient' in a large English psychiatric hospital. He recounts that 'Over the weekend only two of the 54 patients (in his ward) had a visitor. Out of sight, out of mind, with a vengeance'.

Many factors may combine to sever contacts between the patient and his friends and family. Some psychiatric hospitals are still situated at a considerable distance from the conurbations they serve and the cost of travelling to visitors may be prohibitive. Others may be reluctant to visit because of their stereotyped beliefs about mental disorder ('I wouldn't know how to talk to her—suppose I said the wrong thing?'). Apathy and reduced self-esteem on the patient's part may lead to visiting times becoming rituals beset by awkward silences and visitors may soon feel unwanted or unwelcome.

There is also still considerable stigma attached to psychiatric hospitals in the eyes of many members of the public. One young patient known to the author was never visited by his parents who instead provided him with a 'donkey jacket' emblazoned with the logo of a well known construction firm. This the patient was instructed to wear when he visited home at the weekends in order that the fiction that he was working away from home could be maintained for the neighbours' sake.

Loss of personal events (birthdays, anniversaries, holidays) may also occur in the social volume of the long-term unit, and time itself soon loses structure and texture. As Barton comments: 'Isolation, lack of purpose and loneliness beget apathy which in turn causes further isolation' (Barton, 1976).

Over-sedation is also identified as a cause of institutionalization. Laing (1964) has commented that locked doors may be replaced by 'tranquillisers that place the bars of Bedlam and the locked doors *inside* the patient'.

Acutely disturbed patients may be administered large doses of tranquillizers during the few days or weeks after admission to bring much needed relief from the torments of some forms of acute mental disorder. Thereafter the dose may not be reduced as symptoms abate, with the result that the dosage which brought relief during the acute phase now simply sedates and produces lethargy and drowsiness. Medication may not be reviewed as often as it should and it is not uncommon to find patients who have been 'maintained' on the same heavy dose of a tranquillizer for some years. The nursing staff have a responsibility here to draw the attention of senior staff to the patient who is patently over-sedated.

The heavily sedated patient will be easily 'managed' and nursing staff may exert pressure on the doctor to prescribe tranquillizers for the 'difficult' patient.

The *ward atmosphere* is also a causal factor (poor furniture, decoration and lighting, noise, overcrowding, lack of privacy and a general atmosphere of institutional drabness).

Loss of prospects outside the hospital occurs as institutionalization leads to 'disculturation', which is 'an untraining which renders the inmate incapable of managing certain features of daily life on the outside, if and when he gets back to it' (Goffman, 1961). Loss of self-esteem and adoption of the 'sick role' militate against the patient taking up patterns of family life again and resuming his place in his former social background. Fear of rejection, awareness of stigma, loss of job prospects and fear of loneliness may combine to make the patient view discharge fearfully. 'Although some roles can be re-established by the inmate if and when he returns to the world, it is plain that other losses are irrevocable and may be painfully experienced as such' (Goffman, 1961).

Table 13 Factors causing institutionalization (after Barton).

The stripping process
Loss of contact with the outside world
Enforced idleness
Dehumanizing and authoritarian staff attitudes
Loss of personal possessions and personal events
Over-sedation
Sterile ward atmosphere
Loss of prospects

The listing and description of these factors in itself suggests ways of reversing their effect or of preventing their occurrence in the first place.

Rehabilitating the institutionalized patient

Ostensibly nothing could seem more simple. The institutional 'stripping process' leads to institutionalization, so reverse the stripping process—give back that which has been taken away—restore individuality, personal freedoms, dignity, privacy and self-respect, with the ultimate aim of teaching the individual to re-accept responsibility for his or her own life again, and thus attain independence. The realities may be less simple, as ward staff who try to rapidly initiate change will discover. 'Such a view is ingenuous. The fact of the matter is that organisations such as schools and hospitals will, like dragons, eat hero-innovators for breakfast' (Georgiades and Phillimore, 1975). Hall (1983) comments that:

'One of the difficulties commonly faced in initiating a ward based (rehabilitation) scheme is the maze of statutory or merely traditional regulations which has to be traced in order to obtain something quite trivial, such as uncooked food from the hospital kitchens so that patients can cook their own breakfast. The skill required in threading a passage through such mazes is not conventionally taught in medical or nurse training schools so ward staff need a considerable degree of both initiative and persistence'.

Physicists define 'inertia' as 'the tendency of a body to continue doing whatever it is doing', and institutional inertia may be profound.

Awareness of institutional inertia should not become a recipe for inaction however. Hall speaks of the difficulties in *initiating* a ward-based scheme. The difficulties do not lie in the implementation.

A multidisciplinary team approach is essential to planning even a simple ward-based rehabilitation programme. Hospital authorities who may regard a vocal minority as an irritant will often respond to a united front of medical staff, nursing staff, psychologist, social worker, occupational and recreational therapist.

There must be consensus about the aims and objectives of the programme and the means by which these objectives are to be realized, otherwise the programme may suffer from intentional or unintentional sabotage from cynical factions who do not endorse the goals of the rehabilitation team.

Once consensus is achieved, and the appropriate personnel and resources have been allocated, rehabilitation can commence, though the importance of a positive and active rehabilitation philosophy cannot be over-emphasized.

Reversing the stripping process

There is now a wealth of literature on the subject of rehabilitating the psychiatric patient though all adopt the basic approach of gradually returning that which has been stripped away, actively or passively, by institutional living.

Despite the multiplicity of approaches it is still difficult to better the simple and brisk approach advocated by Barton in 1959. Barton suggests eight key steps in rehabilitation.

Re-establish contacts with the family and community in every possible way. This should be done in a systematic way to ensure that each patient on the programme receives his/her share of restored community contacts. Telephone calls and letter-writing hours may be a useful first step. Many patients may have difficulty in composing a letter and may require considerable gentle guidance and assistance from nursing staff. Addresses of relatives will be found in the patient's notes and nurses should try to ensure that the letter is not accusatory or abusive while avoiding the excess of caution which so often perpetuates institutionalization.

Re-training in simple *social skills* may be necessary as social skills atrophy quickly in the long-term unit. There is no substitute for allowing the patient to practise these skills in real life wherever possible. Role-play and rehearsal with feedback of everyday situations (making a purchase in a shop, asking directions, ordering a meal) is undoubtedly valuable but lacks the 'X factor' offered by real life.

Short shopping expeditions, accompanied by the nurse, allow the patient to slowly make the radical adjustments demanded by the greatly different environments of hospital and community. The patient slowly readjusts to people, traffic, the general bustle of community life, handling money, making choices and meeting non-patients.

Visits to the cinema, pubs, park, football match, museum or places of interest identified by the patient are all useful in exercising social skills, restoring confidence and building initiative.

The nurse must avoid the temptation to over-organize these trips into the community, and must resist the temptation to point out obvious solutions, or to discard patients' suggestions out of hand. This is a learning experience for the patient, and tentative attempts to flex atrophied social muscles will quickly be discontinued as the patient bows to the authority and better judgement of the nurse.

Visiting may be made much easier by introducing flexible visiting hours (any time between 9 a.m. and 9 p.m.) and relatives should be encouraged to call in if they are passing and to take the patient out with them wherever possible.

The patient should be encouraged to visit relatives or friends, initially for the day and, as soon as possible, for the weekend.

Carefully structured programmes of daily activity involves structuring the hospital environment so that most of the patient's waking hours involve constructive social learning.

'Untraining' must be replaced by retraining and 'disculturation' must be replaced by 'reculturation'. Base-line measurements should be taken to reveal areas of deficient functioning, and a variety of rating scales are available for this purpose. The NOSIE scale (*Nurse's Observation Scale For Inpatient Evaluation*) is one example and is available in the standard 80 item version and in shorter modifications (Honigfeld and Klett, 1965). (See Appendix 2.)

The NOSIE scale rates the patient on six dimensions—social competence, social interest, personal neatness, irritability, manifest psychosis and retardation, these values being derived from the nurse's scoring of the patient's behaviour over a three day period. Frequency of identified behaviours (e.g. is sloppy, refuses to speak, tries to be friendly with others, sits unless directed into activity) determines scoring (0=never, 1=sometimes, 2=often, 3=usually, 4=always) and the resultant values determine placing on each of the six scales.

Rating instruments of this nature are often made up by individual units, and a simple rating scale is not difficult to compile. Carefully recorded assessment is essential if the efficacy of the rehabilitation measures is to be effectively evaluated.

Social competence may be improved by *social skills training* and real life exposure to the problem area. Practice makes perfect and the nurse should note and warmly reinforce any gains made. Personal neatness may be improved by simple behaviour modification techniques—taking self-help skills (washing, dressing) which have become atrophied, breaking them down into their constituent parts ('chaining') and reinforcing steps towards completion of the *target behaviour* (see Chapter 10). The behaviour modification approach may be organized as a token economy programme (see Chapter 20) where the main ingredient of the ward programme is a specified set of behavioural targets, the performance of which by individual patients is followed by *immediate* reinforcement in the form of a token which can be exchanged for goods or privileges.

In general it seems that the behavioural approach is most appropriate for the more disabled chronic patient (Hall, 1983) though elements of behaviour modification may be usefully employed in any rehabilitation programme. Adaptive behaviours should be increased in frequency by the application of reinforcers, even if these only consist of a smile and a few warm words of approval.

Barton (1976) suggests that 'Each patient needs a well thought out timetable of activities' adding that 'regimentation and organisation . . . necessary in the early stages' will simply perpetuate the disorder if prolonged excessively.

Anthony (1980) suggests that rehabilitation should involve structuring the total patient environment so that the entire day is directed towards a '*total push*' towards rehabilitation. The nurse's every interaction with the patient should be coloured with awareness of the dangers of the 'institutional culture' and should aim at 'normalizing' the environment by regarding each patient as an individual with his/her own likes and dislikes, preferences, strengths, weaknesses and right to personal freedom.

Work therapy of some sort is often identified as part of rehabilitation but the research into this area is not encouraging. Kunce (1970) surveyed the literature on work therapy and concluded that research does not support the idea that work therapy can be therapeutic, a finding substantiated by Anthony (1980).

Dull, boring monotonous tasks have no place in rehabilitation. Monotony and unstimulating routine are *causes*, not cures, of institutionalization. Nevertheless stimulating and creative activities which exercise initiative and reawaken the critical faculties will build initiative and self-esteem. Therefore, industrial or 'work' therapy cannot be disregarded entirely but must be carefully designed for maximum therapeutic effect.

Hobbies and simple creative activities can be organized by the occupational therapist and nursing staff and may include cooking, painting, music and discussion groups aimed at reawakening awareness of current events and life outside the hospital. Activities should realistically reflect those daily activities which will be required at home or in the community at large. Patients may have lost the ability to shop, cook, wash and iron clothes, budget and the multitude of activities involved in running a home in an independent and self-sufficient way.

Access to a washing machine, spin dryer and ironing and cooking facilities is essential. If a domestic kitchen can be simulated as closely as possible then this will be helpful. Most hospitals now have an *assessment and rehabilitation unit* within which the patient's abilities can be assessed and a 'total push' programme, geared to individual needs, can be implemented. Such units encourage the return to self-sufficiency by establishing a domestic, rather than an institutional, atmosphere.

Patients are encouraged to choose and prepare their own food, to tend for their clothing and financial affairs, and to assume increasing responsibility for their total social environment.

Eradication of browbeating and teasing cannot be achieved by legislation. Teaching should be by example. Attitudes are 'caught' not 'taught'. If staff are made fully aware of the dehumanizing effect of failing to respect the dignity and individuality of their patients, this may also prove to be helpful. The problems of overcrowding and under-staffing create an environment which militates against therapeutic nurse/patient relationships, as authoritarian 'management' of patients thrives in such a setting while nurses struggle to cope.

Education of all grades of staff about the dangers of institutionalization is essential in all settings where a large number of inmates receive long-term care.

Loss of personal friends, possessions and events may be combated by encouraging the patient to 'personalize' their room or bed space. Photographs, souvenirs, books and mementoes help mark out a personal 'territory'. Personal clothing should be encouraged wherever possible in an attempt to help provide a personal 'identity kit'.

Birthdays should be celebrated. Case notes contain dates of birth and it is an easy matter for the nurse to compile a list of patients' birthdays and mark these in the ward diary. If the hospital kitchen is contacted a birthday cake is usually cheerfully provided and it is a simple matter to organize the provision of a birthday card and modest gift from ward funds.

Reduction of drugs. Barton (1976) comments that 'It would be foolish to say that all patients should be without drugs, but it seems likely that many are better without them'. Staff should ask themselves whether the patient is receiving drugs for his benefit or for that of the staff. Nurses may be reluctant to '*distranquillize*' patients as they fear that the patient may then become less easy to 'manage'. The drowsy, lethargic patient will not benefit from rehabilitation and excessive or prolonged use of potent sedatives is usually counter productive. Dosages should be reduced and drugs discontinued as soon as is compatible with the judgements of the multidisciplinary team. The doctor is dependent on feedback from the nursing staff to indicate that a patient exhibits marked drowsiness throughout the day, and pressure from the nursing staff often tends to be for increased rather than decreased dosages. A single aggressive incident may be the occasion for nursing requests that tranquillizers be prescribed or dosage increased and the patient may receive the resultant dose for years to come.

Barton (1976) adds that 'In a few cases tranquillisers do seem effective. Too often they get the credit for the effect produced by the enthusiasm and dedication of staff that goes with them'.

Drugs are no substitute for effective nursing care and Lader (1984) has pointed out that many patients habituate quickly to phenothiazine tranquillizers and suggests that the drugs starts to lose efficacy after 6–12 months; the only effects then remaining are unpleasant side-effects.

Adjustments in the ward atmosphere are often necessary, unless the patient is living in a specialist rehabilitation unit. Patient morale is improved by cheerful, homely surroundings, and the opinions of the patients should be sought and acted upon wherever possible.

Awareness of prospects outside the hospital should be encouraged. Prospects of accommodation, employment and social facilities should be displayed on an attractive bulletin board. The disablement resettlement officer, social worker and community psychiatric nurse may have 'surgeries' to stimulate patient interest and provide helpful information.

Discharged patients who have successfully adapted to community life should be encouraged to return for visits, and thus provide incentive. Letters from ex-patients should be encouraged and displayed on the bulletin board.

Voluntary organizations may visit to arrange concerts and other recreational activities and to help provide a breath of fresh air from the 'real world'.

Rehabilitation should, wherever possible, culminate in discharge. There is little point in 'deinstitutionalizing' a patient only to return him to a 'back ward' to regress again.

Discharge may be initially to a *halfway house, hostel* or *group home* but the ultimate target should be complete independence. Rehabilitation not only prepares patients for discharge but improves the quality of life for patients who are never likely to leave. Discharge without adequate preparatory rehabilitation is both pointless and cruel. Inadequately rehabilitated patients may simply drift into another institution (psychiatric hospital, hostel for the homeless or prison) or may lead an aimless vagrant existence on the fringes of society.

The Therapeutic Community

The institutional culture of our large psychiatric hospitals was firmly established in Victorian times.

Kathleen Jones (1972) has pointed out that the Lunacy Act of 1890 promoted the custodial role of the large institutions by its legalistic framework.

'Asylums could only take certified patients; and patients could not be certified until the illness had reached a stage where it was obvious to a lay authority—the J.P. (Justice of the Peace). This made it impossible for the asylums to deal with early diagnosis and the treatment of most mild or acute cases. Their work became largely custodial'

(Jones, 1972).

Patterns of custodial social practices became firmly built into the fabric of the institution and showed a remarkably ability to survive changes in treatment philosophy and mental health legislation.

The large institutions are still with us, as are many residues of custodial practice. Some of these practices seem as monolithic and resistant to change as the buildings in which they are carried out, and they still populate the therapeutic landscape like well-armoured dinosaurs.

During the Second World War, developments in psychiatric theory and practice generated interest in an alternative approach to caring for the mentally disordered. Maxwell Jones was put in charge of a unit which was designed to study and treat neurosis in armed forces personnel and his radically innovative approach gave rise to the philosophy of democratic restructuring of the care setting in a way which led to the establishment of many open and patient-centred care facilities which totally rejected the institutional approach. The concept of the *therapeutic community* was born.

The therapeutic community may be defined as a community in which a conscious effort is made to employ the potential of all staff and patients to create a social environment conducive to personal development and which provides positive social learning experiences.

The therapeutic community offers the opportunity to make *'experiments in living'* and does not promote the surrender of personal autonomy. There is no 'stripping process'. Each person is encouraged to examine and take responsibility for any behaviour which is causing problems, either for himself or others.

The 'social distance' between staff and patients is reduced and there is a levelling of rigid authority structures in favour of democracy and personal accountability.

Free and open communications are central to the

concept. Goffman said of the total institution 'characteristically the inmate is excluded from knowledge of the decisions taken regarding his fate . . . as in concealing diagnosis, plan of treatment and approximate length of stay . . . such exclusion gives staff a social basis of distance from, and control over, inmates' (Goffman, 1961).

In a therapeutic community there is the opening up of new opportunities for the most liberal communication between staff and patients and amongst staff of different grades and disciplines.

Rapoport (1960) has described the set of beliefs which tend to be shared by therapeutic communities:

1 The total social organization in which the patient is involved—and not only the relationship with the doctor—is seen as affecting the therapeutic outcome (the *community* as 'doctor').

2 The social organization is not regarded as a routinized background to treatment, but as a vital force, useful for creating a milieu that will maximize therapeutic effects (for this reason this approach is sometimes called '*milieu therapy*').

3 The core element . . . is the provision of opportunities for patients to take an active part in the affairs of the institution (democratization).

4 *All* relationships within the hospital are regarded as potentially therapeutic.

5 The 'emotional climate' of the institution is accorded significance, and warmth and acceptance are in general regarded as helpful.

6 A high value is placed on communication for its morale-building and therapeutic effects on staff as well as patients (Rapoport, 1960).

Instead of being isolated and powerless figures in a bleak institutional landscape, patients are encouraged to assume full responsibility for their lives and to critically examine their approaches to life in an atmosphere of mutual support and constructive revision of faulty or self-damaging life strategies. Behaviour is placed in a social rather than a medical context.

The background against which this revision of self takes place is seen as being of crucial importance, as the environment of the hospital recreates in miniature the greater social arena.

The approach is multidisciplinary and everyone who comes into contact with the patient in the course of the patient's day (including fellow patients) has a therapeutic potential for promoting social learning.

The emphasis is on *understanding* behaviour rather than simply controlling it. The nurse should ask 'What does this behaviour mean?' rather than 'How can we control this behaviour most easily?'

Independence is maintained and passive adoption of the 'sick role' is discouraged. To this end *nothing is done for patients which they can reasonably be expected to do for themselves or for one another*.

The ward meeting is the functional unit of the community, and open and frank discussion of difficulties is promoted in an attempt to create movement towards solutions. The staff do not always directly intervene to resolve difficulties, and the community discusses the effects of deviant behaviour on the part of a resident. Each individual, staff or patient, is accountable for his/her behaviour to the rest of the community.

Integration of the sexes is an essential step if the community is to realistically recreate the social forces of life outside the hospital in miniature and if an air of 'normality' is to be retained. Segregation is still the custom in some hospitals, male wards being staffed by male staff and female by female, token mixing of the sexes being allowed at occasional recreational functions.

The wisdom of segregation has long been questioned. The report of an early trade union (The Mental Hospital and Institutional Workers Union), published in 1931, observed that 'We are of the opinion that the more general employment of female nurses in certain male wards is calculated to influence beneficially the atmosphere of mental hospitals'.

A single sex community is an unnatural one and does not permit resolution of many of the difficulties in interpersonal relationships which invariably accompany mental disorder.

A major aim should be the stabilization of the adaptive aspects of the person's personality so that the socially maladaptive aspects will gradually be eroded and may eventually atrophy through disuse. The emphasis on personal responsibility is underlined by a shared process of decision-making, with behaviour being discussed by the group, which will impose sanctions and provide rewards and support. The group, is thus seen as a potent factor in treatment, as is everyday feedback from fellow residents.

Such a setting is a demanding one in which to work. Hanvey (1980) has commented that 'such communities demand an almost total commitment from staff, often resembling monks or nuns in their self-containment and dedication. Often staff live in, work hours that any self-respecting trade unionist would disbelieve, and invest most of their waking lives in the growth and development of the community'.

Misconceptions abound about the concept of the therapeutic community. Some staff feel that the abolition of uniforms and the creation of a ward group is synonymous with the creation of a therapeutic community. It is not. Radical restructuring of the social milieu, with attendant restructuring of staff and patient attitudes towards one another, is necessary. It is even more misguided to imagine that the nurse must make the hospital as homely and pleasant as possible, thus creating a 'therapeutic community'. Homely and pleasant surroundings and agreeable social and recreational activities are a first step in rehabilitation, not an end in themselves. Over-emphasis on enhancing the hospital environment, without any other rehabilitative developments, will simply foster dependence and make the patient more vulnerable to the vagaries of life outside the hospital.

The philosophy of the therapeutic community has been embodied in a variety of settings as diverse as psychiatric hospitals, residential homes for emotionally disturbed children and adolescents and the 'Special Unit' at Barlinnie Prison, Glasgow. One of the best known examples is the Henderson Hospital, which treats the intractably sociopathic. An ex-patient describes his experiences of the Henderson Hospital:

'There was an incident when one quite violent male resident was being restrained by a group of us. I hadn't been there very long and so wasn't clued in to the staff policy of non-interference. "What happened to you then?" I demanded of the diminutive Okeke. "Me?" replied the male nurse, "I was frightened. I was taken aback." One of the staff, one of the "runners of the joint", admitted (a) to fear, and (b) that we were better equipped to deal with the situation. So the staff here weren't "tin gods", omnipotent, omniscient, trying to impress, raising themselves up by trying to keep me down. They treated me with respect, I treated them with respect. They treated me as a person, I treated them as people.'

(*Mahoney, 1979*).

Communities like the Henderson Hospital are sometimes viewed with suspicion as bastions of therapeutic heresy. This is unfortunate as the humanistic philosophy of the therapeutic community can be adopted by any mental health care professional in any setting, even if the full range of practices is not immediately feasible. The negative consequences of the custodial approach have been charted by a variety of writers, with horrifying clarity.

Key Concepts

1 Early policies of segregating certified psychiatric patients in large institutions not only produced durable hospitals; it also produced a durable *custodial* approach.
2 Despite the fact that psychiatric care is now offered in a wide variety of settings, a great number of patients continue to receive continuing care in the setting of the large psychiatric hospital.
3 Protracted institutional living may produce a variety of adverse effects which have been collectively described as *institutionalization*.
4 Institutionalization is essentially the end result of the '*stripping*' of freedom, responsibility, social roles and individuality.
5 This '*untraining*' may render the patient unable to resume his/her former roles in society as passive dependence on the institution develops.
6 Institutionalization is most likely to develop in the type of institution described as a '*total institution*' by Goffman, the sociologist.
7 Goffman describes a total institution as 'A place of residence and work where a large number of like-situated individuals, cut off from the wider society for an appreciable period of time, together lead an enclosed, formally administered round of life'.
8 In a total institution the three life areas of work, rest and play take place under the same roof and are subject to the same rules—the life of the inmate is 'totally' organized.
9 The total institution is also characterized by *binary management*, the '*inmate role*', and the '*institutional culture*'.
10 Research suggests that the social dynamics of the institution itself cause many of the problems.
11 The institutionalized patient will be apathetic, submissive, lacking in individuality and interest and may be unable to clearly envisage life outside the hospital.
12 Barton suggests that the features of hospital life responsible for this end state are: loss of contact with the outside world, enforced idleness,

teasing, authoritarian attitudes, over-sedation and loss of prospects, personal possessions and events.

13 Rehabilitation will be necessary before the institutionalized patient can be considered for discharge.

14 Rehabilitation should consist of reversing the 'stripping process' by returning that which has been taken away.

15 Contact with the community must be restored, a programme of daily activity initiated ('total push'), over-sedation discontinued, and awareness of prospects outside the hospital enhanced.

16 Behaviour modification may be helpful in restoring lost self-help and social skills to patients who show marked deterioration.

17 The therapeutic community refers to both a philosophy and a set of associated practices which emphasize autonomy and the provision of positive social learning experiences derived from the community as a whole.

18 No 'stripping process' takes place in a therapeutic community, and personal accountability is retained by all residents.

19 Nothing is done for patients which they can reasonably be expected to do for themselves or for one another.

20 The full range of therapeutic community practices could be implemented in a single ward or unit of a large psychiatric hospital, and the philosophy is appropriate in any setting.

References

Anthony, W. (1980) The Principles of Psychiatric Rehabilitation. Baltimore: University Park Press.

Barton, R. (1976) Institutional Neurosis, 3rd edn. Bristol: John Wright & Sons.

Ennals, D. (1973) Out of Mind. London: Arrow Press.

Genet, J. (1967) The Thiefs' Journal. Harmondsworth: Penguin Books.

Georgiades, N. & Phillimore, L. (1975) The myth of the hero-innovator and alternative strategies for organisational change. In Behaviour Modification with the Severely Retarded. Amsterdam: Associated Scientific Publishers.

Goffman, E. (1961) Asylums—Essays on the Social Situation of Mental Patients and Other Inmates. Middlesex: Pelican.

Gostin, L. (1977) A human condition. Mind, 11.

Hall, J. (1983) Ward based rehabilitation programmes. In Watts, F. N. & Bennett, D. H. (Eds) Theory and Practice of Psychiatric Rehabilitation. Chichester: John Wiley & Sons.

Haney, C., Banks, C. & Zimbardo, P. (1973) Interpersonal dynamics in a simulated prison. International Journal of Criminology and Penology. 1: 69–97.

Hanvey, C. (1980) What is a therapeutic community? Mind out (Journal of the National Association for Mental Health). 43: 11–13.

A History of the Mental Hospital and Institutional Workers Union (1931). Manchester: Express Cooperative Printing Co.

Honigfeld, G. & Klett, C. (1965) The nurse's observation scale for inpatient evaluation. Journal of Clinical Psychology, 21: 65–71.

Jones, K. (1972) A History of the Mental Health Services. London: Routledge & Kegan Paul

Jones, K. & Fowles, A. (1984) Ideas on Institutions—Analysing the Literature on Long-Term Care and Custody. London: Routledge & Kegan Paul.

Kunce, J. (1970) Is work therapy really therapeutic? Rehabilitation Literature, 31: 297–299.

Lader, M. (1984) Inside Out (Journal of the Glasgow Association for Mental Health), 4.

Laing, R. (1964) The Divided Self. Harmondsworth: Pelican.

Lemert, E. (1967) Human Deviance—Social Problems and Social Control. Herts: Prentice-Hall.

Mahoney, N. (1979) My stay and change at the Henderson Therapeutic Community. In Hinshelwood, R. D. & Manning, N. (Eds) Therapeutic Communities—Reflections and Progress. London: Routledge & Kegan Paul

Milgram, S. (1965) Some conditions of obedience and disobedience to authority. Human Relations, 18: 57–76.

Rapoport, R. (1960) Community as Doctor. London: Tavistock Publications.

Rosenhan, D. (1973) On being sane in insane places. Science, 179: 250–258.

Townsend, P. (1962) The Last Refuge—A Survey of Residential Institutions and Homes for the Aged. London: Routledge & Kegan Paul.

Wing, J. & Brown, G. (1970) Institutionalism and Schizophrenia. Cambridge: Cambridge University Press.

8

The Community Environment

A human being is necessarily social. Born helpless and vulnerable, the human creature would not survive without sustenance, care and protection. As development proceeds the network of social relations in which the developing child is involved broadens. The child has little or no control over what is made available for it to experience, and the transmission of social patterns and values is largely one-way.

The process by which the individual learns to 'fit' the culture of the society into which he is born is called the *socialization* process; this does not cease during the lifetime of the individual. Socialization continues from cradle to grave and the largely passive socialization of childhood is gradually broadened by *active* socialization experiences. As we grow older we do not passively absorb life experience but begin to interpret, evaluate and 'sort out' life experiences and our responses to them as personality develops.

Personality and the behaviour arising from it cannot be completely separated from social experience. The actions of individuals can be understood only by reference to the social world in which they take place. Thus the actions of those who become mentally disordered can be usefully viewed within their social setting, and failure to do so may lead to distorted perceptions of mental disorder.

It is not possible to gain an accurate awareness of the social behaviour of the lion by going to a zoo and studying the behaviour of the caged creatures therein. Unnatural environments produce unnatural behaviour. This premise is also true of the hospi-talized person suffering from mental disorder. Much behaviour shown in the hospital is a response to the hospital environment. Hospitals produce 'hospital behaviour' as the patient adopts the 'sick role' and embarks upon a new career as patient which may eventually obliterate those patterns of social behaviour in which clues to the genesis of the mental disorder may be found.

G. H. Mead (1863–1931) was an American philosopher and social psychologist who tried to describe how mind and self arise from social interaction. For Mead, reason and self-consciousness emerge in a single human being by interaction with others: 'the self . . . arises in the process of social experience and activity' and mind is a product of *communication*, 'the language process is essential for the development of the self'—the 'mind' is internalized conversation (Mead, 1934).

Mead also describes the structure of self by dividing it into an '*I*' and a '*me*'. The 'I' is that part of self which is impulsive, free of social constraints and is the most private core of inner experience. It may be difficult to get the 'I' aspect of self clearly into consciousness, unlike the social 'me' which recognizes social values and institutions and is organized around awareness of others. 'I' is private and impulsive. 'Me' is public and conformist.

R. D. Laing (1970) develops this theme by writing of '*true self*' (inner self) and '*false self*' (the aspect of self given over to relations with the outside world and therefore controlled by other people), and adds that 'the self can be "real" only in relation to real people and things'.

Man is a social animal and self only has meaning and reality in its social perspective. Social unity with others is the goal of most human behaviour and the need for a meaningful pattern of human relationships is central to existence.

The psychoanalyst, Erich Fromm (1957) writes of the need of self to find meaningful social expression:

'this awareness of himself as a separate entity, the awareness of his own short life span, of the fact that without his will he is born and against his will he dies, that he will die before those whom he loves, or they before him, the awareness of his aloneness and separateness, of his helplessness before the forces of nature and of society; all this makes his separate, disunited existence an unbearable prison. He would become insane if he could not liberate himself from this prison and reach out, unite himself in some form or other with men, with the world outside'.

To confine our consideration of the mentally disordered to clinical observations made in the hospital setting would be to consider the psychological fish out of the social water which is its natural environment.

Hospitalization may reduce patients to their lowest common social denominator as roles, status and occupation before admission are obscured by the now prevailing state of 'patienthood'. The nurse in the admission ward may tend to see a seemingly homogeneous mass of patients wearing pyjamas, dressing gown and slippers. What she is actually seeing is often a rich and complex sample of humanity—the butcher, the baker, the candlestick maker, the young, the old, the dull, the gifted—persons from a wide range of backgrounds, each with his/her unique life history, each with his/her own social background from which they have emerged and to which they will return. That social background is not merely the meaningless backdrop against which this assortment of social actors have faultily acted out their parts. It is often a dominant factor in the drama of their lives. To neglect it is to lose all clarity of vision.

The nurse should not just focus on the 'patient phase' of mental disorder. The pre-patient and post-patient phases should be considered; life before and after hospitalization are essential dimensions to consider in developing awareness of the life situation of the mentally disordered person.

Mental disorder does not arise in a social vacuum, and increasing awareness of the social causes of mental disorder may enable us to translate the maxim 'prevention is better than cure' into effective practices.

The Individual in Society

George Orwell's novel *1984* portrayed a social climate in which social relationships had all but broken down. Fear and suspicion dogged the footsteps of the inhabitants of his 'future world' and a militaristic bureaucracy rigidly governed every aspect of life. This bleak portrayal of social sterility is a variation on a common theme—the theme that 'progress' may be ultimately dehumanizing and destructive.

On a lesser scale people speak nervously of the 'rat race' and the pressures of urban living, and these anxieties are often organized around a vague feeling that things were once better 'in the good old days'—that the conveyer belt of social change is inexorably carrying us towards a bleak feature. Increase in the incidence of mental disorder is but one of the negative consequences often predicted for the future of urban man. The media pessimistically indicate that abuse of drugs, solvents and alcohol are steadily increasing and that the overall picture is of a social fabric which is becoming distinctly ragged.

Concern with the potentially adverse effects of social change on the individual is one of the oldest themes in the social sciences. In 1893 Erb wrote that

'the demands made on the efficiency of the individual in the struggle for existence have greatly increased and it is only by pulling out all his mental powers that he can meet them . . . all is hurry and agitation; night is used for travel, day for business, even holiday trips have become a strain on the nervous system.'

The founding fathers of sociology not only registered concern about some aspects of social change but offered explanations for them.

Emile Durkheim (1858–1917) suggested that the Industrial Revolution brought about a decay of *mechanical solidarity* which was a social order maintained by powerful collective sentiments and low division of labour. Durkheim suggested that industrialization had led to the creation of a state of *organic solidarity* in which there was complex division of labour, substantial disagreement over social values, and common rules governing behaviour (*norms*). Durkheim suggested that the shift from mechanical to organic solidarity was happening so fast that the division of labour had progressed faster than the moral basis for this division. Society had progressed from a basically agrarian way of life to rapid urbanization and industrialization, and the speed of this transition did not permit the gradual evolution of ideal values and standards of behaviour appropriate to the new industrial setting. The moral basis of society was suffering from 'jet lag'.

Durkheim suggested that the result of this over-rapid transition was major disagreement over appropriate norms—consistent sets of ideal values and standards of behaviour were lacking. This state of 'normlessness' he called *anomie* and he related anomie to many ills of modern society. For the person suffering from anomie, life becomes aimless and the risk of suicide increases as old standards become of little use due to rapidly changing circumstances. Suicide among the separated, divorced, unemployed and the immigrant population may be a reflection of high levels of anomie in these populations.

Ferdinand Tonnies (1855–1936) was a German sociologist who also made major contributions to the literature on social change. He suggested that pre-industrial societies were characterized by intimate and enduring social relationships based upon a clear understanding of each person's place in society, in which family units were large and sprawling and often consisted of three or more generations living in the same locality (the *extended family*). Such a social order he called *Gemeinschaft* (usually translated as 'community') and he emphasized the high value placed on kinship and family solidarity in such a setting. Gemeinschaft socialization usually involved the transmission of meaningful and homogeneous social values via the socialization process.

Tonnies believed that urbanization and industrialization had led to a decay in 'community' values. Society had become large scale, impersonal and calculative. The extended family was dying out to be replaced by the *nuclear family* (a married couple plus their offspring) and children were denied the warmer and broader socialization experiences offered by the extended family. This form of impersonal industrial social life he called *Gesellschaft* (often translated as 'association'). To relate Tonnies to Durkheim we could say that anomie is often a characteristic of Gesellschaft.

Karl Marx (1818–1883) is also regarded as one of the founding fathers of sociology who made major contributions to the sociology of change. For Marx industrial society was characterized by *conflict*, as the vast majority of people had to exist by selling their labour power to the owners of the means of production. The former group he called the *proletariat* and the latter group the *bourgeoisie* and he suggested that such an economic system was based on exploitation of the proletariat leading to increasing conflict between the two groups (or classes).

This view suggests that a social order based upon private ownership of the means of production (capitalism) is both unjust and unstable and that it will not endure but will perish to be replaced by social ownership of the means of production (socialism), as class antagonisms erode the foundations of capitalism.

For Marx, capitalism is characterized by *alienation*; that is, the individual worker feels powerless and unable to control his own destiny. Alienation arises for a variety of reasons:

'first, that the work is *external* to the worker, that it is not a part of his nature, that consequently he does not fulfil himself in his work but denies himself, has a feeling of misery not of well-being, does not develop freely a physical and mental energy, but is physically exhausted and mentally debased. The worker therefore feels himself at home only during his leisure, whereas at work he feels homeless. His work is not voluntary but imposed, forced labour. It is not the satisfaction of a need but only a means for satisfying other needs . . . in work he (the worker) does not belong to himself but to another person'.

(*Marx, 1844*)

For Marx, the urban dweller was alienated man existing in an *atomistic* (fragmented) society.

Max Weber (1864–1920) was a German sociologist whose theories (together with those of Durkheim and Marx) pervade all of modern sociology. Weber disagreed with the Marxian view that heightening class antagonisms would eventually topple capitalism as a social order. Weber rejects the stark Marxian division of society into two diametrically opposed classes (bourgeoisie and proletariat) and instead emphasizes the emergence of *middle class*, and suggests that the quest for *status* dominates urban industrial society rather than the pursuit of class interests. For Weber, the institutions of capitalism are monolithic and resistant to change, and the future is likely to be a bleak bureaucracy.

Thus the effects of social change and the environment on the individual is one of the oldest themes in the social sciences and this is reflected in the writings of the founding fathers of sociology who were concerned, not just with social change, but with its effects.

Madness and the Metropolis

Many studies suggest that the incidence of mental disorder seems directly proportional to the density of living. Mental disorder is more common in towns than in villages and is more common in cities than in towns. As 95% of the population of England and Wales could be defined as living in some sort of urban settlement, the future seems bleak. Initial responses of pessimism may not be justified as urban residence may also partially be effect rather than cause of mental disorder.

City dwellers live closer to hospitals and therefore may be more likely to make use of them (Mangen, 1982) and more likely to turn to a psychiatrist for help. The more intimate atmosphere of the village may create difficulties for the individual who wishes to quietly and anonymously seek psychiatric aid, insofar as the attention of the social 'audience' is more likely to be aroused than in an impersonal urban setting. Consequently some individuals may attempt to deal with mental disorder without formal assistance for fear of evoking stigma.

Urban/rural distinctions are, in themselves, crude and must be more closely examined. There is considerable evidence that large cities have 'pockets of disadvantage' (run-down or deprived areas) which are productive of much mental disorder, while they also have pockets of suburban stability which are no more productive of mental disorder than most villages.

Faris and Dunham (1939) carried out a well-known study of mental hospital admissions in Chicago. They found that the zone of dilapidated housing surrounding the city core produced most admissions and that rates of mental disorder, poverty and delinquency declined steadily the greater the distance from the city centre.

These findings may be partially explained by the suggestion that persons suffering from major mental disorder tend to 'drift' into the cheap rented accommodation offered in city cores as they become progressively more socially disabled.

The 'drift hypothesis' does not completely explain the differences in morbidity between town and country. Rutter et al (1975) examined the rates of psychiatric disorder in inner London and the Isle of Wight and found that psychiatric disorder was twice as common in inner London than on the Isle of Wight. This difference in prevalence applied generally to long-term residents of each area so that a 'drift' to London by the mentally disordered could largely be discounted. The researchers suggested that life in the inner city area was far more productive of stress.

Durkheim's concept of anomie as a potent factor in the aetiology of maladjustment and unhappiness is reflected in the finding that London boroughs with the highest rates of in and out migration, and with the largest number of people living alone, had the highest suicide rates (Sainsbury, 1955) and an examination of suicide rates in a large German city indicated that 'incomplete' households (e.g. one parent families) produced the highest concentration of suicides (Welz, 1979).

Studies of an agricultural district of Sweden showed that men and women who moved to a large city were at greater risk of developing mental disorder than those who remained in rural areas (Hognell, 1966), and a study comparing the prevalence of psychiatric disorder on the Hebridean island of North Uist to that in London revealed a lower prevalence of disorder on the island (Brown et al, 1977).

Several studies suggest that working class women are more vulnerable than middle class women to mental disorder in inner city areas, but no such class difference has been revealed in rural communities (Miles, 1981). Various observers have attempted to identify those aspects of the urban setting which may contribute to mental disorder.

Calhoun (1962), a researcher at the Washington Institute of Mental Health, created an experimental situation to study the effects of overcrowding. He placed a large number of rats in a cage which had a large central area, and two small end pens connected to the main area by small entrances. In the overcrowded centre pen, the normally stable social patterns of the rats broke down and hypersexuality, homosexuality and cannibalism developed in the resultant chaos. In the end pens (each guarded by a dominant male) serenity and order reigned, each being occupied by a rat family who did not overcrowd the space available. Calhoun described the congested central pen as a 'behavioural sink'. This experiment in 'social pathology', with its implications for human communities, aroused much interest among social scientists, though it is always dangerous to draw sweeping inferences from animal experiments.

Fanning (1967) compared the mental health of young housewives living in multistorey flats to that of a comparable group living in houses. The incidence of neurosis in the multistorey dwellers was three times that of the house dwellers and the incidence was twice as high for women living on the top floor as it was for those living on the ground floor, the rate increasing steadily with height above ground level.

Bagley (1974) confirmed that satisfaction was

higher, and consultation rates lower, in a group of house dwellers compared to a similar group living in flats, and another study revealed a rate of neurosis in flat dwellers which was twice that of house dwellers (Hird, 1966).

Life in the environment of the multistorey flat or the concrete desert of the large housing estate may be characterized by lack of amenities, atrophied spirit of community and social isolation—the 'lonely crowd'. A high percentage of residents are liable to be young, working class, nuclear families—a grouping particularly vulnerable to the added stresses of economic recession.

Platt (1983) considered rates for suicide and para-suicide ('attempted suicide') amongst employed and unemployed males in Edinburgh. His results suggest that men out of work for more than a year have a suicide risk nineteen times greater than that of their working counterparts.

Families are the units of which society is constructed and each unemployed 'statistic' reflects a disadvantaged and stressed family unit, unable to compete on equal terms with families untouched by unemployment. Unemployment brings more than loss of income—it brings loss of self-esteem and status. An analysis of New York health records of over 120 years revealed that rates of alcoholism and suicide increased sharply in times of high unemployment (Mangen, 1982). Unemployment may lead to marked feelings of alienation and anomie, with decay, initially of family units, and eventually of entire communities.

Prevention of Mental Disorder

The traditional approach to psychiatry emphasizes treatment given in a hospital in the hope of producing a 'cure' or a reduction of distressing symptoms. Preventive psychiatry aims at preventing mental disorder and consists of three main areas: *primary*, *secondary* and *tertiary* prevention.

Primary prevention aims to reduce the chances of people becoming mentally disordered. Secondary prevention seeks to minimize the effects of already established mental disorder and tertiary prevention seeks to reduce residual effects in an attempt to prevent long-term 'psychological crippling' as a result of mental disorder.

Primary prevention

This involves attempts to modify or reduce those factors in individual or community life which have been shown to increase the risk of mental disorder. This involves counselling, guidance and education of persons and families at risk, for example, immigrants suffering from anomie or young mothers isolated in housing estates or multistorey flats. Single parent families are also at risk as are families affected by unemployment. Clearly the scale of the problem is enormous, and effective primary prevention would involve the deployment of resources on a hitherto undreamt-of scale.

At present many informal voluntary groups offer counselling and support to stressed and vulnerable individuals (e.g. self-help groups for depressed mothers, alcohol or drug abusers, phobics) and the Samaritans and Alcoholics Anonymous spring to mind as prominent examples.

There is already evidence from work in Edinburgh that community action can play an important part in controlling crisis and stress and this has been achieved by the establishment of a multidisciplinary unit in an area where social malaise is at its highest. The unit operates with a team which includes every sub-speciality of social work, both voluntary and statutory, and includes the Citizens' Advice Bureau and representatives of the ministries of social security and employment and the housing department. The unit has attempted to attack the effects of poverty on poorly integrated people and the results have included a reduction in suicide and parasuicide levels, and a reduction in the rates of eviction and of children being taken into care (McCulloch and Philip, 1972).

The concept of the 'walk-in' centre, offering a wide range of advice and support to the stressed, is a promising one and developments in this area should effectively reduce the number of persons requiring in-patient treatment.

Crisis intervention is an approach to primary prevention which suggests that mental disorder may be prevented by offering support and guidance to the person confronted with a seemingly insurmountable problem or crisis.

Caplan, a crisis theorist, has defined crisis as follows:

'a psychological disequilibrium in a person who confronts a hazardous circumstance, that for him constitutes an important problem which he can, for the time being, neither escape nor solve with his customary problem-solving resources' (1964).

Crisis may develop following a marked change in the person's life circumstances and this may generate 'problems in living' which exceed capacity to cope. Such changes may include unemployment, retirement, marriage, having a child, change of job, divorce, separation, bereavement, physical illness or adolescence.

The community psychiatric nurse and the social worker may intervene to offer guidance, counselling and practical assistance (for example, by involving the housing department, disablement resettlement officer, ministry of social security). The aim is to prevent escalation of stress and to promote the development of effective coping mechanisms. The sources of referral may include general practitioners, out-patient clinics, social work departments and the Citizens' Advice Bureau.

Preparation for retirement classes, pre-marriage guidance and advice, marriage guidance counselling and pre-natal classes play a part in primary prevention as do migrant assimilation programmes, groups for the single parent.

Secondary prevention

This aims to minimize the effects of already established mental disorder by detecting it at the earliest possible time in order to prevent illness behaviour becoming firmly established. Secondary prevention utilizes the 'front line troops' of the primary health care team (general practitioners, health visitor and district nurse) who may also be involved in primary prevention. The duration and severity of the disorder may be reduced by effective early intervention, and referral to specialist services (psychiatric out-patient clinics, community psychiatric nurse or social worker).

Tertiary prevention

This seeks to reduce the residual effects of mental disorder and uses positive rehabilitation practices to promote reintegration and independent functioning.

The community psychiatric nurse will spend much time in practices aimed at tertiary prevention, and full use should be made of community agencies and resources.

Hospitalization may lead to loss of self-esteem coupled with difficulty in adjusting to everyday living. Many patients are allowed to make the transition to independent living via a *halfway house* which may be situated in or near the grounds of the hospital. In such a setting there is minimal nursing inter-

vention; nursing staff call in to offer encouragement, support and guidance but patients assume responsibility for organizing their daily living. Patients will buy and cook their own food and attend to all other domestic chores, and most will work in the community, returning to the halfway house in the evening and at weekends.

The *Group Home* is another transitional measure aimed at eventual independence. As the name suggests this is simply a house shared by a small group of ex-patients who run the household relatively independently with occasional visits from 'support staff' (social worker, community psychiatric nurse). Most local authorities cooperate readily in making suitable houses available, and acceptance by local residents is usually high.

Phillips (1966) researched attitudes towards persons suffering from mental disorder and asked respondents how they would feel about having a mentally disordered person as a neighbour. Five hypothetical cases were used and 100% of respondents stated that they would not object to having a phobic-compulsive as a neighbour, 97% had no objection to having a depressed person as a neighbour, 97% did not object to the proposition of a schizophrenic neighbour. Interestingly, the level of acceptance dropped when respondents were asked about their attitudes towards having persons who had been *hospitalized* for these disorders as neighbours (78% were, however, still willing to have a schizophrenic ex-patient as a neighbour).

Younger and better educated persons tend to display more positive attitudes towards ex-psychiatric patients, and one study indicated that age was the most substantial source of variation in attitudes (Whatley, 1968).

Rapid reintegration is important if the 'patient role' is not to be replaced by the role of 'ex-patient'. Consciousness of the need for rapid discharge and reintegration must, however, be coupled with awareness of the need for effective preparation for discharge, adequate provision of community facilities and effective follow-up. Nobody should ever be discharged from hospital without effective individualized planning of care having taken place. Enthusiasm for vigorous discharge policies may have disastrous results if discharge is not carefully planned. The Second Report from the Social Services Committee (1985) comments that 'it (community care) cannot and must not be done on the cheap. If it were the effects on thousands of our most vulnerable fellow citizens could be disastrous.'

Going Home

Those persons returning home after an episode of acute mental disorder will probably have spent only three to four weeks in hospital and their lives will not have been greatly disturbed by hospitalization. The majority of such patients need surprisingly little help in readjusting (Leff and Vaughn, 1972) and attempts to thrust too much care upon many of these persons may actually prolong disorder by impeding the return to independence (Dick, 1981). Discreet monitoring of the phase of readjustment may be carried out by the community psychiatric nurse, (CPN), and patient and family may benefit from referral to an appropriate self-help group (e.g. Alcoholics Anonymous, National Schizophrenic Fellowship, Anorexics Aid, or one of the councils on alcoholism).

The most vulnerable group consists of the recently discharged who have a history of chronic mental disorder (usually schizophrenia) associated with in-patient treatment of some years' duration. In this case, discharge must be preceded by comprehensive rehabilitation (see Chapter 7) and carefully planned provision of community care. Provision of community care raises the role of the CPN who has been described as 'probably the most important single professional in the process of moving care of mental illness into the community' (Second Report from the Social Services Committee, 1985).

The Role of the Community Psychiatric Nurse

Carr et al (1980) identify the following six dimensions of the role of the CPN:

1 *Consultant*—giving advice to other professionals in the community about the type and level of psychiatric nursing required for a given client/client group

2 *Clinician*—delivering nursing care to clients in the community

3 *Therapist*—employing psychotherapeutic and behavioural methods of treatment (e.g. in secondary prevention)

4 *Assessor*—the CPN may assess the care requirements of a given client/client group and may also assess the efficacy of ongoing care programmes

5 *Educator*—of other professions, nursing students and vulnerable groups in the community. Education should not only be about aspects of treatment/care but about the preventive aspects of psychiatry. The potential hazards of mental disorder may be explained in primary prevention programmes (for example, explaining the hazards of drug, alcohol or solvent abuse to schoolchildren)

6 *Manager*—of resources and work priorities, planning and coordination of the development of future patterns of community care

Research indicates that CPNs are often more effective treatment agents than doctors. They are better liked by clients, produced more discharges than did psychiatrists, produced greater satisfaction among clients, and 'neurotic patients treated behaviourally by nurse therapists improved significantly more than did similar patients continuing to have routine treatment from their GPs' (*Nursing Mirror*, 1984).

The CPN has client contact in *hospital*, *home* and *community* and, in the latter setting, liaises with the other members of the primary health care team. Contact with psychiatrist, general practitioner, social worker, health visitor and district nurse is essential if community care is to be effectively provided.

In the *hospital* the CPN meets clients before discharge in order to assess the need for continuing care/treatment after discharge and, importantly, to make the acquaintance of the client so that he/she is a familiar and reassuring presence to the client by the time the first home visit is made. Planning care will involve close consultation with those members of the care team who have been delivering care/treatment during the client's period of hospitalization. Once discharge has taken place the CPN will report back on the progress of clients to the hospital-based team and may also participate in consultations at the out-patient department.

Many hospital-based drug maintenance clinics (depot phenothiazines and lithium salts) are coordinated by the CPN as valuable opportunities for assessing clients' progress are afforded by these departments.

The CPN will also take part in the organization of rehabilitation programmes and will help plan movement from hospital into community (e.g. group homes) by rehabilitated patients.

Conventional psychiatric out-patient departments may come to be replaced by community psychiatric nursing. One set of research findings 'strongly confirm the feasibility of community psychiatric nursing as a replacement for psychiatric outpatient care . . . the nurses clearly became the key workers for their patients' (Paykel and Griffith, 1983). It has also been recommended by the Social Services Committee (1985) that general practitioners refer directly to the CPN.

In the *home* the CPN has an important relationship to both client and the remainder of the family unit. Families are the building bricks of which society is constructed and each family unit tends to develop rhythms, practices and norms which maintain the stability of that unit. This stability may be greatly threatened by mental disorder in any one member of the family. Mental disorder invariably has effects on every member of the family unit, not just the 'patient'.

Role reversal may be necessitated in the case of mental disorder affecting one of the partners parenting a nuclear family—Mum may have to go out to work if her spouse (perhaps the only breadwinner) is hospitalized, or Dad may have to remain at home to look after children of pre-school age if his spouse is hospitalized. Children are likely to be disturbed by the sudden hospitalization of a parent, particularly if this has been preceded by unusual behaviour, and if the remaining parent is stressed to the point of irritability, anxiety or depression. Anomie (normlessness) may prevail as the 'family interior' suddenly becomes unfamiliar or threatening, and support and guidance from the CPN will be of great benefit.

Butterworth and Skidmore (1981) describe the objectives of the first visit by the CPN:

1 *Introduction*—Say who you are, what you do and what you, with the family's help, hope to achieve.
2 *Explanation*—Give truthful details of what has happened to the client and why treatment might be useful.
3 *Information*—Explain probable outcomes and the problems that the family is likely to meet.
4 *Intervention*—Give details of the role you wish to take and the part the family can play in therapy.

Once intervention takes place 'the majority of responsibility for treatment should be handed over to the client' (Butterworth and Skidmore, 1981) insofar as clients must be actively encouraged to assume responsibility for their own lives. Commitment should be elicited from clients and should be reinforced in an ongoing way, the CPN often restricting his/her role to 'pacing' or monitoring change and acting as a resource person.

Clients maintained on medication are more likely to comply with medication regimes if the CPN discusses the client's expectations about medication and ensures that these are realistic. Drugs may be a valuable adjunct to treatment but are not an end in themselves—happiness and adjustment cannot be obtained on prescription.

Troublesome side-effects or signs of over-sedation will be reported by the CPN to the prescribing doctor so that any necessary adjustments in medication may be made.

The CPN will discontinue intervention as soon as is feasible. The length of intervention may vary from a few weeks (e.g. in the case of neurosis, whether this has involved hospitalization or not) to some years (e.g. in some chronic psychoses).

In many cases the CPN will intervene at an early stage in the development of mental disorder to prevent worsening of the person's condition (secondary prevention) and, in many cases, care/treatment is effectively supplied in the community setting without hospitalization ever becoming necessary.

In the broader *community* the CPN may provide valuable inputs into primary prevention programmes by helping to identify vulnerable groups. Such groups may include the unemployed, the recently retired, the recently bereaved, single parent families, immigrants, the divorced/separated, and stressed students. Educative/preventive measures may also be aimed at schoolchildren who are at risk of exposure to a socialization process which positively values alcohol, solvent or drug abuse.

Hollister (1977) suggests that primary prevention should also aim to reduce specific self-defeating behaviours, role failures, relationship breakdowns, emotional over-reactions and other psychological disturbances.

Most primary prevention programmes emphasize the role of stress which may be defined as 'the internal response we experience when subjected to stimuli that threaten our survival or emotional needs' (Justice, 1982). It would be unrealistic to think that all sources of stress (stressors) could be removed from the client's environment. What can be done is to (a) teach effective stress management techniques, (b) teach clients to avoid stressful situations (as in teaching clients to avoid 'trigger' situations which in the past have led to alcohol or drug abuse). Clients should identify their own stress 'thresholds' and should try to avoid exceeding them, and (c) stress-resistance building—building psychological 'strength' so that the person is less likely to experience stress in critical situations.

It is not uncommon for community psychiatric nursing services to be viewed as just another resource available to the hospital. Perhaps it would be more appropriate to view the hospital as a resource available to the community team.

13 The CPN works within the multidisciplinary team and relates to clients, families of clients and 'at risk' groups as well as providing specialist input to health care programmes.

Key Concepts

1 Self is largely the product of social experience.
2 The social experiences of the *socialization* process shape us so that we 'fit' the society into which we are born.
3 Awareness of those social forces which operate on self (both positively and negatively) is important to the understanding of mental disorder.
4 Sociologists have described adverse effects of progressive industrialization e.g. *anomie* (Durkheim), *alienation* (Marx) and decay of *community* (Tonnies).
5 Contemporary studies suggest that the urban setting is more productive of mental disorder than the rural one, though simplistic conclusions should be avoided as other factors may be at work (e.g. *'social drift'*).
6 Urban factors which have been suggested as bearing a positive relationship to mental disorder include overcrowding, decay of 'community', poor housing and high rates of unemployment.
7 Awareness of these factors has enabled identification of vulnerable groups and has led to *prevention programmes*.
8 Prevention may be *primary* (reducing the risk of mental disorder developing in vulnerable groups), and primary prevention may involve *crisis intervention*.
9 *Secondary prevention* aims at minimizing the effects of established mental disorder to prevent the disorder from becoming fully established.
10 *Tertiary prevention* seeks to reduce the residual effects of mental disorder for the prevention of long-term psychological 'crippling'.
11 The community psychiatric nurse is involved in primary, secondary and tertiary prevention and also acts as consultant, clinician, therapist, assessor, educator and manager.
12 The CPN provides inputs in hospital, home and community and communicates with the primary health care team.

References

Bagley, C. (1974) The Built environment as an influence on personality and social behaviour. In Carter, D. V. & Lee, T. R. (Eds) *Psychology and the Built Environment*. London: Architectural Press.

Brown, G. et al (1977) Psychiatric disorder in London and North Uist. *Social Science and Medicine*, **11**.

Butterworth, C. & Skidmore, D. (1981) *Caring for the Mentally Ill in the Community*. Kent: Croom Helm.

Calhoun, J. (1962) Population density and social pathology. *Scientific American*, **206**: 139–148.

Caplan, G. (1964) *Principles of Preventive Psychiatry*. New York: Basic Books.

Carr, P., Butterworth, C. & Hodges, B. (1980) *Community Psychiatric Nursing*. Edinburgh: Churchill Livingstone.

Dick, D. (1981) In Simpson, J. E. & Levitt, R. (Eds) *Going Home*. Edinburgh: Churchill Livingstone.

Erb, W. (1893) In *Civilised Morality and Modern Nervous Illness* (S. Freud 1906). London: Hogarth Press.

Fanning, D. (1967) Families in flats. *British Medical Journal*, **4**: 382–386.

Faris, R. & Dunham, H. (1939) *Mental Disorders In Urban Areas*. Chicago: Chicago University Press.

Fromm, E. (1957) *The Art of Loving*. London: George Allen & Unwin.

Hird, J. (1966) Planning for a new community. *Journal of the Royal College of General Practitioners*, **12**: 33–34.

Hognell, O. (1966) *A Prospective Study of the Incidence of Mental Disorder*. Lund: Scandinavian University Books.

Hollister, W. (1977) Basic strategies in designing primary prevention programmes. In Klein & Goldston (Eds) *Primary Prevention*. Washington, DC: Government Printing Office.

Justice, B. (1982) Primary prevention—fact or fantasy? In *Public Mental Health*. Wagenfeld (Ed.) London: Sage Publications.

Laing, R. D. (1970) *The Divided Self*. Harmondsworth: Penguin Books.

Leff, J. & Vaughn, C. (1972) In Wing, J. K. & Hailey, A. M. (Eds) *Evaluating a Community Psychiatric Service*. London: OUP.

Mangen, S. (1982) *Sociology and Mental Health*. Edinburgh: Churchill Livingstone.

Marx, K. (1844) Mega I/3 In Bottomore, T. B. & Rubel, M. (Eds) *Karl Marx, Selected Writings in Sociology and Social Philosophy. (1961).* Harmondsworth: Pelican.

McCulloch, J. & Philip, A. (1972) *Suicidal Behaviour.* Oxford: Pergamon Press.

Mead, G. H. (1934) *Mind, Self and Society.* London: University of Chicago Press.

Miles, A. (1981) *The Mentally Ill in Contemporary Society.* Oxford: Martin Robertson.

Nursing Mirror (1984) CPNs are more effective than doctors, **158**(4): 6.

Paykel, E. & Griffith (1983) *Community Psychiatric Nursing for Neurotic Patients* (The Springfield Controlled Trial). Royal College of Nursing.

Phillips, D. (1966) Public identification and acceptance of the mentally ill. *American Journal of Public Health,* **56**: 755–763.

Platt, S. (1983) Unemployment and parasuicide in Edinburgh 1968–82. *Unemployment Unit Bulletin,* **10**: 4–5.

Rutter, M., Cox, A., Topling, C., Berger, M. & Yule, W. (1975) Attainment and adjustment in two geographical areas: the prevalence of psychiatric disorder. *British Journal of Psychiatry,* **126**: 493–509.

Sainsbury, P. (1955) *Suicide in London.* London: Chapman and Hall.

Second Report from the Social Services Committee, Vol. 1 (1985) London: HMSO.

Welz, R. (1979) Social and ecological background of attempted suicides in Mannheim. In Hafner (Ed.) *Estimating Needs for Mental Health Care.* Berlin: Springer-Verlag.

Whatley, C. (1968) Social attitudes towards discharged mental patients. In Spitzer & Denzine (Eds) *The Mental Patient.* New York: McGraw-Hill.

9

The Therapeutic Nurse/Patient Relationship

When we treat man as he is
We make him worse than he is.
When we treat him as if he already were
What he potentially could be
We make him what he should be.

Goethe

Psychiatric nursing has been described as essentially 'a human activity' (General Nursing Council, 1982) and the skills required of the psychiatric nurse are those which facilitate the recognition and satisfaction of the interpersonal, emotional, behavioural, cognitive and spiritual needs of patients. These needs will frequently emerge within the framework of the nurse/patient relationship which is potentially the most important factor in treatment.

In the therapeutic nurse/patient relationship, it is the patient's problems and needs and the nurse's interest in alleviating the difficulties associated with these problems that form the basis of the relationship. The skills brought to bear by the nurse are essentially psychotherapeutic skills and the nurse/patient relationship will only be effective if the nurse approaches relationships in a structured way—that is, if she *assesses* needs and problems in a systematic and orderly way, *plans* interventions in a way which shows awareness both of the individuality of her patients and of the range of possible available interventions, *implements* structured and sensitive interactions with definite problem-solving objectives in mind and *evaluates* progress in a way which recognizes growth and development in the relationship and thus ensures that the nurse/patient relationship is a dynamic one (one which moves on continually and does not remain frozen within the constraints of ward routine or of her own value system).

The ability to form therapeutic nurse/patient relationships is rooted in awareness of *communication* skills and these may be further organized into an awareness of *interaction* analysis, the end result being awareness of the components of the therapeutic nurse/patient relationship.

Communication

Communication refers to the exchange of information, feelings, attitudes, beliefs and ideas between persons. Communication is effective when it clearly and accurately conveys the intended messages; effective communication is the basis of all nursing practice. Communication can become ineffective due to difficulties experienced by either the sender or the receiver of messages and it is helpful for the nurse to consider factors facilitating clear communication if she is to be an effective 'sender'. Receiver difficulties may arise when patients are unwilling or unable to consider problematic areas or when the nurse ceases to listen actively because part of her value system has been activated by a patient's statement. Patients may also experience marked 'sender' difficulties because it may be difficult to clearly verbalize problems (due to reduced self-awareness, anxiety, conflict or withdrawal). Interactions alternate between persons so both nurse and patient will be alternately sender and receiver. Before considering sending and receiving skills it is important to consider units of communication and styles of communication.

Communication may be *verbal* or *non-verbal*. Verbal communication consists of what is spoken, and awareness of psychotherapeutic perspectives previously mentioned will help the nurse to consider this sensitively and purposefully.

Non-verbal communication (sometimes referred to as body language) includes gestures, posture, tone of voice, facial expression, eye contact and a host of other channels via which feelings and information tend to 'leak' non-verbally. Verbal communications consist of the *theme* of an interaction but non-verbal communications constitute a *mode* of interaction which may contradict or augment the theme. For example, a patient may verbalize feelings of affection for his father but may clench his fists and frown as he does so—in this example verbal and non-verbal communications are not congruent—an indication of conflict.

Non-verbal communications may have a potent impact on the receiver; often we do not remember *what* was said but we do remember *how* it was said. Sensitivity to non-verbal communications may be developed by simple group exercises. Each student may take a turn as sender while the remainder of the group try to identify the nature of the non-verbal communication sent. Start with facial expressions. Humans have over 200 facial muscles and can communicate the most subtle nuances of feeling by facial expression. Try 'sending' the following feelings by facial expressions alone: happiness, fear, anger, boredom, disbelief, cynicism, amusement, distrust.

Eye contact is also a powerful non-verbal communication. We tend to use eye contact more when receiving (seeking to augment the sender's verbal communications by noting non-verbal cues). Senders should also seek to maintain a measure of eye contact. (As an exercise, try to verbally convey a sincere message while avoiding eye contact: the receiver is likely to regard you as being insincere or untruthful.) Try sending the same verbal message to another student but this time maintain eye contact and smile where appropriate—ask for feedback. Feelings may be clearly communicated using non-verbal channels. Anxiety may be revealed by lip-licking, drying of palms on clothing, foot or finger tapping or head scratching. Even attempts to deceive others tend to be accompanied by a characteristic host of non-verbal leakages.

Morris (1977) identifies the following non-verbal clues which tend to accompany attempts to deceive the receiver: decreased hand gestures, increased frequency of hand–face contacts (chin stroke, lips press, mouth cover, nose touch, cheek rub, eyebrow scratch, ear lobe pull and hair groom gestures, the two most noticeable in this context being the mouth cover and nose touch gestures), increased frequency of body shift movements, increased use of dismissive hand waves and fleeting changes of facial expression quickly suppressed. Non-verbal leakages of the sort described represent unsuccessful attempts to put on a social 'mask', the artificiality of which will be readily apparent to the skilled observer. Our true feelings tend to steadily leak through and contradict the overt message. In the example given above the person attempting to deceive verbally is clearly registering conflict [e.g. mouth covering (an attempt to 'cover up' lies), increased frequency of body shift movements (restless body shifts may signal 'I wish I were somewhere else')].

The receiver may also unintentionally leak disbelief or cynicism by using mouth cover mannerisms as he/she listens to a message which is perceived as dishonest in some way (forefinger resting on upper lip, hand at side of mouth or fingers fanned over upper lip).

It is important to stress that mouth cover mannerisms are not invariably associated with deceit in the sender or cynicism in the receiver—increasing use of the mannerism simply increases the likelihood that this is the case.

Momentary stress is associated with increased frequency of nose-touch mannerisms (touching, rubbing or squeezing the nose), the reasons for this being unclear. Tapping or flapping movements of the foot telegraph restlessness despite verbal expressions of interest, and fist clenching, finger jabbing and kicking movements of the foot indicate aggression. Leg or thigh squeezing indicates tension, and rubbing or stroking of a leg (by hand or by the other leg) is thought to telegraph sexual interest by females (despite non-interested verbalizations).

When two people are feeling relaxed and friendly during an interaction, they tend to adopt similar body postures (postural echoing); they may lean at the same angle, cross their legs in the same direction and nod in agreement with the same rhythm as though they were unconsciously saying 'See, I am just like you'. Morris (1977) suggests that the therapist can help the patient to relax by deliberately adopting a similar posture to him during interactions. Communication is also likely to be improved by this manoeuvre.

Cut-off signals (closing eyes, covering eyes or face) indicate that the sender is under stress and wishes respite for the moment. Ear covering is another cut-off signal (for example, 'I can't hear myself think', or 'stop, I don't want to hear any more of this'). Rejection or conflict may also be revealed by closed body postures (arms folded, legs crossed, trunk turned away) and open postures may signal relaxation, acceptance and willingness to continue the interaction.

The study of body movements is sometimes referred to as *kinesics*, a term introduced by the American anthropologist, Ray Birdwhistell. The study of the way in which people unconsciously structure the space between them is known as *proxemics*, a term coined by another American anthropologist, Edward T. Hall.

Proxemics considers the issue of *personal space*—the invisible portable territory we carry around with us and which we protect against invasion. It is easy to chart your own personal space. Stand immobile, looking straight in front of you, and ask another student to approach you very slowly, first from straight in front. When you feel that he/she has become uncomfortably close say 'stop' and ask a fellow student to mark this point with a chalk mark on the floor. Next have the student slowly advance from right, left and from behind (do not move position), in each case instructing him/her to stop when uncomfortably close. You may move your eyes but not your head. Join up the resultant chalk marks and you have a map of your personal space—the amount of distance you prefer between yourself and others for comfortable interaction. The usual nose-to-nose distance in ordinary conversation is four to five feet and variations of even a few inches either way tend to lead to feelings of discomfort. We all need 'elbow room'.

Personal space violations may be enforced on us involuntarily in crowded public situations and this brings characteristic responses. The next time you are on a crowded tube or bus glance around you. People forced into close proximity with strangers tend to studiously ignore their temporary companions, avoid eye contact and carefully assume neutral facial expressions—floors, ceilings or advertisements may be carefully studied with an intensity usually only displayed by archaeologists scrutinizing a major new find.

When we feel interpersonally or emotionally safe with someone else we do allow entry into personal space. Lovers publicly announce their emotional closeness by holding hands, linking arms, placing arms around shoulders or sitting in close proximity. Think of linguistic expressions of this fact—we speak of being 'close' to someone or 'near' to someone or alternatively we may describe someone as being 'distant' or 'difficult to get close to'.

Some text books enthusiastically recommend field studies of proxemics wherein the student is enjoined to experimentally enter the personal space of a stranger (for example, by sitting close to a stranger on a bus when there are plenty of empty seats elsewhere). This is not recommended—risk of physical injury aside, the resultant misinterpretations may involve the constabulary.

Cultural variations in personal space are dramatic. Western Europeans stand at 'fingertip distance' away from one another; that is, if you extend your arm your fingertips should just about touch your companion's shoulder. Mediterranean people stand at elbow distance and members of Arab cultures

may stand so close that Europeans feel extremely disconcerted and begin to retreat.

Note personal space preferences of your patients during interactions. Do they behave like strangers on the tube? If so, communication is not yet effective. Does personal space preference diminish or increase during an interaction? Diminishing personal space may indicate relaxation and trust and is a good indicator that an effective climate for communication is developing. Lloyd et al (1984) indicate that research findings reliably demonstrate that females are on average better than males in non-verbal receiving and sending ability, this probably being a function of sex-role learning, as there is no sex difference in this respect in pre-school children.

Awareness of the richness of non-verbal cues will enable the nurse to both send and receive more effectively and will enable her to note and explore areas of incongruence. As Morris (1977) says, the aim of the study of non-verbal cues is not to 'dominate one's companions by reading their secret thoughts' but to come to 'a deeper understanding of human interactions'.

Developing Effective Communication

Competence in basic communication skills will be enhanced by increased awareness of communication channels and styles and will enable the nurse to go on to consider interactions arising out of effective communications. Remember that all skills require practice before fluency is achieved and your student group provides excellent opportunities for structured rehearsal and role-play with discussion of feedback.

Verbal and non-verbal communications should be congruent, and communications should clearly and accurately convey the message intended. Having gained competence in communication skills the nurse may begin to use these in a structured way. The following are some simple examples of the application of communication skills.

Initiating a conversation

We have all had experience of this which we bring to the nurse/patient interaction. Try to relax and 'be yourself', having ensured that you have tried to reduce any interpersonal mannerisms which may provoke anxiety or resentment in patients. Introduce yourself and focus on the 'here and now' in a relaxed, friendly and informal manner. It is not helpful to assume that you have the right to use patients' first names on immediate acquaintance. The sensitive nurse develops a 'feel' for interactions and will use first names when it is felt appropriate by both parties. Many people feel devalued by casual use of first names. An adolescent patient may feel distanced and ill at ease if addressed as 'Mr Smith', while an elderly introverted lady may be upset if addressed as 'Mary' by an immediate acquaintance many years her junior. Allow the conversation to develop a rhythm and pace which is comfortable for the patient. Resist the temptation to force things along, allow silences and try not to protract conversations artificially. Remember that the temptation to 'burrow' into intimate areas should be resisted until the patient indicates willingness or interactions have created a climate wherein patients feel safe to disclose such material.

We all have our innermost doubts, fears and anxieties which we will not disclose lightly (if at all) as to do so would make us vulnerable; it would give others the power to hurt us. Entry to these areas cannot be forced but must be granted voluntarily. We all also have intermediate areas—still private and confidential—but perhaps not quite so threatening. Lastly, there is the outer or superficial area or layer of self which consists of material or information about self which is completely non-threatening. Diagrammatically these 'layers' may be shown as follows:

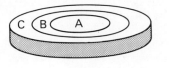

Until patients develop a feeling of trust and security with you, conversations will emanate from area C and may seem trite and superficial (comments about the weather, dietary likes and dislikes, discussions of television programmes). This may arouse feelings of uneasiness in the nurse who may vaguely feel that this patently depressed person should be talking about something more relevant to her present difficulties. Allow the relationship to follow a natural process of evolution. Let the patient relax and come to feel safe with you. Direct questions may simply upset the patient and a series of them may touch

upon a set of psychological 'raw nerves' too soon and provoke anxiety and withdrawal. For example:

> Patient: 'Good morning, nurse. What a terrible day. I hate rainy mornings.'
> Nurse: 'Is that because the weather mirrors your mood?'

Shown diagrammatically:

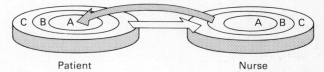

Patient   Nurse

Alternatively the patient may employ this manoeuvre, for example:

> Nurse: 'Hello, Mary, how did you enjoy the film last night?'
> Patient: 'Do you seriously expect me to enjoy films when I'm so depressed that I can't think clearly?'

In this case the patient is 'open for business' interpersonally and the nurse should accept these feelings and work with them.

Patients may ask nurses personal questions and a little self-disclosure is often helpful so long as objectivity is maintained and attention is not diverted away from the patient's difficulties. If patients ask questions which are experienced as too personal the nurse should reflect them back to the patient (why do you feel the need to ask about this area?).

Developing a conversation

Themes may be noted and reflected back to the patient for amplification and development. Empathy will prove essential at this stage just as moralistic or value-laden judgements will prove destructive. The client-centred approach to psychotherapy involves many factors which may be usefully employed by the nurse. Three sets of factors are of particular importance: the *skills*, *attitudes* and *knowledge* of the nurse. Appropriate *skills* include active listening, reflecting, clarifying, providing feedback and supporting. *Attitudes* which will facilitate effective communication include unconditional positive regard, openness, empathy, genuineness, acceptance and trust. *Knowledge* or awareness of processes occurring between persons is also helpful and this area includes awareness of ego states, transactions, games, psychological position, transference and counter-transference relationships, body language and, importantly, awareness of self.

Interaction analysis

As patterns of communication become more effective and productive the nurse will often find it helpful to develop a perspective on the nature of the interactions taking place. Assigning interactions to broad categories enables the nurse to assess both the direction and the likely outcome of a series of interactions, and enables effective evaluation of a given interaction.

Bales (1970) has suggested a system which will enable the nurse to consider the process of interaction purposefully. He suggests four basic categories of interaction behaviour:

1 Positive reactions
2 Attempted answers
3 Questions
4 Negative reactions

Each of these areas is divided into three subcategories (Table 14). Persons who score most

Table 14 The system of categories used in interaction process analysis, considering interpersonal behaviours arising in group settings (Bales, 1970).

A *Emotional area: questions*
1 Shows solidarity, raises other's status, gives help, reward
2 Shows tension release, jokes, laughs, shows satisfaction
3 Agrees, shows passive acceptance, understands, concurs, complies

B *Task area: attempted answers*
4 Gives suggestion, direction, implying autonomy for others
5 Gives opinion, evaluation, analysis, expresses feeling, wish
6 Gives orientation, information, repeats, clarifies, confirms

C *Task area: positive reactions*
7 Asks for orientation, information, repetition, confirmation
8 Asks for opinion, evaluation, analysis, expression of feeling
9 Asks for suggestions, direction, possible ways of action

D *Emotional area: negative reactions*
10 Disagrees, shows passive rejection, formality, withholds help
11 Shows tension, asks for help, withdraws out of field
12 Shows antagonism, deflates other's status, defends or asserts self

highly in the 'attempted answers' category tend to be seen by others as the group leader as their behaviour seems orientated towards achieving the group's goals. High levels of response in the 'positive reactions' category (warm, friendly, emotionally supportive) tend to lead to this type of sender being perceived as the socioemotional leader of the group. The socioemotional leader tends to be better liked than the former type of leader (goal orientated) who may become a source of tension, resentment and animosity.

Heron (1975) offers six basic '*intervention*' categories and describes an intervention as an interaction in which 'the practitioner is offering some kind of enabling service and skill to the client . . . (who) freely elects to avail himself the services of the practitioner . . . as the practitioner freely elects to provide them'. Unlike Bales, Heron focusses primarily on one to one interventions and suggests that awareness of the six categories constitutes a powerful training tool for persons who wish to develop professional intervention skills and 'In particular they aid the development of self-assessment and self-monitoring in the helping professions'.

The categories described by Heron are as follows:

Authoritative

1 Prescriptive—to give advice/evaluations in an attempt to explicitly direct the behaviour of the client
2 Informative—to instruct or inform with the aim of imparting new knowledge to the client
3 Confronting—to give direct feedback and thus directly challenge the restrictive attitudes, belief or behaviour of the client

Facilitative

4 Cathartic—to release tensions by encouraging laughter, crying, trembling or storming, thus enabling the client to abreact painful emotion
5 Catalytic—to be reflective, encourage self-directed problem-solving and elicit information from, to enable the client to learn and develop by self-direction and self-discovery within the context of the intervention but also beyond it
6 Supportive—to be approving, confirming, validating. A supportive intervention affirms the worth and value of the client

The first three categories are described as authoritative (*not* authoritarian) as the practitioner assumes a more overtly assertive role in contrast to the three facilitative categories in which the role of the practitioner is less obtrusive and the interventions are client-centred.

Heron comments that practitioners tend to experience greater difficulty with facilitative interventions, and the lowest level of competence tends to emerge in the handling of cathartic interventions.

The six categories are interdependent though each has relatively pure forms and the main thrust of any given intervention should invariably be clear. The skilled practitioner should be able to move cleanly from one category of intervention to another as the focus of the interaction changes. The six categories may be briefly described as follows:

Prescriptive interventions. These seek to influence or direct the behaviour of the client, especially behaviour that is outside or beyond the practitioner/client interaction. They do not encroach on the self-determining capacity of the client and may include suggestions, advice, recommendations or requests. This type of intervention may usefully be augmented by the practitioner prompting and demonstrating behaviours, and the provision of feedback to the client is helpful.

Heron suggests that this category may include being 'judgemental, critical . . . explicitly seeking to direct behaviour' and the giving of advice is emphasized. There are dangers here. Taylor (1982) observes that

'giving advice is not always a safe practice. If the advice is accepted and the situation remains unimproved or worsens the giver of the advice is likely to be blamed. Instead of giving advice it is more helpful to explore mutually the positive and negative aspects of the possible decisions that are available'.

The ultimate goal of the nurse is to help the client gain confidence in and feel comfortable with his/her *own* ability to make decisions. Given these provisos it can be helpful for the nurse to make suggestions about alternative approaches to current problems. Social skills training provides many examples of the nurse modelling, prompting, shaping and reinforcing adaptive social behaviours until the patient achieves a healthy and comfortable independence.

There are occasions when the nurse may have to make critical interventions. For example, with acutely disturbed patients: 'No, Mr Smith, you cannot punch Mr Jones in the eye/take your clothes off/disturb Mr Johnson like that'.

In the main the emphasis should be on promoting awareness of personal strengths and personal problem-solving abilities. Patients must retain responsibility for their own lives and should not passively and dependently hand over the reins of life to someone perceived as more capable. That route leads to inertia, atrophy and crippling loss of self-esteem.

Informative interventions. These seek to impart new knowledge and information to the client ('I have some information about this and I would like to share it with you and discuss your feelings about it'). Heron (1975) adds that such interventions 'do not suppress but positively enhance the client's needs to participate actively in the learning process in a self-directing manner'. Heron also suggests that this category may include interpretations of the client's experience and behaviour. Unbridled use of interpretation is rarely helpful within the nurse/patient relationship and the combination of interpretation and advice-giving may culminate in the nurse playing destructive 'rescuer' games.

Patients may initially feel cheated or disappointed when the nurse does not offer neat solutions or sweeping advice. Kopp (1974) describes his experience of psychotherapy as follows:

'The patient enters and makes a lunge at me, a desperate attempt to pull me into the fantasy of taking care of him. I step aside. The patient falls to the floor, disappointed and bewildered. Now he has a chance to get up and try something new. If I am sufficiently skilful at this psychotherapeutic judo and if he is sufficiently courageous and persistent he may learn to become curious about himself, to come to know me as I am, and to begin to work out his own problems'.

Not all patients are 'sufficiently courageous and persistent' and these qualities may only emerge from the positive climate created by a series of supportive interventions.

Confronting interventions. These 'reach out to and are supportive of the person while throwing into relief his rigidities and defences so that he can experience his own insight into their role as defences' (Heron, 1975). (Right or wrong, this is the impression you give me—this is how you come across to me—and this is how your approach makes me feel. Perhaps this is feedback you can use.) Such confrontations must be offered in a non-judgemental, non-moralistic and non-punitive way (remember the risk of transference relationships) and they essentially consist of the practitioner reflecting (or 'mirroring') the client's verbal and non-verbal behaviour and offering feedback on it. It should be emphasized that such confrontation does not imply criticism or rejection of the patient as a person, only of certain troublesome feelings, attitudes or behaviour.

Cathartic interventions. These facilitate the discharge of painful, repressed emotions in a way which the patient can handle in a relatively undisruptive way. These emotions may include anger (discharged as 'storming' sounds and movements), grief (tears and sobbing), fears (trembling and shaking) and embarrassment (laughter). The discharge is followed through until distress at that level is cleared. Aids to catharsis include:

1 Reminiscences—the client is invited to recall painful or distressing events (perhaps recounting them in the present tense)
2 Monodrama—the client plays both sides of an internal conflict
3 Relaxation and reverie—accompanied by suitable encouragement
4 Primary contact—gazing into the client's eyes and holding his hands with abundant free attention

Catalytic interventions. These aid the client to learn and develop by self-direction and self-discovery, 'never overstay their welcome and are alive with active empathy' (Heron, 1975). The Rogerian techniques of reflecting and expressing unconditional positive regard—warmth, trust and acceptance—will prove helpful here. Active listening and the giving of abundant free attention create the setting for interventions of this type.

Some Critical Aspects of the Nurse/Patient Relationship

Transference

Psychoanalysis involves working with the transference relationships which develop during therapy but marked transference relationships may constitute a problem within the nurse/patient relationship.

The role and status of the patient may in many ways resemble that of a child. The patient may be uncomfortably aware that he/she has 'failed' interpersonally and may cast the staff into parental roles, expecting from them behaviour appropriate to a father or mother. The nurse who addresses patients from the Parental ego state will rapidly activate feelings of this sort, and the outcome may be unhealthy dependence or hostility.

Some elements of transference are inevitable but heavily established transference relationships may be avoided by picking up transference feelings and reflecting them back to the patient, thus making it clear that *you* are not the locus of these feelings and that they have arisen out of relationships with critical others—they predate the nurse/patient relationship which has simply allowed them to surface.

It is not helpful to simply reject transference feelings; once they have surfaced try to help the patient to see them clearly and facilitate discussion of them. Increased self-awareness is likely if catalytic intervention follows the expression of troublesome transference feelings. Try to avoid the emergence of counter-transference feelings. Adoption of the Adult ego state minimizes the risk of disruptive transference relationships.

Confidentiality

Many persons suffering from mental disorder feel unable to trust others, and one of the ways in which the therapeutic nurse/patient relationship can be helpful consists of the emergence of a climate of trust and acceptance. The nurse should respect confidences of which she may frequently be the recipient and Simpson (1980) comments that 'one of the essential skills in psychiatric nursing is the ability to build a relationship with a patient in which trust is a paramount feature'.

Trust cannot be routinely expected of patients but must be actively earned. The nurse may promote the investment of trust in her by conveying to the patient that she regards all the information she obtains from or about him as being strictly confidential, and it may also be a great relief to relatives to know that nothing about the patient's disorder will be known to anyone except those concerned with treatment. A gentle refusal to discuss other patients' confidences and circumstances will help inspire confidence that the nurse will apply these principles to any confidential material entrusted to her.

On occasion the patient may place the nurse in an untenable position by disclosing information which indicates that an intended course of action on the patient's part may place others or the patient at risk. A reasonable guideline to follow under these circumstances is to indicate to the patient that the nurse has a responsibility to share such information with other members of staff involved in caring for the patient. The nurse may indicate that she accepts that the patient's immediate response may be one of anger or resentment but she may wish to point out that the long-term effects on the patient of such a course of action would be far more damaging than the initial feelings of betrayal.

Aggression

Aggressive behaviour tends to be identified as one of a range of potential 'problems' liable to be shown by patients. In reality aggression can be both constructive and productive and it should not always be viewed in a negative light. The expression of anger serves a purpose. It substitutes a more comfortable feeling for feelings of anxiety and it provides relief from the tension that comes from being frustrated or disappointed, or from a threat to self-esteem (Hays, 1963). It is not helpful for the nurse to respond to an incident of aggressive behaviour by labelling the patient as 'aggressive' or 'violent', thus setting the scenario for a string of self-fulfilling prophecies. Aggression does not usually arise from processes occurring *inside* persons but from processes occurring *between* persons. Altschul and McGovern (1985) comment that

> 'Aggressive or violent behaviour can nearly always be traced to disturbances in the relationships between people. Aggression is not an attribute of a person but a response to a frustrating or frightening experience. It is a feeling most people experience at some time or another'.

Expressions of anger may constitute a powerful cathartic experience and it is important that the nurse stays with it and allows the patient to clear tensions without damage to his self-esteem or that of others. The outcome may be very positive: 'sustained catharsis liberates abundant distress-free attention so that the client is very much alive to the fullness of present time reality' (Heron, 1975).

Expressions of anger may cause the nurse to respond with alarm and may tempt her to control such displays by authoritarian intervention emanating from the Critical Parent ego state. If the anger is allowed to dissipate itself through constructive

channels and the nurse stays and listens and supports with empathy, the result may be a major learning experience for the patient. Verbal hostility may be displaced anger that the patient actually feels for someone else. Quite often the nurse is viewed as a less threatening object for displacement of feelings, though there may be occasions when angry feelings are indeed felt towards the nurse (as when the patient's wishes are in conflict with the objectives of care and treatment).

Often patients feel unable to verbalize emotional tensions and instead express them through disturbed behaviour, a process known as *acting out*. The nurse should not respond to acting out behaviour by simply suppressing it but should recognize it as an indicator of emotional conflict and should encourage the patient to talk about his difficulties (verbalize) instead of acting out.

Remember that many patients experience 'stroke deprivation' and much aggressive behaviour may be designed to elicit negative strokes from others, thus gaining recognition and allaying stroke hunger. The provision of positive strokes by the nurse and her prompting of positive strokes by the patient will greatly reduce this tendency. Ruesch (1957) views acting out as a primitive form of communication (followed on his continuum model by psychosomatic illness and then verbalized feelings).

Anger may find expression verbally or physically. The client who expresses anger or aggression verbally may have made progress if previous expressions of anger were non-verbal.

Again a simple continuum model may help illuminate progress which may be taking place (p. 120):

Acts of physical violence (sporadic) with little coherent expression of emotion→acting out behaviour →negative and destructive verbalizations of anger →constructive expression of anger with exploration of associated feelings.

The therapeutic nurse/patient relationship does not suppress or censor expressions of anger without attempting to understand them. It accepts them, explores them, tries to heighten the patient's awareness of the reasons for them, provides constructive channels for them and thus promotes movement along the above continuum.

When a patient expresses anger towards the nurse the *non-defensive stance* is the most suitable initial response. If the nurse becomes defensive she may rapidly lose complete control of the situation by escalating the defensive behaviour of the patient.

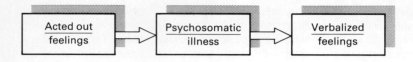

Concerned and supportive responses will often disarm the patient and defuse the situation so that nurse and patient can begin to explore the situation together in an authentic learning experience. The nurse who finds herself the recipient of patients' anger should not always blame herself but should perhaps review her own attitudes if this occurs with disproportionate frequency.

Let us consider two extreme types of approach, both likely to inadvertently provoke anger and aggression: Nurses Saccharine and Vinegar.

Nurse Saccharine

Nurse Saccharine exudes superficial concern for her patients—calls them 'pets', 'poor dears', 'darlings' or 'poor old souls'; she employs a thin veneer of sympathy but does not use empathy, is motherly in a superficial way but never gets close to her patients. She is in fact rejecting and demeaning her patients and is liable to magnify feelings of alienation and anomie.

The author recalls a conversation he had with a male patient who had made a slow recovery from a major cerebrovascular accident. During the patient's hospitalization he was the recipient of the nursing attentions of a staff nurse of the Nurse Saccharine type. The patient (who was both highly intelligent and articulate) was unable to communicate verbally for some time after his stroke and mutely suffered at the hands of his well-meaning nurse. She would sweep into his room, prop him up on his pillows and feed him while maintaining a level of chatter appropriate to a five-year-old ('eat up now, there's a good boy, my—doesn't the stew look lovely, one for the postman, come come now we must clear our plate'). The meal concluded when she (roughly) washed his face, combed his hair and archly enjoined him to 'be a good boy for the nurse now'. She also had a seemingly inexhaustible stock of unhelpful platitudes ('never mind, things will look better in the morning', 'every cloud has a silver lining').

The patient generated absolutely homicidal feelings towards her which he (vainly) tried to communicate with his eyes and he claims that she (inadvertently) provided much of the motivation for his recovery as he would lie awake at night fulminating over murderous fantasies directed towards her, and mentally rehearsing his verbal assassination of her when his speech returned. In the event he was transferred to another hospital and only met her three years later. He met her in the street and (to his consternation and embarrassment) the object of his hostility behaved quite differently outside the hospital setting. She was a vague, nervous and untidy lady who was visibly ill at ease at meeting him. They exchanged polite superficialities and parted, never to meet again, both responding differently outside the victim/rescuer game within which they had interacted previously, he guiltily aware that she was essentially a well-meaning person.

Nurse Vinegar

Nurse Vinegar is authoritarian, rigid, emotionally inhibited and very much the Critical Parent. She would be critical of the behaviour and attitudes of patients (and learners) unless they conformed to her rigid personal value system.

If many patients are admitted in a state of tension which makes them walking time bombs, Nurse Vinegar has an unhappy knack of jumping up and down on the firing pin. Her ego defences will be brittle and, despite the mask of rigid efficiency, she will be easily hurt and therefore will not permit situations which could reach her vulnerable areas to develop. She will tend to be task-orientated and will have difficulty in seeing her patients as individuals (though she will pay lip service to the nursing process as this is perceived as a new part of 'routine'). Her commitment to 'caring' may be more apparent at the verbal level than at the operational level.

These caricatures of Nurses Saccharine and Vinegar are descriptions of extreme types who may be rarely encountered in the 'pure' form. Elements of them may exist in any of us though and will create barriers to effective nurse/patient relationships. Neither addresses patients from the Adult ego state and neither uses empathy. Interpersonally both are (unconsciously) displaying a 'Position Closed' sign and both avoid patients who are interpersonally 'Open for Business' as their interventions tend to be superficial, unsolicited and nurse-centred.

Despite awareness of those factors which generate and provoke aggression, the nurse may occasionally find herself the recipient of physical or verbal aggression through no fault of her own. The patient suffering from schizophrenia may suddenly display violent behaviour (perhaps in response to hallucinatory commands or delusional ideas) and the patient who is admitted under the influence of alcohol or drugs may also display abrupt episodes of disruptive or violent behaviour. When a situation reaches the point where physical assault on staff or patients is probable some points are helpful to remember:

1 Each unit should have a pre-planned way of dealing with such incidents and all staff members should know what it is.

2 The self-esteem of the patient should be protected throughout.

3 Since anxiety and defensiveness are highly contagious, a calm and non-defensive attitude on the nurse's part will help to de-escalate the situation.

4 If physical restraint becomes absolutely necessary, an adequate number of staff members should be available to minimize the chances of injury to staff or patient.

5 Restrain by holding the patient firmly (avoiding pressure on chest, airway or major joints), holding shoulders and applying pressure above and below major joints while talking soothingly and reassuringly to the patient.

6 Discontinue restraint as soon as possible (but be prepared to reapply it).

7 Remain with the patient until he/she is calm and discuss the reasons for the incident (if practicable).

8 Submit incident report with full details including witnesses.

After such an incident, staff and patient should discuss the situation with a view to identifying precipitating factors (and removing or modifying these if possible). The patient will need much reassurance (despite possible production of 'macho' or 'couldn't care less' verbalizations), and the patient should be told that the staff should be approached if these feelings begin again, with a view to talking about tensions productively.

In a few instances aggressive behaviour is not so much a reflection of conflict or tension as a maladaptive behavioural 'mannerism'. Some patients (for

example the sociopathic or schizophrenic) may simply have developed aggressive patterns of responses to a wide variety of interpersonal and environmental stimuli. In this case behaviour modification will help reduce the frequency of aggressive responses—behaviour is determined by its consequences—and the staff should ask 'Am I maintaining this aggressive behaviour by inadvertently reinforcing it?' Remember that nursing time and attention may be the most potent reinforcers of all. Is this patient ignored most of the time and only reinforced (by nursing time and attention) for episodes of disturbed behaviour? If so, reinforce episodes of calm and rational behaviour by paying attention to these episodes (note them and warmly reinforce them verbally and ensure that they incur nursing time and attention). Aggressive verbalizations should not be reinforced (I'll come back when you feel more relaxed). Make it clear that you are not rejecting the patient—only the disturbed behaviour.

Some aspects of the ward environment will increase the likelihood of aggression, notably the absence of effective communications between staff and patients. Ward groups provide a forum whereby tensions and frustration can be constructively expressed. The staff should make it clear that someone will always be available should a patient wish to talk about his/her difficulties. Boredom and rigid ward routines may create tensions and simultaneously deny the opportunity to ventilate them.

Responding to the Patient who is Withdrawn or Uncommunicative

It is not helpful to force nursing attention on the withdrawn patient. There may be much anxiety, depression or loss of self-esteem underlying withdrawal and these troublesome feelings will simply be intensified by unsolicited nursing intervention.

In many cases the withdrawn or depressed patient will benefit if the nurse simply spends time with the patient without forcing conversation. If the patient is sitting in a quiet corner of the ward the nurse may ask permission to share this quiet corner for a few minutes as she quietly writes up notes or records (try to respect personal space which may be very large in this case). The patient becomes accustomed to the presence of the nurse and will relax in her presence and may eventually feel like speaking. Positive strokes from the nurse are important (smiles, warm greetings, placing an arm around shoulders on entering or leaving the room). Try not to force the pace; it is more helpful to create a climate of trust and acceptance. Shared activities will be helpful (board games, walks, table tennis etc.). In this instance the nurse is offering her friendship rather than her therapeutic skills, though these may be gently employed later as trust is gained and the patient expresses willingness to talk. Try not to underestimate the interpersonal stresses experienced by the person who is low in self-esteem and confidence and who is experiencing high levels of anxiety. Simply entering a room full of strangers (day room, dining room, occupational therapy department) may be an intimidating experience for such a patient.

It can help if one nurse per shift is assigned to such a patient to slowly win trust and restore confidence. Taxing experiences (involving mixing with others) will be much less traumatic if the patient is accompanied by a familiar and trusted nurse.

Remember the risk of dependence and try to gently steer the patient in the direction of social independence as quickly as is compatible with psychosocial integrity.

Clare (1976) summarizes the role of the psychiatric nurse well when he describes her as 'in a special way the patient's constant companion, confidante, therapist and friend'.

Key Concepts

1 Psychiatric nursing is essentially a human activity based on the relationship between nurse and patient.
2 The nurse/patient relationship may be the most important factor in treatment.
3 The nurse/patient relationship centres around the knowledge, attitudes and skills of the nurse, all of which are used to help the patient improve personal functioning.
4 Knowledge of psychotherapeutic principles and dimensions of communication are the basis of the therapeutic nurse/patient relationship.

5 Communication may be verbal or non-verbal and awareness of the latter enables the nurse to respond more effectively to patients' needs.
6 Awareness of patterns of communication enables the nurse to practice her own communication skills.
7 The effective psychiatric nurse is a skilled communicator.
8 Practice is essential before competence in communication skills is gained; an ounce of theory followed by a ton of practice is essential.
9 Awareness of communication patterns enables the nurse to progress on to the consideration of *interactions*.
10 Interactions have been analysed in the group setting (Bales) and in the one to one setting (Heron).
11 Heron's six category *intervention analysis* provides a useful summary of possible categories of structured interaction.
12 The nurse will find it helpful to consider her own interaction style as well as that of her patients—revision of transactional analysis should help here.
13 The *attitudes* brought by the nurse to each interaction are important: helpful attitudinal components include *warmth, trust, acceptance* and *unconditional positive regard*.
14 Unhelpful attitudes involve use of the nurse's own value system and any tendency to moralize or become judgemental.
15 Helpful *skills* are largely those involved in the client-centred (Rogerian) approach and include *reflection, clarification, empathy* and *active listening*.
16 Confidentiality is an essential component of the nurse/patient relationship and trust must be actively earned.
17 *Transference* feelings should be reflected back to the patient for exploration as there is a risk of *dependent transference*.
18 Aggression is not always negative as it may ventilate troublesome tensions, and lead to *cathartic* experiences and an increase in self-awareness.
19 Aggression should not be rigidly controlled but should be therapeutically channelled where possible.
20 The withdrawn patient should not be 'jollied along' but should be gently and sensitively reintroduced to interpersonal life.

References

Altschul, A. & McGovern, M. (1985) *Psychiatric Nursing, 6th edn*. London: Baillière Tindall.

Bales, R. (1970) *Personality and Interpersonal Behaviour*. New York: Holt Rinehart & Winston.

Clare, A. (1976) *Nursing Mirror*, **143**: 61–62.

General Nursing Council (England and Wales) (1982) *Training Syllabus for the Register of Nurses (Mental Nursing)*. London: General Nursing Council.

Hays, D. (1963) Anger: a clinical problem. In Burd & Marshall (Eds) *Some Clinical Approaches to Psychiatric Nursing*. London: Macmillan.

Heron, J. (1975) *Six Category Intervention Analysis. Human Potential Research Project*. University of Surrey: Centre for Adult Education.

Kopp, S. (1974) *If You Meet the Buddha on the Road, Kill Him!—A Modern Pilgrimage Through Myth, Legend, Zen and Psychotherapy*. London: Sheldon Press.

Lloyd et al (1984) *Introduction to Psychology*. New Zealand: Fontana.

Morris, D. (1977) *Manwatching—a Field Guide to Human Behaviour*. London: Jonathan Cape.

Ruesch, J. (1957) *Disturbed Communication*. New York: W. W. Norton.

Simpson, R. (1980) Confidentiality in psychiatric nursing. *Nursing Times*, **76**(19): 835–836.

Taylor, C. (1982) *Essentials of Psychiatric Nursing, 11th edn*. St Louis: C. V. Mosby.

10

Behavioural Concepts and Nursing Intervention

The single most characteristic thing about human beings is that they learn. Learning is so deeply ingrained in man that it is almost involuntary.

Jerome Bruner

Many psychotherapeutic approaches centre around exploration of the inner experiential world of the patient. The patient reveals troublesome thoughts, feelings and emotions to the therapist who interprets them in the hope that the patient will develop insight into problem areas and, armed with a new clarity of vision, become able to conquer them. Psychoanalysis and related approaches are classic examples of the *interpretive* approach to inner conflicts and there are other insight-directed schools of thought in psychotherapy.

Interpretive approaches are the province of the expert and the nurse should resist the temptation to interpret the patient's experiences and feelings. Without the appropriate specialist knowledge base, interpretive approaches may do more harm than good.

An alternative approach, in which the psychiatric nurse may become actively involved, is the *behavioural* approach which focusses on behaviour rather than the inner world of private experience. Though behavioural approaches concentrate on behaviour, a reduction in the level of troublesome behaviours is usually associated with an attendant improvement in thinking and feeling.

Behaviour

The word 'Behaviour' is used rather loosely by the lay person, who may vaguely speak of 'good behaviour' and 'bad behaviour'. The psychologist uses the word behaviour to refer to *those activities of an organism which can be observed*. Unlike the private world of thoughts and feelings, behaviour is public and observable. If we say 'John felt angry as he swept the floor' we have only identified one behaviour in this statement. Feeling angry is an inner experience which can only be reported by the person concerned. Anger is not directly observable. Sweeping the floor *is* a behaviour as it *can* be directly observed by an outsider.

A person reads a book, eats breakfast, brushes his teeth, talks, blushes, laughs and cries. All of these are forms of behaviour in that they may be observed, and their incidence measured, by the observer.

Behaviourism

The American psychologist John B. Watson was the first to advance the view that behaviour rather than inner experience should be the area of study of psychology. He advanced this view in the early 1900s and since then the scientific study of behaviour has become a rapidly developing field with many implications for workers in the field of mental disorder.

His viewpoint has become known as *behaviourism*, and its adherents as *behaviourists*. Before the advent of behaviourism, psychology had consisted of the study of mental experiences in an attempt to unravel the mysteries of the mind, and many psychological theories were founded on woolly and highly subjective speculation of a vaguely philosophical nature. Behaviourists insisted that only by studying what animals and people do—their behaviour—could psychology become a truly objective science.

While behaviourism did much to counter the introspective speculations of early psychologists, the important and fascinating study of the mental processes of the individual has continued, this area of study being known as *cognitive* psychology. Cognitive psychology has included study in the areas of perceptions, thinking and ideas.

Behaviourism and Psychiatry

Behaviourists have largely rejected the concept of mental illness and instead describe mental disorder as learned behaviour. They point out that not only useful behaviours are learned. We do not always profit from experience but may learn behaviours that are either useless or harmful—so-called *maladaptive behaviours*.

Behaviourism rejects the notion of 'underlying causes' and suggests that the symptom *is* the neurosis. Eysenck (1960) has stated that if you 'get rid of the symptom—you have eliminated the neurosis'.

Behaviourists are also critical of concepts like 'insight' and 'the unconscious mind' and instead focus on how behaviour is learned and maintained.

Wolpe (1976), writing from this viewpoint, has defined neurosis as 'a persistent unadaptive habit acquired by learning in anxiety generating situations, with anxiety usually its central feature'.

The view that mental disorder consists of learned maladaptive behaviour has given rise to *behaviour therapy* which bases its interventions on the assumption that maladaptive behaviour can be *unlearned* and displaced by learning more adaptive responses to problem situations.

Behaviour therapy must be approached by acquiring an understanding of the underlying learning theories.

Learning

Learning may be defined as 'relatively permanent changes in behaviour that occur as the result of prior experience' (Hilgard et al, 1979). Learning takes place under a variety of circumstances, but perhaps the simplest form of learning is *associative learning*—the type of learning which involves making a connection or *association* between two events in the environment.

Associative learning may take place as a result of either *classical* or *operant conditioning*.

In classical conditioning the individual learns that two *stimuli* usually go together, that one usually precedes the other. For example, a baby learns that the sight of his bottle (one stimulus) is associated with the taste of milk (second stimulus). In operant conditioning the individual learns that some *response* made leads to a particular *consequence*. For example,

the baby learns that raising the bottle to his mouth (response) brings milk (consequence).

Both operant and classical conditioning have important applications to the treatment and understanding of mental disorder.

Classical conditioning

The study of classical conditioning began with a series of experiments by the Russian physiologist, Pavlov, at the turn of the century.

Pavlov noted that a hungry dog will salivate at the sight or smell of meat; that is, the *stimulus* of the sight of food produces the *response* of salivation. This response occurs naturally; it is not necessary to arrange any learning for it to occur. Pavlov therefore referred to the food as an *unconditioned stimulus*, and the response of salivation as an *unconditioned response*.

When a bell or buzzer is sounded before giving food, the animal comes to *associate* the bell with the imminent arrival of food and will eventually salivate in response to the stimulus of the bell. Dogs do not naturally salivate at the sound of bells. Pavlov's experimental subjects had *learned* to do so by a process of associative learning. In this experiment the bell became a *conditioned stimulus* and the response of salivation became a *conditioned response*.

Repeated pairings of the conditioned stimulus (bell) and the unconditioned stimulus (food) strengthen or *reinforce* the conditioned response (salivation).

If the conditioned behaviour is not reinforced, the conditioned response gradually diminishes and will eventually disappear; that is, it will undergo the process of *extinction*.

J. B. Watson used this stimulus/response model of learning to experimentally produce phobic responses. He conditioned his own child to become afraid of furry animals by frightening him with a loud noise every time he played with a favourite furry toy. The child came to associate the toy with the unpleasant stimulus of the loud noise—the noise had become a conditioned stimulus producing the conditioned response of fear.

It has been suggested that many common phobias may have arisen in this way, as maladaptive responses of anxiety become produced in response to previously neutral environmental stimuli (Eysenck and Rachman, 1961).

The child in Watson's famous experiment eventually showed fear of all furry objects, even including hearth rugs and men with beards; that is, his fear had *generalized*. Generalization of anxiety may be a feature of many neurotic disorders as more and more environmental factors are perceived as threatening.

Classical conditioning may not only produce maladaptive behaviours; it may also be used to eradicate them.

In the procedure of *aversion therapy* a problem behaviour is linked with an unpleasant stimulus in the hope that extinction of the behaviour will occur. The alcoholic may be given a glass of his favourite drink coupled with an emetic or electric shock in the hope that he will come to associate alcohol with the conditioned response of nausea or pain, thus removing the pleasurable associations alcohol once had for him. The sexual deviant may be given electrical shocks as he views slides of his aberrant type of sexual behaviour, thus substituting unpleasant associations for pleasant ones and hopefully conditioning an aversion to the problem behaviour. Thus, classical conditioning of any kind is a form of learning by association.

Operant conditioning

Many behaviours do not appear in simple response to external stimuli. *Operant behaviours* are simply 'emitted' by the organism and do not occur in response to any particular stimulus.

The basic principle governing the level of operant behaviour is that *behaviour is determined by its consequences*. Behaviour which is rewarded (reinforced) will tend to increase in frequency while behaviour which is devoid of rewarding consequences will tend to decrease in frequency. This principle tends to be zealously applied by parents and teachers who will reward desirable behaviour and punish undesirable behaviour.

The American behaviourist B. F. Skinner demonstrated that animals placed in a modified cage (the 'Skinner Box') rapidly learned to depress levers when the lever-pressing response was reinforced by the delivery of a pellet of food. The animals' lever-pressing response was not *produced* by reinforcement but was simply increased in frequency. Left alone in the cage animals move around restlessly and, by chance, occasionally press the lever. As lever-pressing is associated with the delivery of food, the frequency of the response increases dramatically.

Thus operant conditioning refers to increasing the probability of a response by following the occurrence of the response with reinforcement. In this way, operant conditioning of any kind is a form of learning by consequences.

A *positive reinforcer* is a rewarding stimulus that, when presented after a response, increases the frequency of the response. A *negative reinforcer* is a stimulus that, when *removed* following a response, increases the probability of the response. Electric shock and painful noise qualify as negative reinforcers if they can be turned off once the desired response is made.

Negative reinforcement is not synonymous with punishment. Punishment is a situation where an aversive stimulus is delivered every time an undesired response is made, thus *decreasing* the frequency of the undesired behaviour. If an animal were to be given an electric shock every time it depressed a lever, then the response could be said to be punished by introducing the aversive stimulus. The response, in this case, would decrease in frequency and would probably undergo the process of extinction.

Seligman (1973) has suggested that the 'learned helplessness' seen in reactive depression and many long-term psychiatric patients, characterized by apathy and submissiveness, may be due to a lack of negative reinforcement; in other words repeatedly unsuccessful attempts to evade unpleasant environmental stimuli may lead to a chronic 'give-up reaction'. 'Learned helplessness' is not situation-specific. When placed in another environment, where reinforcement is available, the patient may still not respond as he has learned that responding is not worth the effort.

Similarly an individual will learn to be helpless if he is rewarded regardless of what he does. An example of this is the pop star who is extravagantly praised whether his performance merits it or not. After a while he stops responding and becomes depressed (Mackay, 1975).

Seligman (1973) is thus proposing that reactive depression results when reinforcers are not made contingent upon responding.

Behaviour Therapy and the Psychiatric Nurse

The fact that the acquisition and extinction of behaviours (both adaptive and maladaptive) may be determined by the availability of reinforcers is obviously one of great interest to the psychiatric nurse, and may make her view her interactions with patients in a different light.

Reinforcement takes many forms and the nurse's time, attention and sympathy may be one of the most potent reinforcers of all. If the reinforcer of nursing attention is randomly given, the result may be that undesirable behaviours are inadvertently strengthened and desirable behaviours may be weakened.

The author recalls a vivid example which took place in the 'refractory' ward of a large psychiatric hospital. Peter, an acutely disturbed teenage schizophrenic, often lashed out impulsively at staff or fellow patients. When such an incident occurred the well-meaning charge nurse invariably responded by placing a calming arm around Peter's shoulder, giving him a cigarette and sitting with him, talking soothingly, for some time. In other words Peter was being reinforced (cigarette, time, attention and sympathy) for behaving aggressively. Small wonder that incidents of this nature steadily increased in frequency as Peter's stay in the ward progressed. The situation was reviewed and staff were instructed to make reinforcers contingent upon his occasional calm and relaxed episodes, which were infrequent. The staff now spent time with Peter when he was calm and relaxed and registered their approval of these periods. Aggressive episodes were treated by quietly and firmly leading Peter to his bed in a side ward where he was asked to remain for ninety minutes, without nursing contact.

After a few weeks of this selective reinforcement the aggressive incidents decreased sharply in incidence and relaxed behaviour predominated.

The author also recalls Agnes, an elderly lady who was suffering from an agitated depression. She would have episodes of weeping and self-recrimination during which she announced that she would be 'better off dead' and described herself as a 'bad' and 'hopeless' person. She had behaved like this for two years but would occasionally have 'good' days when she read, knitted contentedly or watched television with fellow patients, chatting as she did so. The nursing staff tended to leave the patient to her own devices during her 'good' spells but invariably responded to her tearful outbursts by offering tea, time and attention, thus inadvertently reinforcing them.

After reassessment of the situation the staff commenced a policy of quietly and gently leading Agnes to her room when she repeated this behaviour and leaving her there till she was calm. Relaxed and contented episodes were reinforced by spending time with the patient and approvingly commenting on her improved frame of mind. In two or three weeks Agnes was contentedly attending the occupational therapy department and was rarely seen to become upset. The 'good' days now predominated.

Obviously it is essential that the depressed patient be allowed to 'talk through' troublesome thoughts and feelings with an attentive and caring nurse but it may be a great disservice to the patient to reinforce residual feelings of hopelessness which have persisted long after the acute depressive episode has passed.

In the case of both Peter and Agnes the reduction of the problem behaviour had many added advantages. The gains generalized as fellow patients now saw them as less 'alien' and more approachable and consequently involved both patients in more social activities.

There is much more to the therapeutic nurse/patient relationship than a simple application of the principles of operant conditioning but an awareness of these principles may prevent basic errors of approach.

More structured use may be made of the principles of operant conditioning. Ayllon and Azrin (1968) described how long-term psychiatric patients, who had become deficient in basic 'self-help' and social skills, could be retrained using the *token economy programme*. In this approach to rehabilitation the desired 'target behaviours' are identified and each is assigned a value in tokens, which can be exchanged for privileges or for goods (sweets, foodstuffs, cigarettes, books, magazines) at a 'token shop' which may be set up in a room off the ward.

As it is imperative that reinforcement should follow the desired response immediately, the patient is given the appropriate number of tokens as soon as he completes the desired task. Typical target behaviours may include washing, cleaning teeth, acceptable standard at tidiness check, appropriate meal time behaviour, making own bed, bathing, shaving and socializing appropriately with others.

As in the previous examples the resultant gains may be generalized as the patient becomes more socially acceptable to others and gains confidence as a result.

Structured approaches of this sort are usually coordinated by the clinical psychologist but the active participation of a nursing staff aware of the underlying principles is essential, and the psychiatric nurse may opt to take a post-registration course in behaviour therapy.

Workers in the field of mental handicap have made extensive use of operant conditioning techniques to improve functioning in the area of self-help and social skills, and have reduced the incidence of maladaptive behaviours by identifying and removing their reinforcers.

We have said that a basic principle of operant conditioning consists of increasing the frequency of desired responses by arranging rewarding consequences for them. In the case of the severely handicapped child or the institutionalized chronic schizophrenic, one could wait indefinitely for the appearance of suitable behaviours to reinforce.

In this case it is necessary to break the target behaviour down into simple steps or stages and reinforce successive approximations towards the target. This is referred to as the *shaping* of behaviour. Each step must be small as a too advanced step in the chain of behaviours will prevent success from occurring. Imitative prompts are useful in the shaping of behaviour. As always, reinforcement of success must be immediate and unmistakeable.

The shaping of behaviour

Example 1. As an example we may consider the reinstatement of the simple self-help skill of shaving. This may be broken into a series of simple steps (*chained*) and immediate reinforcement offered as each step is mastered. Reinforcement may take the tangible form of a sweet or cigarette but should always be accompanied by verbal praise and encouragement, which may prove potent reinforcers in themselves.

Our example of the target behaviour of shaving may be chained as follows:

1 Seat the patient in front of the mirror and ask him to place a towel around his neck. Demonstrate the behaviour and prompt the patient to attempt it by placing the towel in his hands and guiding it to his neck. Repeat until the patient succeeds and reinforce immediately. Finish shaving the patient yourself.

2 The patient will now be expected to progress a step further in the chain before reinforcement takes place.

Start by asking the patient to put the towel in place and remind him by demonstrating if need be. Comment approvingly when he does so and

immediately progress to the next step in the chain—applying lather. Place the brush in his hand and ask him to lather it, demonstrating the required behaviour and guiding his hands if need be. Promptly reinforce the behaviour as soon as it appears.

3 Approvingly supervise the patient through steps 1 and 2 and now ask him to lather his chin, again guiding his hands if need be and repeating until the behaviour is completed without assistance. As before, reinforce immediately and complete the chain.

4 Reinforcement is now contingent on the patient shaving the more easily accessible parts of his face (cheeks). Prompts and guidance are again given if necessary, the preceding parts of the chain having been completed without assistance.

5 The patient is now required to complete steps 1–4 without assistance and progress to shaving all necessary facial areas, supervised and encouraged by nursing staff.

6 Washing face.

7 Drying face. The chain is now complete and the target reached.

It may be argued that it would be simpler to teach the patient to use an electric razor but the above sequence has the advantage of also teaching use of soap and towels and using the bathroom, and is thus more likely to produce generalization in the area of personal hygiene.

Progress through the chain may be rapid though some days may have to be devoted to each step, depending on the patient's abilities.

The author successfully used the above chain with a small group of institutionalized schizophrenics who had gradually lost self-help skills over the years as the staff attended to their personal hygiene because they were 'too slow' and 'didn't make a good job of it'.

Example 2. The reinstatement of the skill of making a bed. The same principle of breaking the target behaviour into undemanding steps and immediately reinforcing desired responses is used. The above behaviour may be chained as follows:

1 Strip bed

2 Put bottom sheet in place

3 Tuck in bottom sheet

4 Place top sheet in place and tuck in

5 Add blankets

6 Add pillow

7 Add counterpane. Chain complete and target reached

It will be apparent that many self-help skills can be easily restored using this simple procedure and the resultant successes may provide considerable reinforcement for the nurse.

As an exercise you should attempt to 'chain' some simple self-help skills (for example, cleaning teeth, dressing, polishing shoes and bathing).

Gains in the area of self-help skills may produce valuable generalization as the patient becomes more acceptable to others and gains in confidence and self-esteem.

Punishment

Active punishment is not used in behaviour modification as it is not only ethically dubious but it is less effective than reinforcing desired behaviours. The patient rapidly learns that no response = no reinforcement.

Behavioural Treatments of Neurosis

By far the greatest amount of space in the literature of behaviour therapy has been devoted to the treatment of the neuroses in general and to phobias in particular.

Wolpe (1958) devised a technique called *systematic desensitization* which has become the treatment of choice for phobias and other anxiety responses and is taught to conquer the resultant feelings of anxiety.

The patient is taught a 'response antagonistic to anxiety' which often consists of training in muscular relaxation. Once the patient learns to induce a state of *relaxation*, with associated feelings of calmness, this can be used to cancel out or 'inhibit' feelings of anxiety.

The patient is asked to construct a '*hierarchy*' of anxiety-evoking situations, assisted by the therapist, ranked in ascending order from the least to the most anxiety-evoking. He is then asked to imagine the lowest item on the hierarchy while in a state of deep relaxation. Should he manage this, without becoming significantly anxious, the next item is presented and so on until the top of the hierarchy is reached without the patient experiencing the anxiety previously associated with this image. Should the patient become overwhelmingly tense during treatment, he indicates this to the therapist (usually by raising a finger) and is then asked to think about the item lower down the hierarchy and tackle the difficult step after more relaxation.

Desensitization may also be offered *in vivo*, that is in the real life situation, and, in some cases, this may be more effective than desensitization by use of the imagination.

Another approach is *flooding* wherein the patient is exposed to the most feared situation in real life and taught to master the resultant feelings of anxiety.

These treatments are often offered to the out-patient by the clinical psychologist with the participation of the psychiatric nurse, who may help teach relaxation techniques and may accompany the patient in real life exposure to feared situations.

Behavioural methods of treatment will be discussed more fully in the sections on the treatment of specific mental disorders.

Key Concepts

1 Behaviourism is a philosophical approach to psychology which contends that, if it is to be scientific, psychology must concentrate upon observable *behaviour* rather than private subjective events such as thoughts, images, and ideas.
2 Behaviour refers to '*those activities of an organism which can be observed*'.
3 Behaviour may be learned by the processes of *classical* or *operant conditioning*.
4 In classical conditioning the individual pairs or *associates* two events and learns that the two usually go together.
5 In operant conditioning the individual learns that some response made leads to a particular *consequence*.
6 Desired responses may be increased in frequency by arranging rewarding consequences for them, while undesired behaviour may be decreased in frequency by ensuring that it is not followed by rewarding consequences.
7 The principles of operant conditioning underlie the approach of *behaviour modification* which is used to shape behaviour in the fields of psychiatry and mental handicap.
8 Once a desired *target behaviour* has been identified, it can be reached by *chaining* the behaviour and *reinforcing* successive approximations to it.
9 Reinforcement must be immediate.
10 Gains made in one area may '*generalize*', or spread, to others.
11 Maladaptive behaviour may be inadvertently

reinforced by providing the potent reinforcers of nursing time and attention.

12 The *token economy* is a structured approach to rehabilitation based on the principles of behaviour modification.

13 Behaviour therapy includes many other approaches (for example, *systematic desensitization* and *flooding*, which are treatments sometimes used to deal with phobias).

14 In systematic desensitization in imagination, the patient gradually learns to overcome his phobic anxiety by imagining previously anxiety-provoking scenes whilst relaxed or comfortably hypnotized.

15 In flooding, the patient is exposed to the situation identified as most anxiety-evoking, without a hierarchical approach, and is taught to master the resultant anxiety levels.

References

Ayllon, T. & Azrin, N. (1968) *The Token Economy: A Motivational System for Therapy and Rehabilitation.* New York: Appleton-Century-Crofts.

Eysenck, H. J. (1960) *Handbook of Abnormal Psychology.* London: Pitman Books.

Eysenck, H. J. & Rachman, S. (1961) *The Causes and Cures of Neurosis.* London: Routledge and Kegan Paul.

Hilgard, E., Atkinson, R. & Atkinson, R. C. (1979) *Introduction to Psychology.* New York: Harcourt Brace Jovanovich.

Mackay, D. (1975) *Clinical Psychology. Theory and Therapy.* London: Methuen.

Seligman, M. (1973) *Helplessness. On Depression, Development and Death.* San Francisco: W. H. Freeman.

Wolpe, J. (1958) *Psychotherapy by Reciprocal Inhibition.* California: Stanford University Press.

Wolpe, J. (1976) *Theme and Variations. A Behaviour Therapy Casebook.* Oxford: Pergamon Press.

11

The Process of Nursing

> . . . the desire to help another person does not mean that
> we have the ability to do so . . . (it must) be developed
> in relation to the circumstances of daily life
>
> *Dorothea Oram*

The 'process of nursing' is the term used to describe an expression of the planned philosophy of individualized patient care, which tries to see past the diagnostic 'label', and considers the patient as a whole person.

It emphasizes the importance of comprehensively assessing the patient's needs, and planning individualized nursing interventions designed to meet them.

Nursing has been defined as

> 'primarily assisting the individual (sick or well) in the performance of those activities contributing to health, or its recovery, that he would perform unaided if he had the necessary strength, will or knowledge. It is likewise the unique contribution of nursing to help the individual to be independent of such assistance as soon as possible'
>
> (*Henderson, 1966*).

In psychiatric nursing it is perhaps particularly important to help the patient gain the necessary 'strength, will and knowledge' to enable him to regain normal functioning, and it is also essential that the psychiatric nurse is conscious of the importance of helping the individual to become 'independent of such assistance as soon as possible'. The psychiatric nurse must learn to 'let go' as soon as it is practicable, despite the fact that this 'letting go' may seem contrary to her basic 'nursing instincts'.

The nurse may be regarded as a temporary substitute for what the patient lacks to make him 'complete', 'whole', or 'independent' (Henderson, 1966) and movement towards these goals should motivate the whole range of nursing activities.

The process of nursing is an expression of the philosophy used to promote growth, or movement, in these directions.

Why the Process of Nursing?

Chapman (1983) has commented that 'nursing is still task-orientated, largely based on the medical model, and hidebound by tradition' (Chapman, 1983).

The term 'task orientation' refers to the fact that much of traditional nursing consisted of reducing patient care to a series of tasks, designed to maximize physical comfort, and organized around the patient's diagnostic 'label'. These tasks would then be assigned to members of the ward team and there would be sporadic outbursts of nursing activity as tasks were completed. A wave of activity would take place as pressure areas were cared for, medicines administered or dressings done.

The organization of patient care was dominated by inflexible 'ward routine' and waves of activity would be initiated at the start of each shift as the nurse in charge allotted tasks to members of the ward team. The junior nurse was expected to quickly familiarize herself with 'ward routine' and organize her nursing activities around it.

Such a regime creates the risk that the nurse may come to see the patient in terms of the number and type of tasks he was likely to generate, rather than seeing him as a person. It also creates the risk that the criterion of the nurse's efficiency may come to be the speed with which she performs allotted tasks and familiarizes herself with routine, thus placing routine before patients.

The patient's day was thus dominated by the rhythms of ward routine, as were the nurses' perceptions of her role.

Nurse/patient interactions tended to be fragmentary and disorganized in such a setting, as nurse/patient contact tended to be high during the completion of tasks and low between waves of task completion activity. Nurses were not encouraged to develop an awareness of the physical, psychological and social effects of the patient's illness but instead the critical dimensions of the patient were often seen as the physical problems he presented, each being responded to by the performance of the appropriate nursing task.

Nursing care was considered as being satisfactory when tasks were matched with problems and, often, little consideration was given to areas of psychological and social functioning which did not generate appropriate nursing tasks.

Peaks of nursing activity were often interspersed with troughs of low patient-centred activity. Much lip service has been paid to the principle of 'talking to patients' though, in practice, many nurses felt uneasy at the prospect of anything other than superficial interactions, as the roles of nurse and patient may be psychologically and socially distanced.

The Patient Role

Jourard (1964) has commented that, despite lip service to the principle of establishing empathy with patients, much nursing activity seemed aimed at getting patients to 'conform to the roles they are supposed to play in the social system of the hospital, so that the system will work smoothly, work will get done faster, and the patients will be less of a bother to care for'.

The submissive nature of the patient role is often well-illustrated in psychiatric nursing when the 'ideal patient' may be approvingly described as being 'clean, quiet and cooperative'.

Patients may be ill-informed about diagnosis, treatment and nursing care, with the result that needless levels of anxiety and resentment may develop. Task orientation does not lend itself to the establishment of empathy with the patient, and the result may be that hospitalization is experienced as dehumanizing and alienating.

Nurse will Make it Better

Or will she? Illich (1976) has discussed the potentially harmful effects of medical care and discusses three categories of *iatrogenesis* (damage caused by the medical system). He describes 'clinical iatrogenesis' (physical damage inadvertently caused by doctors during treatment), social iatrogenesis (the addiction of people to medical care as a solution to all their problems) and 'structural iatrogenesis' (the destruction of the patient's autonomy, along with the expropriation of his/her responsibility for individual health care).

Social iatrogenesis, as reflected in the patient's tendency to 'medicalize' all life problems and seek medical solutions to non-medical problems, may be intensified by overprotective nursing, particularly in the field of psychiatry. The end result may be the patient who responds to all life crises and difficulties by seeking prescriptions for antidepressants or anxiolytics instead of attempting to cope with the causes of stress, and arriving at lasting and adaptive solutions.

Structural iatrogenesis has been widely described in psychiatry where long-term institutional care may lead to the syndrome of 'institutionalization', characterized by loss of autonomy and individuality. Inflexible ward routines and authoritarian nursing attitudes have been identified as critical factors in the development of this state (Barton, 1976).

Nursing interventions based on the task-orientated approach, however well-intended, may create the risk that high levels of anxiety and dependence are created in the patient, who may also develop distorted perceptions of his/her own health status.

Task orientation denies the 'wholeness' of the patient and incorporates dangerous 'blind spots' in respect of vital areas of psychological and social functioning.

What has perpetuated task orientation for so long? Old habits die hard. Chapman (1983) has commented that 'The adherence to tradition highlights that nurses are the greatest hindrance to progress in nursing'.

What is so Different about the Process of Nursing?

It has been said that 'The Process is not new in nursing; the "good" nurse has always used it' (Roper et al, 1981). In other words nurses have often assessed patients' needs in a comprehensive fashion and have planned nursing care accordingly, evaluating the efficacy of the care plan as they implemented it. What was lacking was an analytical approach to solving patient's problems and a method of ensuring that all members of the care team were aware, not only of the problems identified, but of the stratagems agreed upon to reduce them.

A key component of the process approach is the systematic and orderly assessment of the needs of the patient and the careful selection of nursing interventions appropriate to those needs. Once identified, the nursing interventions are carefully organized as an individualized *nursing care plan* and the success of the plan is monitored, or evaluated, in an ongoing way.

The nursing care plan should take account of the fact that health has three dimensions—physical, psychological and social—and needs in all three areas should be met where possible.

The process of nursing thus has four components:
1 Assessment
2 Planning
3 Implementation
4 Evaluation
It is a philosophy of nursing, and the instrument of its application is the nursing care plan.

All aspects of the plan should be clearly and carefully documented and must be readily available to all staff involved in the patient's care, and all care given should be recorded.

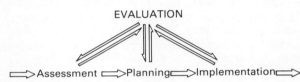

Figure 9 The process of nursing.

Assessment

Roper (1976) listed twelve *activities of living* in respect of which patients may have actual or potential health problems and with which they may therefore require assistance. The twelve activities of living (ALs) listed are as follows:

1 *Maintaining a safe environment*

Has the patient any sensory deficit (poor eyesight, poor hearing or any loss of sensation)? Are adjustments in the patient's environment necessary due to confusion or suicidal feelings?

2 *Communication*

Does the patient communicate freely or is he withdrawn and uncommunicative. Is the content of his speech coherent and rational or does it reflect underlying thought disorder? Is he anxious or suspicious? Does he maintain eye contact? Are his non-verbal communications congruent with his verbal ones? Can he read and write? Remember that communication can be affected by mood, level of intelligence, personality traits and current awareness of reality.

3 *Expressing sexuality*

Do the patient's attitudes reflect an appropriate level of psychosexual maturity? Does the patient express sexual fears or anxieties? Does the patient express disordered sexual thoughts or feelings?

4 *Working and Playing*

What is the patient's occupation? Where does he work? Are there any indications of difficulties in the work situation? What are his hobbies and interests? Is he socially active or isolated? Are difficulties in interpersonal and social relationships apparent? Does he have many friends?

5 *Sleeping*

Does the patient suffer from insomnia? Does he feel refreshed or unrefreshed on waking? Does he suffer from 'early morning waking'? Is his mood worse in the mornings? Does he take sleeping tablets? Does he waken during the night? At what time does he usually retire to bed? What factors increase or decrease his sleep? Does he suffer from nightmares?

6 *Eating and drinking*

Does the patient take an adequate diet? Is there any evidence of anorexia or food refusal? Does the patient express delusional beliefs about his food? Is there any indication of excessive alcohol consumption or loss of control over alcohol consumption? Is the patient well-nourished or undernourished? Does he eat alone or with others? Is the patient able to eat and drink independently?

7 *Personal cleansing and dressing*

Is there evidence of self-neglect or loss of interest in personal hygiene? Does the patient express an interest in his/her appearance? Is there any loss of self-help skills in relation to cleansing and dressing? Does the patient require assistance with cleansing and dressing due to confusion? Does the patient's clothing reflect financial hardship?

8 *Breathing*

Does the anxious patient complain of difficulty in breathing or 'tightness in the chest'? Does he have any pain or discomfort associated with breathing? Does the patient smoke? If so, how many a day? Is he smoking more or less lately? Does he have anxieties associated with smoking?

9 *Eliminating*

Does the patient experience frequency of micturition? Does he have constipation associated with low food/fluid intake? Does he express delusional beliefs about bowel function?

10 *Mobilization*

Is the patient physically active/overactive/inactive? Does the patient with cerebral pathology have any paralysis/anaesthesia/muscular pain or discomfort?

11 *Controlling body temperature*

Is there any evidence of flushing, excessive perspiration, goose flesh or shivering? Is there any evidence of pyrexia or hypothermia in the confused patient who may not be able to express any associated feelings of discomfort? Does the drug addict or alcoholic who may have been 'living rough' have any evidence of infection, as evidenced by pyrexia?

12 *Dying*

Does the patient express fears of death unjustified by his physical condition? Does he express suicidal or homicidal feelings? Is the patient preoccupied by fears of death? Remember that the elderly patient with chronic brain failure may develop terminal illness and require the specific nursing care appropriate to the dying patient; in other words, the nurse should ensure that he is permitted to die with peace and dignity.

In the above, the original AL model has been retained in outline but the emphasis has been shifted towards the sort of areas of psychosocial dysfunction that the psychiatric nurse may expect to encounter. Many patients in the psychiatric hospital will have actual or potential physical problems.

The AL model also touches upon areas of psychosocial functioning though it requires modification if it is to be used as a framework for assessment in the psychiatric hospital, as it was primarily intended for use in non-psychiatric areas.

Many, if not most, of the patients in the psychiatric hospital may be in a good state of physical health, however, and it may then be more appropriate to consider the psychological and social areas of functioning (psychosocial functioning) in greater detail in order to identify actual or potential problems.

Assessing psychosocial needs

One way of considering human behaviour is based on the assumption that each individual has a wide range of physical, psychological and social *needs*, and that our range of behaviour is primarily concerned with meeting these needs.

A need is a deficiency state which gives rise to *drives* aimed at fulfilling the need. For example a deficiency of food and water would constitute a *need* which would give rise to the drive to eat and drink, thus satisfying the need.

During a period of illness, however, the patient's ability to meet his own needs may be impaired, and they may remain unsatisfied.

Abraham Maslow, an American humanistic psychologist, suggested that needs are the primary influence on human behaviour and further suggested that human behaviour is best understood by developing awareness of unsatisfied needs (Maslow, 1970).

Maslow suggested a method of studying needs by arranging the main human needs in a hierarchical structure of five need systems, arranged in ascending order.

At the bottom of his hierarchy he placed the *basic physiological needs* (hunger, thirst and related needs) followed by *safety needs* (need to feel secure and out of danger) *belongingness and love needs, esteem needs*, and, at the top of the hierarchy, *self actualization needs* (needs to find self-fulfilment and realize one's potential) (Figure 10).

Maslow suggested that needs at lower levels must be satisfied before we can progress up the hierarchy to satisfy needs at higher levels. If the satisfaction of higher needs is blocked the individual may return to behaviours that fulfil needs at a lower level.

If we imagine a castaway on a desert island, his immediate and most pressing need would be to find food and water to satisfy his basic physiological needs.

He may then progress to building a shelter to fulfil his safety needs. Once he has ensured food, water and shelter he may well be afflicted with loneliness, may feel the need for the company of others; in other words, he may become conscious of the fact that his belongingness needs are unsatisfied. He may then partially meet this need by capturing and domesticating wild animals or birds, and making pets of them, and then move further up the hierarchy to satisfy his esteem needs by showing ingenuity and competence in making his island more 'liveable' by

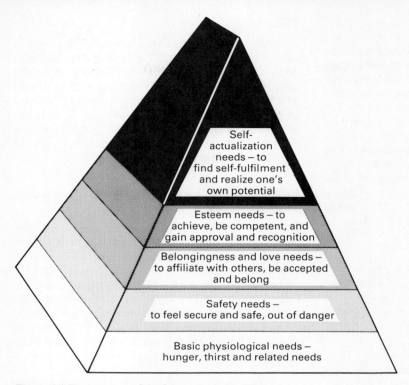

Self-
actualization
needs – to
find self-fulfilment
and realize one's
own potential

Esteem needs – to
achieve, be competent, and
gain approval and recognition

Belongingness and love needs –
to affiliate with others, be accepted
and belong

Safety needs –
to feel secure and safe, out of danger

Basic physiological needs –
hunger, thirst and related needs

Figure 10 The structure of the five need systems (Maslow).

cultivating crops, diverting water sources and otherwise making his mark on his environment. Should a storm suddenly destroy his shelter and imperil his crops he would, however, revert to the lowest level of the hierarchy as the satisfaction of basic needs was again threatened.

So it is with mental disorder. The storm of stress may destroy psychological and social equilibrium and the individual may revert to satisfying lower level needs in a suddenly threatening world.

For example the patient suffering from depression may develop a negative view of self and be unable to effectively satisfy belongingness needs—self-esteem is often noticeably low in depression. The result may be that the patient is unable to effectively reach the next level of esteem needs and this may generate the drive to search for approval from others. Remember that what other people think of us may determine, to a greater or lesser extent, what we think of ourselves.

Chronic anxiety may lead to fixation at the level of satisfying safety needs, at the expense of success in the higher areas of belongingness and esteem.

The patient tormented by delusions of persecution may revert to the level of only effectively satisfying basic physiological needs. His feelings of threat may be so overwhelming and preoccupying that his needs for belongingness and esteem are completely blocked, and this may be reflected in his poor relationships with others and his high levels of tension and dissatisfaction.

This is not to say that any need is ever completely satisfied, though the individual must at least partially fulfil a lower need level before progressing to the satisfaction of higher need levels.

Only when basic and safety needs are met is the individual able to expand his behaviour to include relationships with others. Fixation at lower need levels is a noticeable feature of many mental disorders, and successful treatment and nursing care may enable the patient to resolve the difficulties leading to behavioural stagnation, thus enabling progress to the satisfaction of higher need levels.

In assessing this area of functioning the nurse should take a comprehensive 'nursing history' and should consider the following points:

1 *Patient's perception of his own level of functioning*. What does he complain of? What troubles him? What does he feel unable to do? Has there been a discernible change in the level of psychosocial functioning of late?—if so, how has it manifested itself? What does he wish he were able to do? How are his relationships with others—at home/work/socially? Is he socially active or inactive? Does he identify any sources of stress? Have there been any recent crises or changes in life circumstances? Are his expressions of self-image positive or negative? What does he like and dislike about himself? Does he consider himself to have a problem or problems? Does he see himself as 'sick'? What is his attitude towards his current difficulties? Does he see himself as being in need of help?

2 *Nurse's perception of the patient's functioning*. Objective assessment is important and value judgements should be avoided. The modified activities of living model may prove useful in providing points of reference.

3 *Others' perception of the patient's functioning*. How do 'significant others' (family, spouse, friends) feel about the patient's level of functioning? Is there social/domestic stress? Do they express anxieties or doubts about his thinking, mood or behaviour? What does he complain of to them? What changes have they noticed? Are they supportive of him? Is he insightful about his difficulties? How has his behaviour affected the family unit?

By gathering information from the above sources the nurse should be able to compile a clear profile of the patient's level of functioning and may thus identify both actual and potential problems. It is essential that accurate assessment is made as soon as possible in order that the nursing care plan takes account of all problem areas to produce intervention that is both appropriate and effective. Assessment lets us decide upon the direction care should take and, if assessment is patchy or incomplete, care may be directed towards the wrong areas.

The above principles of assessment may be incorporated in a simple assessment form (see Appendix 2) and in the patient's 'nursing history'.

Assessment may now be followed by the planning of nursing care objectives, and these should be structured in the form of a nursing care plan which should also be incorporated in the nursing history.

Planning

Planning of nursing care should involve drawing up a list of clear statements of the expected outcomes of care—the nursing objectives. Where possible, discussion with the patient and his family should take place to establish realistic objectives of patient care. Objectives should, where possible, be stated in observable or measurable terms so that subsequent evaluation may be effective. Planning should involve consideration of:

1 *Identification of nursing interventions appropriate to the patient's needs*

That is, the selection of routes by which nursing goals or objectives may be reached. For example, the objective of restoring lost self-help skills may be aimed at by deciding upon a simple programme of behaviour modification. Deficient communication skills may be aided by involving the patient in ward discussion groups. The confused and disorientated patient may be involved in reality orientation groups. The patient who is lacking in social skills may be given assertive training.

2 *Selection of a suitable environment*

Does the patient require high levels of nursing observation? (for example, the confused or suicidal patient) Would a measure of quiet and privacy be more appropriate initially (for example, in the case of the patient undergoing drug or alcohol withdrawal or the acutely anxious patient) or would the patient benefit from the presence of others? (for example, the withdrawn or uncommunicative patient) Would the patient benefit from occupational, industrial or social therapy?

3 *Consideration of available personnel*

Has assessment revealed problems with which the social worker or community psychiatric nurse or recreational therapist may be able to help? Is nursing coverage appropriate in terms of numbers, level of preparation and previous experience?

Having selected appropriate environment, personnel and nursing interventions the nursing care plan can then be prepared to utilize these resources for the patient's benefit.

The nursing care plan should identify the planned

nursing activities in sufficient detail and in clear and unambiguous language so that any other nurse, on reading the plan, would be aware of and could carry out the planned nursing activities.

Continual revision of the nursing care plan will be required as additional data is collected from ongoing assessment or if it becomes apparent that nursing interventions are not producing the expected outcome. The nursing care plan must not become static, otherwise nursing care will simply stagnate, and progress towards care objectives will slow down or cease altogether.

The nursing care plan, and its revisions, should also be incorporated in the nursing history and must be available to all nursing staff.

Implementation

The third stage in the process of nursing is implementation, or actually carrying out the prepared plan. A day-to-day record of implementation should be kept and it should record the following facts:

Which activity was carried out
When the activity was carried out
Who carried out the activity
The patient's responses to the activity

The recording sheets should also be placed in the nursing history so that a clear record of the implementation of the nursing care plan is compiled.

All team members should have an opportunity to discuss their contributions and any observations they have made. The progress of the nursing care plan should also be discussed with the patient so that he is kept 'in the swim'. Relatives should also be informed of progress and the basis of the care plan should be explained to them.

Evaluation

Evaluation is the process of determining whether the objectives of nursing care have been realized. Evaluation should be continuous and begins from the moment the nurse begins to interact with the patient. Evaluation should occur simultaneously with all nursing care though more formal and structured evaluation, involving as many team members as possible, should be undertaken at a stated time or in response to changing circumstances. If expected outcomes are not being reached the possible reasons

should be discussed and the nursing care plan reformulated if necessary. The opinion of the patient and relatives concerning the outcomes should also be considered.

Examples of objectives which may have been successfully realized include:

Decrease in maladaptive behaviours
Increase in adaptive behaviours
Reduction of feelings of unhappiness, aggression, insecurity or anxiety
Increase in feelings of efficiency, autonomy, self-esteem and confidence
Positive attitudinal change

The patient may discard the 'sick' or dependent role and show evidence of having developed positive interpersonal stratagems for coping with the stresses of everyday living. This may be coupled with heightened awareness of the self-damaging consequences of past behavioural patterns.

Behavioural changes are visible, and can thus be readily evaluated. Changes in mood and thinking may be reported by the patient, though associated behavioural change may be apparent.

Key Concepts

1 The process of nursing is an expression of the philosophy of individualized patient care, which tries to see past the diagnostic 'label' and considers the patient as a whole person.
2 Nursing is more than a series of tasks.
3 The process of nursing consists of the following four components: *assessment, planning, implementation* and *evaluation*.
4 The instrument of the application of this philosophy is the *nursing care plan*.
5 Assessment takes account of the three components of health—*physical, psychological* and *social*.
6 Assessment may be organized around the framework of the twelve activities of living.
7 Psychosocial functioning may be further assessed by identifying any 'behavioural stagnation' arising from incomplete or blocked *need satisfaction*.
8 Assessment should generate the production of nursing *care objectives*, which should be stated in clear and unmistakeable language using, where possible, observable or measurable terms.

9 The second phase, planning, entails matching appropriate nursing interventions to the care objectives, thus formulating the nursing care plan.
10 The nursing care plan must be available to all nursing staff so that all are aware of the planned activities.
11 The third stage in the process is implementation, or actually carrying out the prepared plan.
12 The nursing care plan must not become static, otherwise nursing care will simply stagnate, and progress towards care objectives will slow down or cease altogether.
13 Evaluation should be continuous and should involve as many team members as possible.
14 The process of nursing is not an end in itself but is a means towards the end of patient-centred care.

References

Barton, R. (1976) *Institutional Neurosis, 3rd edn.* Bristol: Wright.

Chapman, C. M. (1983) The paradox of nursing. *Journal of Advanced Nursing*, **8**: 269–272.

Henderson, V. (1966) *Basic Principles of Nursing Care.* Geneva: International Council of Nurses.

Illich, I. (1976) *Limits to Medicine.* Harmondsworth: Penguin Books.

Jourard, S. M. (1964) *The Transparent Self.* New York: Van Nostrand.

Maslow, A. (1970) *Motivation and Personality, 2nd edn.* New York: Harper & Row.

Roper, N. (1976) *Clinical Experience in Nurse Education.* Edinburgh: Churchill Livingstone.

Roper, N., Logan, W. W. & Tierney, A. J. (1981) *Learning to Use the Process of Nursing.* Edinburgh: Churchill Livingstone.

III

THE AFFECTIVE DISORDERS

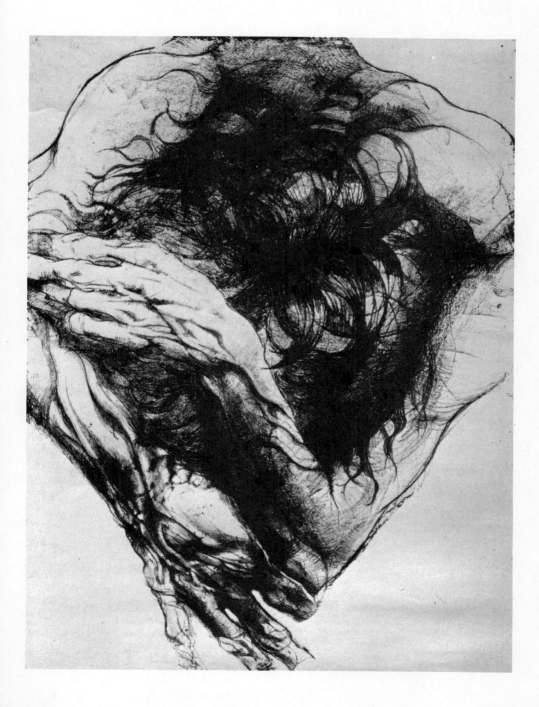

12

Depression

> I was much further out than you thought
> And not waving but drowning
> I was much too far out all of my life
> And not waving but drowning
>
> *Stevie Smith*

Depression is a disorder in which mood and vitality are lowered to the point of distress. Self may seem worthless and the world meaningless and there may be pervasive feelings of misery, hopelessness and despair. The depressed person may brood over past failures or losses, real or imagined, and the future may seem hopelessly bleak. The risk of suicide is often high.

Depression may be a reaction to a significant *loss*, whether this takes the form of loss of a loved one, loss of security or stability (as in unemployment, divorce, failed examinations) or loss of well-being associated with a painful, threatening or chronic illness. Relationship problems are a contributory factor in 50% of depressions involving young women and here it may be a response to the loss of an idea; for example, infidelity may bring about the loss of the idea that the patient was loved to the exclusion of others, with an attendant loss of security.

Depression occurring as an unusually prolonged or intense reaction to loss is called *reactive* or *exogenous* depression and is classified as a neurosis, thus being often called *neurotic depression*.

Particularly severe depression may also arise *without* any discernible cause in external events, seeming to arise from 'within' the patient. This type of depression is called *endogenous* depression (Gk. *endos*—within) and is classified as a psychosis, thus being referred to as *psychotic depression*.

In endogenous depression genetic and biochemical factors are important, as opposed to environmental events, though these may act as precipitating factors. Delusions are not uncommon in endogenous depression and these often reflect underlying despair and torment as they take the form of feelings of guilt, sin, worthlessness, poverty or hypochondriasis. Feelings of self-blame and self-punishment prevail and the mood may be one of abject misery.

Endogenous depression may be part of an overall disorder of mood in which depression alternates with mania—*bipolar affective psychosis* (manic-depressive psychosis) or mood may be persistently lowered or elevated, without alternations between the two extremes—*unipolar affective psychosis*.

Opinion is divided as to whether the distinction between neurotic and psychotic depression is a valid one. Many clinicians view the field of depressive disorders as a spectrum or continuum, with reactive depression at one extreme, moderate and mixed depressions in the middle, and psychotic depression at the other, the suggestion being that patients may move from one extreme towards the other.

How Common is Depression?

Depression is one of the commonest states known to mankind and was described in antiquity, for example the description of King Saul's melancholy contained in the Old Testament.

About one in ten of the population will suffer from depression (Ingram et al, 1981) and women are twice as likely to be affected as men (Paykel and Rowan, 1979). The prevalence of depression is higher in younger women and tends to decrease with age, while the opposite pattern is found in males, where the prevalence is lower in young men and increases with age (Weissman and Myers, 1978). Reactive depression is twice as common as endogenous depression and the overall incidence of depression in the UK seems to be rising (Dally and Harrington, 1975).

Risk Factors for Depression

Sex

The higher incidence of depression in women has been noted in many studies, and various explanations have been offered. Women may complain more readily of depression than men and may be more prepared to discuss troublesome feelings and seek treatment. This may be in keeping with the artificially created role of the 'weaker sex', and may reflect a socialization process which ascribes to women an essentially passive and dependent gender role.

Women's life circumstances may also make them more vulnerable, as in the case of young married women, especially those with young children, who suffer a degree of social isolation in their roles of 'housewife' and 'mother' which may supersede all social roles obtaining before marriage. The role of 'housewife' may be accompanied by low prestige, lack of companionship, lack of social fulfilment and worries about financial matters and child rearing.

An American study of depressed hospitalized women revealed that women who had employment outside the home recovered more quickly than housewives (Mostow and Newberry, 1975), and another study suggests that women in employment outside the home present fewer symptoms (and recover more quickly) than housewives (Nathanson, 1975).

A confiding and sympathetic relationship with a sympathetic partner, be it husband or boyfriend, is thought to reduce the likelihood of depression developing, and the absence of such a relationship increases the risk. In marriages where the husband is the dominant partner and the wife is relegated to a secondary role the wife must do most of the adjusting, and self-esteem and satisfaction are likely to diminish, thus increasing vulnerability to depression.

Biological explanations have also been offered for the higher female incidence of depression, and vulnerability increases during the pre-menstrual period and after childbirth or hysterectomy (Miles, 1981) though it may be difficult to separate the latter two events from their symbolic social significance and thus ascribe a purely biological basis to them. The concept of pre-menstrual tension also remains a rather contentious one and there is debate about the usefulness of the concept.

Fertility is reduced by about 30% in women with major mood disorders when compared to the rest of the female population (Winokur, 1981).

Age

The female risk of depression seems to decrease with age while the male risk increases. Suicide rates are higher for elderly males while parasuicide rates are highest for young females. Endogenous depressions tend to have a later age of onset than reactive types.

A number of studies suggest that the incidence and prevalence rates of depression in women reach a peak at the age range 35–45 years and there is no evidence of an increase in incidence associated with the menopause (Boyd and Weissman, 1982).

Social class

Depressive disorders seem to be concentrated in working class women, especially those with children under six years of age. One study of depressed women (Brown and Harris, 1978) revealed clinical depression in 23% of working class women compared with only 6% of middle class women in the population studied. There was no class difference in risk of developing depression among women without children. This study further indicated that middle class women seem surprisingly protected against depression once they have children, while areas of life difficulty tend to last for much longer with working class women.

Stressful life events experienced by working class women were more numerous and more severe and the study went on to list four vulnerability factors which increase the risk of depression. These were:
1 Lack of a close confiding relationship
2 Loss of a mother before the age of 11 years
3 Having three or more children under the age of 14 years living in the house
4 Lack of employment outside the home (Brown and Harris, 1978).

These findings are supported by studies which indicate that working class marriages are more likely to be characterized by lack of communication and intimacy (Komarovsky, 1967) and by segregation of marital roles, that is separate leisure activities, social relationships and separate duties (Bott, 1957).

Bipolar affective disorder (manic-depressive psychosis) seems to occur more frequently in the upper socio-economic classes (Boyd and Weissman, 1982) unlike schizophrenia, which seems to occur more frequently in the lower socio-economic classes.

This anomaly of distribution may be partially due to diagnostic bias and it has also been suggested that it may arise as a result of a particular personality type predisposing both to the disorder and to a rise in the social scale (Boyd and Weissman, 1982). Patients with bipolar disorders are more likely to be highly educated than patients with depression alone (Winokur, 1981) and increased drive in bipolar disorder may account for this level of educational attainment and the resultant potential for a rise in social class.

Family history

There is much evidence to suggest a genetic component in the affective psychoses insofar as both unipolar and bipolar disorders show familial trends. The disorder, or the predisposition to it, may be transmitted on the X chromosome (the sex chromosome). A father can only contribute his X chromosome to a daughter (female chromosomal arrangement is XX) whereas to a son he gives his Y chromosome (male chromosomal arrangement is XY). As a woman has two X chromosomes and a man has only one, women are roughly twice as likely as men to develop unipolar or bipolar affective disorder. X chromosome 'markers', like colour blindness, have been used in studies which suggest 'X-linkage' in the transmission of the affective psychoses, though these findings remain contentious.

Twin studies show concordance rates of 70% for monozygotic twins and 20% for dizygotic twins, compared to an incidence of 1% in the general population and 10–15% in first relatives (Ingram et al, 1981). These findings further support the case for the importance of genetic factors, though, if the disorder were to be exclusively determined, genetically one would expect concordance rates of 100% in monozygotic twins. A predisposition or vulnerability to the disorder may be transmitted, unlike the disorder itself which may not be transmitted.

No relationship between reactive (neurotic) depression and family history has yet been clearly demonstrated and it seems improbable that reactive depression is substantially determined genetically.

Personality type

Depression seems more likely in persons with the following personality characteristics: Likelihood to break down under stress, lack of energy, insecurity, introversion, sensitivity, tendency to worry, social 'awkwardness', unassertiveness, dependency and obsessionality (Boyd and Weissman, 1982).

These characteristics may reflect social stresses and pressures as well as the influence of heredity. Childhood experiences may contribute substantially to the formation of these traits. For example, there is evidence that a disruptive, hostile and negative environment in a child's home constitutes a risk factor for depression (Boyd and Weissman, 1982).

The Chemistry of Depression

Heredity often expresses itself biochemically, and the possible importance of biochemical factors in depression was demonstrated when it was revealed that the drug reserpine often caused depression. Reserpine depletes the brain of compounds called *monoamines* which are involved in the transmission of nerve impulses. 'Reserpine depression' is most likely to arise in patients treated with reserpine who have a past history of depression and it is possible that the drug somehow activates a tendency already present in the patient.

The group of antidepressant drugs known as *monoamine oxidase inhibitors* act by increasing the concentration of monoamines, and there is some recent evidence that electroplexy (which relieves major depressions) does likewise (Trethowan and Sims, 1983). Tricyclic antidepressants also increase monoamine concentrations, while the drug lithium seems to control mania by reducing the level of monoamines.

Research into the chemistry of depression continues though there is some debate as to whether reported fluctuations in cerebral chemistry are the cause or the effect of depression.

'Learned helplessness'

The psychologist Seligman (1975) demonstrated that a state of passive 'helplessness' may be experimentally induced in dogs exposed to electric shocks which they cannot escape. This 'learned helplessness' was carried into later situations by the dogs and they failed to escape electric shocks when this was made possible. Seligman suggests that this resembles human depression which may also result from situations in which there is helplessness and threat outside the subject's control.

Miscellaneous factors

Depression is not uncommon after severe attacks of influenza but is usually both mild and of short duration. Some widely used drugs may also induce depression (e.g. some oral contraceptives, barbiturates, methyldopa, benzhexol and dexidrine) though the likelihood of a depressive response to these agents is increased if there is a past history of depression; that is, the drugs may simply act on a predisposition to the disorder. Anti-Parkinsonism drugs may cause depression (e.g. benzhexol) but in this case it may be difficult to separate the effects of the drug from responses to the illness or responses to the hospitalization which may precede the use of the drug.

In summarizing the possible aetiological factors in depression it seems that genetic factors are involved in endogenous depression and that these factors may be expressed biochemically. Social factors (loss, deprivation, stress, hardship) seem to be more critical in reactive depressions though they may also serve to precipitate a latent endogenous depression.

Prognosis for Depression

Depression does not cause permanent damage or mental deterioration and, in general, a person who has been severely depressed for a very long time can be expected to make a complete recovery (Watts, 1973). Many effective treatments are available, though early recognition and treatment are important if the risk of suicide is to be reduced and if the individual and her family are to be spared extreme distress.

Symptoms of Depression

The symptoms of reactive and endogenous depression overlap insofar as both have many features in common—the core symptoms of depression. Reactive depression is a neurosis, so insight is retained and delusions are absent, whereas endogenous depression is a psychosis, so insight may be lost or impaired and delusions, rarely hallucinations, may be present.

Depression has physical, psychological and social effects and these manifest themselves as follows:

Physical

Activity is reduced and the patient may spend much time brooding morosely. Facial expression is sad and careworn and the patient may stare bleakly into space and reply slowly and haltingly to questions. The tone of voice may be flat and monotonous and there may be a marked 'dullness' to responses. On occasion the patient may be seen to wring his/her hands and utter exclamations of despair. The patient may also be seen to rock monotonously back and forth and may pick at the skin or gnaw the lower lip. General appearance reflects the patient's lack of interest, and clothing may be unkempt and personal hygiene neglected. The eyes have a dull and lacklustre appearance and nutritional state may be poor. Movements are often tired and despondent and the patient may seek a quiet corner of the ward where he/she may sit in a state of wretched isolation. The very company of fellow patients may be irksome and social or group activities are avoided.

Endogenous depressions may assume either a retarded or agitated form and, in the latter, restlessness and purposeless activity may be noticeable. In retarded forms psychomotor retardation may be extreme and the patient may spend much time lying in bed in an almost stuporous extreme of depression.

In some cases there may be attempts to overcome the depression and the patient may smilingly deny depression—the so-called 'smiling depression'. The depressive smile is tight and wan, and expressed claims of adjustment have a hollow and superficial ring. Between 'smiles' the face reveals deeply etched signs of tension and depression, and shows of enforced gaiety rarely last for long.

The patient may experience feelings of *depersonalization* and *derealization*, that is, the patient may feel the self or the environment to be strangely unreal. Patients may describe these feelings by saying that voices seem to filter through faintly, as though through an auditory 'fog', and may add that they feel strangely divorced from their environment, as though they were spectators at some strange and meaningless game.

Derealization and depersonalization added to overall loss of drive and vitality and feelings of abject misery increase the likelihood of the patient shunning the company of others and engaging in conversation slowly and hesitantly.

In some depressive states elements of anxiety or agitation may coexist with the core symptoms of depression, and the patient may complain of aches and pains, palpitations, tachycardia, blurred vision, dizziness, dry mouth, headache or nausea. Restlessness and anxiety may become extreme and the risk of suicide is increased in this situation.

Beck depression inventory

This inventory measures feelings and behaviours common in depression and relates them to the overall level of depression.

Read over the statements grouped with each letter, *A–U*. Pick out the statement within each group that best describes the way you feel today, that is, right at this moment. Circle the number next to the statement that you have chosen in each group. If two or more statements in a group describe the way you feel equally well, circle each one. Be sure to read over all of the statements in each group before you decide on one.

A Sadness
  0 I do not feel sad.
  1 I feel blue or sad.
  2a I am blue or sad all the time and I can't snap out of it.
  2b I am so sad or unhappy that it is quite painful.
  3 I am so sad or unhappy that I can't stand it.

B Pessimism
  0 I am not particularly pessimistic or discouraged about the future.
  1 I feel discouraged about the future.
  2a I feel I have nothing to look forward to.
  2b I feel that I won't ever get over my troubles.
  3 I feel that the future is hopeless and that things cannot improve.

C Sense of failure
  0 I do not feel like a failure.
  1 I feel I have failed more than the average person.
  2a I feel I have accomplished very little that is worthwhile or that means anything.
  2b As I look back on my life all I can see is a lot of failures.
  3 I feel I am a complete failure as a person (parent, husband, wife).

D Dissatisfaction
  0 I am not particularly dissatisfied.
  1a I feel bored most of the time.
  1b I don't enjoy things the way I used to.
  2 I don't get satisfaction out of anything anymore.
  3 I am dissatisfied with everything.

E Guilt
  0 I don't feel particularly guilty.
  1 I feel bad or unworthy a good part of the time.
  2a I feel quite guilty.
  2b I feel bad or unworthy practically all the time now.
  3 I feel as though I am very bad or worthless.

F Expectation of punishment
  0 I don't feel I am being punished.
  1 I have a feeling that something bad may happen to me.
  2 I feel I am being punished or will be punished.
  3a I feel I deserve to be punished.
  3b I want to be punished.

G Self-dislike
  0 I don't feel disappointed in myself.
  1a I am disappointed in myself.
  1b I don't like myself.
  2 I am disgusted with myself.
  3 I hate myself.

H Self-accusations
  0 I don't feel I am any worse than anybody else.
  1 I am critical of myself for my weaknesses or mistakes.
  2 I blame myself for my faults.
  3 I blame myself for everything bad that happens.

I Suicidal ideas
  0 I don't have any thoughts of harming myself.
  1 I have thoughts of harming myself but I would not carry them out.
  2a I feel I would be better off dead.
  2b I feel my family would be better off if I were dead.
  3a I have definite plans about committing suicide.
  3b I would kill myself if I could.

J Crying
  0 I don't cry any more than usual.
  1 I cry more now than I used to.
  2 I cry all the time now, I can't stop it.
  3 I used to be able to cry but now I can't cry at all even though I want to.

K Irritability
  0 I am no more irritated now than I ever am.
  1 I get annoyed or irritated more easily than I used to.
  2 I feel irritated all the time.
  3 I don't get irritated at all at the things that used to irritate me.

L Social withdrawal
  0 I have not lost interest in other people.
  1 I am less interested in other people now than I used to be.
  2 I have lost most of my interest in other people.
  3 I have lost all my interest in other people and don't care about them at all.

M Indecisiveness

0 I make decisions about as well as ever.
1 I try to put off making decisions.
2 I have great difficulty in making decisions.
3 I can't make decisions at all anymore.

N Body image change

0 I don't feel I look any worse than I used to.
1 I am worried that I am looking older or unattractive.
2 I feel that there are permanent changes in my appearance and they make me look unattractive.
3 I feel that I am ugly or repulsive looking.

O Work retardation

0 I can work about as well as before.
1a It takes extra effort to get started at doing a task or job.
1b I don't work as well as I used to.
2 I have to push myself very hard to do anything.
3 I can't do any work at all.

P Insomnia

0 I can sleep as well as usual.
1 I wake up more tired in the morning than I used to.
2 I wake up 1–2 hours earlier than usual and find it hard to get back to sleep.
3 I wake up early every day and can't get more than 5 hours sleep.

Q Fatiguableness

0 I don't get any more tired than usual.
1 I get tired more easily than I used to.
2 I get tired from doing anything.
3 I get too tired to do anything.

R Anorexia

0 My appetite is no worse than usual.
1 My appetite is not as good as it used to be.
2 My appetite is much worse now.
3 I have no appetite at all anymore.

S Weight loss

0 I haven't lost much weight, if any, lately.
1 I have lost more than 5 pounds.
2 I have lost more than 10 pounds.
3 I have lost more than 15 pounds.

T Somatic preoccupation

0 I am no more concerned about my health than usual.
1 I am concerned about aches and pains or upset stomach or constipation.
2 I am so concerned with how I feel or what I feel that it's hard to think of much else.
3 I am completely absorbed in what I feel.

U Loss of libido

0 I have not noticed any recent change in my interest in sex.
1 I am less interested in sex than I used to be.
2 I am much less interested in sex now.
3 I have lost interest in sex completely.

From Beck, A. T.: Depression: causes and treatment, Philadelphia, 1967, University of Pennsylvania Press. **Scoring:** 0–9 = normal range; 10–15 = mild depression; 16–19 = mild to mod. depression; 20–29 = mod. to severe depression; 30–63 = severe depression.

Appetite may be greatly reduced (especially in endogenous forms) and weight loss may be extreme. Anorexia is variable in reactive forms and may not be a problem. In some cases compensatory overeating occurs, particularly in milder reactive depressions, and in this case it seems that the patient is attempting to provide rewards, or pleasurable experiences, in an otherwise bleak and unfulfilling world.

Sleep disorders are common in depression and may contribute greatly to overall feelings of wretchedness. *Early insomnia* is common in reactive depression; that is, the patient has difficulty in sleeping in the early part of the night. There is difficulty in falling asleep, with restlessness, broken fitful sleep and excessive dreaming. This type of sleep is unrefreshing and the patient awakes feeling fatigued and tense.

Early morning waking

This is common in endogenous depression and this term refers to the patient's tendency to wake early in the morning and to be unable to fall asleep again. Mood will be at its lowest on waking and the patient may be accustomed to watching the dawn break while smoking endless cigarettes and drinking cup after cup of coffee. At this time, while the world is still asleep and darkness still reigns, problems seem even larger than in the light of day and the patient's sense of hopelessness and despair may become overwhelming. Suicide risk is high at this time.

Libido, or sexual drive, is greatly reduced in depression and this may be one of the earliest presenting symptoms in the young married woman. If the husband has not recognized or accepted that his wife is suffering from depression, this loss of interest in sexuality may provoke considerable domestic friction which, in turn, may worsen the depression.

There may be a degree of menstrual irregularity, with amenorrhoea in some cases, and fertility is reduced.

Constipation may develop, often arising from low dietary intake, but compounded by the overall lethargy and sluggishness of depression. In endogenous depression intractable constipation may nurture delusional beliefs about bowel function. The patient may believe that his/her bowels are 'blocked' or 'rotten' or are afflicted with cancer.

Psychological Effects of Depression

Lowering of mood may be profound. The patient feels depressed, miserable and careworn. Concentration is poor and the patient may appear vague and indecisive in conversation. Loss of drive and interest are apparent and the patient may express little interest in discussion of his/her difficulties, or may attempt to minimize or dismiss them.

In reactive depression mood tends to improve with congenial company, only to deteriorate again when the patient is alone. In this case the patient may experience a lowering of mood as the day goes on, whereas in endogenous depression mood is lowest in the morning and improves as the day goes on (*diurnal variation*).

Thinking is often slow and difficult and there may be *poverty of thought* in extreme cases. In some cases the patient may show a morbid preoccupation with death or disease and there may be a marked hypochondriacal content to speech.

Intelligence and memory are well preserved, though psychomotor retardation and poor concentration may lead to poor intellectual performance and patchy amnesia.

Thought disorder may be noticeable in endogenous forms and the patient may express delusions of *guilt, sin, unworthiness, poverty* or *hypochondriasis. Nihilistic* delusions may also be expressed in endogenous depression and the patient may refuse food on the grounds that his bowels have rotted away or that he is already dead. Delusional thinking in endogenous depression usually has the underlying themes of guilt and self-punishment and the patient may dwell on his imagined sinfulness and unworthiness, citing imaginary crimes and misdemeanours to support this view.

Hypochondriacal delusions may be explained by the patient as evidence of his sins being punished by unspeakable and incurable diseases, these often being identified as a punishment from God. If strong feelings of guilt are coupled with agitation, suicide risk is particularly high.

The theme of retribution for imagined sins may be coupled with *paranoid* ideas, the patient despairingly exclaiming that his sinfulness is apparent to all, and he/she may suggest that others are to play an active role in the justly deserved punishments which are to come.

In some very severe cases of agitated endogenous depression mothers have been known suggest suicide pacts to husband and children, and some have harmed or killed their children in an attempt to expiate sins or to spare the children any more time in the unendurable agony of a flawed existence.

Reproaching auditory hallucinations may occur in endogenous forms, but are rare.

Social Effects of Depression

Loss of drive and interest leads to neglect of family and friends. The depressed housewife may cease shopping, cooking and housework and may neglect to send her children to school. This may cause considerable friction with her spouse, and angry husbands may see such women as 'lazy' or 'apathetic' or 'neglectful' or 'irresponsible' and may embark upon heated recriminations. Loss of libido will further contribute to a domestic and marital climate of deterioration and resentment, which will worsen an already deepening depression.

Impaired concentration and loss of drive and interest will lead to a record of poor work performance and mounting absenteeism, thus escalating the depression further.

Previously valued social interests and hobbies will be neglected and the depressed person may show unwillingness to go out or to mix with friends. Sometimes frantic attempts are made to overcome the mounting sense of despair and the depressed person may make attempts to 'fight back' by embarking upon a forced campaign of social activities. The depressed young woman may spend much money on clothes, cosmetics and the hairdresser and become an inveterate 'party goer' in an attempt to overcome the steadily increasing weight of depression. Solace may be sought in sexuality and the depressed young woman may 'sleep around' as a palliative against despondency. Such sexual encoun-

Table 15 Clinical features of depression.

Core symptoms (common to all depressive states)	Variations from core symptoms (endogenous depression)	(reactive depression)
Physical		
Patient appears sad and careworn. Libido decreased. Anorexia and insomnia common. Weight loss may be marked, though compensatory over-eating may occur. Associated feelings of anxiety common and patient may complain of aches and pains, palpitations and headaches. Fertility reduced.	Menstrual irregularity or amenorrhoea may occur. Early morning waking may occur (peak suicide risk). Marked anorexia common.	Early insomnia common. Sleep is fitful and unrefreshing. Anorexia also common, but over-eating occurs in some cases.
Psychological		
Reduction of vitality. Loss of drive, energy and interest. Concentration is poor and indecisiveness or indifference common. Mood is persistently low. Intelligence and memory are well preserved though psychomotor retardation may impair intellectual performance.	Insight lost or impaired. Delusional thinking may be apparent and this usually has a theme of self-blame and self-punishment. Hallucinations may occur but are rare. Mood lowest in morning. (Diurnal variation).	No loss of insight. No delusional thinking. Mood becomes worse as the day goes on.
Social		
Loss of drive and interest may lead to neglect of family, friends, occupation and previously valued social activities. The environment may be perceived as meaningless in severe cases and this may lead to social disengagement.	Pervasive feelings of misery and despair rarely respond to interventions by well-meaning friends.	Mood may lift in the company of others only to lessen when the patient is alone again.

ters are often governed by a search for acceptance, reassurance and human warmth rather than a genuine interest in sex or the person concerned. Attempts to escape into sexuality may further fuel feelings of guilt and worthlessness and may add to overall social disorganization and loss of control.

Escape may be sought in alcohol or illicit drugs, and vulnerability to lasting dependence may become high.

Spending sprees and neglect of financial responsibilities may occur and bills may accumulate, unopened and unpaid.

The depressed person's family may be driven to extremes of distress and often try to ascribe the depression to some tangible factor (overwork, relationship problems or studying) thus often confusing cause and effect, though contributory factors may assume these forms.

Attempts to fight back in the way of seeking solace in alcohol, frantic socializing, sex or other erratic departures from the pre-depressive lifestyle are unsuccessful and become more sporadic until they are usually abandoned.

As the depression deepens the person may become more and more dependent on others (particularly in reactive forms) and the depressed person may make progressively more and more demanding claims on the time and company of others, often displaying a childlike and unreasonable refusal to consider the inconvenience and impracticality of many suggestions made.

As the depression deepens further, these approaches are discarded and the world seems progressively more and more meaningless. Despair and withdrawal now tend to predominate.

Differential Diagnosis

Primary or 'true' depressive disorders must be distinguished from *secondary* depressions, that is depressions due to physical illness or associated with, and secondary to, another psychiatric disorder.

Many drugs induce depressive responses and, in

this case, the response may be transient in that discontinuation of the drug will remove the depressive symptoms. In some cases the drug seems to precipitate a latent depression which will persist after the drug has been discontinued.

In myxoedema, reduced thyroid function leads to lethargy, loss of vitality, irritability and, sometimes, paranoid delusions. This group of symptoms may mimic primary depression, and differential diagnosis is important. Parkinson's disease and Addison's disease may also mimic primary depression as both may cause lethargy, irritability and depression.

In young adults depression may be an early sign of schizophrenia, and many organic states, especially cerebral tumour or arteriosclerosis, may present with depressive symptoms. If the presenting features of depression are mainly physical, extensive physical examination and investigation should take place to exclude an underlying physical illness.

Accurate diagnosis is important if the family is to be spared much distress and if the risk of suicide is minimized by early intervention and treatment.

Treatment of Depression

In reactive depression arising from loss it is important that the patient be allowed to work through grief responses (the 'grief work') and over-zealous use of antidepressant drugs may prevent this process from occurring fully, thus preventing complete adjustment to the loss, and driving the depression 'underground'. An awareness of this fact must also be coloured by an awareness of the risk of suicide, and the importance of a supportive nurse/patient relationship as a major factor in treatment cannot be over-emphasized.

Treatment in depression may be physical (drugs and electroplexy) or non-physical (psychotherapeutic techniques).

Physical treatment

Anti-depressant drugs

There are three major groups of drugs used in the treatment of depression: *tricyclic antidepressants*, *monoamine oxidase inhibitors* and *lithium salts*.

Tricyclic antidepressants. These drugs are so called because their chemical formula contains three rings (tricyclic=three ringed) and because they are thought to act by blocking reuptake of neurotransmitters. The most widely used drugs of this type are:

Amitriptyline (Tryptizol)
Nortriptyline (Aventyl)
Protriptyline (Concordin)
Imipramine (Tofranil)
Clomipramine (Anafranil)
Desipramine (Pertofran)
Doxepin (Sinequan)

These drugs differ slightly in their effects. Amitriptyline and doxepin are more sedative in their effects and are thus suitable for depressions with an element of agitation. Protriptyline may have a slightly energizing effect and may thus be more suitable for retarded depressions.

Tricyclics may take 2–3 weeks to have maximum effect and patients should be reassured during this period as they may feel that drug therapy is failing. As tricyclics take effect, psychomotor retardation tends to improve before mood starts to lift, creating a high risk period for suicide. During intense depression, psychomotor retardation may be intense and patients may lack the volition to make a suicidal attempt. As psychomotor retardation lifts, but mood initially remains low, agitation may appear and risk of suicide increases. Mood does not lag far behind psychomotor retardation in lifting, however, and agitation should subside at this time.

Side-effects of tricyclic therapy include: dry mouth, retention of urine, dizziness, constipation, hypotension and, rarely, jaundice or blood dyscrasias. The nurse should be aware of side-effects and should report those which become troublesome to the medical staff.

Monoamine oxidase inhibitors. These are usually not the first choice in treatment because of potentially serious side-effects. They act by inactivating the enzyme monoamine oxidase, which normally 'mops up' excess of monoamines in the brain. Thus monoamine levels mount, exerting an energizing effect.

Examples of these drugs are phenelzine (Nardil) and tranylcypromine (Parnate). Side-effects include: hypotension, anorexia and insomnia, but the major potential problem is the possibility of acute episodes of hypertension, causing violent headache, palpitations and collapse. Hypertensive episodes may be precipitated by an interaction between the amino acid *tyramine* and monoamine oxidase inhibitors. Foods rich in tyramine should therefore be avoided by patients receiving this treatment. Foods which *must* be avoided are identified to the patient and include:

Cheeses
Pickled herrings
Red wines
Sherry
Fermented sausages
Fermented meats
Meat extracts

Many other drugs interact adversely with MOIAs to cause hypertension. These include:

Amphetamines
Oral hypoglycaemics
Levodopa

The nurse must be alert to the dangers of hypertension and careful observation, coupled with immediate reporting of adverse reactions, is important.

Lithium. Lithium is a naturally occurring substance which belongs to the same chemical group as sodium and potassium. It was first used experimentally in the treatment of affective disorders (disorders of mood) in 1949.

Lithium is extremely effective in bipolar and unipolar affective disorders and has a prophylactic effect in stabilizing mood. Patients maintained on lithium have fewer, and less extreme, mood swings and the drug is effective in the treatment of both manic and depressive extremes of mood.

The most widely used preparation is lithium carbonate (Priadel, Camcolit), though the nitrate and acetate are said to be equally as effective.

The drug is potentially toxic and there is a narrow margin between the therapeutic dose and toxic dose levels which give rise to troublesome side-effects. It readily crosses the blood/brain barrier and causes slowing of EEG rhythms. It is excreted almost entirely by the kidneys.

If lithium concentration in the body becomes too high, the following side-effects may develop:

Weight loss
Diarrhoea
Tremors
Slurred speech
Vomiting
Confusion
Restlessness

Convulsions
Stupor
Coma
Circulatory collapse and death

Blood levels of lithium must be carefully maintained within the therapeutic range and below the level at which side-effects may start to occur. Serial estimation of plasma lithium levels is necessary to stabilize a patient on the drug. (For advice to the patient receiving lithium therapy, see Chapter 14).

Electroplexy

Electroplexy produces good results in 70–80% of patients with major depressive disorders (Clare, 1976) and may rapidly control the symptoms of endogenous depression, but it has little effect in reactive depression. The best results are obtained in patients showing:

Severe depression with retardation
Sudden onset
Good premorbid personality
Prominent guilt feelings and delusions
Early morning waking
Worsening of symptoms in the morning (Granville-Grossman, 1971)

Like tricyclic therapy, electroplexy may cause psychomotor retardation to lift before mood, temporarily increasing suicide risk until mood lifts.

Electroplexy is also effective in reducing manic extremes of mood which may appear in bipolar affective disorders.

Electroplexy may be used effectively during the initial period of tricyclic treatment to raise mood during the 2–3 week period which elapses before the drugs take effect.

Non-physical treatment

A variety of psychotherapeutic approaches have been used effectively in the treatment of depression and may be particularly effective in the treatment of reactive depressions. The nurse may play an active role in many of these treatments which include:

Group psychotherapy
Relaxation therapy
Social skills training
Behaviour modification
Social, occupational, industrial, music and art therapies
Psychodrama

These approaches, and the nurse's role in them, will be discussed more fully in the chapter on the nursing care of the depressed patient, though it must again be emphasized that a therapeutic nurse/patient relationship is one of the most important therapeutic constants during the depressed patient's stay in hospital.

Key Concepts

1 Depression is a disorder in which mood and vitality are lowered to the point of distress.
2 Depression may be *reactive* (neurotic) or *endogenous* (psychotic).
3 Reactive depression is a reaction to a discernible event in life circumstances, that is a *loss* of some kind. Its causes are external to the patient and it is therefore sometimes called *exogenous* depression.
4 Endogenous depression arises from within the patient and has no discernible cause in life circumstances. Genetic and biochemical factors seem to play an important part in its development.
5 Endogenous depression may constitute one extreme, or pole, of a *bipolar* affective disorder (manic-depressive psychosis) or may exist on its own, as may mania (*unipolar affective disorder*).
6 One in ten of the population will suffer from depression and women are twice as likely to be affected as men.
7 Depression is common in young, working class, married women with young families, who have no employment outside the home.
8 Endogenous depression has a *familial* tendency and twin studies show high concordance rates.
9 Genetic predisposition towards depression may express itself biochemically and studies reveal abnormalities of monoamine concentration.
10 Depression does not cause permanent damage or mental deterioration and prognosis, in most cases, is good.
11 All depressions carry a risk of suicide and this is most marked in agitated endogenous depressions associated with feelings of guilt or blame.
12 Depression has physical, psychological and social effects and the overall picture is one of loss of drive, vitality, interest and libido, with the added problems of delusional thinking and loss of insight in many endogenous attacks.
13 Primary depressions must be distinguished from depressions secondary to physical illness or to associated mental disorder.
14 Treatment of depression may be physical (anti-depressant drugs, electroplexy) or non-physical (psychotherapeutic approaches) and the two are often combined.
15 The major antidepressant drugs fall into three categories: *tricyclics*, *monoamine oxidase inhibitors* and *lithium salts*.
16 The patient on monoamine oxidase inhibitors must avoid foods rich in the amino acid tyramine if major hypertensive side-effects are to be avoided.
17 There is a narrow margin between therapeutic and toxic levels of lithium, and serial estimation of plasma concentration is used to ensure the appropriate dose range for the patient.
18 Electroplexy is effective in most cases of endogenous depression but is less so in reactive depression.

References

Bott, E. (1957) *Family and Social Network*. London: Tavistock Publications.

Boyd, J. & Weissman, M. (1982) In Paykel, E. S. (Ed.) *Handbook of Affective Disorders*. Edinburgh: Churchill Livingstone.

Brown, G. & Harris, T. (1978) *Social Origins of Depression*. London: Tavistock Publications.

Clare, A. (1976) *Psychiatry in Dissent*. London: Tavistock Publications.

Dally, P. & Harrington, H. (1975) *Psychiatry and Psychology for Nurses*, 5th edn. London: Hodder & Stoughton.

Granville-Grossman, K. L. (1971) Convulsive therapy. In Granville-Grossman (Ed.) *Recent Advances in Clinical Psychiatry*. London: Churchill Livingstone.

Ingram, I., Timbury, G. & Mowbray, R. (1981) *Notes on Psychiatry*, 5th edn. Edinburgh: Churchill Livingstone.

Komarovsky, M. (1967) *Blue Collar Marriage*. New York: Vintage Books.

Miles, A. (1981) *The Mentally Ill in Contemporary Society*. Oxford: Martin Robertson.

Mostow, E. & Newberry, P. (1975) Work role and depression in women. *American Journal of Orthopsychiatry*, **45**: 538–548.

Nathanson, C. (1975) Illness and the feminine role. *Social Science and Medicine*, **9**: 57.

Paykel, E. & Rowan, P. (1979) In Granville-Grossman (Ed.) *Recent Advances in Clinical Psychiatry*. Edinburgh: Churchill Livingstone.

Seligman, M. (1975) *Helplessness*. San Francisco: W. H. Freeman.

Trethowan, W. & Sims, A. (1983) *Psychiatry*, *5th edn*. London: Baillière Tindall.

Watts, C. (1973) *Depression. The Blue Plague*. East Sussex: Priory Press.

Weissman, M. & Myers, J. (1978) Rates and risk of depressive symptoms in a United States urban community. *Acta Psychiatrica Scandinavica*, 57: 219–231.

Winokur, G. (1981) *Depression. The Facts*. Oxford: Oxford University Press.

13

Nursing the Depressed Patient

In a real dark night of the soul it is always three
o'clock in the morning.

F. Scott Fitzgerald

Depression often presents special challenges to the
nurse. The depressed patient often feels that self is
worthless and that life is meaningless, and these feelings may be coupled with the belief that the situation
is hopeless. This negative view of self and environment often results in the patient becoming isolated
in a state of passive misery in which little interest is
shown in self or others and social activities are shunned. Much time may be spent brooding over the past
while the present slips away unnoticed. The future,
when it is considered, seems barren and threatening. The risk of suicide may be high.

The nurse should avoid light-hearted attempts to
minimize the patient's feelings, however well-
meaning these attempts may be. Suggestions to the
effect that the patient should 'cheer up' or 'look on
the bright side' will simply indicate a lack of understanding of the patient's predicament and may
deepen feelings of depression.

In order to offer the depressed patient effective
nursing care, a comprehensive nursing history
should first be taken. Table 16 reveals some of the
problems experienced by depressed patients and
this may help the nurse to envisualize the effect
depression has on the patient's ability to cope with
everyday living.

Nursing Assessment of the Depressed Patient

Reference has already been made to the negative
view of self which often prevails in depression. The
patient may describe self as worthless or hopeless
and may make frequent reference to real or

Table 16 Symptoms occurring in hospitalized depressed
patients.

Symptoms	Patients showing symptoms (%)
Reduced energy level	97
Impaired concentration	84
Anorexia	80
Initial insomnia	77
Loss of interest	77
Difficulty starting activities	76
Worrying more than usual	69
Subjective agitation	67
Slowed thinking	67
Difficulty with decision-making	67
Terminal insomnia	65
Suicide ideation or plans	63
Weight loss	61
Tearfulness	61
Movements slowed (subjective perception)	60
Increased irritability	60
Feels will never get well	56

Symptoms were considered present if they represented a
change from level of functioning. From Baker et al.
Comprehensive Psychiatry (1971).

imagined failures, errors or misdeeds. In endogenous forms, hypochondriacal ideas may be
expressed freely and self-blame and self-
depreciation may be noticeable.

Stressful life events may be identified by the
patient and these may play a causative role in
reactive depression or may act as a precipitating
factor in endogenous depression. Suicidal ideas or
feelings may be expressed by the patient, and the
nurse must not dismiss these but should listen to
them carefully, noting (a) the intensity of these feelings, (b) their frequency (how often does the patient
feel like this?), (c) their duration (how long do these
feelings last?) and (d) 'trigger factors' (are these
feelings triggered by any particular situation? do

they tend to arise at any particular time of day?), (e) how long has the patient been feeling like this? (f) has the patient discussed these feelings with anyone else? (g) has the patient made any suicide attempts? (h) has the patient made any suicidal plans? and (i) what reduces these feelings?

The nurse must always remember that the absence of suicidal verbalizations does not always mean that suicidal *feelings* are absent.

Table 16 reveals that 63% of the hospitalized depressed patients studied had experienced suicidal feelings. Many suicidal patients will actively deny the presence of these feelings and may present the world with the brittle façade of the 'smiling depression'.

The patient may also complain of insomnia, anorexia, loss of energy, loss of interest in self and environment, irritability, poor concentration and difficulty in starting or sustaining activities.

Agitation and worrying are common problems (see Table 16) and the patient may complain of indecisiveness, poor memory and general inability to cope with the demands of daily living. Loss of libido may add to the general feelings of malaise and tension and the patient may feel a profound sense of inadequacy.

Nursing Perceptions of the Patient's Functioning

Assessment of the patient's ability to cope with activities of daily living will provide a useful framework for assessment, though it must be stressed that this framework is by no means exhaustive. Rigid adherence to any assessment framework may simply reduce the patient to a 'parcel of problems' and may deny the individuality and uniqueness of each patient. This approach does, however, provide a basis for the systematic and orderly assessment of patients' needs, which, in turn, will enable an individual care plan centred around each patient's unique pattern of needs, to be constructed.

The activities of living model was introduced in Chapter 11 and may be applied to the assessment of the depressed patient as follows:

1 *Maintaining a safe environment*

Adjustments in the patient's environment may be necessary due to the risk of suicide (see Table 17)

and it may be necessary to impose restrictions regarding bathing and the use of sharp instruments. Discreet but careful observation is necessary.

2 *Communication*

The patient may be dull and vague in conversation and may even find conversation irksome. Table 16 reveals that 67% of the depressed patients studied suffered from slowing down of thought processes and 77% experienced loss of interest. These two factors often combine to create market communication difficulties in depression.

Underlying delusions may be apparent in endogenous depression (delusions of sin, guilt unworthiness, hypochondriasis, poverty).

In reactive depression some patients may be anxious to discuss troublesome thoughts and feelings, particularly if tricyclic antidepressants have alleviated psychomotor retardation.

3 *Expressing sexuality*

Loss of libido is usually present and this may fuel hypochondriacal feelings.

4 *Working and playing*

There may be a history of failing efficiency and interest, both at work and in leisure activities. The patient may have become isolated and withdrawn and may shun company, preferring isolated corners of the ward.

5 *Sleeping*

The patient may have complained of insomnia, and observation of the sleeping pattern may reveal *initial insomnia* or *early morning waking*. Early morning waking may be associated with depressive ruminations and suicidal feelings of despair. T. S. Eliot captured these feelings poignantly:

'Lying awake, calculating the future,
Trying to unweave, unwind, unravel,
And piece together the past and the future,
Between midnight and dawn, when the past is all deception,
The future futureless.'

The nurse should ask the following simple questions:

Table 17 Assessing the degree of suicidal risk.

Behaviour or symptom	Intensity of risk		
	Low	Moderate	High
Anxiety	Mild	Moderate	High or panic state
Depression	Mild	Moderate	Severe
Isolation/withdrawal	Vague feelings of depression, no withdrawal	Some feelings of helplessness, hopelessness, and withdrawal	Hopeless, helpless, withdrawn and self-deprecating
Daily functioning	Fairly good in most activities	Moderately good in some activities	Not good in any activities
Resources	Several	Some	Few or none
Coping strategies	Generally constructive	Some that are constructive	Predominantly destructive
Significant others	Several who are available	Few or only one available	Only one, or none available
Psychiatric help in past	None, or positive attitude toward	Yes, and moderately satisfied with	Negative view of help received
Lifestyle	Stable	Moderately stable or unstable	Unstable
Alcohol/drug use	Infrequently to excess	Frequently to excess	Continual abuse
Previous suicide attempts	None, or of low lethality	None to one or more of moderate lethality	None to multiple attempts of high lethality
Disorientation/disorganization	None	Some	Marked
Hostility	Little or none	Some	Marked
Suicidal plan	Vague, fleeting thoughts but no plan	Frequent thoughts, occasional ideas about a plan	Frequent or constant thought with a specific plan

From Hatton, Corrine, Sharon Valente, and Alice Rink, 1977. *Suicide; Assessment and Intervention.* New York: Appleton-Century-Crofts.

What helps the patient to sleep?

Which environment is most conducive to sleep?

Does the patient identify any factors which prevent or disturb sleep?

Does the patient sleep during the day, thus preventing the re-emergence of a healthy sleep cycle?

If the patient suffers from early morning waking, does he/she prefer the company of the night nurse for a chat and warm drink at this time?

6 Eating and drinking

Is there evidence of dietary neglect? Does the patient complain of anorexia? Where and when does the patient prefer to eat? Has the patient any special dietary requirements or strong dietary likes or dislikes? Does the company of fellow patients deter the patient from eating?

Remember that Table 16 reveals that 80% of patients studied experienced anorexia. Is there evidence of alcohol or drug abuse? (both of which markedly increase the intensity of suicide risk in depression). Does the patient drink excessive amounts of coffee or tea? (Coffee and tea are stimulants and will add to feelings of tension and will exacerbate insomnia—a milky drink is preferable at night.)

7 Personal cleansing and dressing

Is there evidence of self-neglect? Does the patient express an interest in his/her appearance? Does the patient respond to comments about his/her appearance? Does the patient attend to his/her personal hygiene (a) adequately? and (b) without prompting? How does the patient respond to prompts from nursing staff about cleansing and dressing (positively or negatively?)

8 Elimination

Does the patient suffer from constipation/dehydration associated with low dietary intake before admission? Does he/she express delusional beliefs about bowel function? (common in endogenous depression).

9 Mobilizing

Is the patient isolated and inactive? Does he/she spend most of the day seated in an isolated corner of the ward or lying in bed?

10 Dying

Does the patient express suicidal feelings or discuss suicidal plans? Does he/she refer to death/dying frequently?

The above framework may serve to quickly identify actual or potential problems liable to be encountered in nursing the depressed patient. It is by no means fully comprehensive, however, as many of the difficulties described are manifestations of powerful underlying psychological tensions or deficits. The patient may show fixation at a low level of the hierarchy of human needs described in Chapter 11. The depressed patient may be threatened by overwhelming suicidal ideas which lead to fixation at the level of safety needs.

Hypochondriacal delusions may add to the feeling that the patient is never secure and safe but is continually threatened. The result of fixation at the level of safety needs will be that the patient cannot progress to the next level in the hierarchy of needs (belongingness and love needs,) but is too preoccupied by feelings of threat and danger to deal with belongingness needs and consequently neglects them, becoming isolated and preoccupied.

If much time is spent contemplating the futility of existence, and considering ways of ending it, well-meaning attempts at involving the patient in social

or recreational activities may be rejected irritably. The patient may feel imprisoned by loneliness and tormented by guilt and anxiety. In such a state, suicide may seem a welcome release to the patient. The diary kept by a depressed young American girl contained the following description of her feelings three weeks before her suicide:

> 'Not a tear, not a sigh, not a spark of anger—only quiet despair, and madness. I can feel myself slipping—my mind is—is going. It is blank, except for the tormenting thoughts I have. If only I could forget—complete oblivion would be a blessing.'
>
> (*Cavan, 1928*)

Self-esteem is often intolerably low in depression and this may reflect fixation at the level of belongingness and love needs, as chronic difficulties are being experienced at this level of the hierarchy. The patient who feels a helpless and unwanted failure, unable to gain acceptance by others, will suffer massive loss of self-esteem which may be apparent in self-depreciatory attitudes and feelings of discomfort in most social situations. Loss of self-esteem may also be apparent in the patient's difficulty with decision-making (experienced by 67% of patients described in Table 16). This indecisiveness may simply reflect the patient's poor opinion of his/her own abilities and may be further indicated by the patient dwelling on past failures (real or imagined). Chronic fixation at this level may lead to deeply seated feelings of inadequacy and unworthiness. These feelings were graphically described by a young depressed woman as follows:

> 'A frown instead of a smile can ruin my day. I lack faith in my own abilities, I'm eager to attempt unwanted tasks but really expect to fail. My frustration can lead to my making brusque statements which are upsetting to others but I'm immediately apologetic.'
>
> (*Stanway, 1981*)

In other words, the depressed patient becomes programmed to respond with a sense of failure. The need for reassurance may be profound and the patient may show a tendency to become overly dependent on those individuals providing reassurance. If positive growth is to take place, these vital feelings of self-esteem must be generated by self, not others, though the nurse can do much to facilitate movement in this direction.

Others' Perceptions of Patients' Functioning

Another source of useful information is to be found in the patient's 'significant others' (spouse, parents, siblings, friends, workmates)—that is, others who play a significant part in the patient's life.

The patient may have concealed some information lest he/she appear foolish or 'bad' in the nurse's eyes. More information may be omitted by the patient as he/she feels it to be irrelevant or simply overlooks it. An informal chat with visitors may complete the assessment profile of the patient's psychosocial functioning. It may emerge that a previously relaxed and loving wife and mother has become increasingly tense and solitary. Family and friends may have become progressively neglected, and performance at work may have become poorer. Loss of interest and drive may have manifested itself in neglect of self and household and mounting irritability. There may also be a history of well-meaning friends attempting to 'cheer her up' or 'take her out of herself' or perhaps admonishing her and urging her to 'pull herself together'. A background of mounting social and marital disintegration may become apparent and it may emerge that not a single member of the family unit remains unscathed by the patient's depression.

The nurse should try to ascertain whether the spouse has clearly grasped the nature and extent of the partner's disorder—whether it is accepted or rejected. Is the spouse now clearly aware of the nature of the depression? Is he/she prepared and willing to cooperate in treatment with understanding?

Stress factors which may have played a causative or precipitating part may be revealed by the spouse (unemployment, financial hardship, relationship difficulties, housing problems) and the social worker may be able to help alleviate some of these factors if they are identified at assessment. Discussing the patient's depression with significant others may reveal the need for much simple explanation of the effects of depression which may help reduce high anxiety levels in members of the patient's family. It should be emphasized that depression does not cause lasting damage and that most cases respond well to treatment. Family members may be further heartened by the awareness that they can play a positive part in helping the patient towards recovery.

A day in the life of a depressed person

The following is an account of a typical day in the life of a hypothetical patient suffering from depression:

5 a.m. Awakened from a restless sleep. Disturbing dreams frequently interrupted sleep. Felt fatigued and tense on awakening and was unable to get back to sleep. Got out of bed and made coffee. Sat at window smoking and drinking coffee and looking out at the sleeping city. The world still dark and silent. Time passed slowly—glanced at the clock continually. Felt tense and miserable. Brooded over past and contemplated the future bleakly. Paced up and down room for a while trying to see solutions. None apparent. Sense of despair deepened. Conscious of own heart beating—pulse seemed irregular—checked it frequently. Had more coffee and smoked another cigarette. Tried to read, but couldn't concentrate. Couldn't remember which day it was. Been off sick for two months now—can't face thought of returning to work.

Sky lightening now and several house lights apparent—people going to work. World seems strangely divorced from me—only this room seems real. Everything happening outside house could be a dream—perhaps it is. Birds singing outside now—life seems to roll on remorselessly and meaninglessly.

8 a.m. Got dressed—didn't wash—feel very cold now—sat at electric fire and smoked another cigarette. Another day—so much time and no purpose to any of it. Must tidy this room sometime.

9 a.m. Post arrived—three brown envelopes—probably bills—and a handwritten envelope. This was a letter from Andrew at work. Usual inane and inconsequential chatter about work—who cares about promotions?—he bores me—if he comes calling again I still won't open the door—I can recognize his silhouette through the frosted glass. Work is so important to these people—still, I suppose I really should get another medical certificate—they might sack me. Perhaps I should try to get a job elsewhere.

10 a.m. Lay on the sofa and tried to sleep, but couldn't.

11 a.m. I wish someone interesting would call. I could collapse and die here and no-one would ever know. Perhaps I will go to the shops later.

1 p.m. Forgot to take my tablets again—they just make my mouth dry and make me feel nauseated. Still I suppose they might help.

2 p.m. Went into kitchen to make something to eat. What a mess—I must buy some washing-up liquid and do the dishes sometime.

4 p.m. Have to get out—will go shopping.

6 p.m. Went to supermarket—forgot to get almost everything I went out for— must be careful with money now. Street crowded with rude, busy people—everyone seems to hurry so much—where are they all going? Cold day—raining—saw some people from work and hid in a doorway to avoid them and the inevitable questions and the prying eyes. Life seems so ugly and trivial now.

7 p.m. Made something to eat, but didn't seem to have any appetite—must tidy this kitchen sometime.

8 p.m. Watched television for a while, but simply found it irritating—my mind wanders continually—can't concentrate.

9 p.m. The late evening anxiety arrived again—felt that I was going to die—my heart was racing and I felt faint—had to get out—fresh air helped a little and I returned home feeling defeated, tense and miserable.

10 p.m. Went to bed—hope I sleep well tonight.

The above account is constructed from statements made by several patients who clearly conveyed crushing feelings of despair and hopelessness which made life seem dreary and oppressive. The risk of suicide is high in such a situation and ability to cope with activities of living is grossly impaired.

Factors that Improve or Worsen Depression

Caro et al, (1983) considered Western 'common-sense' ideas about factors which improve or worsen depression by interviewing a large number of 'non-patients' (Table 18). They concluded that it would be difficult to fault the list of factors identified from a

Table 18 Factors affecting depression.

	% (of people suffering)
Factors worsening depression	
Being alone	24
Thinking about problems	18
Unwanted obligatory socializing	14
Parties and social gatherings	12
Something going wrong generally	10
Problems	10
Being rejected	8
Too much to do	8
Things going wrong at work	6
People	6
Unwanted activity	4
Sympathy	2
Having to make a decision	2
Factors improving depression	
Seeing people—friends	36
Attributing the depression to a cause	34
Rectifying the situation causing it	26
Doing something—keeping busy	24
Listening to music or records	22
Sleeping	20
Doing something constructive or creative	18
Reading something	16
Seeing a film	16
Getting moral support—reassurance	12
Doing something to take your mind off it	10
Talking to someone	10
Working	8

Adapted from Caro, Miralles & Rippere (1983).

psychological point of view, though the positive strategies identified could have included emphasizing areas of psychological strength, improving nutritional state and taking exercise.

Planning Nursing Care for the Depressed Patient

Consideration of problems (actual or potential) revealed at assessment will enable the nurse to match these with appropriate nursing strategies. Assessment of activities of daily living will readily reveal areas of impaired functioning which lend themselves to nursing intervention, but the nurse must never forget the pervasive feelings of hopelessness, failure and low self-esteem which may influence the patient's every action. The nurse must also be alert to the fact that many depressed patients will attempt to manipulate the nurse in order to obtain approval and reassurance in a way that is both irrational and unrealistic. Depressed patients must be gently, but firmly, brought to the realization that the nurse cannot, and will not, assume responsibility for the patient's life. The role of the nurse is to provide a psychological climate conducive to recovery and to support and guide the patient during the process of recovery. Depressed patients may see the nurse as a critical source of moral authority to be cajoled, threatened or placated by token displays of 'good behaviour'. The nurse should reject the role of critical parent and must resist the temptation to play parental 'games' with the unreasonable or unrealistic depressed patient.

Maladaptive behaviours must not be inadvertently reinforced, but the nurse must be available to help the patient do 'grief work', and suicidal verbalizations should never be dismissed lightly.

The Grieving Process

Bowlby (1973) described four phases in the grieving process:

1 *Denial*. The person experiencing a loss cannot believe what has happened; the loss seems unreal. He appears to be in control and intellectual responses may be appropriate, but emotional responses are forced into the background causing a steady rise in emotional tensions. Men may be particularly reluctant to allow the emotional aspect to surface and may attempt to maintain a 'stiff upper lip'.

2 *Sensation of loss*. Distress associated with the loss is now experienced. Feelings of helplessness, frustration and numbness may appear, often coupled with feelings of anger and injustice. Weeping will occur at the thought of the loss and may be frequent and intense.

3 *Restitution*. Mourning begins in the third phase. Concepts about the loss are restructured and there may be much repetitive discussion of the loss. In the case of bereavement, the deceased person may be idealized and there may be identification with the positive traits of the person who has died. Feelings of guilt or hostility may also emerge and the bereaved person may become preoccupied with the loss and show a lack of concern and consideration for others. A jumbled mass of memories and ideas, often carrying a powerful emotional charge, are being sorted out during this phase and the bereaved person needs the opportunity to discuss these.

4 *Resolution*. This is marked by a return of interest in others and reconciliation with the fact that loss has occurred. Resolution usually takes six to twelve months but may sometimes extend for as long as two years.

Even after healthy resolution, significant reminders of loss (birthdays, Christmas or the anniversary of the loss) may precipitate intense feelings of loss.

The above four phases do not occur only as a response to bereavement, but also in any situation involving loss. The nurse may help patients do 'grief work' by listening carefully and by recognizing the intensity of grief. Patients must be allowed privacy when preferred, and the nurse should encourage healthy and open expression of grief to enable the patient to work towards resolution.

Maladaptive Responses to Loss

In selecting suitable nursing interventions the nurse should also be aware of *maladaptive* responses to loss. Instead of progressing steadily towards resolution, some patients may become fixated at the early levels of the grieving process. Feelings of guilt, self-reproach or hostility may become marked, or the patient may assume self-defeating and destructive attitudes of helplessness and despair, resulting in a chronic 'give-up reaction'. While it is an important part of the nurse's role to guide the patient through the grieving process by encouraging '*grief work*', it is not helpful to reinforce sterile and negative approaches to life. Thus the nurse should give of her time and attention to the patient who has suffered loss, but has yet to complete 'grief work'. The nurse should *not* reinforce delusional feelings associated with depression by responding to them with time and attention. They should be quietly and firmly ignored while positive, adaptive utterances and actions should be encouraged and reinforced.

There is no value in the nurse becoming as upset as the patient in the belief that this will somehow help. If this occurs we now have two upset people instead of one. The nursing approach should be gentle, but firm and consistent, and any gains made by the patient should be emphasized and reinforced, thus creating a climate of positive growth to replace the previous one of despair, self-defeat and self-pity.

Assisting the Depressed Patient

Activities of living

Assessment will have revealed problems in this area, and planning care now involves establishing *objectives* of care and the necessary *actions* whereby the resultant care plan can be implemented.

1 *Maintaining a safe environment*

High suicide risks may be identified by referring to Table 17. The nurse should attempt to identify sources of danger in the ward environment. Vigilance is important with respect to drugs. Depressed patients may pretend to swallow tablets so that they can be hoarded for a suicidal attempt. Tablets may be stolen from the medicine trolley if there is even momentary inattention on the part of the nurse. Fellow patients may be persuaded to hoard their tablets, or patients with access to the grounds may be persuaded to bring a bottle of aspirin or codeine for 'headaches'.

Anything sharp is potentially dangerous and wrist-slashing is a widely used method of attempting suicide. Razors, knives, scissors, nail files, broken bottles or light bulbs may be used. A window may be broken and the wrist lacerated against the broken edges.

The depressed patient may try to unobtrusively leave the ward—and thus the hospital—the better to complete a suicidal plan undisturbed.

Discreet, but constant vigilance is essential and the nurse should beware of attempts of 'emotional blackmail' on the patient's part. (Why must you escort me to the bathroom—don't you realize how degrading it is? I can't be followed around for the rest of my life—please show me that you trust me!) If suicidal potential is high, the nurse must never yield to entreaties of this sort, which may be genuine or may be manipulative. Risks cannot be taken. The cost of error is too high.

2 *Communication*

Hauck (1973) has identified common themes in the communications of depressed patients and suggests suitable positive responses to them. Self-blame is common in depression and the patient may describe himself/herself as stupid/ignorant/bad/a failure.

The depressed patient may gain comfort from reflecting on the fact that we all, on occasion, commit acts which could be described as bad/stupid/a failure, but this does not make us a bad or stupid person! We can all learn from the mistakes we will inevitably make, but must learn to judge the act rather than the person making it.

Table 19 Maintaining a safe environment.

Problem	Objective	Action
Risk of suicide	Render environment safe for patient	Remove/protect sources of danger

Table 20 Communication.

Problem	Objective	Action
Patient withdrawn and uncommunicative	To establish healthy patterns of awareness and interaction	Spend time with patient. Encourage group activities. Listen attentively to patient
Patient demanding and over-dependent	Encourage patient to set limits on behaviour and assume responsibility	Behaviour modification
Patient expresses destructive feelings of self-pity and defeat	To promote an increase in self-esteem	Identify, reinforce and prompt positive responses
Patient expresses depressive delusions	To reduce incidence of delusional verbalizations	Define reality of situation. Do not reinforce delusional verbalizations

The depressed person should also realize that self-worth is not determined by external achievement and competence. Achievement does not always bring happiness. There are many 'successful' and miserable people. Being accepted by fellow patients and by nursing staff on the basis of positive aspects of self may promote awareness of this important fact. Ellis (1962) also points out that nearly all instances of unhappiness are due to internal thoughts rather than external events.

Depressed patients may have developed the habit of defining various environmental factors as 'very upsetting' and will then proceed to make themselves 'very upset' whenever these often inevitable events occur. We may be unable to change life, but we can work on our responses to it!

Ellis (1962) also stresses that any quest for perfection or absolute control over the exigencies of life is hopeless and is likely to produce despair and inefficiency. To err is human because people are fallible. Perfection should not be sought in self or others—or even in life. The world is one of probability and chance. People should learn from their wrong decisions instead of waiting for perfect solutions—which do not exist. Hospitalization will afford the depressed patient the opportunity to make 'experiments in living' and to work on faulty or self-destructive approaches to life.

Alternative strategies for living will not be created in an interpersonal vacuum, or suddenly fall from a clear blue sky. The depressed patient must be encouraged to communicate with others, and group activities can provide a suitable setting. The group setting may be an informal social or recreational one or may take the form of a social skills training group or a supportive psychotherapeutic group discussion. Inaction does not lead to growth. Introspective brooding will simply lead to inertia. The depressed patient must be gently encouraged to mix with others and to identify and discuss problem areas. The nurse may provide informal social skills training by providing feedback and by modelling appropriate responses in a variety of simple situations (e.g. having a chat or sharing a task or game). This will heighten patient awareness of both positive and negative aspects of 'presentation of self'. The nurse should also listen attentively and should try to avoid answering too many direct questions for the patient, thus creating dependence. 'Question reflection' reduces the risk of inertia and dependence. For example, the patient may ask 'Why do I feel so uncomfortable in the presence of strangers?' and the nurse should resist the temptation to analyse behaviour (and offer solutions) but should 'reflect' the question by saying 'Why do *you* think you feel uncomfortable?'

The patient should be encouraged to assume responsibility for his/her behaviour and it may be useful to have a daily 'audit' of the patient's behaviour by saying 'Well—what went well for you today? What gave you a feeling of success or improvement? Do any of your problems seem a little smaller today? What do you feel a little more confident about today? What did you enjoy today?' The depressed patient may be slow or reluctant to identify gains, and the nurse may point out any advances (however minor) she has observed and discuss these to promote self-esteem and confidence.

The 'audit' should also realistically review any persisting difficulties: 'What went wrong today—and why? What do you still need practice at? What do you still want to improve on? What do you still avoid or feel unable to do?' Simple and realistic assessment of these areas can lead to productive attempts at solving interpersonal problems if the nurse guides, supports and motivates. Try to finish the 'audit' on a positive note by stressing the day's most noticeable achievement, remembering that what seems trivial to the onlooker may be of major importance to the depressed patient.

Identify and reinforce any gains made. Depressed patients often respond well when the nurse demonstrates awareness and approval of gains. It is often helpful when the nurse can genuinely and warmly say 'What a difference when you smile' or 'It's so different talking with you when you are relaxed like this—so much more enjoyable' or 'You did that really well!' Discussion of the patient's occupation, hobbies and interests may lead to a therapeutic 'role reversal' whereby the nurse may learn from the patient. The patient may gain confidence and self-esteem from describing and explaining his job, hobbies and interests, thus realizing that there *are* areas where he is knowledgeable and successful.

Do not reinforce delusions by attempting to reason with the patient or by reprimanding him/her. It is more helpful to quietly and firmly say 'I'll come back when you feel better and want to talk about something else'.

Reinforce rational verbalizations by recognizing them and praising them. For example: 'What a pleasant change it is talking to you when you feel better/calmer'.

3 Expressing sexuality

The depressed patient may worry about loss of libido and this, in turn, may fuel feelings of anxiety or hypochondriasis and add to overall feelings of failure. The nurse should explain that loss of libido will disappear as depression lifts and should emphasize that it has no organic cause and will not cause any damage or have any residual effects.

4 Working and playing

The depressed patient may also benefit from occupational or art therapy. These activities stimulate creativity and may generate a feeling of achievement. Creative activities also allow the patient to express psychological tensions, and work produced may be used as a focal point for discussion.

The patient should not be forced into group activities, but should be gently and firmly encouraged to spend time with others. Time spent with the nurse on a one-to-one basis may help prepare the patient for meeting others.

Simple non-demanding activities are best initially, and games which involve some exercise are helpful (e.g. table-tennis, badminton). Exercise can have a stimulating effect and will also improve appetite and sleep. Even watching television in the company of others may be a first step. Ensure that the patient is not troubled by well-meaning, but over-congenial, fellow patients.

Social skills training can take place in a group setting or may be provided as the nurse prompts, guides and provides feedback in the course of everyday activities.

Reinforce any gains made and chain simple tasks for the very depressed patient (Chapter 10.)

5 Sleeping

Many depressed patients lie abed during the day as they feel lethargic and lack interest. The nurse should attempt to ensure that this does not happen and should encourage exercise. The patient should be weaned from sleeping tablets where possible and should be discouraged from smoking or drinking tea or coffee excessively before bedtime. A warm milky drink is more appropriate. Provide a warm, safe, distraction-free sleeping environment. If the patient wakes early, a nurse should be there to sit with the patient and reduce the feelings of misery often experienced at this time of day by the depressive.

6 Eating and drinking

The depressed patient often picks at food or complains about it and may eat very little.

Small portions of attractively served food will help, and the nurse should ascertain whether the patient prefers to eat alone or in the company of others. Feelings of inadequacy and loss of confidence may make meal-times spent with others an

Table 21 Expressing sexuality.

Problem	Objective	Action
Loss of libido with associated anxiety	To reduce anxiety	Explain reasons for loss of libido

Table 22 Working and playing.

Problem	Objective	Action
Loss of drive and interest with associated difficulty in starting activities	To restore confidence and improve overall level of social functioning	1 Group activities 2 Social skills training 3 Behaviour modification

Table 23 Sleeping.

Problem	Objective	Action
1 Initial insomnia	To establish a healthy sleep	Prevent sleeping during day
2 Early morning waking		Encourage exercise. Discourage excessive smoking or tea/coffee drinking

ordeal for the patient, and meals may be best provided with some privacy initially. Fluid balance should be charted until intake becomes stable at 2.5–3 litres daily.

7 Personal cleansing and dressing

The depressed patient may unobtrusively neglect personal cleansing and may become so dirty and neglected in appearance that other patients avoid him/her, thus intensifying feelings of rejection. The nurse must be very firm in this area and should ensure that the patient bathes and attends adequately to personal hygiene. Be prepared for irritable responses and lack of cooperation but try to avoid becoming over-authoritarian. Prompt appropriate cleansing behaviour and try to make these activities as attractive as possible. Encourage visitors to bring in some scented soaps and talcs, and warmly reinforce any progress made by the patient. Allow the patient to soak in a warm bath for as long as is desired. This will have a relaxing effect, and patients often feel like talking when relaxing in the bath. Relatives should be asked to bring in as big a variety of clothing for the patient as possible and a new dress or hair-do can work wonders for the patient's morale.

8 Elimination

Constipation associated with low dietary intake is a common problem but will usually respond well to a regime of moderate exercise coupled with copious oral fluids and some dietary roughage. The alleviation of chronic constipation will greatly improve the patient's overall sense of well-being. Adequate oral fluids will also reduce the risk of urinary tract infection which is also potentiated by poor personal hygiene.

9 Mobilizing

Studies suggest that exercise alleviates depression (Winokur, 1981) and short walks in the hospital grounds (escorted by the nurse) may dramatically improve the patient's sense of well-being. The patient may be resentful of suggestions of exercise at first, but time spent in the fresh air is soon enjoyed, and looked forward to, by most patients.

10 Dying

Patients' suicidal feelings should never be 'swept under the carpet' but must be acknowledged and dealt with. The very act of discussing these feelings openly may reduce their intensity for the patients.

Table 24 Eating and drinking.

Problem	Objective	Action
Anorexia Low fluid intake	Restore healthy intake. Improve nutritional state	Provide balanced diet. Chart fluid intake and encourage oral fluids

Table 25 Personal cleansing and dressing.

Problem	Objective	Action
Neglect of personal hygiene and dress	To re-establish adequate level of self-care	Behaviour modification

Table 26 Elimination.

Problem	Objective	Action
1 Constipation 2 Risk of urinary tract infection associated with low output	To restore healthy eliminatory patterns	1 Exercise, fluids and roughage if required 2 Encourage oral fluids

Table 27 Mobilizing.

Problem	Objective	Action
Lethargy	To initiate healthy patterns of activity	Encourage exercise

Table 28 Dying.

Problem	Objective	Action
Expression of suicidal feelings or plans	To help the patient to reduce troublesome impulses towards self-harm by improving coping strategies	Plan coping strategies with patient

Try to identify 'trigger factors' with the patient, that is events or situations which worsen these feelings, and make a pact with the patient to the effect that you will try to reduce these 'triggers'. Assure the patient that you will always be available to listen at times of peak stress and that you will stay with the patient until these feelings abate. This will help reduce the feelings of isolation and helplessness which potentiate suicidal feelings.

Be aware that suicide risk is at a peak 10–21 days after commencing tricyclic medication and after the first electroplexy treatment. In both these cases mood is still low, but psychomotor retardation will have started to lift so that the patient may now have the volition to actively pursue a suicide plan.

Evaluation of the Care Plan

This should take place every time nursing intervention takes place. The nurse should ask 'Is this approach working? Should I now modify this approach in the light of feedback now available. Are we realizing our care objectives?'

Evaluation should lead to positive growth or movement in the care plan as function gradually returns. Do not become over-confident or start to develop the plan too quickly. Self-esteem is very fragile in depression and the patient is quick to respond with a sense of failure to minor setbacks. The pace must be realistically tailored to the individual patient's abilities.

Preparation for Discharge

This involves discussing the stresses that discharge may create for the patient, and the family should be fully involved and advised of the role that they may play in helping the patient to adjust to the demands of everyday living again. Talking to medical and nursing staff at visiting times should have armed relatives with a new awareness of the effects of depression and should have prepared them for the sometimes demanding business of helping the patient recovering from depression to readjust to the home environment.

Relatives will often have experienced much stress as they watch a family member slide deeper into depression. Visiting the intensely depressed patient will have contributed to feelings of anxiety, often needlessly tinged with guilt, and it is important that patient *and* family receive the support of social worker and community psychiatric nurse.

The community psychiatric nurse will usually introduce herself to patient and family before discharge takes place, and her support and guidance will play a critical role in the months after discharge. The social worker may offer invaluable advice and assistance with social factors which may have acted as causative or precipitating factors (e.g. financial or housing difficulties).

The disablement resettlement officer may also visit before discharge and may advise the patient about the availability of re-training schemes and courses.

The nurse should discuss discharge with the patient and should offer support and encouragement. Addresses of useful support groups in the community may be given to the patient (Appendix 5). While in hospital the depressed patient will have become accustomed to spending the day in an atmosphere of support and in the company of others. The prospect of discharge—returning him/her to a situation without immediate support, and to the resumption of the responsibilities which hospitalization has temporarily eased—may be very anxiety-evoking for the patient.

Assurance that regular visits will be paid by community staff will reduce tensions, and this availability of support must be emphasized.

Time may also weigh heavily on the hands of the discharged patient and there may be fears that the depression will assert itself again. Simple advice about structuring everyday life may be helpful in the short term. Time should not be spent aimlessly, as an existence like this may prove to be a fertile breeding ground for tension and depression. The patient may be advised to establish a simple time-table for the week. (For example: Monday—shopping, Tuesday—visit a friend or family member, Wednesday—evening at home, Thursday—have a friend or family member round to visit, Friday—evening at home, Saturday—arrange a rewarding event, perhaps a simple treat like a special meal or a trip to the theatre or cinema with friends, Sunday—go for a walk, vary the route each week, quiet evening at home afterwards). Exercise, adequate diet and meeting people should be emphasized. Any difficulties should be tackled immediately and should not be allowed to accumulate. Keeping a diary and reading will also help to lend pattern and structure to life, and hobbies and interests should be encouraged.

At all costs the patient must avoid reverting to a pattern of aimless drifting and mounting tensions and should, by now, be capable of identifying those roads which lead to depression. Effective treatment and nursing care should have provided the patient with an effective 'mental map' of the landscape of depression. Adequate community support will provide the patient with the will to avoid returning to the darker corners of this landscape.

Key Concepts

1 Careful assessment of the depressed patient will enable the compilation of the 'nursing history' essential to the construction of the effective care plan.

2 Assessment must include careful consideration of the patient's abilities to cope with activities of living.
3 All available sources of information should be used in constructing the nursing history.
4 It is particularly important that suicide risk is assessed carefully (see Table 17).
5 The nurse must help the patient to work through the *grieving process* if this is yet to be completed.
6 Residual feelings of guilt, unworthiness or failure should not be reinforced.
7 Sympathy is no substitute for *empathy* when nursing the depressed patient.
8 A nursing 'audit' of the patient's progress will help the patient to develop clearer perspectives in the current life situation.
9 Social skills training and behaviour modification are useful throughout the implementation of nursing care.
10 Measures aimed at improving physical state will also improve psychological well-being.
11 Do not force the pace of nursing interventions. Patience is essential.
12 Be prepared to continuously evaluate and revise the care plan.
13 Community support for patient and family should be discussed before discharge.

References

Bowlby, J. (1973) *Attachment and Loss: Separation, Anxiety and Anger, Vol. 2*. New York: Basic Books.

Caro, I., Miralles, A. & Rippere, V. (1983) What makes depressed people feel worse? and what's the thing to do when you're feeling depressed? *Behaviour Research & Therapy*, **21**(5): 477–495.

Cavan, R. S. (1928) A Suicide Diary. In Kaplan, B. (Ed.) *The Inner World of Mental Illness (1964)*. London: Harper & Row.

Ellis, A. (1962) *Reason and Emotion in Psychotherapy*. New Jersey: Lyle & Stuart.

Hauck, P. (1973) *Depression*. London: Sheldon Press.

Stanway, A. (1981) *Overcoming Depression*. Feltham: Hamlyn Publishing.

Winokur, G. (1981) *Depression: The Facts*. Oxford: Oxford University Press.

14

Mania

Mania (the Greek word for madness) is a psychotic disorder whose main feature is an abnormal elevation of mood. It is the polar opposite of depression and is grouped with the depressive disorders as an *affective disorder*, that is a disorder of *affect* or mood.

The affected individual may also suffer from depressive attacks, this combination of alternating bouts of mania and depression being known as *bipolar affective psychosis* or *manic-depressive psychosis*. Sometimes there is a history of mania (or endogenous depression) without any alternation between the two extremes of mood. Where only one extreme of mood recurs, the patient is said to suffer from *unipolar affective psychosis*, though mania is more common as part of a bipolar disorder. Unipolar mania is much less common than unipolar depression.

Mania is the rarest of the major psychoses and the risk of developing this disorder is less than one half that of developing schizophrenia; only one individual in two hundred will develop the disorder in the course of their lifetime (Krauthammer and Klerman, 1979).

Mania is more common in women and may be slightly more common among single and divorced persons (Krauthammer and Klerman, 1979). The disorder also seems to be slightly more common in persons of the Jewish race, negroes and the upper socioeconomic classes (Boyd and Weissman, 1982).

First attacks occur between 20 and 35 years, though these may be mild and may pass unrecognized (Trethowan and Sims, 1983).

The cyclical alternation between mania and depression observed in bipolar disorders led early French psychiatrists to name this condition 'folie circulaire' (circular madness) and a minority of bipolar disorders do tend to present with a relatively regular cycle, with short intervals of weeks or months between episodes (Gelder et al 1983).

It is important to distinguish true mania from mania due to secondary causes. Secondary causes of mania include treatment with tricyclic antidepressants (thought to trigger underlying mania), amphetamines, corticosteroids, L-dopa and isoniazid. More rarely, a secondary mania has been reported in association with acute and chronic brain failure, influenza, encephalitis, multiple sclerosis and cerebral tumours (Krauthammer and Klerman, 1979).

Mania is thought to be associated with the *cyclothymic* personality which is prone to mood swings and which also displays a tendency towards extremes of mood, though it is difficult to ascertain whether cyclothymic traits are a prodromal symptom of the disorder or whether mania is more likely to develop in cyclothymic individuals. There is some evidence that the mood and energy changes in bipolar patients precede the development of the first definite affective disorder by some years (Waters, 1979).

Clinical Features

As depression is a combination of misery and loss of vitality so mania, its polar opposite, is a combination of elation and increased energy in which there is an acceleration of mental and physical activity in contrast to the generalized 'slowing down' of depression.

Mood is elevated and the patient feels euphoric, excited and optimistic; there is boundless energy with pressure of thoughts and flight of ideas. Grandiose delusions may be apparent and speech will be rapid and garrulous, the patient flitting from one subject to another, often with bewildering speed. Insight is almost invariably lacking and the patient may announce that he has 'never felt better' or that he feels 'on top of the world'. Dress is liable to be garish, and strange combinations of bright colours are often preferred. Female patients may wear an excess of hastily applied make-up so that they resemble a crudely painted doll. Physical overactivity will also be marked and may prevent sleep or adequate dietary intake. Behaviour is likely to be erratic, impulsive and disinhibited and the patient may laugh, joke and burst into snatches of song. Libido is increased and sexual advances may be made to complete strangers. Elation may be punctuated by flashes of irritability or aggression and the patient will not respect the privacy of others or show any regard for social convention, tending, in consequence, to be very interfering. In extremes of mania there is a risk of exhaustion and collapse.

Sim (1974) describes a patient who showed marked hyperactivity coupled with almost superhuman energy. The patient was running through some back streets when he met a youth on a motor cycle who was impressed by his running and offered to pace him. The results were so impressive that the motor cyclist suggested that they go along to a sports event which was being held locally. The manic individual enthusiastically agreed and entered several 'invitation' races, rolling up his trousers and running in his socks. He won several prizes. On the way home, and still full of energy, he passed the grounds of a well-known athletic club and decided the cinder track needed rolling. He then broke into a shed, got out the heavy roller (normally pulled by two men) and pulled it twice around the track. Next he decided to paint the railings, so he got brushes and paint and went round a large section of the ground. On returning home he climbed up a drain pipe and gained entry by an upper window.

Table 29 lists the symptoms of mania and compares them to those of depression.

Table 29 Clinical features of manic-depressive illness.

	Manic phase	Depressed phase
Mood	Elated, euphoric, optimistic, jovial, excitable, sardonic, impulsive	Depressed, miserable, wretched
Activity	Accelerated, boundless energy, restless	Retarded, reduced, listless, lacking in energy
Behaviour	Disinhibited, erratic, impulsive, may be anti-social or aggressive	Indecisive, hesitant, lacking in initiative
Thought	Pressure of thought and flight of ideas	Slow, laboured and repetitive
Speech	Rapid, garrulous, may be incessant speech with rhyming and punning. Speech obscene or disjointed at times	Slowed, laconic and monotonous
Concentration	Marked distractibility	Impaired, difficult to gain and hold attention
Memory	Hypermnesia (increased memory, often for trivial or irrelevant detail)	Often impaired
Delusions	Grandiose delusions may be expressed, patient may feel omnipotent	Delusions of sin, guilt, unworthiness, self-reproach or hypochondriasis may be expressed
Sleep	Overactivity may prevent sleep	Insomnia (usually early morning waking)
Appetite	May be increased but overactivity often prevents adequate intake	Usually reduced
Libido	Increased (hypereroticism)	Reduced—may be frigidity, impotence or amenorrhoea
Insight	Almost invariably lacking	Usually lacking but recurrent attacks may bring some insight
Variability	No particular pattern	Usually worse in mornings

Varieties of Mania

Manic states are classified according to the degree of mood elevation present. *Hypomania* is now the most commonly encountered clinical form of mania (Trethowan and Sims, 1983). The term literally means 'little mania' and refers to a mild manic state characterized by elevation of mood, restlessness, increased energy, flight of ideas and loss of inhibition. The patient is excessively cheerful and excitable and may behave impulsively. Hypomania may shade off into mania proper.

Rarer manic states include *chronic mania*, acute delirious mania (*Bell's mania*)—an extremely acute form which may culminate in physical exhaustion and death—and *manic stupor*, in which mood elevation is combined with marked psychomotor retardation (the patient may sit motionless and unresponsive, but with a broad grin on his face). The latter three states are now fortunately very rare.

Schizophrenic symptoms may co-exist with the features of mania to produce the mixed clinical picture referred to as a *schizo-affective state*. A survey of 18 studies carried out since 1921 revealed that 'schizophrenic' symptoms were reported in 20–50% of manic patients (Pope and Lipinski, 1978), and differentiation between the two disorders may be difficult. Recent discussions of the differentiation between schizophrenia and bipolar psychoses suggest that schizo-affective disorders should be viewed as variants of affective disorder rather than close relatives of schizophrenia (Tyrer and Shopsin, 1982).

The X-ray-like technique called positron-emission tomography reveals abnormal patterns of glucose metabolism in the brain and has produced some evidence of difference in these patterns between manics and schizophrenics. Some manics show evidence of increased glucose metabolism in the right temporal lobe if they are in the midst of an attack, while low-competence schizophrenics show decreased glucose metabolism in the frontal cortex (Meyer and Salmon, 1984).

Aetiology

There is now much evidence to suggest that there may be a biological basis for mania. Lithium salts often have a dramatic effect on the disorder, and the shift from mania to depression is associated with increased blood levels of calcium and phosphorus, the same phenomenon also being discernible when some depressives move towards agitation (Meyer and Salmon, 1984). A mutant protein (Duarte protein) has been found with increased frequency in brain specimens taken at autopsy from individuals with affective disorder and/or alcoholism (Nurnberger and Gershon, 1982).

Biochemical abnormalities may be transmitted genetically and there is clear evidence that affective disorder, or the predisposition to it, may be determined genetically. No exact mode of inheritance has been identified, though in at least 10% of cases one or other parent has had an attack of mania or depression, and up to 25% of the children of one manic-depressive patient may be affected (Trethowan and Sims, 1983), though it should be remembered that affective disorder may also be related to family environment, race or culture as well as to heredity.

Children are thought to be at increased risk of a bipolar disorder with a clear manic component if (a) there is a family history of bipolar disorder, (b) they have shown disturbances of affect, particularly hyperexcitability, (c) they show significantly higher ability on verbal (rather than visual-motor) items on the Wechsler Intelligence Scale for Children and (d) there is evidence of EEG irregularity in the frontal lobes of the brain (Kestenbaum, 1979).

Psychoanalysts have viewed mania as a relief phase with denial of underlying depression, the belief being that the patient attempts to obtain relief from feelings of guilt and the need for punishment, thought to be basic to depression, by completely denying these feelings and assuming the fragile and brittle euphoria of mania (Lewis, 1981).

Behaviourists suggest that certain manic behaviours are indicative of patterns of high reinforcement and the extinction of inhibition (Meyer and Salmon, 1984) and it certainly seems plausible that some manic behaviours are *maintained* by social reinforcers since the humorous, disinhibited hypomanic may seem amusing to others who may provide much reinforcement in the form of laughter, approbation and incitements to further behavioural excesses.

Treatment

Lithium, usually administered as the carbonate, reverses the symptoms of mania in 70–80% of cases

(Meyer and Salmon, 1984) though it takes about a week to have any effect. Haloperidol is often used to reduce troublesome symptoms until the lithium starts to take effect.

Principles of lithium treatment—advice to the patient

Lithium is an effective drug which prevents troublesome swings in mood in many patients but *the margin between the therapeutic dose and the toxic dose is narrow* and it is therefore important that patients understand and adhere to medication regimes. The following principles should be emphasized to patients:

1 Lithium tablets must be taken *regularly* each day, *even if no signs of mood disturbance are present*. Neglect of medication routine greatly increases the risk that mood will rapidly destabilize.

2 If a tablet intake is forgotten, *the patient should not try to make up by taking more tablets the next time.*

3 Containers of clear plastic with separate compartments for each day of the week may be used as an aid to remember the regular tablet intake.

4 If mood becomes unstable, despite careful adherence to medication regime, *the doctor should be consulted* as it may be necessary to increase the dosage or commence supplementary treatment.

5 Lithium is taken in one or two daily doses (e.g. morning and evening) and the tablets should be washed down with ample amounts of water.

6 Blood samples are taken once a week during the first few weeks and thereafter at longer intervals. The last lithium dose should be taken 12 hours (11–13 hrs) before the blood sample is taken. *Blood sampling is essential* to ensure that the appropriate plasma concentrations are being reached.

7 Early side-effects may occur during the first 1–2 weeks of treatment (nausea, loose stools, stomach ache and fatigue in arms and legs). These side-effects usually disappear as treatment continues.

8 Possible later side-effects are hand tremor, goitre (swelling of the neck due to enlargement of the thyroid gland), myxoedema (sluggishness due to reduced metabolism as the activity of the thyroid may be reduced), polyuria (increased production of urine), polydipsia (thirst with increased fluid intake), weight gain, pimples, psoriasis and oedema.

9 Deficiency of water or sodium (salt deficiency) increase the risk of lithium poisoning. The patient should be advised to be alert to the following risk situations: heavy sweating, fever, vomiting, diarrhoea, narcosis, surgery, low salt diet, slimming, treatment with diuretics. *The patient must consume ample amounts of water and salt.*

10 Signs of impending lithium poisoning include apathy, sleepiness, decreased ability to concentrate, muscle weakness, heaviness of the limbs, uncertain gait, coarse and possibly irregular tremor, tremor of the jaw, slight muscle twitches, indistinct speech, nausea, vomiting, stomach ache and diarrhoea. *If the doctor cannot be contacted, treatment should be stopped temporarily.*

11 Owing to risk of damage to the unborn child, women in lithium treatment should use contraceptive measures. In most cases it is advisable that lithium treatment is stopped when a woman plans to become pregnant and as soon as an unplanned pregnancy is discovered.

12 Lithium treatment is discontinued during the days around the delivery, and women receiving lithium treatment should not breast feed their babies.

13 Should the patient be admitted to hospital for any reason, the receiving doctor should be advised immediately that the patient is receiving lithium therapy.

14 Lithium may interact adversely with codeine, morphine, amphetamines and some antirheumatic drugs.

15 Lithium does not change the effects of alcohol but many patients receiving lithium will also be receiving tricyclic antidepressants which will cause drowsiness if any more than very moderate amounts of alcohol are consumed.

16 The patient receiving lithium should understand the drug and should participate fully in his treatment management, just as a diabetic patient understands and is actively involved in the administration of his insulin.

17 It should be emphasized that disorders of mood are eminently treatable and that careful adherence to the principles of treatment will prevent relapse in most cases.

Electroplexy may prove effective for patients who are unresponsive to drug therapy and is also indicated in mixed states of mania and depression when treatment of the manic component does not improve the depressive symptoms, which may even be worsened (Dowson and Roth, 1983).

Supportive psychotherapy and the involvement of the psychiatric social worker also play an important part in treatment, and the family may need considerable support and guidance as the behaviour of the manic patient may have strained the resources of the family unit to breaking point. The parents of one manic girl had resorted to the desperate expedient of taking her for walks in the early hours of the morning in the hope that she would tire herself out. They were also confronted with very considerable debts accumulated by their daughter who had become recklessly extravagant. Both parents had lost weight, and the father's attendance at work had suffered as he was often too exhausted to attend, in consequence of his daughter's refusal to distinguish between night and day. Relations with neighbours had become very strained as the daughter would put on her record-player at full volume during the night and would shout ribald or obscene remarks at neighbours when she met them.

Manic patients may have to be admitted to hospital compulsarily due to gross lack of insight. There is also a major risk that the patient will have fallen foul of the police due to reckless or irresponsible behaviour, often of a sexual or aggressive nature.

One male patient, brimming with confidence and energy, stripped to his underwear in a crowded city street, announcing that he intended to run from Glasgow to Edinburgh in record time. This action rapidly caused a major traffic jam and attracted a large crowd of onlookers, rapidly followed by the constabulary who only succeeded in arresting the would-be marathon runner after sustaining a remarkable catalogue of injuries.

Once admitted, there is a great risk that the patient will impatiently attempt to leave hospital, the better to attend to ill-conceived and extravagant schemes.

Prognosis and Duration

A study of 2000 hospitalized manics revealed that only 14 (0.7%) had symptoms persisting for longer than five years and also indicated that the most frequent duration of symptoms was four months (Wertham, 1928), though later studies suggested high rates of chronicity (56% and 45% respectively) (Poort, 1945; Bratfos and Haug, 1968).

This startling variation in recurrence rates may be possibly explained, at least in part, by rather elastic diagnostic criteria and ineffective follow-up. Studies suggest that the proportion of patients recovering from an initial attack depends strongly on the length and efficiency of follow-up (Winokur et al, 1969).

The risk of recurrence may be high in some patients although personality and social functioning may be good between episodes. Early recognition of recurrence is essential as severe episodes may produce chronic social and vocational impairment.

Key Concepts

1 Mania is a psychotic disorder characterized by abnormal elevation of mood.
2 Mania (like depression) is an *affective disorder* (a disorder of mood).
3 Mania commonly forms part of a *bipolar affective psychosis* (manic-depressive psychosis) in which there is cyclical alternation between mania and depression.
4 Mania is the rarest of the major psychoses and is more common in women.
5 Mania is often associated with the *cyclothymic personality* (prone to mood swings).
6 Mania is the opposite of depression; the patient feels euphoric, confident, optimistic and brimming with physical and psychological energy.
7 Delusions of grandeur may occur and there is pressure of speech and flight of ideas.
8 *Hypomania*, a lesser degree of mood elevation, is more common than acute mania.
9 Research suggests that there are powerful genetic influences in this disorder and that these are probably expressed biochemically.
10 Treatment often consists of *lithium*, which is very successful in stabilizing mood in most cases, though electroplexy may be used in drug-resistant cases.
11 Course and prognosis are variable as many manic episodes tend to recur, though effective community support and follow-up reduces the chances of relapse.

References

Boyd, J. & Weissman, M. (1982) Epidemiology (of affective disorders). In Paykel, E. S. (Ed.) *Handbook of Affective Disorders*. Edinburgh: Churchill Livingstone.

Bratfos, O. & Haug, J. (1968) The course of manic-depressive illness. *Acta Psychiatrica Scandinavica*, **44**: 89–112.

Dowson, J. & Roth, M. (1983) Mania. In Berrios, G. & Dowson, J. H. (Eds) *Treatment and Management in Adult Psychiatry*. London: Baillière Tindall.

Gelder, M., Gath, D. & Mayou, R. (1983) *Oxford Textbook of Psychiatry*. Oxford: Oxford Medical.

Kestenbaum, C. (1979) Children at risk for manic-depressive illness. Possible predictors. *American Journal of Psychiatry*, **136**: 1206–1208.

Krauthammer, C. & Klerman, G. (1979) The epidemiology of mania. In Shopsin, B. (Ed.) *Manic Illness*. New York: Raven Press.

Lewis, H. (1981) *Freud and Modern Psychology*. New York: Plenum Press.

Meyer, R. & Salmon, P. (1984) *Abnormal Psychology*. London: Allyn & Bacon.

Nurnberger, J. & Gershon, E. (1982) Genetics. In Paykel, E. S. (Ed.) *Handbook of Affective Disorders*. Edinburgh: Churchill Livingstone.

Poort, R. (1945) Catamnestic investigations on manic-depressive psychosis. *Acta Psychiatrica et Neurologica*, **20**: 59–74.

Pope, H. G. (Jr) & Lipinski, J. F. (Jr) (1978) Diagnosis in schizophrenia and manic depressive illness: a reassessment of the specificity of schizophrenic symptoms in the light of current research. *Archives of General Psychiatry*, **35**(7): 811–828.

Sim, M. (1974) *Guide to Psychiatry, 3rd edn*. Edinburgh: Churchill Livingstone.

Trethowan, W. & Sims, A. (1983) *Psychiatry, 5th edn*. London: Baillière Tindall.

Tyrer, S. & Shopsin, B. (1982) Symptoms and assessment of mania. In Paykel, E. S. (Ed.) *Handbook of Affective Disorders*. Edinburgh: Churchill Livingstone.

Waters, B. (1979) Early symptoms of bipolar affective psychosis. *Canadian Journal of Psychiatry*, **24**: 55–60.

Wertham, F. (1928) A group of benign chronic psychoses. *American Journal of Psychiatry*, **9**: 17–78.

Winokur, G., Clayton, P. & Reich, T. (1969) *Manic-Depressive Illness*. St Louis: C. V. Mosby.

15

Nursing Care of the Overactive Patient

Table 30 Disorders in which overactivity may occur.

Unipolar affective psychosis (manic type)
Bipolar affective psychosis
Hypomania
Schizophrenia (e.g. catatonic elation state)
Drug abuse (e.g. amphetamines and their derivatives)
Acute brain failure (e.g. delirium tremens)
Hyperkinetic syndrome of childhood
Chronic brain failure of old age
Some hysterical reactions

The arrival of the manic patient will create abrupt and dramatic changes in the climate of the ward community. The patient will interfere with the activities of patients and staff alike, will rapidly make the acquaintance of everyone encountered, and may rapidly threaten to disrupt the fragile equilibrium of fellow patients. The patience and energy of nursing staff may be strained to the extreme and realistic limits must be quickly set to the patient's behaviour if the well-being of fellow patients is to be preserved.

The overactive patient may be too restless to eat or sleep adequately, may show complete disregard for social conventions and the privacy of others and, may make a self-appointment as an honorary member of the nursing staff. The overactive patient's potential for creating chaos should not be underestimated.

Despite displays of boisterous and disinhibited behaviour, the overactive patient is vulnerable. If the prevalent mood is one of boundless optimism, enthusiasm and energy, the patient may be readily exploited by others as money and personal possessions are freely given away and the patient is readily incited to further behavioural excesses by unscrupulous patients who may find his/her manic antics amusing. There is often also a serious risk of exhaustion, malnutrition and injury incurred during episodes of impulsive and reckless behaviour.

The main aims of nursing intervention should therefore be to safeguard the patient (and fellow patients), to impose limits on the patient's behaviour and to promote the development of more appropriate behavioural patterns.

Assessment of the effects of hyperactivity on the patient's approach to activities of daily living will reveal many problems (actual and potential) towards which nursing care may be directed, though the nurse should not forget that the family of the patient will also have been taxed to the extreme and will consequently need much support from the hospital staff. The family should be made aware of the objectives of care and treatment and, where possible, involved if the risk of future relapse and strain on the family unit is to be minimized. The family will also prove to be a useful source of information about the appearance, extent and effects of the patient's disorder, as the patient is unlikely to give a reliable account of social and interpersonal functioning before admission.

The patient is unlikely to offer any complaints but may insist that 'things have never been better'. The mood of elation, coupled with optimism and lack of insight, may lead to the patient refusing treatment and being low on cooperation with the nursing staff. Hospitalization is likely to be accepted reluctantly and mutinously by the patient who not only does not feel unwell but is liable to be hatching improbable and extravagant schemes which require his presence elsewhere.

The overactive patient may have a markedly irritant effect on some of his fellow patients and continuous nursing observation is important if violent altercations are to be avoided. If anything, the hypomanic patient is more at risk in this respect as he is likely to be perceived as a nuisance by fellow patients, whereas the manic patient is more likely to be seen as having a major psychological disorder.

The nurse should remember that the euphoria displayed by the manic patient is fragile and may rapidly be replaced by flashes of irritability or aggression as the patient is restless, impatient and intolerant of frustration. Fortunately, the patient is also likely to be highly distractible so that aggressive episodes may often be quickly defused by directing the patient's attention on to another subject.

Nursing interventions appropriate to common problems associated with overactivity may be summarized as in Tables 31–39.

1 Maintaining a safe environment

The overactive patient lacks internal controls, so external controls should be imposed by the nurse if escalation of potentially harmful behaviours is to be avoided. This may take the form of setting clear limits to the patient's behaviour, and nursing staff should firmly ensure that these are observed. Clearly defined limits provide a framework within which the patient is freer to function more appropriately and to learn more socially acceptable ways of behaving. Behavioural limits must be acceptable to fellow patients as well as to staff. There is little point in compromising over behaviours which are distressing or threatening to the other patients in the ward and which perpetuate an atmosphere of tension and uncertainty. The nurse must clearly communicate her expectations of the patient and frequent reminders will be necessary.

Despite the need for firmness and consistency the nurse should try to avoid excessive limit setting as this may provoke hostility, resentment and retaliatory excesses in behaviour.

The nurse may offer the patient a choice of alternative behaviours ('You cannot hit Mr A. but you can tell me why you feel angry or come for a game of table tennis with me').

The nurse must always explain the reason for limits to the patient and frequent reminders will be necessary, though the nurse should try to ensure that these do not sound like nagging.

The principles of behaviour modification should be incorporated into the nursing approach and the nurse must ensure that rational behaviours are reinforced while maladaptive behaviours are not. It is all too easy to inadvertently reinforce inappropriate behaviours in the patient with elevated mood. The patient may be playful, humorous and witty and the nurse must avoid registering any 'appreciation' of outlandish behaviour as the patient will be quick to detect reinforcing smiles. All ward patients must be reminded that the patient should not receive any amused or appreciative feedback as this will simply serve as an incitement to further behavioural excesses. The nurse may have to actively ensure that the overactive patient is not furtively incited to further extremes by fellow patients.

Careful observation is important as the patient is liable to be both impulsive and unpredictable in his behaviour. A moment's inattention could have major consequences. The patient may display a reckless disregard for both his own safety and that of others, and sources of danger may be disregarded. The author recalls a patient who noticed a bird's nest lodged in a gutter some sixty feet above the ground. The patient, who had been talking about his boyhood 'bird-nesting' activities, promptly scaled a drain-pipe and proceeded to investigate the roof-top for further ornithological finds and was only persuaded to descend after much difficulty.

Overactive patients who become depressed are at high risk of suicide; the patient's mood must be monitored carefully and warning signs of depression or agitation reported promptly.

The elated patient may quickly become belligerent and physically aggressive, and the nurse should ensure that he does not impose his unwelcome attentions excessively upon fellow patients as the risk of violence may then become high.

2 Communication

The overactive patient may experience flight of ideas and this will be reflected in pressure of speech. In extreme cases conversation may become incoherent

Table 31 Maintaining a safe environment.

Problem	Objective	Action
Risk of harm to self or others arising out of impulsive, suicidal or aggressive behaviour	To maintain a safe environment and reduce the incidence of potentially harmful behaviours	Set acceptable limits on patient's behaviour Behaviour modification Careful observation Remove/safeguard sources of danger

Table 32 Communication.

Problem	Objective	Action
Pressure of speech Distractibility Inappropriate or obscene language	To promote rational and appropriate patterns of communication	Shaping of verbal responses Social skills training Behaviour modification

and punctuated by snatches of song, obscenities or ribald remarks. Many patients show an astonishing memory (*hypermnesia*) often for trivial or unimportant details. Distractibility may be marked and it may be difficult to sustain the patient's attention long enough for effective communication. Disinhibition may lead to the patient making offensive or rude comments to fellow patients, and comments on the appearance of others may be made with startling candour. Jokes and punning or alliterative speech may be prominent.

Grandiose delusions may be expressed in mania and this may be reflected in a penchant for ill-conceived and extravagant schemes. If unchecked, the patient may attempt to organize a programme of recreational activities for the ward which would make the last days of Pompeii seem like a Sunday school picnic. Startling sexual suggestions may be made to complete strangers; female patients are more likely to indulge in this behaviour.

The patient should be approached frequently, but for short periods of time at first. Conversation should be simple and should emphasize the here and now, that is ward life and activities of daily living. Limits should be set upon inappropriate topics and the nurse may shape verbal responses in appropriate directions by refusing to respond to inappropriate greetings or suggestions and by persistently prompting rational utterances. Simple elements of social skills training may be useful in shaping interactional patterns, and the patient's attention should be drawn to the social consequences of inappropriate verbal content ('I'm going now because I find that sort of conversation foolish/distasteful/unpleasant'). Rehearsal of simple adaptive patterns of verbalization may be helpful ('Let's try greeting one another again but this time try to be more relaxed' or 'Let's go and join in a conversation but this time try not to interrupt so much'). The patient should be encouraged to try to listen more attentively and to discuss the effects of his utterances/behaviour on others.

Overactive patients may discover a real or imagined physical or personality defect in some other person, often a nurse, and may delight in repeatedly calling attention to this defect, often in an offensive or sarcastic way. Nursing the manic patient is not an occupation for the over-sensitive. Such utterances should be quietly ignored and the nurse must attempt to maintain her equanimity, difficult as this may be.

Maladaptive verbalizations should not be reinforced by devoting time and attention to them, but rational episodes should be noted and warmly reinforced by nursing time and attention or privileged recreational activities. The Premack Principle may be used to select high intensity behaviours which may then be selectively used as rewards for rational behaviour (a low intensity behaviour). Thus the nurse may discover that a hyperactive patient enjoys playing table tennis and that he spends as much time playing it as he can. This would be a suitable high intensity behaviour (something the patient enjoys doing a lot of) to remove and only return in carefully metered amounts as a reward for calm and rational behaviour (low intensity in the case of most overactive patients).

A firm, kind low-pitched voice is most effective and the nurse should avoid loud demanding tones which may quickly provoke aggressive behaviour. Quiet persuasion will be more effective than commands and the nurse should suggest things to the patient rather than seem to issue abrupt instructions ('Come along now Mr A.—time for your bath' may generate resistance but 'Why don't I run a nice hot bath for you and get you the soap your wife brought in' may have the desired effect).

As limits are gradually internalized the staff may relinquish their own external controls and return the responsibility for control to the patient.

3 Expressing sexuality

Loss of inhibition coupled with increased libido may prove a formidable combination in generating inappropriate sexual behaviours. Exhibitionism, masturbation in public places and promiscuous sexual gestures towards others may cause difficul-

Table 33 Expressing sexuality.

Problem	Objective	Action
Inappropriate sexual behaviours	To reduce these in incidence	Behaviour modification

ties. Limits must be clearly and firmly set and it must be made apparent to the patient that participation in valued social and recreational activities is dependent upon the absence of such inappropriate behaviours. The patient who persists in any of these activities should be removed from the setting generating the inappropriate response, the nurse verbally registering disapproval, and should be given time to reflect upon the undesirable consequences of this behaviour in a quiet room. Reinforcing responses of shock, alarm or disgust should be avoided by the nurse.

4 *Working and playing*

The overactive patient shows heightened responsiveness to environmental stimuli. Turning on the radio may be enough to prompt him to leap to his feet and enthusiastically sing and dance to the music. The patient may prove to be disruptive if allowed to participate in group activities in the occupational or industrial therapy department too soon after admission. He will interfere, criticize and make improbable suggestions to fellow patients, rapidly exhausting their tolerance and patience and imposing an undesirable degree of strain upon them. The mood may be one of infectious jollity and exuberance which some fellow patients may initially find attractive. This behaviour is sustained at such a pitch, however, that initial responses of amusement tend to be short lived. The author remembers a manic patient who would burst into song in the early hours of the morning or switch on the ward lights at 3 a.m. to tell his long-suffering fellow patients a joke that he had just remembered. The result on the dynamics of the ward population was interesting.

Previously hostile or uncooperative patients suddenly aligned themselves with the staff in the face of the 'common enemy', and withdrawn patients joined the remainder of the ward population, if only to sit in a strained silence balefully regarding the offender who was warbling operatic arias as he rearranged the ward furniture.

The nurse should seek appropriate outlets for the excessive energy of the overactive individual; games such as table tennis and badminton will allow harmless dissipation of energy. The element of competition should be removed as this will cause the elated patient to become over-stimulated and excited. It is best if the nurse says 'Let's not bother keeping a score' or 'I can't remember the score'.

An exercise cycle is an excellent means of allowing the patient to safely work off energy, though the nurse should ensure that the patient does not 'overdo' it.

Simple group activities provide the opportunity to promote more adaptive patterns of social interaction and should be preceded by nursing reminders of limits applying in these situations coupled with rehearsal of appropriate approaches to others.

5 *Sleeping*

The overactive patient may be too restless to sleep. His thought processes will remain accelerated at night and time spent in bed may seem a waste of time to him. There is a danger of exhaustion and debilitation if adequate sleep is not ensured as the overactive patient will ignore fatigue signals from his body and will continue to push himself beyond safe limits. His overactivity is also likely to disturb the sleep of fellow patients.

Table 34 Working and playing.

Problem	Objective	Action
Patient over-stimulated by social and recreational activities resulting in an increase in overactivity	To ensure that appropriate channels are provided for the productive or harmless dissipation of excess energy	Provide a safe environment which takes account of the patient's tendencies but still allows an appropriate degree of activity and self-expression

Table 35 Sleeping.

Problem	Objective	Action
Overactivity preventing sleep	To ensure that the patient has adequate sleep	Remove distracting stimuli and administer hypnotics as prescribed

The sleeping environment should be a quiet, well-ventilated room and a night light will reduce distracting patterns of shadow. Coffee and tea should be avoided near bedtime as both have a stimulant effect; a milky drink is more appropriate. Naps during the day should be discouraged and hypnotics administered as prescribed.

6 Eating and drinking

Lack of adequate nutrition may lead to complete exhaustion in the patient who is too 'busy' to stop to eat. Meals may be commenced but are often quickly discarded as the patient is too distractible to concentrate on eating. Meals should not be served in the dining area as this will contain too many distractions for the patient, and food should be cut into bite-sized portions by the nurse before offering the meal. The overactive patient needs a high calorie intake as he is consuming energy in prodigous amounts and is likely to ignore feelings of hunger. The availability of snacks which the patient can eat 'on the move' will provide essential calories, and food should be available at all times. Sandwiches, Complan, Build-Up and similar food supplements are useful, though the nurse should remember that intractable constipation due to low residue may ensue. The risk of constipation may be reduced by offering pieces of fruit or by adding natural bran to milky drinks.

Water or fluids should be offered every hour as fluid loss is accelerated in overactivity. The patient should be weighed daily under standard conditions to ensure that major weight loss is not occurring.

Patients receiving lithium therapy should be encouraged to maintain an average daily fluid intake of 3–4 litres and should avoid excessive use of salt.

7 Personal cleansing and dressing

The elated patient may show a preference for garish colours and improbable combinations of items of clothing. Make-up may be excessively and clumsily applied by the overactive female patient, thus making her a potential object of ridicule by fellow patients. Clothing worn may be quite inappropriate to prevailing weather conditions, and the patient may be reluctant to change clothing as often as is compatible with maintaining personal hygiene as favourite items of clothing may be clung to tenaciously. The female patient with increased libido may wear revealing items of clothing thus increasing the risk of sexual exploitation by unscrupulous fellow patients.

It is often helpful to establish a system of 'clothing checks' whereby the patient has acceptable standards identified during discussion with the nurse and is thereafter expected to conform to these standards at routine checks in which the nurse

Table 36 Eating and drinking.

Problem	Objective	Action
Inadequate dietary intake due to restlessness	To ensure adequate intake	Provide high calorie snacks and monitor intake and weight

Table 37 Personal cleansing and dressing.

Problem	Objective	Action
Inappropriate dressing and inadequate cleansing	To establish appropriate patterns of cleansing and dressing	Identify acceptable standards and shape behaviour towards these

should ensure that clothing is appropriate to climate and social setting. Acceptable standards at checking should be reinforced with praise and the opportunity to indulge in preferred recreational activities. Failure to reach unacceptable standard (unfastened zips and buttons, soiled or inappropriate clothing) should lead to clear reminders of agreed standards and may lead to short periods of non-participation in desired activities.

Cleansing may present problems as the patient feels too busy to attend to personal hygiene, and close supervision with careful prompting may be necessary. Impaired judgement may lead to the patient reducing the bathroom to a shambles during cleansing activities, and lack of supervision may lead to the bathroom acquiring a certain Venetian character as taps are left running, with resultant flooding. Manic patients may decide to wash their hair in the lavatory bowl and a patient nursed by the author used a lavatory brush to wash his back before admission and was admitted with multiple lacerations which were heavily infected and slow to respond to treatment.

8 Elimination

The risks of constipation and dehydration associated with low intake have already been mentioned but it should be emphasized that the overactive patient may ignore difficulties of this type, even disregarding discomfort arising from faecal impaction or retention of urine. Nursing vigilance is therefore necessary, and intake and output may be charted to identify the possibility of complications arising from eliminatory irregularities.

Lithium therapy tends to cause frequency of micturition but many overactive patients are too 'busy' to attend to the urgent demands of a distended bladder. In this situation there is a risk of spasm of bladder neck and retention.

9 Mobilizing

The nurse should set limits on the amount of time spent by the patient in energy-consuming activities, and should attempt to ensure a quiet, calm and non-stimulating environment. A calm and consistent nursing approach is helpful and the nurse may capitalize on the patient's distractibility by diverting attention away from physical activities into conversation.

Nursing the overactive patient may be tiring for the nurse and will demand all of her reserves of patience, observation and ingenuity.

Barile has described non-productive reactions which may be generated in the nurse by the always demanding and sometimes onerous task of nursing the overactive patient. The nurse may find herself (a) encouraging outlandish behaviour because of unconscious anxiety about regressed behaviour, unconscious anger at the patient or envy of the patient's attention-getting behaviour, (b) responding when the patient is angry or critical by being angry or hostile in return, leading to excessive setting of limits or other unconsciously retaliatory behaviour, or (c) becoming frustrated and confused, as these patients often do not respond readily to nursing intervention. This may lead to inconsistent approaches (Barile, 1984).

Table 38 Elimination.

Problem	Objective	Action
Potential risk of constipation, faecal impaction or retention of urine	To promote healthy patterns of elimination	Monitor intake and output Ensure adequate intake of roughage and fluids

Table 39 Mobilizing.

Problem	Objective	Action
Generalized overactivity creating risk of exhaustion	To reduce potentially hazardous patterns of overactivity	Set limits Reduce excessive environmental stimuli Prompt and shape adaptive activity patterns

Lyon (1978) has cautioned against excessive use of limit setting or the tendency to regard limit setting as an end in itself. Limit setting merely lowers overactivity to the point where the patient can begin to learn from the whole experience of the disordered episode, can gain heightened awareness of the nature of the disorder and can restore lost self-esteem and impaired social functioning.

Preparation for discharge should ensure planning of careful follow-up visits by the community psychiatric nurse and the psychiatric social worker, and the family should be educated as to early warning signs of future relapse. Winokur et al (1969) have pointed out that patients who receive adequate community support and follow-up are less likely to suffer relapse of affective disorder.

Key Concepts

1 The overactive patient is usually admitted to hospital because the overactivity is harmfully affecting the patient, usually his/her family and sometimes society.

2 A major nursing aim is to rechannel the overactivity into less harmful areas.

3 The overactive patient lacks internal controls, making it necessary for the nursing staff to impose external controls initially if further harm is to be prevented.

4 As internal control is gradually re-established, the nursing staff should phase out external controls.

5 The overactive patient may have a very disruptive effect on the ward community, and nursing staff should safeguard the other patients from the effects of the patient's overactivity, as well as safeguarding the patient in question.

6 It will be necessary to set limits on many of the patients' behaviours but *limit setting* should not be regarded as an end in itself.

7 The ward environment should be rendered safe for the patient and should also be quiet and non-stimulating.

8 The patient will show disregard for danger, hunger, thirst, fatigue and cold, so careful nursing observation is important to safeguard the patient's well-being.

9 The overactive patient has impaired judgement and must be safeguarded by the nurse against exploitation (sexual, financial or social).

10 Behaviour modification will prove effective in shaping many overactive behaviours in desirable directions.

11 Effective planning for discharge and community support and follow-up will reduce the likelihood of further relapses.

References

Barile, L. (1984) The client who is overactive. In Lego, S. (Ed.) *American Handbook of Psychiatric Nursing*. Philadelphia: J. B. Lippincott.

Lyon, G. (1978) Limit setting as a therapeutic tool. In Backer, B. et al (Eds) *Psychiatric/Mental Health Nursing*. Berks: Van Nostrand Reinhold.

Winokur, G., Clayton, P. & Reich, T. (1969) *Manic-Depressive Illness*. St Louis: C. V. Mosby.

16

Anxiety

Fear has many eyes and
can see things underground.

Miguel Cervantes

The word 'anxiety' is probably derived from the Latin 'anxietas', meaning disquiet, and refers to the constellation of physical and psychological responses generated by the organism in response to threat, be the threat real or imagined. Anxiety may also be generated in response to threats to self-esteem or by the emergence of a situation in which one feels pressurized to perform beyond the limits of one's abilities.

Freud differentiated between *objective anxiety* and *neurotic anxiety*. Objective anxiety is a realistic response to perceived danger in the environment, whereas neurotic anxiety arises from *unconscious* conflict within the individual. Objective anxiety may also be described as *fear* as it is a response to a recognizable source of danger, and may be regarded as adaptive in most situations as it increases the individual's alertness and ability to respond to danger. Fear mobilizes our '*fight or flight*' responses, which are orchestrated by the sympathetic nervous system, and the resultant state of physical and emotional tension is familiar to most people. Fear responses are part of everyday life and only become maladaptive when they are prolonged in duration or increased in intensity to the point of causing incapacity.

Neurotic anxiety was thought by Freud to arise from unconscious conflict between the Id and the constraints imposed by the Ego and Super-Ego. In this case the threat to the individual comes from *within*. Powerful Id impulses (mainly sexual and aggressive) constitute a threat to the psychological equilibrium of the individual as they insistently urge actions which are not compatible with personal or social values. Strong feelings of hostility towards a parent may conflict with the belief that one should love one's parents, thus generating high levels of anxiety in response to this threat to personal and social equilibrium.

Freud saw anxiety as the raw material from which neuroses are constructed; all neuroses may be considered as maladaptive responses to anxiety.

Given the important part played by anxiety in the architecture of all neuroses there are, nevertheless, some neurotic states in which the component of anxiety predominates and in which anxiety presents as the major clinical problem. These neuroses are collectively referred to as *anxiety states* and are probably the commonest mental disorders.

Coping with Anxiety

Sustained anxiety is a very unpleasant emotion and the anxious individual tends to use various methods of reducing this uncomfortable state.

There may be a direct and rational effort to remove or reduce the anxiety-evoking stimuli. The student who is experiencing chronic study difficulties and examination failures, despite working to capacity, may reluctantly decide to terminate an uncomfortable situation, which is productive of much anxiety, by changing or restructuring his/her course. It is not always possible to deal directly with sources of anxiety in this way. Many troublesome and persistent feelings of anxiety have their origins in a variety of interpersonal and social factors, which may interact in a complex fashion, making identification of 'trigger factors' less easy. In this situation the individual may *defend* against anxiety rather than deal directly with the causes. Simple examples of *defence*, as opposed to *coping*, would include attempts to 'deaden' anxiety with alcohol or tranquillizers. Excessive alcohol consumption may often indicate attempts to 'self-medicate' against anxiety.

Commonly the individual may defend against anxiety by using defensive strategies which reduce a threatening reality by distorting it. Freud used the term *defence mechanisms* to describe strategies aimed at preserving self-image by resorting to self-deception. Defence mechanisms are unconscious

179

attempts to maintain psychological equilibrium and are used by normal, neurotic and psychotic individuals.

A number of these mechanisms have been described, but some of the commoner are as follows:

Repression

Threatening thoughts, feelings or ideas are denied access to consciousness or action. Anxiety-evoking memories may also be conveniently buried deep in unconsciousness, as in the case of humiliating mistakes or failures. Feelings of hostility or homosexuality may also be repressed, as to allow them access to consciousness may be too anxiety-evoking. In repression, these sources of anxiety have not been *removed* but simply thrust deep into unconsciousness, where they may continue to generate considerable tensions. Repression is also called 'motivated forgetting'.

Rationalization

Rationalization consists of giving rational explanations for irrational behaviour. For example, a person may fail to obtain a greatly desired promotion and respond with cheerfulness (irrational behaviour) by announcing that 'I didn't really want the job anyway' (rational explanation). A mother may vent her anger and frustration on her child by spanking it (irrational behaviour) and by announcing that 'it was really for the child's own good' (rational explanation). The tendency to 'save face' by seeking to explain erratic behaviour or by justifying failures is widespread and is not, in itself, evidence of neurosis.

Projection

This refers to the tendency to protect ourselves against recognizing our own undesirable qualities by assigning them in exaggerated amounts to others. A woman may project her own unacceptable sexual feelings for another man into him and believe that he is constantly trying to seduce her. The husband who has insistent tendencies towards infidelity may accuse his wife of desires in this direction. The person with a tendency to be rude or unkind may be persuaded that his colleagues abound in these qualities. Thus, any unkind treatment of these others is justified as he is simply giving them what they deserve.

Normal individuals may use projection frequently, but it may come to characterize most interactions in the paranoid psychoses.

Reaction formation

This consists of the expression of motives which are the opposite to those actually possessed. Thus, the individual who has a strong fascination with pornography may publicly criticize material of this sort, and the person who may inwardly fear their own tendencies towards cruelty may publicly criticize blood sports.

The author recollects a patient who, in a group therapy session, listened to a fellow patient's account of how a stranger had made homosexual overtures to him. This account triggered an explosive tirade against homosexuals which reduced the remainder of the group to stunned silence. This patient frequently and venomously expounded his belief that homosexuals were 'everywhere', and that 'no-one is safe where they are concerned'. He stated that he had never been molested personally in any way, but added angrily that he would make sure that he never was.

The mother motivated by unconscious feelings of hostility towards her child may publicly be overindulgent and may frequently declare her love and affection to anyone who can be persuaded to listen.

It should not be assumed that motives publicly expressed are always the opposite of those possessed privately. Many individuals become members of 'anti' groups in a conscious and rational declaration of belief. What tends to characterize the reaction formation is a tendency to 'protest too much', often with a strong emotional charge attached to these repeatedly expressed declarations.

Displacement

If a drive (e.g. sexual or aggressive) cannot be either reduced or safely expressed, then it may be directed against a substitute object. The ward sister who has been criticized by a superior may displace her feelings of anger onto a junior nurse (who may, in turn, displace them onto her boyfriend).

Feelings of anger or resentment may commonly be displaced onto inappropriate objects. The workman who has been given a 'dressing down' by a superior may angrily slam doors afterwards, be snappy with workmates and may angrily kick a tin can on the way home. On arriving home, he may kick the cat or find fault with his spouse or children.

Sublimation

This mechanism allows the re-direction of unacceptable drives into socially acceptable channels. Strong and insistent urges of a sexual nature may find expression in creative activities such as art, poetry or music.

The unfulfilled need to give maternal care may find expression in caring for the sick, or in devoting much time and energy to the care of a pet cat or dog.

Freud considered that civilization arose as man sublimated his sexual instincts into the arts and sciences, creating neurosis as a by-product. He further considered that neurosis arose when unconscious tensions became greater than the individual's capacity for sublimation.

Suppression

The *only* defence mechanism employed consciously. It consists of attempts to thrust threatening thoughts or feelings out of consciousness, as in anticipating or remembering a stressful event. Its use is revealed by statements like 'I'm just not going to think about it any more', or 'I'm just going to put it out of my mind', or 'I'm just going to forget it ever happened'.

This mechanism tends to be singularly unsuccessful in reducing anxiety.

Defence mechanisms and adjustment

The use of defence mechanisms is not, in itself, evidence of neurosis. We all use defence mechanisms at times, and moderate use of them may constitute a useful palliative against the stresses of everyday life.

Use of defense mechanisms becomes maladaptive when their use becomes a fixed and rigid response to every minor stressful event. Excessive and inflexible use of these mechanisms may be very apparent in many mental disorders where they distort reality and militate against effective social learning and problem solving.

Classification of Anxiety States

Anxiety may arise as a secondary feature of mental disorder. For example, anxiety may be prominent during the early stages of schizophrenia when the patient is bewildered by strange perceptual experiences.

In paranoid or hebephrenic schizophrenia, the delusional content may be so terrifying as to cause responses of panic. Many organic states are marked by high levels of anxiety. Cerebral arteriosclerosis may present with a marked component of anxiety, and the bizarre perceptual disturbances of delirium tremens may lead to overwhelming feelings of panic referred to as 'the horrors' by many alcoholics.

Where anxiety arises in the absence of such conditions, and seems to arise from an inability to cope with the stresses of everyday living, the term *primary anxiety state* (or primary anxiety neurosis) is used to describe the resultant disorder. The primary anxiety state may be *free-floating* or *phobic*. Free-floating anxiety (non-situational anxiety) is generalized and is not attached to any specific situation or identifiable fear. It may occur in attacks or exist as a persisting state. The patient is troubled by persistent feelings of dread or apprehension which may amount to feelings of impending doom, and panic attacks may occur.

In phobic anxiety there is abnormally intense dread of specific objects or situations, that is the patients suffer from exaggerated and irrational fears which lead to avoidance of the feared object or situation. These fears are often of things which most people fear or dislike to some extent but, in the case of phobic anxiety, the fear has become exaggerated to the point where it interferes with the ability to cope with everyday life.

Phobias tend to be related to objects (animals, insects, dirt, 'germs' or disease) or situations (open spaces, closed spaces, heights, travel, crowds).

In practice, pure states of free-floating or phobic anxiety are uncommon and the two types often exist together. Free-floating anxiety has a tendency to attach itself to objects or situations, thus assuming phobic dimensions.

How Common are Anxiety States?

Anxiety states are probably the commonest mental disorders and accounted for 27% of patients who consulted general practitioners for psychiatric problems, in one London practice studied (Kedward and Cooper, 1966).

Figures derived from general practice suggest that two-thirds of patients with anxiety states are women, but among psychiatric in-patients, the sexes were equally divided (Marks, 1981). The latter finding suggests that men may tend to suppress anxiety more than women, and may come to treatment only when severely incapacitated. In the UK the prevalence of anxiety states has been estimated at 2–7% of the population (Marks, 1981) and the age incidence suggests that anxiety states are largely a feature of young adult life. The mean age of onset of symptoms is around the early twenties and, in several series, the mean duration of symptoms before treatment was about five years (Marks, 1981). Anxiety that begins for the first time over the age of 40 is commonly part of a depressive state rather than a primary anxiety state. Anxiety *symptoms* are much commoner than anxiety states, and one American study revealed their presence in 15% of normals studied (Schwab et al, 1979), especially among the poor, old, widowed or separated.

Aetiology of Anxiety States

This is an area marked by considerable differences of opinion.

The Freudian view is that anxiety is generated by *conflict* between powerful Id impulses; the restraining influences of the Ego and Super-Ego have already been mentioned. Freud emphasized the origins of conflict in the unconscious mind but, in practice, many individuals have some idea of the areas involved, though they may be unable to clearly specify the issues involved. Perhaps the general public is more 'psychology conscious' than was the case in Freud's time, and thus many people may struggle to identify the roots of their anxieties in areas which would not be considered by their grandparents.

Predisposition to anxiety may be genetically influenced insofar as many critical personality traits may predate the onset of the disorder by some time. Eysenck suggests that the unstable introvert confronted by stress will either become chronically anxious (anxiety state), morbidly preoccupied by self (neurotic depression) or will develop ritualistic techniques for reducing his anxiety (obsessive-compulsive state) (Eysenck, 1957).

Eysenck has emphasized hereditary variables of temperament but this viewpoint does not exclude the importance of learned behaviour in the genesis of anxiety.

Anxious children are often borne of anxious parents who unintentionally communicate their insecurity and fear to their offspring who may eventually develop numerous irrational fears and a basically dependent and immature personality.

Consider a small child happily playing in the garden while his mother sits nearby and reads. The child stumbles and grazes his knee and immediately goes frowning to mother who has not noticed the incident. Mother notices the abrasion and cries out in alarm, gathering the child to her bosom as she rushes for the first-aid box. The child is now alarmed, perhaps terrified, and cried in distress as mother has clearly signalled that this is a distressing and upsetting experience. Similar incidents may now evoke distress responses in the child as he is learning that these are appropriate responses to perhaps trivial incidents.

Mother models distress responses and reinforces her child for emulating them by using the potent reinforcers of time, attention, affection and sympathy.

Feelings of insecurity in children may be further intensified by inconsistent responses from parents who may themselves be maladjusted. Maladaptive behaviours modelled by parents often include 'making mountains out of molehills', 'getting into a flap' over trivial occurrences, etc.

Fear of animals, the dark, strangers, etc., may be deeply implanted by the overprotective mother, and this will foster anxiety-proneness by denying the child adequate experience in handling the stresses of everyday life. The maladjusted mother who is temperamentally unsuited to handling the stresses associated with motherhood may be particularly fearful and overprotective with her first child and may have gained in confidence by the time siblings arrive, as the anticipated disasters failed to materialize. Rutter et al (1970) found 'neurotic' disturbances more frequently in eldest children and less frequently in younger.

Single terrifying experiences in childhood may crystallize into lasting phobias in adult life, the origins of which the patient cannot remember. Such a phobic fear may *generalize* as fear is produced in response to objects which resemble the initial fear-evoking stimulus. In a classic experiment J. B. Watson (1920) demonstrated that an 11-month-old child (little Albert) learned to be afraid of a white rat because of its association with a fear-producing stimulus. When the boy was first shown the rat he reached for it, showing no fear and behaving in a completely relaxed fashion in its presence. After a while, the presentation of the rat was paired with a fear-producing stimulus. Every time the child touched the rat he was frightened by a loud, unexpected, sound. The boy quickly developed a fear of the rat and this *generalized* to other furry objects, including his mother's fur neckpiece and men with beards (Watson and Rayner, 1920).

Avoiding the feared object is reinforcing, as it reduces fear, and thus situations that were productive of anxiety in childhood may continue to be avoided in adulthood as the avoidance behaviour of the phobic is persistently reinforced.

Clinical Features of Anxiety

Anxiety has marked physical and psychological effects and the former may be so severe as to suggest physical illness to the uninformed observer. The psychological effects are diverse and unpleasant and include feelings of dread and apprehension. The patient feels that 'something terrible is going to happen', and this sensation of impending doom may provoke panic attacks. The patient may worry incessantly and suffer from an inability to relax coupled with fatigue and irritability. Concentration

is poor and the patient is absent-minded and restless. Acute episodes of anxiety may occur during sleep, giving rise to nightmares, and initial insomnia is common.

Psychological tension is equalled by the high level of physical tension which may affect every body system (Table 41), giving rise to a variety of alarming symptoms including 'palpitations', tension, headaches, perspiration, tachycardia, nausea, tremors and frequency of micturition. Hypochondriacal preoccupations become common, and intolerance of strong stimuli such as bright lights or noise may lead to eccentric behaviour such as wearing dark glasses in dim winter weather. Analgesics may be consumed in large amounts to medicate against a host of aches and pains. Many patients suffer from an overwhelming feeling that collapse and death are imminent during acute attacks, as they fear that their heart is about to stop. Some patients become preoccupied with cardiac function and may often be seen to clutch their chests or check their

Table 40 Psychological symptoms of anxiety.

Feelings of tension and impending catastrophe—patient feels that something terrible is about to happen
Worry or apprehensiveness
Inability to relax
Restlessness
Feeling of being unable to cope
Poor concentration and absent-mindedness
Fatigue and nervous exhaustion
Irritability
Early (initial) insomnia
Nightmares
Panic attacks
Phobias
Depression
Depersonalization
Derealization
Hypochondriacal preoccupations
Feelings of insecurity, inferiority and helplessness
Occasional episodes of talkative euphoria

Table 41 Physical symptoms of anxiety.

Cardiovascular system Tachycardia, palpitations, dropped beats, chest pain, flushing, faintness, raised or lowered blood pressure.
Respiratory system Increased respirations, shortness of breath, yawning, sighing, tightness in chest.
Gastrointestinal system Nausea, vomiting, belching, diarrhoea, dyspepsia, 'butterflies in stomach', abdominal pain, dry mouth, loss of weight, anorexia, or increase in appetite, constipation, dysphagia.
Urinary system Frequency of micturition, stress incontinence.
Nervous system Tension, headaches, blurring of vision, tinnitus, clonic jerks, tremor, dilated pupils, migraine.
Endocrine system Increased adrenal and thyroid function.
Musculoskeletal system Aches and pains, teeth clenching, increased muscular tension and weakness, akathisia (the 'jitters'—inability to keep still).
Reproductive system Decreased libido, increased menstrual flow.
Skin Perspiration, pallor, blushing, cold clammy palms.

pulse. They may complain of a feeling like a tight band around the chest and suffer from frequent 'palpitations'. These fears may lead to the development of a *cardiac neurosis* (*Da Costa's syndrome*), and patchy amnesia coupled with chronic tension may lead the patient to fear that he is losing his sanity.

Phobias

A phobia is an *irrational fear of an object or situation* which tends to lead to *avoidance behaviour*; that is, the patient avoids the fear-evoking object or situation and will often go to elaborate lengths to avoid confronting the 'trigger' object or situation. The resultant feelings of incapacity may cause both personal distress and social disruption.

All of us find certain objects or situations somewhat unpleasant—we may dislike spiders, heights or enclosed spaces and feel uncomfortable when confronted by the 'trigger' stimulus. There is a marked difference, however, between adaptive fears or strong dislikes and a phobia. Most people would feel uncomfortable when standing at the edge of a high building and would perhaps avoid such a situation wherever possible. This response of tension is quite adaptive as such a situation is potentially dangerous and should not be confused with a truly phobic fear of heights. The patient may be unable to ascend staircases in department stores or even be unable to use the upper deck of buses— both situations where there is *no* risk and where the fear must be regarded as irrational. In phobias there is an intense *dread* of the situation, which may give rise to overwhelming feelings of panic or impending collapse.

The phobic patient may use the defence mechanism of *rationalization* in an attempt to justify exaggerated feelings of fear. Phobic fear of dogs may be rationalized by describing them as 'dangerous'; fear of spiders may be justified by describing them as 'disease carriers'. These rationalizations do not stand up to close examination however. Many of them contain elements of truth, but this has been distorted out of recognition.

Some phobias may cause little social disruption. For example, the person with a phobic fear of snakes is unlikely to unexpectedly encounter these animals in the UK. Many common phobias do cause much suffering and social disorganization however. The

Table 42 Some examples of phobias and their names.

Animals—Zoophobia
Bacteria—Bacteriophobia or microphobia
Bees—Apiphobia or melissophobia
Being afraid—Phobophobia
Being alone—Autophobia or monophobia
Being buried alive—Taphophobia
Being stared at—Scopophobia
Birds—Ornithophobia
Blood—Haematophobia
Blushing—Erythrophobia
Cancer—Cancerophobia
Cats—Ailurophobia
Childbirth—Tocophobia
Children—Paediophobia
Corpses—Necrophobia
Crowds—Ochlophobia
Darkness—Nyctophobia
Death—Thanatophobia
Dirt—Mysophobia
Disease—Pathophobia
Dogs—Cynophobia
Dreams—Oneirophobia
Enclosed spaces—Claustrophobia
Fire—Pyrophobia
Flying—Aerophobia
Foreigners or strangers—Xenophobia
Heights—Acrophobia
Heart disease—Cardiophobia
Horses—Hippophobia
Illness—Nosophobia
Insanity—Lyssophobia
Insects—Entomophobia
Light—Photophobia
Lightning—Astrapophobia
Marriage—Gamophobia
Men—Androphobia
Mice—Musophobia
Nakedness—Gymnophobia
Open spaces—Agoraphobia
Pain—Algophobia
Reptiles—Batrachophobia
Ridicule—Katagelophobia
Satan—Satanophobia
Sexual intercourse—Coitophobia
Sharp objects—Belonophobia
Sleep—Hypnophobia
Speed—Tachophobia
Spiders—Arachnophobia
Syphilis—Syphilophobia
Thunder—Keraunophobia
Travel—Hodophobia
Venereal disease—Venereophobia
Water—Hydrophobia
Women—Gynophobia
Worms—Helminthophobia

The above list merely gives some examples of phobias and it is not necessary that the nurse attempt to memorize the list, or even sections of it. It is provided to give some indication of the range of phobic stimuli. The use of Latin/Greek names is not essential, for example it is quite acceptable to speak of 'a phobia of bees' rather than apiphobia.

agoraphobic housewife may become housebound as she fears to leave the home; as a result she will be unable to work, shop, go on holiday, visit friends and relatives, take the children to school or enjoy leisure activities outside the home. The resultant strains on the family unit may be intense.

Phobic anxiety may assume the form of the *monophobia*, that is the fear of a *specific* defect or situation, and many animal and social phobias are included in this category.

Phobic anxiety may also be *diffuse* as it extends to a variety of related situations to produce the *complex* or *multiple* phobia. Agoraphobia is included in this category as the patient's fears often include crowded public places, open spaces, deserted streets, travelling and using public lavatories. Multiple phobias appear to be much more common than monophobias (Trethowan and Sims, 1983), though the true prevalence of monophobias may be difficult to estimate as they may never occasion treatment if the subject of the phobia is so uncommon as to be easily avoided. An extensive range of phobias has been identified (Table 42), but it is unlikely that the nurse will encounter most of these in the psychiatric hospital. Many do not occasion treatment and most of those that do so will respond to out-patient treatment. Some phobias can be very destructive in their impact (e.g. agoraphobia) and the nurse may well be involved in in-patient treatment in these cases.

Agoraphobia

Agoraphobia is probably the most common phobia and its incidence appears to be increasing. Half a million people are known to be suffering from agoraphobia in the UK and 10 persons per 1000 can expect to have agoraphobic symptoms, if not the fully blown phobia (Vose, 1981).

The term 'agoraphobia' is often misinterpreted as meaning a fear of open spaces, which is an oversimplification of the facts. The word agoraphobia is derived from two Greek words: 'agora'—meaning a market place or place of assembly, and 'phobos'—meaning terror and flight.

It therefore literally translates as 'fear of the market place', and refers to a phobic fear of public places of assembly. Agoraphobia has also been called 'street fear' and describes the condition where the patient fears to leave the security of home and has a particular dread of impersonal public places like supermarkets and crowded streets.

On leaving home the agoraphobic will gradually develop mounting feelings of terror which may often culminate in a panic attack. One sufferer vividly describes such an attack. 'When panic struck me, all common sense, reasoning and normality were blown to the winds in a blinding sheet of terror, which deprived me of the ability or will to think, move or breathe properly. I felt, (and was), as white as a sheet, with every drop of blood appearing to have drained from my body; mouth dry and hands and body clammy with cold sweat.' (Vose, 1981)

During such a panic attack (which may arise in any phobia) there is an overwhelming sense of vulnerability and loss of control. Strong feelings of depersonalization may arise—the legs become 'jelly like'; 'palpitations', overbreathing and a sense of impending disaster crowd in.

Claustrophobia

Claustrophobia is a fear of enclosed spaces, and feelings of discomfort in such situations are common and must be distinguished from a true phobia.

Most of us would find being crushed in a crowd unpleasant, but the claustrophobic's fears may result in an inability to enter lifts, cars, buses, aircraft or any small room. Even closing the door in a large, spacious room may cause apprehension in a sufferer.

Claustrophobia is less common than agoraphobia, and sufferers do not present for treatment as frequently as agoraphobics. An element of claustrophobia may develop in association with agoraphobia.

Animal phobias

These are not uncommon and may include fear of cats, dogs, rats, mice and snakes, though the most common seem to be phobias of insects and birds (closely followed by phobias of rats and mice) (Whitehead, 1980).

Most are not incapacitating and those which do cause some incapacity fortunately tend to respond well to behaviour and therapy.

School phobia

This may be a cause of persistent truanting, and must be distinguished from the sometimes intense dislike of school shown by many children. The child may feign illness to avoid school and will display the physical and psychological features of anxiety at the prospect of attending school. This phobia is commonest in the age group 11–12 years, that is around the period of the move from primary to secondary school, and is slightly more common in boys (Whitehead, 1980). Treatment usually consists of a blend of behavioural techniques and psychotherapy, and this combination is most likely to produce a lasting result to the problem.

Social phobias

In 1621 Barton, in *The Anatomy of Melancholy*, described Hippocrates thus:

'Through bashfulness, suspicion and timourness, will not be seen abroad; loves darkness as life and cannot endure the light . . . He dare not come in company for fear he should be misused, disgraced, overshoot himself in gesture or speech, or be sick; he thinks everyman observes him'.

Social anxieties may be monophobic (fear of trembling or blushing) or multiple (a diffuse blend of fears of seeming foolish/being taken ill/vomiting/eating in public/meeting strangers).

Social skills may deteriorate badly in response to underlying fears of this kind, and anticipatory anxiety prior to entering a feared situation may lead to some of the fears being partially realized as the patient blushes, trembles or feels nauseated. Relaxation techniques and social skills training can be extremely effective in reducing phobias of this type.

How do Phobias Arise?

It has been suggested that phobias arise as the result of a process of conditioning. Watson demonstrated that little Albert had *learned* his fear of furry objects as he came to associate them with an unpleasant stimulus. Phobias may be the result of unpleasant experiences in early life, the initial causative event often being forgotten.

The psychoanalytical view is that phobias are indicative of conflict in the unconscious mind. A fear of heights may reveal unconscious impulses of self-harm, while a fear of sharp objects may reveal unconscious feelings of aggression, the sharp objects being potential weapons. A fear of snakes may be identified as revealing high levels of unconscious

sexual anxiety, as the snake is symbolic of the penis. Thus the psychoanalyst will view the phobia as the symbol of repressed fear.

Differences of opinion about the aetiology of phobias may be of academic interest but have little real significance for clinical practice, as efficient treatments have long been identified and tend to be widely adopted.

Who is Likely to Develop a Phobia?

Phobias are relatively widespread in their distribution, and the seeds of phobic disorders may be detected in most of us insofar as phobic *symptoms* are extremely common. It has been suggested, however, that phobic anxiety is commoner in females and that the female preponderance is greater for animal phobias and agoraphobia while social phobias appear to occur about equally between men and women (Marks, 1981).

Table 43 Anxiolytic drugs ('minor tranquillizers'—reduce tension, agitation and anxiety and many have a mild muscle-relaxant effect).

Examples—drugs	Trade name	Average dosage
Diazepam	Valium/Atensine	6–40 mg/day
Chlordiazepoxide	Librium	15–100 mg/day
Oxazepam	Serenid	45–120 mg/day
Medazepam	Nobrium	15–40 mg/day
Lorazepam	Ativan	1–10 mg/day
Clobazam	Frisium	10–30 mg/day
Ketazolam	Anscon	15–45 mg/day
Nitrazepam	Mogadon	5–20 mg/nocte
Flurazepam	Dalmane	15–30 mg/nocte
Temazepam	Normison/	
	Euhypnos	10–20 mg/nocte
Clorazepate	Tranxene	15–45 mg/day

Site of action Mainly in the limbic system and reticular formation. Probably black transmission at the synapse.

Uses
1 Anxiety state
2 Sleep problems
3 Muscle tension
4 Alcohol withdrawal (usually Chlordiazepoxide)
5 Status epilepticus (IV Diazepam)

Side-effects
1 Habituation—may cause serious withdrawal symptoms
2 Drowsiness—especially in the elderly
3 Slow reaction time
4 Decreased libido
5 Respiratory failure (IV Diazepam)
6 Ataxia

Research also suggests that phobic responses may be commoner in psychosexually immature woman and that the rate of marriage is significantly higher among female phobics than in the general population (Mayer-Gross et al, 1977). The latter finding may indicate an urgent need for security and support. Many phobias, however, arise in individuals with previously normal personalities.

Prognosis

Most phobias respond favourably to psychological methods of treatment which are particularly effective when applied to monophobias. Multiple phobias may take longer to respond, and a small number of these only will culminate in a chronic and seemingly intractable state of phobic anxiety.

Key Concepts

1 Anxiety consists of a blend of physical and psychological responses to *threat*, be the threat real or imagined.

2 *Objective anxiety* is a realistic response to perceived danger in the environment and is adaptive in most situations.

3 *Neurotic anxiety* arises from *inner* threat generated by conflict in the unconscious.

4 Anxiety is the raw material from which all neuroses are constructed, and neurosis may be regarded as a maladaptive response to anxiety.

5 In some neuroses the individual attempts to reduce anxiety by developing ritualistic techniques (obsessive compulsive neurosis), in others the individual becomes morbidly preoccupied with self (neurotic depression), and in others the anxiety itself predominates (anxiety state).

6 Anxiety states are probably the commonest mental disorders and arise when stress exceeds capacity to cope.

7 High levels of anxiety may be associated with excessive use of *defence mechanisms*, though use of these is part of everyday life and is not in itself evidence of neurosis.

8 Anxiety states may be *phobic* (anxiety attached to a particular object or situation) or *free-floating* (anxiety is unattached and the patient cannot offer any particular explanation for it).

9 Anxiety states are widespread in their distribution but tend to be commonest in young females.

10 Anxiety may be *learned* behaviour, as the maladjusted mother communicates her anxieties to her child producing an anxiety-prone adult.

11 Anxiety has a wide range of distressing physical symptoms which indicate sympathetic arousal.

12 The psychological effects of anxiety may be equally diverse and may cause much psychosocial disruption.

13 Phobias are relatively common and a phobia may be defined as an 'irrational fear of an object or situation'.

14 Phobias may be highly specific fears (*monophobias*) or vague and widespread fears (*multiple phobias*).

15 Agoraphobia is the most common multiple phobia and may be very incapacitating.

16 Most phobias respond favourably to psychological methods of treatment and prognosis is usually good.

References

Eysenck, H. (1957) *Dynamics of Anxiety and Hysteria.* London: Routledge & Kegan Paul.

Kedward, H. & Cooper, B. (1966) Neurotic disorders in urban practice. *Journal of the College of General Practitioners,* **12**: 148–162.

Marks, I. (1981) *Cure and Care of Neuroses.* Chichester: John Wiley & Sons.

Mayer-Gross, W., Slater, E. & Roth, M. (1977) *Clinical Psychiatry, 3rd edn.* London: Baillière Tindall.

Rutter, M., Tizard, J. & Whitmore, K. (1970) *Education, Health & Behaviour.* Essex: Longman.

Schwab, J. et al (1979) *Social Order and Mental Health.* New York: Brunner-Mazel.

Trethowan, W. & Sims, A. (1983) *Psychiatry, 5th edn.* London: Baillière Tindall.

Vose, R. (1981) *Agoraphobia.* London: Faber & Faber.

Watson, J. & Rayner, R. (1920) Conditioned emotional reactions. *Journal of Experimental Psychology,* **3**: 1–14.

Whitehead, T. (1980) *Fears and Phobias.* London: Sheldon Press.

17

Nursing the Anxious Patient

The fears we know are of not knowing.

W. H. Auden

The effects of anxiety are usually experienced as being very distressing by the patient. The essential feature is chronic autonomic overactivity, characterized by sweating, 'palpitations', nausea, faintness and a feeling of impending catastrophe. There is an overall state of physical and psychological tension which is reflected in impaired social functioning.

Anxiety may be generalized (*free-floating*) or related to specific situations (*phobic*). Free-floating anxiety is more or less constantly present but may fluctuate in intensity, as graphically described by Wordsworth:

'My apprehensions come in crowds,
I dread the rustling of the grass.
The very shadows of the clouds
Have power to shake me as they pass.'

The experience of chronic anxiety may be grossly incapacitating, and patients are liable to be exhibiting high levels of distress on admission, the very experience of admission often tending to heighten already severe anxiety levels.

Anxiety states are psychoneurotic responses so that patients usually have acute awareness of disorder which also heightens distress levels. Many patients fear that they are 'going mad' and thus need much support and reassurance. The marked physical symptoms of anxiety may have led to deep-seated hypochondriacal fears; 'palpitations' may generate fears of heart disease and headaches may induce fears of a brain tumour.

Physical, psychological and social symptoms overlap and interact ominously, and effective nursing care addresses itself to problems in these three areas. Effective nursing care will rapidly reduce anxiety levels and will help the patient to formulate effective coping stratagems, thus restoring self-confidence and self-esteem.

The main aims of nursing care may be summarized as follows:

Physical symptoms: relaxation therapy, breathing exercises, dietary modifications
Psychological symptoms: supportive psychotherapy, meditational exercises
Social symptoms: behaviour rehearsal and assertiveness training

Physical Symptoms

These respond well to simple nursing interventions, often to the considerable surprise of the patient. It is helpful for the nurse to maintain a calm, confident and relaxed approach throughout, as anxious patients are often quick to respond adversely to any signs of indecision or hesitance on the nurse's part. Relaxation therapy will help to quickly and dramatically reduce troublesome symptoms and is easily taught by the nurse. The patient may be taught to relax both body and mind by practising a simple sequence of relaxation exercises. Basic relaxation programmes run as follows:

1 Lie down and arrange yourself comfortably.
2 Close your eyes gently. Become aware of your body and how it feels.
3 Concentrate on your breathing—slow and gentle—breathing through your nostrils and making exhalations last as long as inhalations.
4 Tighten the muscles of your feet and legs—as tight as you can—be aware of the tension.
5 Slowly let the tension go—let your feet and legs feel heavy and relaxed—be aware of the relaxation—study it.
6 Using this technique of tension and relaxing continue up the body, concentrating progressively on thighs, buttocks, abdomen, back, chest and shoulders, hands, lower and upper arms, neck and facial muscles (relax the jaw and let it sag slightly).
7 Once the whole body is relaxed, become aware of your breathing again. Relax the whole body further, aiming for deeper and deeper levels of relaxation.

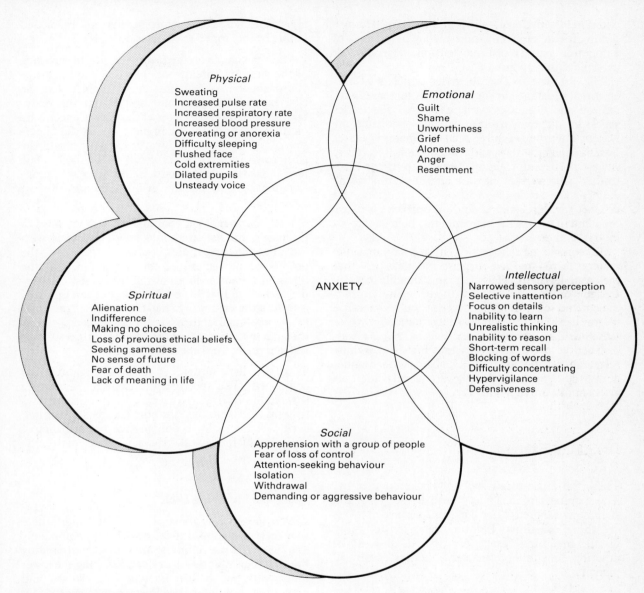

Physical
Sweating
Increased pulse rate
Increased respiratory rate
Increased blood pressure
Overeating or anorexia
Difficulty sleeping
Flushed face
Cold extremities
Dilated pupils
Unsteady voice

Emotional
Guilt
Shame
Unworthiness
Grief
Aloneness
Anger
Resentment

ANXIETY

Intellectual
Narrowed sensory perception
Selective inattention
Focus on details
Inability to learn
Unrealistic thinking
Inability to reason
Short-term recall
Blocking of words
Difficulty concentrating
Hypervigilance
Defensiveness

Spiritual
Alienation
Indifference
Making no choices
Loss of previous ethical beliefs
Seeking sameness
No sense of future
Fear of death
Lack of meaning in life

Social
Apprehension with a group of people
Fear of loss of control
Attention-seeking behaviour
Isolation
Withdrawal
Demanding or aggressive behaviour

Figure 11 The symptoms of anxiety.

8 Lie quietly for several minutes.
9 When you are ready, slowly bring your body back to a state of readiness. Open your eyes gently and do not sit up until you are quite ready.

Relaxation therapy should be taught twice daily until the patient becomes fluent in the techniques. This usually takes 7–10 days. Continue once daily thereafter, whether the patient feels stressed or not.

It is not helpful to practice relaxation therapy after a heavy meal, and ideally a quiet, distraction-free room without harsh lighting should be used.

Biofeedback equipment may be used as an aid to relaxation therapy and consists of pieces of apparatus which provide biological information, not usually available, to the individual as 'feedback' from his body, thus enabling him to gauge the efficacy of his relaxation exercises. Most biofeedback equipment consists of a simple meter (powered by a flashlight battery) which measures a given index of autonomic activity (muscle tension, heart rate or galvanic skin response).

The simplest is a small meter which measures electrical resistance in the skin. This increases with tension and decreases with relaxation. Electrodes are fastened to two fingers of the dominant hand (the patient must be reassured that the meter operates from a small battery and cannot cause electrical shocks). The information derived from the electrodes is converted into an audible tone by the meter. The tone increases with tension and decreases with relaxation, and the objective is to use the mind to silence the machine, this being achieved by trial and error.

As competence is gained in relaxation many patients learn—to their surprise and pleasure—that they can learn to effectively and quickly control anxiety responses, with resultant gains in self-esteem and self-confidence which should generalize to previously troublesome social situations.

Before discharge, patients may be given a self-instruction audio cassette with which to continue relaxation practice at home. The Lazarus technique, designed to produce deep levels of relaxation, is given in full in Appendix 1.

Breathing Exercises

These are a useful adjunct to relaxation therapy. The respirations in anxiety tend to be rapid and shallow and there is often a chronic pattern of 'over-breathing'. Chaitow (1983) suggests the following useful breathing exercises, which should be described in simple terms easily understood by all patients:

Three-stage breathing

Practise this lying on your back. If the lower back does not comfortably touch the floor then either bend the knees or place a cushion under them:

1 Rest your hands on the upper part of the chest and breathe in slowly so that this part of the chest rises slightly. Exhale and ensure that all air has been expelled before allowing the inrush of fresh oxygenated air to again expand this part of the chest. Repeat 5–10 times. The hands are passive, just rest-

ing on the chest and sensing the rhythmic rising and falling of the upper chest cage.

2 Place the hands on the lower ribs just to each side of the sternum (breast-bone) so that the fingertips almost touch on exhalation. As you inhale, feel the ribs expand outwards and away from the body, taking the hands apart from each other. Concentrate on the exhalation being complete so that the fingertips come, once again, towards each other and the ribs crowd in towards the centre of the body. The next inhalation again produces the sideways expansion of the rib cage as the air fills the lungs. Repeat 5–10 times.

3 Rest your hands on your abdomen at the level of the navel. Inhalation should now commence with the abdomen expanding outwards to allow the downward movement of the diaphragm and the filling of the lower lobes of the lungs. As this happens, the hands will be felt to be pushed upwards (towards the ceiling). Exhalation reverses this, and as the diaphragm returns to its high domed position, the abdomen flattens and the hands return to their starting position. Repeat 5–10 times.

Thus the three individual stages of breathing are completed. The speed of the exercises should be slow and unhurried. After practising for some days they may be combined into the complete breathing cycle which should accompany the performance of the individual stages once these have been mastered.

Complete breathing cycle

Lie on the floor as above. Place your hands where they feel most comfortable. Breathe out completely and then start the complete breathing by expanding the abdomen slightly (as in stage 3), filling the lower lungs with air before allowing the lateral and upwards expansion of the lower ribs to enable that part of the lungs to fill as well. Finally, complete the inhalation by expanding the upper ribs forwards to fill the upper lungs and air passages. This slow filling of the whole chest cavity with its maximum capacity of air should take a count of between 8 and 15 seconds, depending on capacity and control. There should be no straining or tension during the full breathing cycle. If you feel laboured or tense during the exercise, then shorten the time.

Exhaling reverses the procedure with the upper passages emptying first, then the lower ribs collapsing gently back to the resting position, and finally with the expanded abdomen relaxing and the 'used' air from the lower lobes of the lungs being exhaled. Try to see the process as a bellows emptying. The last air should be expelled with a slight contraction of the abdominal muscles to take them just beyond their resting position. Pause, with no air in the lungs, for no more than 2–3 seconds. The re-filling of the lungs following the same slow pattern is then almost automatic as the air rushes in to fill the vacuum thus created. Inhalation and exhalation should take the same length of time. Repeat this 5–10 times or perform the exercise just once or twice in any appropriate situation.

All breathing should be through the nose, and the exercise should be followed by resting for a few minutes whilst breathing in a natural and uncontrolled way.

Overbreathing of a panting and spasmodic nature is common during 'panic attacks' or episodes of acute anxiety. The result is often excessive loss of carbon dioxide due to hyperventilation. The patient may then feel faint and light-headed which will heighten feelings of impending collapse or death. Re-breathing of carbon dioxide (using a paper bag) will quickly reduce these troublesome feelings, and the patient should be gently prompted to relax during rebreathing. Allow the patient to hold the paper bag and prompt him/her to remove it every 2–3 respirations. One to two minutes of rebreathing usually reduces feelings of faintness and panic. Once faintness subsides, discontinue rebreathing and gently prompt the patient to practise a few complete breathing cycles.

During panic attacks patients are acutely aware of increased respirations and heart rate and are often extemely distressed by these, thus worsening both. It is helpful if the nurse maintains a calm and relaxed manner and points out that that patient's heart and lungs are no more active than they would be after a period of healthy exercise (e.g. jogging, playing tennis).

The value of calm and reassuring attitudes on the part of the nurse cannot be over-emphasized.

Exercise within the patient's capabilities has several advantages: it distracts the patient's attention from introspective brooding or worrying, and it helps to restore natural patterns of breathing. This natural state of relaxation which follows physical exercise is often profoundly calming. Exercise may take the form of keep-fit classes, jogging, a brisk walk in the fresh air or use of the exercise cycle.

Teaching the patient relaxation therapy and breathing exercises will produce benefits other than symptom control. Self-image may be negatively revised as a result of medication (I have messed up my life—I can't cope without these tablets—without these tablets I wouldn't be normal). Anxiolytic drugs also lead to dependence and they are not a long-term solution. Research has indicated that drugs are no more effective than supportive counselling, and also notes that drug therapy may have marked negative side-effects (Zitrin et al, 1978). The acquisition of new self-help skills (relaxation, breathing exercises) tends to positively revise self-image (I am now stronger than before—I can now control these problems by myself—I can face the future armed with new resources).

Given the problems of anxiolytic medication as a long-term solution, it is also true that anxiolytic drugs may be useful as a first-aid measure. Some patients may be so panic-stricken that effective communication is almost impossible; intravenous diazepam may then be the approach of choice. Short-term anxiolytic medication (7–10 days) also makes the patient amenable to psychotherapeutic intervention where incapacitating levels of anxiety may have made this impossible without medication.

Diet

Anxiety commonly causes gastrointestinal symptoms (nausea, vomiting, food intolerance, dyspepsia, anorexia) and it is important to ensure that an adequate diet is taken. High sugar consumption may lead to reflex hypoglycaemia characterized by irritability, fatigue, dizziness and reduced stress threshold, and consumption of caffeine-rich foods will intensify the symptoms of anxiety. Poor diet has been called 'the primary stress factor' (Chaitow, 1983) and dietary re-education will not only help correct current deficiencies but will help raise stress threshold. The consumption of 'junk food' (with its inevitable additives, colourings, flavourings and anti-oxidants) has also been associated with erratic behaviour and mood instability in both children and adults.

Patients may be advised to avoid foods which are *low* in fibre, *high* in fat, *high* in salt and sugar, *mainly* processed, packaged and canned, and, in particular, *high* in caffeine.

Depressed persons may self-medicate by drinking lots of coffee because of its stimulant effect, and anxious or stressed individuals may inadvertently heighten stress levels by consuming caffeine-rich foods. The commonest dietary sources of caffeine are shown in Table 44.

Table 44 Caffeine content in various beverages.

Beverages (180 ml or 8 oz)	Caffeine content (mg)
Brewed coffee	80–140
Instant coffee	60–100
Decaffeinated coffee	1–6
Leaf tea	30–80
Tea bags	25–75
Instant tea	30–60
Soft drinks	15–80
Cocoa	10–50
Chocolate (1 oz)	20
Caffeine-containing analgesics	30–50 per unit

Reducing caffeine intake may initially cause mild withdrawal (headache, irritability) but will soon reduce tension levels and improve overall feelings of well-being.

The patient should be encouraged to eat foods which are *high* in fibre, *low* in fat, and *easy* on salt and sugar, and *plenty* of salads, fruit and vegetables should be eaten.

Psychological Symptoms

Feelings of dread, of impending doom, hypochondriacal feelings, irritability and impaired concentration also respond well to simple nursing interventions. The patient may be taught simple meditational exercises, and supportive psychotherapy will prove effective.

Meditational exercises bring about a variety of helpful physiological changes; the EEG pattern becomes marked by the alpha waves associated with relaxation, and heart rate and blood pressure fall. The aim of meditation is to divert the conscious mind from everyday thought processes, thus inducing a state of tranquil detachment which is physically and psychologically refreshing. A sitting or kneeling position is adopted and the spine must be kept straight. The eyes are closed gently and all muscles (from feet to face) are relaxed. Breathing should take place through the nose and should be slow and unhurried. As each slow nasal exhalation occurs, the subject should inwardly repeat a key word in a slow droning manner so that each mental repetition of the word lasts as long as each exha-

lation. Suitable words include 'one', 'calm' or—classically—'om'.

As the exercise continues, deeper and deeper levels of calm and relaxation will be attained. Continue for 10–20 minutes before becoming aware and slowly getting up. Do not try to force relaxation during meditation—it will come naturally. Let any distracting thoughts or images flow through your mind rather than try to actively dispel them. The unhurried tidal rhythms of your breathing and the hypnotic effect of repeating your chosen word will soon subdue irrelevant mental activity.

Relaxation therapy should be practised before meditational exercises are commenced and the person should be able to practise effective physical relaxation before turning to meditation. After a week or two of relaxation exercises, a meditation session may be added daily to a relaxation sequence until the person is eventually practising 5 minutes of relaxation followed by 10 minutes of meditation twice daily.

Psychotherapy in anxiety has been described as 'the treatment of choice in every case' (Stafford-Clark and Smith, 1983) and every nurse/patient interaction provides opportunities for effective supportive psychotherapy. Active listening may help the patient talk out areas of tension, and use of reflection will increase self-awareness.

Nelson-Jones (1983) suggests three specific approaches to helping stressed or anxious clients to confront and handle problematic situations.

1 Clients may be encouraged to explore their standards relating to stressful situations by such means as discussing ways in which people's thoughts can affect their feelings and behaviour. It is helpful here to remember the comments made by Albert Ellis (1962) that people often define situations as 'very upsetting' and then proceed to make themselves 'very upset' whenever they encounter them. Life is one situation of probability and chance. We cannot control the vagaries of life but we can work on our responses to them. Ellis goes on to comment that unhappiness is not so much caused by external events but by our internal responses to them.

Self-defeating verbalizations and unrealistic or irrational feelings may be identified and reviewed in an atmosphere of warmth and support. The client who has set unrealistically high personal standards should be gently encouraged to work comfortably within his/her own sphere of personal competence. Brooding over past failures (real or imagined) will sabotage the present needlessly—the past need not be a predictor of the future. Each day brings its own new and unique opportunities, and clients should be encouraged to live comfortably in the here and now.

2 Clients may use their newly acquired relaxation and meditational skills to approach previously troublesome situations with confidence. 'Trigger' situations which evoked anxiety in the past should be considered and discussed, and alternative approaches should be considered.

3 The client may be supported as new skills are practised in real life situations. Rehearsal and role-play with feedback will help the client to become calmer and more in control, and gains will steadily generalize. Assertiveness training will be useful for some clients and will produce an increase in social competence and a decrease in feelings of tension or inadequacy.

Troublesome *social* symptoms will respond well to assertiveness training and behaviour rehearsal, and some clients will also be offered behaviour therapy (e.g. for phobic anxiety). The nurse may help the client who is receiving behaviour therapy by providing the necessary training in muscular relaxation and by providing support and feedback as therapy progresses.

In the case of patients receiving systematic desensitization in imagino (ascending the hierarchy in imagination), the psychologist or nurse therapist may wish the nurse to accompany the client in vivo (in real life) as conquered areas are tackled by the patient. Thus the nurse may accompany the agoraphobic on short shopping trips, reporting back on her progress and providing support and encouragement.

The client throughout any treatment approach to chronic anxiety should be gently reminded that:
Making mistakes is OK
Being proud of yourself for any reason is OK
Liking yourself is OK

Problems with activities of living

Tables 45–56 give a brief summary of possible problems with activities of living and possible interventions.

1 *Maintaining a safe environment*

Intolerable levels of stress may create a risk of suicide or parasuicide, and careful assessment of risk should be made. The agitated patient who is experiencing insomnia, anorexia and hypochondriacal feelings is a high risk. Risk is further heightened by poor response to medication and negative view of life circumstances. It is helpful to provide 'safety valves' for the patient (if you can't sleep or want to talk *at any time* come and tell me—we can talk as long as you want and about anything you want).

Careful but discreet observation and removal/ protection of obvious sources of danger may be necessary.

Once progress is made with self-control of troublesome symptoms (via relaxation, breathing and meditational exercises), risk should reduce.

2 *Communication*

Alarming surges of autonomic activity may preoccupy the patient to the detriment of rational constructive thinking and verbalization. It is helpful to encourage the patient to interrupt build-ups of

Table 45 Maintaining a safe environment.

Problem	Objective	Action
Risk of suicide/parasuicide	To reduce this risk	Provide 'safety valves' for patient—render environment safe

Table 46 Communication.

Problem	Objective	Action
Inability to verbalize feelings clearly—disordered, irrational or self-defeating verbalizations	To facilitate patterns of constructive communication—to increase self-awareness	Supportive psychotherapy—emphasis on active listening and reflection with discussion of lifestyle

tension by *thinking* rather than by surrendering to waves of troublesome feelings. Physical touch may be useful in calming the patient, and a calm, confident tone of voice will help the patient to sit, think and concentrate (Adult ego state) rather than feel or act impulsively and illogically (Child ego state).

Sensitivity to non-verbal indicators of anxiety (tremor, hand-wringing, foot or finger tapping, lip biting, restless pacing) is helpful, and these non-verbal cues may be reflected back to the patient in an effort to identify 'triggers' (What are you feeling? Are you anxious? What brought on these feelings? What were you doing when they arrived? i.e. time, context, people, events, expectations).

Note and reinforce gains and increases in interpersonal competence.

3 *Expressing sexuality*

Loss of libido is common in anxiety and some patients may develop hypochondriacal fears of organic disease associated with this. Simple explanation that this dysfunction is purely physiological (*not* pathological), and that it will abate as tension does, is helpful.

4 *Working and playing*

The nervous and fearful patient may feel dispirited or alarmed at the prospect of group activities. A gently tailored programme of gradual reintroduction to group activities (of a non-competitive and non-threatening nature) should accompany training in relaxation and meditation. Returning strengths should find social exercise in simple group discussions and shared activities.

Specific areas of difficulty will benefit from simple *social skills training*. For example: 'I can't initiate or sustain conversations well'—'OK, let's work on that: introduce yourself to me and tell me a little about yourself' (modelling, prompting and feedback will help). 'Let's try that again but this time smile and look at me as you introduce yourself—like this.'

Assertiveness training will also help many clients ('if you disagree, say so, politely but firmly—practise saying 'no'—make your point when appropriate').

5 *Sleeping*

Relaxation and meditation techniques dramatically reduce insomnia and no other intervention may be needed. Caffeine intake should be reduced and no caffeine should be taken before bedtime. Cigarette smoking actually increases tension and heavy smoking should be discouraged, especially before bedtime. Exercise during the day will also promote healthy tiredness towards the end of the day. Discourage naps during the day.

6 *Eating and drinking*

The value of diet in the management of chronic stress has already been discussed and patients will

Table 47 Expressing sexuality.

Problem	Objective	Action
Loss of libido—sexual fears	To reduce anxiety associated with transient sexual dysfunction	Explain basis of dysfunction and reassure

Table 48 Working and playing.

Problem	Objective	Action
Reduced efficiency and blunted social skills	To help restore healthy patterns of social interaction	Group activities, behaviour rehearsal, social skills training

Table 49 Sleeping.

Problem	Objective	Action
Insomnia	To re-establish a healthy sleep cycle	Relaxation therapy, dietary modification, exercise

Table 50 Eating and drinking.

Problem	Objective	Action
Food intolerance Anorexia Imbalanced or inappropriate diet	To promote healthy and regular eating habits	Dietary education Light healthy diet

Table 51 Personal cleansing and dressing.

Problem	Objective	Action
Neglect of hygiene or obsessional preoccupation with it	To help restore appropriate patterns of cleansing and dressing	Prompting, shaping and reinforcement of appropriate responses

Table 52 Breathing.

Problem	Objective	Action
Hyperventilation Unhealthy breathing patterns	To restore healthy patterns of breathing	Teach three-stage breathing and complete breathing cycle

benefit from short educative sessions. A light balanced diet will reduce gastrointestinal symptoms and these will reduce as competence in stress management increases.

Alcohol consumption should be discussed. In moderate amounts, alcohol may reduce tension, but immoderate consumption will sharply increase it.

7 *Personal cleansing and dressing*

The patient who is incapacitated by acute anxiety is liable to neglect cleansing and dressing, thus adding to overall feelings of disorganization and helplessness. Chronic levels of moderate anxiety may be associated with the emergence of obsessional traits in relation to cleansing and dressing, and time-consuming repetitive rituals may emerge. Neglect will respond to firm and gentle prompting with verbal reinforcement of gains. Encourage visitors to help by asking them to bring in favourite items of clothing, soaps and perfumes, and to praise improvements. Limit-setting should be used in response to obsessional behaviours, and many patients report that relaxation before cleansing and dressing reduces obsessional urges. A warm bath will promote relaxation.

8 *Breathing*

9 *Elimination*

In acute anxiety there may be marked intestinal hurry with diarrhoea. A low residue diet will be appropriate until relaxation exercises have been mastered and autonomic activity decreases. In chronic anxiety there may be constipation associated with anorexia and, in this case, a high fibre diet may be commenced immediately.

Hypochondriacal fears should elicit explanation that changes in eliminatory pattern are physiological, not pathological, and that they will quickly respond as stress levels fall.

10 *Mobilizing*

In acute anxiety the patient may be restless and over-active, and attempts may be made to flee the ward during panic attacks. Reassurance, relaxation and breathing exercises will help the patient to gain control of these troublesome feelings.

Underactivity may be associated with the inertia and psychological paralysis of chronic anxiety. Relaxation and meditation will again help, and graduated physical exercise is invaluable.

11 *Controlling body temperature*

These are further examples of physiological responses which the patient may misinterpret as

Table 53 Elimination.

Problem	Objective	Action
Diarrhoea Constipation Hypochondriacal fears about bowel function	To stabilize bowel function and reduce eliminatory anxieties	Dietary modification Explanation Relaxation

Table 54 Mobilizing.

Problem	Objective	Action
Overactivity (acute anxiety) Underactivity (chronic anxiety)	To restore appropriate levels of motor activity	Relaxation Exercise

Table 55 Controlling body temperature.

Problem	Objective	Action
Flushing and sweating	To allay discomfort and fears associated with these	Relaxation Explanation Warm bath

Table 56 Dying.

Problem	Objective	Action
Fears of death	To reduce these	Explanation Supportive psychotherapy

being pathological. Explanation and reassurance will help, and the patient who is sweating profusely may need additional oral fluids and regular access to a warm bath (which will also promote relaxation).

12 *Dying*

The host of alarming physical symptoms to which the anxious patient is subject may induce fears of disease or death. Fear of heart disease is common (due to tachycardia, tightness in the chest and 'palpitations'). Explanation about 'fight and flight' responses may accompany training in relaxation, and deep-seated fears should be allowed expression and discussion during nurse/patient interactions. Fears will gradually subside as general well-being improves, though the nurse should never underestimate the torment they can cause to stressed patients.

In conclusion we should note that anxiety is one of the commonest manifestations of mental disorder. It is the raw stuff of which all neuroses are constructed and may emerge as a facet of any mental disorder.

The techniques mentioned for reducing stress and anxiety will therefore be a useful addition to the therapeutic repertoire of any nurse and will prove helpful in a wide range of situations. Before teaching these techniques to patients the nurse should master them herself by careful practice. Nursing can be a stressful occupation, and practice of these techniques will raise and strengthen stress thresholds.

Key Concepts

1 Anxiety has marked physical, psychological and social symptoms which tend to interact and reinforce one another.
2 Distressing autonomic symptoms may fuel *hypochondriacal* fears.
3 Physical symptoms respond well to *relaxation* and *breathing exercises*, augmented by *exercise* and *dietary modification*.

4 Psychological symptoms respond well to *psychotherapy* and *meditational exercises*.
5 Effective care adds to self-esteem and self-confidence by developing new strengths in the patient and by heightening self-awareness.
6 Social difficulties may be helped by *social skills training*, especially assertiveness training and behaviour rehearsal and practice.
7 The stress-proofing techniques mentioned may be usefully acquired by the nurse by simple practice.

References

Chaitow, L. (1983) *Relaxation and Meditation Techniques*. Northants: Thorsons.

Ellis, A. (1962) *Reason and Emotion in Psychotherapy*. New Jersey: Lyle & Stuart.

Nelson-Jones, R. (1983) *Practical Counselling Skills*. New York: Holt, Rinehart & Winston.

Stafford-Clark, D. & Smith, A. (1983) *Psychiatry for Students, 6th edn*. London: George Allen & Unwin.

Zitrin, C. et al (1978) Behaviour therapy, supportive psychotherapy, imipramine and phobias. *Archives of General Psychiatry*, **35**: 307–316.

IV
ANXIETY EXPRESSED AS ILLNESS OR RITUAL

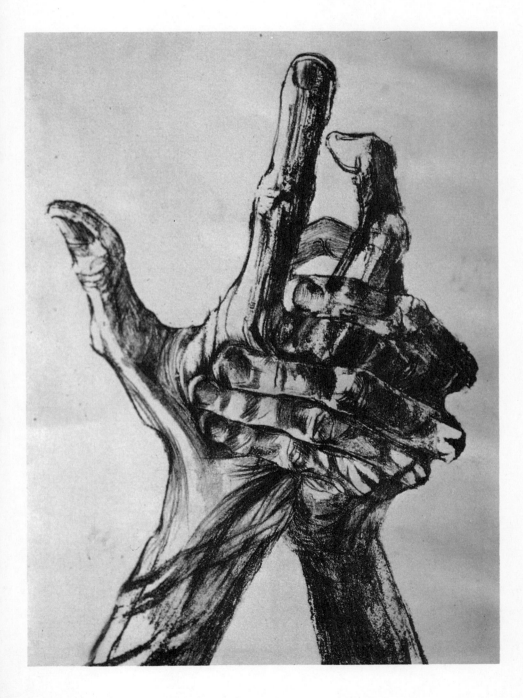

18

Hysteria

Hysterical states represent the attempt, never fully conscious and often completely unconscious, to obtain relief from intolerable stress by the exhibition and experience of symptoms of illness. Hysteria may permit escape from an intolerably stressful situation due to the almost universal custom of making life easier, at least temporarily, for those who are ill. It is part of our social ethic that we should feel sorry for sick people, should try to be helpful to them and should free them from many of their normal responsibilities for the duration of the illness. Thus hysterical reactions may produce relative *gains* and advantage for the patient if the hysteria permits escape from a stressful role or conflict situation. Thus hysteria will only develop if there is both *stress* and an *illness-rewarding situation* that produces many secondary gains for the patient.

Hysteria must not be confused with *malingering*, which is the deliberate and fully conscious faking of illness. The underlying cause in hysteria is *unconscious conflict* which the patient is unable to resolve; the resultant manifestations of illness are very real to the patient and may cause considerable incapacity and distress.

The development of the concept of hysteria sheds interesting light on early psychiatric thinking and reveals areas of prejudice and myth which have persisted, albeit in adulterated form, to the present day.

The word hysteria is derived from the Greek word 'hystera', meaning womb or uterus, and the Ancient Greeks were firmly persuaded that the uterus was capable of wandering around the abdominal cavity, causing emotional disturbance as it did so. Thus hysteria has ancient links with femaleness and there is little doubt that the unfortu-nate women persecuted as witches included many hysterics in their ranks.

In 1817 John Haslam, the apothecary to Bethlem, wrote: 'In females who become insane the disease is often associated with the peculiarities of their sex' (Skultans, 1979). This theme of sexual stigma was enthusiastically developed by the Victorians who carefully described the alleged medical vulnerabilities of the 'weaker sex'. The Victorians believed that only women could suffer from hysteria, suggesting that it arose from an 'irritation' of the sexual organs. This Victorian preoccupation with sexual function produced many bizarre medical theories, some of which persisted well into the twentieth century, and many of which form a part of contemporary sexual mythology.

In 1842 an eminent French physician produced a three volume treatise on 'involuntary seminal emissions' and warned that masturbation could 'menace the future of modern societies' and in 1863 a Scottish physician introduced the term 'masturbatory insanity', believing masturbation to be a common cause of insanity (Szasz, 1973), a belief which is sadly far from dead as evidenced by the frequency of anxious letters on this subject appearing in the 'advice columns' of popular magazines. Alarmed Victorian fathers promptly invested in a variety of bizarre devices designed to prevent this dangerous practice in their offspring. One such item, which was widely sold, consisted of a spiked ring which was placed around the penis and held in place by a lockable belt. Victorian fathers could thus lock this horrific gadget in place on their hapless offspring and complacently retire to bed in the smug awareness that any unseemly nocturnal tumescence would have a painful and bloody conclusion.

In 1869 Kahlbaum, a German psychiatrist famous as an early classifier of 'mental diseases', gave the name 'catatonia' to a condition he believed to be caused chiefly by excessive masturbation and in 1882 Krafft-Ebing published the famous *Psychopathia Sexualis* (the first systematic study of psychosexual disorders) which insisted that masturbation led to homosexuality (Szasz 1973).

During the last quarter of the nineteenth century,

menstruation was even held to be a pathological condition, being regarded as 'proof of the inactivity and atrophy of the uterus' (Skultans, 1979).

The Victorian ethic of hard work, sobriety, prudence and sexual discretion emphasized social and personal equilibrium, and this equilibrium must have been jarred by unruly and turbulent sexual feelings. Cognitive dissonance must have been particularly marked in response to female sexuality as it was popularly believed that healthy women did not experience sexual feelings and submitted to sexual advances only in response to maternal instincts, though this refinement was thought to be confined to middle class ladies, the labouring classes being 'wanton and sexually depraved' (Skultans 1979). The 'medicalization' of female sexuality not only restored order but permitted control and led to horrific psychiatric excesses.

In 1885 hysteria was treated by surgical removal of the ovaries in Paris, by surgical removal of the clitoris in London and Vienna, and by means of cauterization of the clitoris in Heidelberg. As late as 1905 a prominent American psychiatrist was recommending the treatment of masturbation in children by cautery to the spine and genitals and in 1918 Ernest Jones, a pioneer British psychoanalyst, insisted that 'true neurasthenia will be found to depend on excessive onanism (masturbation)' (Szasz, 1973).

Psychiatry came of age as a discipline during an era of sexual guilt, repression and misogyny and this is reflected in much of the content of early psychoanalytical writing. Freud incorporated much Victorian morality into medicine by claiming that masturbation was pathological in the adult and led to neurosis. He also suggested that hysteria was a defence against repressed ideas and feelings, which were usually sexual.

In his Studies On Hysteria (1925), Freud (and his colleague Breuer) suggested that hysterics suffer from painful, traumatic memories which do not 'wear away' normally but remain an active and *unconscious* force motivating behaviour ('what cannot be remembered cannot be left behind'). Since negative unconscious memories cannot be expressed normally, their emotional energy is 'dammed up' to be converted into the physical symptoms of hysteria. The main aim of therapy was seen to be getting the patient to relive the original traumatic experience (usually under hypnosis), thus releasing the pent-up emotions which were causing the symptoms.

Freud also proposed a *seduction theory*, according to which repressed memories nearly always revealed seduction or sexual molestation by a parent or adult while the patient was still a child, though he later modified this theory by suggesting that the seduction was often a fantasy event rather than a physical one. Repressed memories or wishes about seduction were then thought to give rise to hysterical symptoms after puberty.

The theories of Freud and his contemporaries powerfully influenced twentieth century psychiatry and much early psychiatric theory in general, and beliefs about sexuality in general and hysteria in particular, arose from this strange Victorian blend of sexual superstition, fear and prejudice, liberally spiced with misogyny.

As late as 1940 the medical regulations of the US Naval Academy at Annapolis prescribed that candidates be rejected by the examining surgeon 'for evidence of masturbation' (Szasz, 1973).

The bedrock of psychiatric theory contains many strange fossils, some of which continue to warp later theoretical strata.

Ironically, later psychotherapeutic approaches emphasized the tension relief associated with orgasm (whether self-induced or not) and viewed it as a desirable palliative against stress—the maxim then seeming to be 'an orgasm a day keeps the psychiatrist away'.

At the present time many writers consider the concept of hysteria to be a somewhat dubious one. Feminist writers have irately dismissed the concept of hysteria as a product of male sexual guilt and fears, manufactured by psychiatrists as convenient evidence of female 'inferiority'. Some psychiatrists have suggested that the term may come to be abolished completely (Trethowan and Sims, 1983), though use of the term persists, largely due to its clinical usefulness.

It would perhaps be unfortunate if the term were to be abandoned altogether, though great caution should be exercised in using it. The adjective 'hysterical' is a convenient epithet of abuse for men to use in describing female behaviours of which they disapprove, and tends to conjure up images of a histrionic female making selfish and irrational demands of her long-suffering spouse as she reclines dramatically on a chaise-longue (rather like the heroine in a Puccini opera).

The clinical realities differ radically from the conventional myths. Hysteria may affect men as well as women, and this fact was recognized by Freud, though hysterical states involving physical symptomatology (as opposed to mental symptomatology) remain much more common in women (Meyer and Salmon, 1984).

In recent decades there has been a decreased incidence of classical hysteria in Western societies, though disorders of this sort are more common in Mediterranean peoples and remain common in parts of the Third World (Sainsbury, 1980). No more than 1–2% of referrals are now diagnosed as suffering from hysteria (Trethowan and Sims, 1983), though a hysterical overlay may be present in many common psychiatric disorders.

Classification of Hysterical Disorders

Hysterical disorders include *dissociative* (mental) and/or *conversion* (physical) symptoms, a history of chronic multiple complaints (*Briquet's syndrome*), and hysterical personality disorder. There are also a number of rare and exotic hysterical manifestations.

Dissociation hysteria

In dissociative responses, unpalatable ideas or memories are completely cut off from consciousness so that the patient is no longer aware of them. The result is often *hysterical amnesia*, or loss of memory for unpleasant images which threaten the patient's pride, well-being or happiness. Memory in hysterical amnesia usually returns spontaneously within 24 hours or so (Trethowan and Sims, 1983) and if the amnesia is prolonged, malingering is a distinct possibility.

Hysterical *fugue* is a specific form of hysterical amnesia in which people are unable to recall their prior identity and wander away and assume an entirely new identity. Fugue is literally 'a flight', often from a painful or threatening situation, and the patient is often found bewildered, far from home, with no memory of what he has been doing.

One patient, a successful executive, disappeared for two weeks and was found working as a cook's assistant in the kitchen of a 'fast food' snack bar. It emerged that, two days before his fugue episode, his wife had told him that she was leaving him for another man and he had simply dissociated from the severe stress he anticipated would occur when she left him (Meyer and Salmon 1984).

Fugue states are the commonest dissociative phenomena encountered in clinical practice (White and Dowson, 1983) and may also occur in depressive states or as the sequel to a major epileptic seizure. In day-dreaming and pathological lying there is also a degree of dissociation. Somnambulism, or sleep-walking, was until recently considered to be a dissociative phenomenon but has been reclassified as a sleep disorder consisting of a learned behaviour that was not quelled at onset (Meyer and Salmon 1984).

Table 57 Differentiation between hysterical and epileptic seizures.

	Hysteria	Epilepsy
Onset	Often gradual. Patient may choose safe place to fall	Sudden onset. Patient may be injured in fall
Consciousness	Retained	Lost
Sequence	No sequence. Generalized twitching or flailing of arms and legs	Sequence of aura, tonic, clonic, coma and recovery stages
Pupils	Remain normal	Dilated
Setting	In the presence of an audience	May occur at any time and in any place
Response to painful stimuli	Patient responds to painful stimuli (pinching of ear lobes or pressure on supraorbital notch)	No response—sensation slowly returns as coma state wears off
Duration	Seizure often improbably prolonged	Clinic stage lasts 2–3 minutes
Convulsive movements	Increase in response to attempts at restraint	Restraint does not affect movements
Incontinence	Does not occur	Double incontinence may occur

Conversion hysteria

In conversion hysteria, mental tensions are converted into *physical* symptoms as opposed to the mental symptoms of dissociative states.

The range of possible symptoms is very wide and may include hysterical seizures (though these are readily distinguished from those of organic origin). (Table 57), paralysis and loss of sensation (the latter often failing to correspond to any known distribution of nervous pathways), deafness, blindness, aphonia (inability to speak, or mutism), fainting attacks, anorexia, frigidity, impotence, dysmenorrhoea, vomiting, visual disturbances and skin rashes. Almost any symptom is possible and pain may be complained of in almost any site, though headaches and vague abdominal pains predominate. There may be dysphagia due to localized oesophageal spasm (globus hystericus), and retention of urine or faeces may occur.

Hysterical blindness may occur after the person has witnessed a very traumatic event and is a defence against re-experiencing such anxiety (the rock opera 'Tommy' is based on such an occurrence); in hysterical paralysis the resultant disability may extricate the person from an anxiety or guilt-evoking situation. Hysterical paralyses were reported from a variety of combat situations in both world wars and a variety of conflicts since. Consider the teenage fighter pilot in World War II—to continue flying was to court the ever-increasing possibility of death; to refuse to fly was to risk being labelled as a coward. Hysterical paralysis of a limb arose in a number of individuals trapped in such a conflict-arousing situation, and the resultant disability resolved the situation by enabling the person to exit from the stressful situation without experiencing colossal loss of self-esteem or increase in anxiety.

The Bible provides a description of symbolic hysterical paralysis and aphonia:

> If I forget thee, O Jerusalem, let my right hand forget her cunning. If I do not remember thee, let my tongue cleave to the roof of my mouth.
> (Psalm cxxxvii, 5, 6)

In one case a single woman had to look after her ageing and cantankerous mother, at considerable social and personal cost. She felt unable to express the resultant feelings of hostility, as these were socially unacceptable, but often secretly 'wished her away'. This conflict between desire and duty caused her considerable stress. She felt very guilty when the old lady fell in the garden and broke her hip, this incident coinciding uncannily with her less charitable thoughts. The daughter developed a paralysis of her right hand—the one she had thought of pushing her mother with. This paralysis freed the daughter from the conflict-arousing situation as she was now unable to look after her mother (Haslam, 1982).

In another case a rather extroverted girl was disappointed at being rejected for nurse training when she left school. She incurred considerable 'loss of face' and resentment as she now found herself nursing disappointment instead of patients. She was taken to hospital after a fall but was found only to be suffering from simple bruising. She complained of loss of movement and sensation in one of her legs and showed no response when the affected limb was pricked with a sterile needle. After admission she was noticed to be able to sit up in bed from a lying position, which movement requires the use of the thigh muscles as an anchor, and treatment by psychotherapy removed the paralysis (Haslam, 1982).

The above examples highlight the fact that *hysterical 'illnesses' are communications by the weakened or stressed, in the language of illness*. 'Body language' is being used to communicate distress, and treatment must facilitate the verbal expression of that which is being conveyed non-verbally.

Many patients with conversion symptoms display a strange bland indifference to what seems to be a serious symptom (la belle indifference) in contrast to the responses of anxiety and tension one would expect under the circumstances.

Florid conversion symptoms such as paralysis, blindness and deafness are now uncommon and most commonly encountered symptoms are pain, dizziness, headaches and muscle spasms (Watson and Buramen, 1979).

Briquet's syndrome

This refers to polysymptomatic, polysystemic conditions without organic origin (*chronic multiple complaint disorder*), and involves the production of a variety of conversion symptoms over a period of years. The gain involved often appears to be the gratification from gaining concern and attention from others or the reinforcement of fantasized 'sick roles'. The symptoms are true conversion symptoms in that they are produced quite unconsciously and without any element of conscious deception.

Hysterical personality disorder

This is characterized by excessive dependence on others, a labile mood, inability to sustain satisfactory close relationships, a tendency towards attention-seeking behaviour, craving for appreciation, suggestibility and theatricality. The individual is often sexually immature and there may be underlying frigidity despite displays of flirtatious behaviour. Individuals with such traits are liable to episodes of self-injury, and may develop conversion or dissociative symptoms in response to stress. Stress threshold tends to be low.

Uncommon Hysterical Reactions

The variety of hysterical responses seems to be almost endless, and many exotic manifestations have been described. These include the following:

Ganser's syndrome (hysterical pseudomentia)

In its complete form, this syndrome consists of clouding of consciousness accompanied by conversion symptoms and, above all, a tendency to give approximate answers to questions. When asked to identify the sum of two plus two the patient may answer—five. When asked how many legs a dog has the patient may answer—three. It is usually encountered in those in some sort of predicament—for example, prisoners on remand—and is very uncommon. Few cases last very long—usually less than a month—and spontaneous remission is likely. There is little agreement as to whether Ganser's syndrome should be regarded as psychosis, hysteria or malingering (Lazarus, 1964).

Munchausen syndrome

This is named after a fictitious German baron famed for the number of exaggerated tales associated with him. It consists of a plausible presentation of physical symptoms used in order to achieve multiple hospitalizations. This syndrome differs from Briquet's syndrome in that there is active and deliberate fabrication. The symptoms of Briquet's syndrome are produced unconsciously, those of Munchausen's syndrome are produced consciously, and usually arise from a basically hysterical personality.

Patients with Munchausen's syndrome accurately feign disease and are sometimes known as 'hospital hobos' or 'hospital tramps'.

Pallis and Vanji (1979) in a journal article called 'McIlroy Was Here' traced the travels of a famous Munchausen sufferer, Stewart McIlroy, through 68 different hospitals, with at least 207 known admissions in England, Ireland, Scotland and Wales. He used a variety of fake names and was only traced by records of the intricate scar pattern on his abdomen. McIlroy had thousands of X-rays and blood tests and 48 lumbar punctures, and his body was crisscrossed with scars from exploratory operations (Pallis and Vanji, 1979).

This 'hospital addiction' is fortunately rare and probably arises from a compulsion to repeat reinforcing situations arising in a 'care setting'. It is commoner in males and usually arises during the early twenties.

The couvade syndrome (sympathetic pregnancy)

This refers to a psychogenic disorder in which the father (or more rarely the children) 'comes out in sympathy' with a pregnant woman by developing abdominal swelling, early morning sickness, nausea, cravings and dyspepsia. Acute abdominal swelling is uncommon and is probably caused by depression of the diaphragm accompanied by lordosis (exaggerated forwards curvature of the lumbar spine). The abdominal swelling disappears under anaesthesia, only to reappear as soon as consciousness is regained. The abdominal swelling developed by a serving soldier resembled that of an eight months pregnancy (Enoch and Trethowan 1979) and it has been suggested that the symptoms may arise from a blend of envy and concealed homosexuality (Meyer and Salmon 1984).

Women may occasionally exhibit many signs of pregnancy when they falsely believe themselves to be in this condition (*pseudocyesis*), and the abdominal distention in these cases is also produced by diaphragmatic compression and lordosis.

Mass hysteria

Epidemic, or mass, hysteria has been described for many centuries and is most likely to occur in closed communities. There were many instances of outbreaks arising in convents in medieval times and the disorder is most likely to affect young girls around the age of puberty. The first person affected may have a genuine illness; the epidemic then spreads rapidly, often causing overbreathing, dizziness, fainting and assorted aches and pains. Alarming outbreaks of this sort occasionally occur in schools and may affect both sexes.

In closed female communities the cause is most likely to be repressed sexuality. In his account of mass hysteria arising in a medieval convent (The Devils of Loudon), Aldous Huxley described florid hysterical manifestations arising in a community of nuns. These manifestations always coincided with the arrival of a handsome young priest. Huxley's novel is based on historical accounts of events arising in the convent at Loudon, and the mass hysteria only terminated with the execution of the priest concerned (he was charged with witchcraft).

Multiple personality

This is a rare dissociative state in which the patient is dominated at any one time by two or more distinct personalities which are dissociated from one another and are often very dissimilar. One well-known case described Eve White, a serious and conscientious young mother, who developed an ancillary personality—Eve Black, who was flirtatious, irresponsible and impulsive. The personality Eve Black was completely aware of the existence of Eve White but Eve White did not suspect Eve Black's existence until they met in the therapist's consulting room. The two personalities produced different results on electroencephalograms, personality tests and handwriting analysis. Eve Black was very different from Eve White, being vain, shrewd, childish, egocentric and devoted to cruel pranks. Later, a more mature third personality emerged who called herself Jane (Sizemore and Pittillo, 1977). Two similar cases have been described, though it is perhaps noteworthy that all three cases were described in America, and the last case was described in 1954. There is a risk that the psychotherapist might (unwittingly) selectively prompt some utterances and not others, and may select the patient's behaviour and feelings, assigning some to one extreme and some to another, thus suggesting an ancillary personality to the patient. This condition may thus simply be the product of therapeutic manipulation.

Possession states

In medieval times hysterical women were frequently thought to be witches possessed by evil spirits, or communing with them, and were burned. Such superstitions seem to die hard. In 1975, in South Yorkshire, a 31-year-old man returned home after an all night exorcism 'to rid him of demons', and brutally killed his wife to rid her of evil spirits (Enoch and Trethowan, 1979). Within a month a clergyman carried out an 'exorcism' on a prostitute 'possessed of evil spirits of mocking and lying' in front of a mass congregation, television cameras and pressmen, with, it was reported, 'the full approval of the Bishop' (*The Guardian*, 1975). In 1979 two Roman Catholic priests in West Germany were charged with causing the death of a woman who starved to death while they were trying to drive out the 'devils' which possessed her (Enoch and Trethowan, 1979).

It is tempting to dismiss these unfortunate events as the result of the activities of the credulous or feeble-minded, but there is considerable evidence that many hysterical disorders may result in manifestations readily mistaken for 'possession' by the misguided or credulous. Many Third World immigrants come from cultures in which belief in possession is very strong, and such states may form an integral part of religious ceremonies during which dissociative responses are common and are viewed as having religious significance. *Glossolalia*, or automatic speech, in which the mouth speaks without the person knowing or willing what is said, may occur in dissociative states and may suggest possession to the startled and uninformed observer. The words spoken during glossolalia are not true language but *pseudo-language* which may be mistaken for a foreign tongue. Glossolalia often occurs during the mass hysterical reactions which are induced by the heightened emotional state of Pentecostal religious ceremonies, and is mentioned in the Bible. Some hysterical reactions take the form of dissociative trances in which glossolalia is common and may be accompanied by facial tics. Some such patients may even claim to be possessed, and there is a possibility that such hysterical 'possessions' allow dramatic relief of unbearable tensions. Claims of 'possession' may, of course, also be made by the schizophrenic patient.

Hysterical acting-out behaviour has also been responsible for claims of *poltergeist* activity, especially if these claims are accepted by an alarmed and credulous family. One such case has been described by Enoch and Trethowan (1979) and involved an adolescent girl whose family accepted her explanation of the 'manifestations', though these never occurred when strangers were present. The family described 'cold winds' and 'strange pushes', objects were claimed to have mysteriously moved, and strange noises and knockings abounded. The disturbances ceased when the daughter was placed in a new school.

Compensation neurosis

Genuine physical injury may trigger deep-seated dependency needs, especially if it is followed by sympathy, freedom from responsibilities and the possibility of monetary compensation. The injury may also trigger off feelings of conflict or anxiety, and more symptoms may be produced by the mechanism of conversion to produce a 'compensation neurosis' in which elements of malingering are sometimes blended with true conversion symptoms. If there is a lengthy period of time between the injury and indications of a settlement satisfactory to the patient, then the risk of compensation neurosis is increased. Hysterical reactions of this type may sometimes arise when there is no litigation or claim for compensation.

Treatment

Hysteria essentially consists of communications by the weakened or stressed in the language of illness, and the resultant symptoms may be physical (conversion) or mental (dissociation), or a blend of both. 'Body language' is being used to communicate distress, so treatment must therefore facilitate the verbal expression of that which is being conveyed non-verbally. Sources of stress should be identified and, where possible, removed or reduced.

Treatment should involve discussions with the family and other significant figures in the patient's life, and bargains and compromises may be necessary. Supportive psychotherapy will help the patient review faulty responses to stress and generate more adaptive strategies for the future.

The classical treatment of hypnosis consisted of psychoanalysis and/or hypnosis in an attempt to uncover unconscious causes of conflict, and both are still sometimes used, though psychoanalysis can be very time-consuming and may thus confirm feelings of chronic incapacity.

The power of suggestion may be effective in relieving many hysterical reactions, and this may be responsible for many cases of 'faith healing'. 'He cures most in whom most have faith', said Galen in 200 AD and studies report dramatic relief of chronic

neurotic symptoms associated with embracing a variety of cults, both Christian and non-Christian.

Nursing Care

Hysterical symptoms may be transparent to all but the patient. However, the nurse should remember that they are unambiguous signals of intolerable distress, and should therefore beware of any tendency to treat them lightly or regard them with contempt. A conversion symptom should be dealt with in much the same way as a delusion, that is by accepting the patient's need for the symptom but also by being careful not to reinforce it. The nurse must avoid being drawn into lengthy discussions of the patient's symptoms but instead should focus attention on healthy patterns of activity and interaction with others.

Assessment of the patient may uncover problems in the following areas:

Maintaining a safe environment. This may involve the nurse safeguarding the patient who has conversion symptoms manifesting themselves as sensory deficit. There may be visual disturbances ranging from blurring of vision to complete blindness, though the latter is now unusual. Hysterical paralysis or anaesthesia necessitates care of pressure areas, and joint exercises should be carried out.

Communication. This should gently but firmly promote decision-making with the hysterical patient, and gains and successes should be noted and reinforced. While avoiding attempts at an analytical or interpretive approach, the nurse should promote careful exploration of the patient's life strategies in an attempt to heighten self-awareness and the formulation of healthier responses to stress.

Talking with the hysterical patient is very important as it encourages the patient to verbally communicate stress and consider coping responses, instead of responding with non-verbal 'illness behaviour'. Many patients will display considerable resistance to exploratory dialogues of this sort, preferring to cling tenaciously to the defences of the sick role, and are reluctant to part with secondary gains associated with 'illness'.

The nurse who does not play her part in this 'illness game' may initially be regarded with annoyance and disfavour. Child-like recriminations and accusations may be directed against her by the patient who feels neglected or rejected, as attention is not focussed on her physical symptoms. Much patience and perseverence may be called for in this situation and the nurse must resist any tendency to assume the role of 'critical parent'. It is essential that the nursing approach be a concerted one, based on team discussion of the patient's difficulties. It would be disastrous if a well-meaning nurse were to respond positively to the patient's 'illness behaviour' and thus unwittingly subvert the objectives of the nursing care plan.

Communications should always incorporate persistent but gentle reminders that loss of function due to conversion symptoms is recoverable.

Expressing sexuality. This may be a difficult area for the patient due to psychosexual immaturity or conversion symptoms resulting in vaginismus and dyspareunia. The male patient may suffer from impotence, and discussions of sexual attitudes and activities should direct the patient's attention towards psychological causes and away from 'physical' causes. Highly extroverted patients are more liable to experience hysterical vaginismus, unlike introverted patients whose vaginismus is more likely to be a straightforward anxiety reaction (Lazarus, 1964). Discussion of sexual situations should emphasize that 'frigidity' does not necessarily imply deficient sexual ability or feelings (many women who are completely frigid in heterosexual situations are capable of self-induced orgasm) (Lazarus, 1964). Sexual difficulties are most likely to be the result of tensions arising from distorted attitudes or expectations about relationships, though simple sexual misconceptions may also be responsible, as may fear of pregnancy.

Psychosexual immaturity in the hysterical female may also manifest itself in seeming sexual precocity, leading to flirtatious behaviour and attitudes. The hysterical personality may also be marked by a tendency towards displays of emotional attachment which are intensely expressed but shallowly felt. The patient may be 'in love with being in love' but relationships are often unstable and stormy. In rejecting this behaviour nursing staff should make it clear that they are not rejecting the patient—simply the behaviour.

Working and playing. This should promote the development of coping strategies. Atrophied social skills and lowered self-esteem may respond favourably to simple group activities, and social skills

training will allow the patient to rehearse and practise faulty social behaviours. Fellow patients may be avoided, and invitations to participate in group activities declined, the patient preferring the seclusion of her 'sick bed'. It is not helpful to coerce the patient into group activities as this is likely to produce even more 'illness' as a defence against stressful nursing demands. Try to discover the patient's preferred recreational activities, her interests, her likes and dislikes, and structure small-scale activities around these. Simple one-to-one activities (a chat, board games) may help to win trust and establish confidence initially. The hysterical patient may be considerably disabled socially, so introduction to group activities should be gently graduated but progressively more demanding.

Group activities should be followed by a short, informal and confidential 'post mortem' with the nurse. This will help to identify areas of persisting social difficulty which may become the target of future practice and rehearsal. Try to conclude these sessions on a positive note by commenting on achievements and gains (however minor) as the hysterical patient may be quick to respond negatively to real or imagined setbacks. The nurse must also be firm, however, and persisting maladaptive behaviours must not be reinforced.

Sleeping. This may be difficult due to insomnia or nightmares, and the nurse's first line of approach should be to ensure that the environment is conducive to sleep. A warm bath or a milky drink will promote healthy sleep while the use of hypnotics may simply serve to further 'medicalize' the patient's life.

Eating and drinking. This may present problems as the 'ill' patient picks listlessly at food and displays anorexia consonant with the debility suggested by conversion symptoms. Many hysterical patients will baulk at eating a full meal but will cheerfully eat snacks between meals or ask visitors to bring in chocolates and sweets which are ingested in quantities hardly consonant with anorexia. Snacks and milk-based food supplements should be available and the nurse must avoid confrontations over uneaten meals. A casual and cheerful approach to meals will not reinforce illness behaviour associated with 'anorexia'. In some cases the anorexia will be genuine, so the nurse must ensure that dietary intake is adequate. The patient may ask visitors to bring in 'invalid foods', and the nursing staff should dissuade them from doing so while offering reassurance about the monitoring and maintenance of dietary intake. The patient may also have been in the habit of consuming inordinate amounts of vitamins and 'health supplements' and may protest about their unavailability in hospital. A brief but firm chat with the doctor will underline the fact that only pre-scribed medications should be taken. The author vividly recalls a patient who arrived clutching a carrier bag containing an assortment of 'health foods' that would have taxed the digestive tract of an alligator. The patient was in the habit of consuming a cocktail of substances including ginseng, royal jelly, iron, seaweed extract, pollen tablets, amino acid tablets and every vitamin known to the pharma-copoeia (to say nothing of a few 'discovered' by the manufacturers of 'health foods').

Personal cleansing and dressing. This may reflect obsessional traits associated with the hysteria and the nurse must firmly set limits on time-consuming behaviours of this type.

Elimination. This may be problematic due to con-stipation associated with low dietary intake; natural bran may be added to soups and puddings to alleviate this problem.

Mobilizing. This may present problems if the patient has hysterical paralysis. Passive movements of limbs may be used initially, though progress to active movement should be as quick as is compatible with avoiding undue distress. The patient should be invited to use a walking aid for a few days and should then progress to walking gently supported by the nurse's arm, though the patient should be advised that, if he tends to fall, the arm support will not be sufficient. The progression should be towards independence (support from furniture and walls and then no means of support). Trust exercises will help here. For example, the nurse may hold both the patient's outstretched hands and may then ask the patient to close her eyes while she is guided and gently supported around the room. Guidance may then be reduced to one hand. The patient is then asked to stand unsupported while the nurse remains close by. All gains should be warmly praised and the nurse should not allow immediate 'give up' reactions from the patient.

Throughout implementation of the care plan the nurse must remember that the patient's hysterical defences must not be abruptly stripped away from her and that the diminished ego reserves of the patient must not be overtaxed by a programme which is too demanding. If these precautions are not observed there may be a risk of suicidal gestures, as the patient is still grappling with intolerable stress but now has no neurotic defences against it. The effective programme returns strength and function as it slowly erodes maladaptive defences.

At all costs the patient must not be allowed to simply drift along trapped in the 'sick role' like a fly trapped in medical amber. Hysterical symptoms are often of great value to the patient and will be parted with reluctantly. Perseverence is important, though progress may be slow and painful. Eventually the person behind the 'illness' will emerge, often blinking painfully at the harsh light of interpersonal 'day'.

Key Concepts

1 Hysteria consists of the *communication* of distress in the language of illness.
2 The symptoms are the result of *unconscious conflict*.
3 Hysteria should not be confused with malingering, which is a conscious and deliberate attempt to fake illness.
4 Hysterical reactions to stress may produce physical symptoms (*conversion hysteria*) or mental symptoms (*dissociative hysteria*).
5 Conversion symptoms are almost endless in their range but may include paralysis, anaesthesia, blindness, deafness, mutism, seizures, 'sick headaches' or vague but distressing pains.
6 Florid conversion symptoms are now uncommon in the industrial West but are more common in Mediterranean peoples and may be relatively common in underdeveloped Third World countries.
7 Dissociative symptoms usually take the form of *amnesia* or *fugue states*, both of which are attempts to blot out or deny a threatening reality.
8 The nurse is unlikely to encounter a classical hysterical reaction in the in-patient population but may well encounter a depression or anxiety state with a hysterical overlay.
9 Treatment consists of reduction of stress factors, encouraging verbal expression of distress and shaping adaptive strategies to enable the patient to cope with future stress.

10 The nurse must not reinforce 'illness behaviour' but must gently and firmly encourage the patient to gain in self-awareness, verbal communication and social skills.

11 Nursing intervention must not abruptly strip the patient of the defences provided against stress by the hysterical reaction. Defences should only be gently removed as areas of strength are given in return.

References

The Guardian (1975) April 16.

Enoch, M. D. & Trethowan, W. H. (1979) *Uncommon Psychiatric Syndromes, 2nd edn*. Bristol: John Wright.

Haslam, M. T. (1982) *Psychiatry*. London: Heinemann.

Lazarus, A. (1964) Treatment of chronic frigidity. In Eysenck (Ed.) *Experiments in Behaviour Therapy*. Oxford: Pergamon Press.

Meyer, R. & Salmon, G. (1984) *Abnormal Psychology*. London: Allyn & Bacon.

Pallis, A. & Vanji, A. (1979) McIlroy was here: Or was he? *British Medical Journal*, 1: 973–974.

Sainsbury, M. (1980) *Key to Psychiatry, 3rd edn*. Australia: Australia & New Zealand Book Co.

Sizemore, C. & Pittillo, E. (1977) *'I'm Eve'*. New York: Doubleday.

Skultans, V. (1979) *English Madness. Ideas on Insanity 1580–1890*. London: Routledge and Kegan Paul.

Szasz, T. (1973) *The Manufacture of Madness*. London: Paladin.

Trethowan, W. & Sims, A. C. (1983) *Psychiatry, 5th edn*. London: Baillière Tindall.

Watson, C. & Buramen, C. (1979) The frequencies of conversion reaction symptoms. *Journal of Abnormal Psychology*, 88: 209–211.

White, C de B. & Dowson, J. (1983) In Berrios, G. & Dowson, J. H. (Eds.) *Treatment and Management in Adult Psychiatry*. London: Baillière Tindall.

19

Obsessive-Compulsive Neurosis

> 'It is an accustomed action with her to seem thus washing her hands: I have known her continue in this a quarter of an hour.'
>
> *Shakespeare: Macbeth, Act V, Scene 1*

Obsessive-compulsive neurosis is an uncommon mental disorder in which unwelcome thoughts persistently intrude into consciousness and give rise to the urge to carry out repetitive actions.

The preoccupying ideas or thoughts are referred to as *obsessions* and the repetitive actions, which the patient feels compelled to carry out, are referred to as *compulsions*. Obsessions and compulsions are combined as the salient features of obsessive-compulsive neurosis.

Obsessions are usually repetitive, often unpleasant, always unwelcome, and are accompanied by feelings of emotional tension. Obsessional ideas are recognized by the person as being inappropriate, senseless or alien to the person's nature but are also experienced as being uncontrollable. They may take the form of repetitive checking or counting of numbers, or saying words and phrases in the head, these sometimes being obscene, philosophical or completely meaningless. One patient mentally repeated the phrase 'This is not the way to do it', tapping his fingers to accent the rhythm of the words. Snatches of a song may be inwardly repeated, or elevated and degrading thoughts may follow one another (*contrast ideas*). Thus an elevated religious idea may be immediately followed by a grossly sexual one and these contrasting ideas may force their way into consciousness with great force and frequency, to the great distress of the patient. The patient may fear that he will utter his intrusive ideas aloud in an inappropriate place and a minister plagued by obscene ruminations feared that he would inadvertently utter obscenities from the pulpit.

Obsessive ruminations often give rise to *compulsions*, that is an action, or series of actions, which the person feels compelled to carry out. While recog-

nizing the irrationality of compulsive behaviours, patients describe strong feelings of tension or discomfort which arise if the compulsive actions are not carried out.

A man of 37 years old has described a steady increase of obsessional symptoms over 12 years. He worked as an engineer but was becoming progressively more inefficient at his job because every time he had to count numbers he felt compelled to check his figures more than 20 times. He developed elaborate rituals which involved getting into lifts, walking alongside another person and even getting in and out of his car, that required a great deal of checking and touching. Sometimes it would take him 45 minutes to leave his car after arriving in the car park. He became increasingly miserable and despondent about his inability to cope with everyday living (Sims, 1983).

The sequence of compulsive behaviours generated may develop into elaborate and lengthy rituals. One patient took 2½ hours to shave, much of this time being taken up in checking the exact setting of the razor, and in making sure that all the adjustable parts were screwed to an exact degree of balance and tension. Similarly, when punching his time card to clock in or out of work, the card had to be taken back six to a dozen times to make quite sure that it had been correctly punched (Stafford-Clark and Smith, 1983).

Rituals may be an ineffective attempt to relieve anxiety, as unconscious or semi-conscious anxieties are often the raw stuff from which obsessive-compulsive neuroses arise. Lady Macbeth repeatedly washed her hands to cleanse them of the contamination she felt she had acquired as the initiator of a murder, and thus symbolically reduced the guilt she felt.

The nurse should not underestimate the degree of suffering and misery caused by obsessive-compulsive states and should be aware of the extent to which these disorders can impair everyday social functioning.

Obsessional preoccupations which become the driving force behind compulsive rituals are usually one of three kinds:

211

1 *Sexual.* These preoccupations are connected with the fear of impregnating women, if the patient is a man, or of becoming pregnant if the patient is a woman. Thus an obsessional male may be compelled to wash out the bath with disinfectant three or four times before and after taking a bath to avoid insemination of the bath or bath water which might impregnate the next woman to use the same bath.

A highly intelligent woman of 45 years old contrived to undergo a hysterectomy in the hope that this would remove her fear of becoming pregnant by contact with articles which might have been handled by a man (Stafford-Clark and Smith, 1983).

2 *Aggressive.* These preoccupations are connected with a fear of causing injury or doing harm to self or others. Thus the obsessional mother may have exaggerated fears about sticking a nappy pin into her baby and may develop complicated nappy changing rituals to reduce these fears. The mother with a fear of harming her children may develop elaborate rituals involving locking up knives and hiding the key, perhaps inwardly repeating obsessional phrases as she does so.

3 *Contaminatory.* These anxieties may give rise to complicated rituals designed to reduce the risk of contamination by dirt or germs. Washing and dressing may become an exhausting and protracted affair in which parts of the body are washed in careful sequence, teeth are brushed with so many strokes in one direction and so many in the other, underarm deodorants are applied with similar obsessional care, and clothing is folded and refolded before being put on. Compulsive hand washing may take place with great frequency throughout the day, and there may be great preoccupation with neatness, cleanliness and orderliness.

Compulsive behaviours arising from these three basic anxieties tend to be of two types: (a) *washing* and (b) *checking* behaviour, though these may be combined.

There is a possibility that compulsive behaviour becomes a firmly established conditioned response arising from the conditional stimulus of the obsessional thought, which, in itself, is an attempt to control threatening emotions.

Aetiology

Obsessional ideas and compulsive rituals are a prominent part of the games and fantasy life of young children and are certainly not pathological in this context. Children's games often involve behaviours like trying to avoid stepping on cracks in the pavement or fallen leaves, or touching railings and counting them as they walk along the street.

The obsessional (or *anankastic*) personality often predates the onset of obsessive-compulsive disorders, though this personality type is relatively common and the majority will not develop overt disorder. The anankastic personality is characterized by rigidity and lack of adaptability. The individual is formal, precise and pedantic and is often conservative and authoritarian. Neatness, order, conformity and regularity will be highly valued by the anankastic, and this battery of response may be construed as arising from inner feelings of insecurity, disorder, anxiety and personal guilt.

Anankastic features may be modelled by parents who over-emphasize neatness and cleanliness to their infant offspring—perhaps starting with overstrict potty training. The child may become firmly persuaded that clean=good and dirty=bad, and these feelings may generalize so that untidiness, lack of conformity, lack of discipline, or routine are perceived as 'bad' and anxiety-evoking.

A measure of anankastic traits may be a positive advantage in certain occupations. One would hope that a bank manager, accountant or lawyer would be meticulous and would pay scrupulous attention to detail. The anankastic nurse will be punctual, conscientious, and attentive to detail, will adhere rigidly to the procedure manual and respect authority, and will react sharply to 'slackness' or 'inattention' in her subordinates. Her ward will be neat and tidy but her relationships with her patients and colleagues are unlikely to be relaxed and cordial. Anankastics are often awkward in the interpersonal sphere. People cannot be arranged as neatly and readily as objects and are often distinctly inconsistent.

Obsession-compulsion assessment

This questionnaire has been devised by doctors at the Institute of Psychiatry, London. It is used to make a preliminary assessment of the degree of difficulty suffered by obsessional compulsive patients:

> Please answer each question by putting a circle around the 'T' or the 'F' (True or False) following the question. There are no right or wrong answers, and no trick questions. Work quickly and do not think too long about the exact meaning of the question.

1 I avoid using public telephones because of   T/F
   possible contamination
2 I frequently get nasty thoughts and have   T/F
   difficulty in getting rid of them.
3 I am more concerned than most people   T/F
   about honesty.
4 I am often late because I can't seem to get   T/F
   through everything on time.
5 I don't worry unduly about   T/F
   contamination if I touch an animal.
6 I frequently have to check things (e.g.,   T/F
   gas or water taps, doors, etc.) several
   times.
7 I have a very strict conscience.   T/F
8 I find that almost every day I am upset by   T/F
   unpleasant thoughts that come into my
   mind against my will.
9 I do not worry unduly if I accidentally   T/F
   bump into somebody.
10 I usually have serious doubts about the   T/F
   simple everyday things I do.
11 Neither of my parents was very strict   T/F
   during my childhood.
12 I tend to get behind in my work because I   T/F
   repeat things over and over again.
13 I use only an average amount of soap.   T/F
14 Some numbers are extremely unlucky.   T/F
15 I do not check letters over and over again   T/F
   before posting them.
16 I do not take a long time to dress in the   T/F
   morning.
17 I am not excessively concerned about   T/F
   cleanliness
18 One of my major problems is that I pay   T/F
   too much attention to detail.
19 I can use well-kept toilets without any   T/F
   hesitation.
20 My major problem is repeated checking.   T/F
21 I am not unduly concerned about germs   T/F
   and diseases.
22 I do not tend to check things more than   T/F
   once.
23 I do not stick to a very strict routine when   T/F
   doing ordinary things.
24 My hands do not feel dirty after touching   T/F
   money.
25 I do not usually count when doing a   T/F
   routine task.
26 I take rather a long time to complete my   T/F
   washing in the morning.
27 I do not use a great deal of antiseptics.   T/F
28 I spend a lot of time every day checking   T/F
   things over and over again.
29 Hanging and folding my clothes at night   T/F
   does not take up a lot of time.
30 Even when I do something very carefully I   T/F
   often feel that it is not quite right.

It has been suggested that heredity may play a part in the transmission of obsessive-compulsive disorders, as up to one-third of the relatives of patients show varying degrees of obsessionality (Trethowan and Sims, 1983), though these findings may be rather suspect as learning within the family could satisfactorily account for these figures and no control group was used. Minor obsessional traits are relatively common in the general population and the criteria used in the study of pathological obsessionality should not be too elastic or results are bound to be misleading.

Freud suggested that obsessional symptoms result from repressed impulses of an aggressive or sexual nature; this proposition relates neatly to the turbulent sexual fantasies of many patients and their preoccupation with their own sexual and aggressive impulses. Freud also suggested that obsessional symptoms may be associated with regression to the anal stage of development; this would provide an explanation of the obsessional patient's preoccupation with excretory functions and dirt, and with compensatory over-emphasis on cleanliness and neatness. Attractive as they may be, these theories remain unconfirmed by objective evidence at the present time.

Obsessional symptoms first occur commonly between the ages of 10 and 15 years; in nearly a quarter of obsessional neurotics, the disorder has become established by the age of 15 years, and by the age of 30 three-quarters of cases have become manifest. Development is usually insidious with about seven years between onset and psychiatric referral (Sims, 1983).

Precipitating factors include critical life events like marriage, pregnancy and childbirth, and bereavement. Relationship difficulties, conflict situations and physical illness may also precipitate the disorder. Symptoms may wax and wane in intensity as episodes of stress lead to exacerbations.

Factors associated with prognosis are described in Table 58, though fully developed obsessive-compulsive states tend to have a poorer prognosis than other neurotic reactions (Ingram et al, 1981).

Incidence

The reported incidence of obsessive-compulsive neurosis in groups of psychiatric patients ranges from 0.1% to 4.6% (Rachman and De Silva, 1978).

Table 58 The prognosis of obsessive-compulsive neurosis

Factors associated with good prognosis
Mild symptoms
Absence of compulsions
Depressed mood
Obvious precipitating factors
Absence of previous personality disorder
Short interval between referral and onset
Episodic form of disorder
Short duration with early onset

Factors associated with poor prognosis
Single marital status
Obsessions starting in childhood and occurring
   continuously or repetitively throughout adolescence
Insidious onset
Impaired insight
Previous obsessional personality
Persistent and troublesome compulsive behaviours
Progressive worsening of symptoms over the years

Treatment

Treatment of obsessive-compulsive neuroses requires relearning adaptive patterns of behaviour, with or without associated use of drugs. Behavioural approaches to treatment are often particularly useful.

Drugs

Clomipramine (Anafranil), a tricyclic antidepressant, may reduce the intensity of obsessive-compulsive symptoms, particularly if there is associated depression, though studies suggest that symptom relief is not always dependent on the presence of a depressed mood, indicating that the drug may have a primary effect on the symptoms of this disorder (Rack, 1980). The latter finding is debatable as studies have also revealed that clomipramine did not have a detectable effect on rituals after a two year follow-up period (Mawson et al, 1982). It has been suggested that antidepressants may facilitate behavioural treatments by relieving troublesome mood states (Dowson, 1983).

Drug treatment has also involved other antidepressants (doxepin, amitriptyline, imipramine and mianserin), benzodiazepines, chlorpromazine and haloperidol, though in general, medication has not been markedly effective in the treatment of obsessive-compulsive disorders (Marks, 1978).

Psychotherapy

Supportive psychotherapy has an important role in the treatment of this disorder (Dowson, 1983) and may produce important symptom relief in addition to encouraging the patient to actively seek solutions to problem behaviours. The nurse has an important part to play here as she may encourage a problem-solving approach and constructive examination of approaches to daily living.

While supportive psychotherapy may impart therapeutic momentum, there is no convincing evidence to confirm the efficacy of interpretive psychotherapy based on psychoanalytical principles (Rachman and Hodgson, 1980).

Electroplexy

This may alleviate symptoms which are secondary to endogenous depressive states but its value in obsessive-compulsive neurosis is, at best, limited and short lived (Dowson, 1983).

Psychosurgery

This has the reputation of being successful in intractable cases, but recent reviews of psychosurgical research indicate that it is not often effective (Trotter, 1976; Rachman and De Silva, 1978).

Behaviour therapy

A variety of behavioural techniques have been used in the treatment of obsessive-compulsive disorders and these include many simple techniques which may be effectively used by the nurse, though it must be emphasized that the use of these techniques should be sanctioned by discussion with the other members of the care team.

Thought stopping

This is a simple behavioural technique which often proves effective in reducing both the frequency and intensity of obsessional thoughts. The patient is seated with his eyes shut and he is instructed to give free rein to his obsessional thoughts. When they are flooding his mind he signals to the therapist who shouts 'stop'. The patient is instructed to keep his mind blank after the 'stop' signal or to imagine some pleasant scene. The signal interrupts the obsessional train of thought abruptly and the patient is instructed to imagine the therapist's voice shouting 'stop' when obsessional thoughts intrude in future.

Self-administered aversive stimuli (snapping an elastic band against the wrist) will also interrupt obsessional trains of thought and may prove to be a simple but effective 'first aid' measure.

Exposure

Exposure to the situation triggering the urge to carry out compulsive behaviours often proves effective. For example, the patient plagued by the impulses towards compulsive hand washing is asked to repeatedly contaminate his hands (for example, by touching the sole of his shoe) and is then prevented from carrying out his compulsive ritual (*response prevention*). The therapist may also demonstrate the required behaviour (*modelling*) by contaminating his own hands and then carrying on with normal activities without washing his hands. The three ingredients of modelling, exposure and response prevention may prove to be very effective, and Marks (1981) has reported that exposure was followed by lasting improvement in rituals for up to three years in a series of more than 200 patients. This improvement generalized, allowing the patients to lead a fuller and happier social life. Marks suggests that when rituals are present without depression, exposure is then the treatment of choice.

Nursing care

The nurse must remember that obsessive-compulsive states can be remarkably resistant to any form of treatment; an approach must therefore be adopted which is realistic and not too hurried. Problems may be encountered in the following areas:

Maintaining a safe environment. Obsessive-compulsive states may cause intense misery and torment to the patient, and suicide risk may be high. The nurse should therefore ensure that a *safe environment* is maintained, and careful but discreet observation is important. Assessment of the patient may reveal intense feelings of torment with associated suicidal feelings or plans. Any previous history in suicidal attempts or self-mutilating behaviour should be noted as increasing the suicidal risk. A history of unsuccessful treatment also augments suicide risk.

Communication. This may be affected by the neurosis as the patient may be tense and preoccupied and consequently reluctant to communicate freely. Recreational and diversional therapy will help the patient to relax and will create a setting which will facilitate the development of a therapeutic nurse/patient relationship. The nurse should focus on the patient, not his symptoms, during interaction and the nurse should remember that the tense and anxious obsessive-compulsive patient may have little tolerance for frustration. It is necessary that communication proceeds at a pace which is comfortable for the patient and a calm quiet approach is desirable. The obsessive-compulsive patient often has difficulty in expressing thoughts and feelings and simple social skills training exercises may prove to be very helpful.

Expressing sexuality. This may reveal an element of sexual preoccupation in the patient's thinking, and compulsive behaviours may be generated in response to these. Supportive psychotherapeutic discussion may help to defuse the patient's anxieties associated with disturbed sexual imagery.

Working and playing. These will often be problematic areas for the patient. Compulsive rituals may have badly impaired efficiency, and occupational, industrial and recreational therapy will help the patient to regain some of the lost rhythms of daily activity. Listening to music, doing crossword puzzles and playing board games will provide distraction from obsessions and compulsions and may thus help restore lost self-esteem and confidence. Limits must be clearly set on ritualistic behaviour, and the teaching of thought-stopping techniques will be helpful here. It is also essential to protect the patient from the ridicule of his fellow patients who may be amused or intrigued to witness ritualistic behaviour. Behaviour modification will also be useful insofar as abstinence from ritualistic behaviour should be noted and warmly praised. Rituals should not be inadvertently reinforced by responding to them with undue nursing attention.

Sleeping. This may be difficult as tormenting obsessional thoughts or the urge to carry out compulsive behaviours may prevent sleep. Sleeping during the day, even napping in an armchair, should not be permitted if insomnia is a problem, and thought-stopping techniques may prove to be particularly useful in helping the patient to sleep. Relaxation exercises may prove to be particularly effective if combined with thought-stopping for the obsessive-compulsive insomniac. The provision of an environment conducive to sleep is also important and the appropriate factors can only be established after consultation with the patient (What helps you sleep? What disturbs your sleep?).

Eating and drinking. These may also be problem areas if the patient has compulsive rituals associated with eating. There may be a risk of malnutrition, and dietary intake should be carefully monitored. Insisting that the patient eats at set times or in a set place may simply intensify anxiety and thus worsen ritualistic behaviour. Elasticity of approach is helpful here and the patient should be allowed to eat where and when he feels like it initially. Ready availability of food is important.

Personal cleansing and dressing. This may be a major focus for ritualistic behaviour and thus for therapeutic intervention. Exposure and response prevention may usefully focus around these times and the nurses must firmly set limits on compulsive behaviour, reinforcing and recording gains.

Elimination. This may be beset by contaminatory fears with associated compulsive cleansing rituals. Again the nurse must firmly monitor and regulate these activities and set clearly defined limits to problem behaviours. Uncontrolled hand washing may lead to severe dermatitis and the nurse should ensure that visits to the lavatory are not the occasion for intense compulsive outbreaks.

The nurse should remember that interruptions of ritualistic behaviour may generate intense feelings of hostility in the patient and he/she should be prepared for resentful or aggressive verbalizations.

Progress may be slow but the nurse must curb any feelings of impatience and must avoid any tendency to 'force the pace'. Support and encouragement are essential and should be constantly provided. The family should be informed of the treatment and nursing regime and should be involved wherever possible, as many obsessive-compulsives improve in the controlled environment of the hospital only to deteriorate again after discharge if social support is not available.

Key Concepts

1 Obsessive-compulsive neurosis is an uncommon but extremely distressing mental disorder which may be very resistant to treatment.
2 It consists of a blend of *obsessions* (unwelcome but persistently intrusive thoughts) and *compulsions* (actions which the patient feels compelled to carry out).
3 Compulsive behaviours may develop into lengthy and elaborate *rituals*, which greatly impair efficiency and well-being.
4 Obsessional preoccupations may be *sexual, aggressive* or *contaminatory*.
5 Compulsive behaviours usually consist of *washing* or *checking*.
6 The *anankastic* personality type is often associated with the disorder and may be rooted in parental attitudes which over-emphasize discipline, cleanliness and comformity.
7 Obsessional characteristics are 'normal' in children.
8 Freud suggested that obsessional symptoms may reflect repressed impulses of a sexual or aggressive nature associated with regression to the anal stage of development.
9 Treatment may consist of drugs, psychotherapy and behaviour therapy, though psychosurgery has been used in intractable cases.
10 Nursing care must set limits on ritualistic behaviour and may usefully incorporate behavioural techniques.
11 Behavioural techniques used include *exposure, thought stopping, response prevention, modelling* and *behaviour modification*.
12 There may be a high suicide risk and nursing approaches must take account of this.

References

Dowson, J. (1983) Management of obsessive-compulsive disorders. In Berrios, G. & Dowson, J. H. (Eds) *Treatment and Management in Adult Psychiatry*. London: Baillière Tindall.

Ingram, I., Timbury, G. & Mowbray, R. (1981) *Notes on Psychiatry, 5th Edn.* Edinburgh: Churchill Livingstone.

Marks, I. (1978) Behaviour psychotherapy of adult neuroses. In Garfield & Bergin (Eds) *Handbook of Psychotherapy and Behaviour Change*. New York: John Wiley.

Marks, I. (1981) *Cure and Care of Neuroses*. New York: John Wiley.

Mawson, D., Marks, I. & Ramm, L. (1982) Clomipramine and exposure for chronic obsessive-compulsive rituals. *British Journal of Psychiatry*, **140**: 11–18.

Rachman, S. & Hodgson, R. (1980) *Obsessions and Compulsions*. Herts: Prentice-Hall.

Rachman, S. & De Silva, P. (1978) Abnormal and normal obsessions. *Behaviour Research and Therapy*, **16**: 233–248.

Rack, P. (1980) The chemotherapy of obsessive-compulsive disorders. *Pharmacological Medicine*, **1**(2): 22.

Sims, A. (1983) *Neurosis in Society*. London: The Macmillan Press.

Stafford-Clark, D. & Smith, A. (1983) *Psychiatry for Students, 6th Edn*. London: George Allen & Unwin.

Trethowan, W. & Sims, A. (1983) *Psychiatry, 5th Edn*. London: Baillière Tindall.

Trotter, S. (1976) Federal commission O.K.'s psychosurgery. *A.P.A. Monitor*, **7**: 4–5.

V
SCHIZOPHRENIA

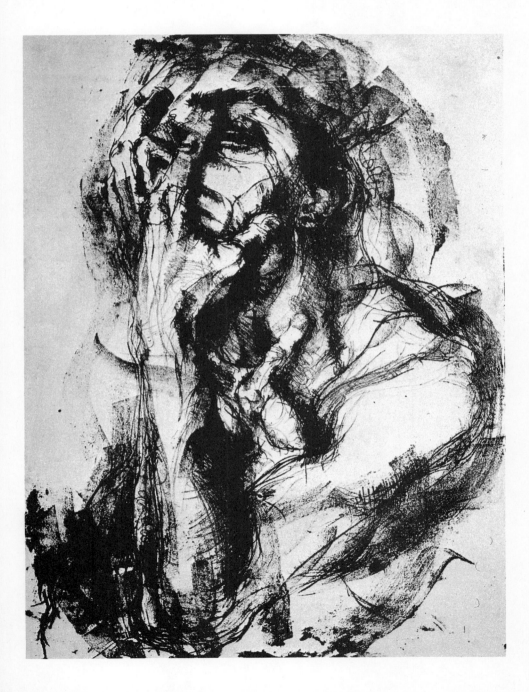

20

Schizophrenia

Of all mental disorders, schizophrenia probably causes more fear and misunderstanding than any other. It resembles most closely the layman's concept of 'true madness' as many sufferers retreat into a distorted, and sometimes fantastic, inner world of jumbled thought processes and bizarre perceptual experiences wherein they may seem completely estranged from human understanding. The term 'schizophrenia' may suggest 'split personality' to the layman, a sort of Jekyll and Hyde division of personality. This is quite untrue. The personality in schizophrenia may fragment or deteriorate, but does not 'split' clearly to produce a double or multiple personality, despite the fact that the word schizophrenia does literally mean 'splitting of the mind'. Double or multiple personality is a very rare hysterical phenomenon and is quite dissimilar in presentation from schizophrenia. The schizophrenic suffers from impaired '*reality testing*' and eventually seems to view reality through a strangely distorting lens. The inner world of the patient becomes populated by strange delusional ideas and this alien landscape is often illuminated with frightening intensity by vivid hallucinatory experiences. Clear consciousness and intellectual capacity are usually maintained, though disturbances of thought, perception, and mood may be marked.

The disorder seems to strike at the very foundation of personality and, in severe cases, may seem to reduce it to ruins, though recognizable 'fragments' remain apparent to family and friends. Schizophrenia is very variable in course and outcome, and may range from acute, but short-lived, forms occurring in reaction to stress (*reaction schizophrenia* or *schizophrenic reaction*) to an insidious and progressive

form which tends to run an unremittingly downhill course (*nuclear* or *process* schizophrenia).

How Common Is Schizophrenia?

The estimated risk of developing schizophrenia at some time in life varies from 0.7–3.0%, with an average risk of 0.8% (8 persons per 1000 of the population), the variations in prevalence arising out of international differences in the definition of schizophrenia.

Psychiatrists in the USA have a broader definition of schizophrenia and tend to diagnose it more often than their British counterparts who, in turn, diagnose manic-depressive psychosis more often.

The disorder tends to develop in adolescence, but may do so insidiously so that diagnosis of schizophrenia reaches a peak in the age group 20–39 years. All persons younger than 20 years are considered not to have reached the peak risk period, and persons who are older than 39 years are considered to have passed the peak risk period.

Variations in reported international incidence rates may be marked. Using an incidence rate expressed as the number of new cases in a given period per 100 000 of the population, an average incidence rate of 21.8 cases per year has been established, though surveys have in recent years suggested higher rates from the following countries: England, 30.6; Ireland 52.0; Germany, 53.6; and the USA 72.0 (Tsuang, 1982).

These seeming variations may be reflections of differing diagnostic criteria rather than true indications of morbidity. Using more stringent criteria a recent survey suggested an incidence rate of 11–14 cases per year per 100 000 in England (Tsuang, 1982).

Schizophrenia accounts for some 15% of admissions to psychiatric hospitals, for 45% of the hospital population, and for the majority of long-stay patients (Ingram et al, 1981).

The disorder is slightly more common in males than in females and onset is usually earlier in men,

221

whereas women have higher rates in the older age groups.

What Causes Schizophrenia?

The cause of schizophrenia is as yet unknown, though many predisposing and precipitating factors have been identified. The influences of heredity and environment seem to be closely entangled in the aetiology of schizophrenia, and the effects of both, and their interaction, have been closely studied.

Heredity

Research seems to provide strong evidence that there are important genetic factors in the aetiology of schizophrenia. The closer the blood relationship of a person to a schizophrenic, the higher the risk of schizophrenia. The brothers and sisters of schizophrenics have a risk of developing the disorder which is ten times higher than that of the general population. For children of schizophrenics the risk is 15 times the general population risk (12.3%). If both parents are schizophrenic the risk increases to about 40%. The risk to uncles and aunts, nephews and nieces, grandchildren, and half-brothers or sisters is approximately three times that of the general population (Tsuang, 1982).

There is also a possibility that what is being transmitted is not faulty genes, but faulty child-rearing practices (see Chapter 2), and that schizophrenic children are borne into stressful and deprived environments similar to those which caused mental disorder in their parents.

Twin and adoption studies have been used in an attempt to distinguish hereditary influences from environmental ones.

Two important studies of adopted children suggest that the higher frequency of schizophrenia in the children of schizophrenic parents cannot be ascribed entirely to child-rearing practices. Heston and Denny (1968) studied the life history of 47 adopted children born to schizophrenic mothers and revealed an incidence of approximately 11% for schizophrenic disorder in the adopted children compared to an incidence of 0% in 50 children of non-schizophrenic mothers used as a control group.

A Danish study suggested a 19% incidence of schizophrenia in the children of schizophrenics who had been adopted and brought up away from their parents, though the same study indicated the remarkably high incidence of 10% in the adopted children of a control group of non-schizophrenics. This suggests that the diagnostic criteria used in this study may have been rather elastic (Heston and Denny, 1968).

A further test from the same Danish study suggested that children of 'normals' reared by schizophrenics did not show a raised incidence of schizophrenia, thus casting some doubt on 'family pathology' models.

Twin studies provide further evidence of the presence of a critical genetic component. Identical twins, who develop from the same egg (monozygotic twins) are more likely to develop schizophrenia than fraternal twins, who develop from different eggs (dizygotic twins); that is, the *concordance* rate is higher for monozygotic than for dizygotic twins (Table 59).

Table 59 From Gotesman and Shields (1973)

Country	Percentage of concordance	
	Monozygotic twins	Dizygotic twins (same sex)
Japan (1961)	60	18
Norway (1967)	45	15
Denmark (1969)	56	26
Finland (1971)	35	13
USA (1972)	43	9
UK (1972)	58	12

The fact that about half of the MZ twins studied were *not* concordant for schizophrenia is incontrovertible evidence that the disorder is not *entirely* hereditary, otherwise concordance rates would be 100%. It seems that what is inherited is not the disorder itself, but a predisposition towards it. This predisposition may or may not manifest itself as schizophrenia, depending on the presence or absence of precipitating factors which may well be environmental.

The Chemistry of 'Madness'

It has long been recognized that certain drugs mimic psychosis in their effects; that is, they are said to be *psychotomimetic*. Mescaline and lysergic acid diethylamide (LSD) produce states which mimic psychoses in many important respects, the so-called *model psychoses* (see Chapter 2). Mescaline is structurally similar to the neurotransmitter *dopamine*— (neurotransmitters are chemicals present in minute amounts in the nervous system which facilitate the passage of nerve impulses)—and it was considered that schizophrenics may suffer from an abnormality of dopamine production, either from producing abnormal dopamine molecules, or from producing dopamine in excessive amounts. It was also noted that many tranquillizing drugs, which effectively dampen psychotic symptoms, block dopamine receptor sites, whereas amphetamine has the opposite effect. Amphetamine abuse is often characterized by schizophrenic-like symptoms, and amphetamines worsen the symptoms of schizophrenia. It has also been observed that disulfiram (Antabuse) raises dopamine levels and can induce psychotic reactions, and is therefore contraindicated in schizophrenia (Smythies, 1975). While dopamine levels seem to be *raised* in schizophrenia, they are *lowered* in Parkinson's disease, and the tremor and rigidity of this condition often shows dramatic improvement when large doses of dopamine are given. Parkinson's disease and schizophrenia thus seem to be 'biochemical opposites', yet schizophrenia has been reported in association with Parkinson's disease (Clare, 1976) suggesting that schizophrenia cannot be simply explained in terms of raised dopamine levels alone.

Schizophrenia has also been attributed to vitamin deficiencies, sensitivity to wheat protein (as found in coeliac disease), allergies, virus infections and a wide range of abnormalities of body chemistry—all without the production of convincing evidence that would bear close experimental scrutiny. Research continues and opinion is divided about the importance of biochemical factors, or as to whether these are cause or effect of the disorder.

Smith (1982) has commented that '. . . even if important biochemical abnormalities were to be found exclusively in schizophrenia, the illness could not be viewed simply as a disorder of metabolism, primarily without psychological meaning'.

Neurophysiological Findings

It has been demonstrated that a relatively high number of schizophrenics are left-handed, indicating that the right cerebral hemisphere may be dominant in schizophrenia (Tsuang, 1982). (The brain consists of two identical hemispheres, each controlling movements on the *opposite* side of the body. For example, in the *right*-handed person, the *left* hemisphere is dominant and controls actions of the *right* arm, leg and eye.)

The observation that the *right* side of the brain may be dominant in schizophrenia is interesting because the right side of the brain is considered to be associated with emotions, whereas the left side usually contains the language centres. Some types of temperal lobe epilepsy involving the right side of the brain may produce marked emotional disorder. These observations remain largely unsubstantiated by detailed research at the present time.

The technique of computerized axial tomography (the CAT scan)—a sophisticated X-ray technique whereby a three-dimensional picture of the brain may be assembled—reveals enlargement of the cerebral ventricles in about 40% of chronic schizophrenics though the relevance of this finding, and whether or not it is cause or effect of the disorder, has been disputed (Trethowan and Sims, 1983).

Another finding is that about 70% of schizophrenics reveal an 'eye tracking dysfunction'; that is, their eyes follow movement jerkily. This dysfunction also occurs in 45% of immediate relatives of schizophrenics and it has been suggested that it may provide a useful 'marker' in the study of the genetics of schizophrenia (Tsuang, 1982). This defect may, however, simply indicate impaired attention rather than an underlying neurophysiological defect.

Psychological and Social Factors

So far we have considered processes arising *inside* persons, but discussions of schizophrenia have also considered processes occurring *between* persons in an attempt to shed light on the elusive causes of this disorder.

Consideration of the interpersonal approach to schizophrenia is inseparable from the prolific writings of R. D. Laing, already briefly introduced in Chapter 2.

Laing suggests that there may be some 'method in madness' in that schizophrenia may consist of 'normal responses to an abnormal situation' (Laing and Esterson, 1964), the 'abnormal situation' being distorted family dynamics, which in turn mirror the distortions in society as a whole. Laing suggests that the behaviour and feelings of schizophrenics are 'much more socially intelligible than has come to be supposed by most psychiatrists'.

Laing considers the families of schizophrenics to be characterized by confused, distorted and irrational relationships, which eventually generate the essentially protective responses of schizophrenia in the hapless children of 'schizophrenogenic' parents. Bombarded by the contradictory demands of 'double bind' situations (see page 17) and dazed by the distorted and irrational demands of the family, the schizophrenic eventually recoils from this threatening 'reality' into the safety of psychotic withdrawal and fantasy. Laing suggests that a salient characteristic of the 'schizophrenogenic' parent may be *denial* of the reality of the victim child's experiences, a denial which may not only be rigidly controlling, but irrational. For example, puritanical parents may tell their daughter not merely that she should not act on her sexual desires, or even that she ought not to have them, but that she *does not have them*.

A further theme in Laing's work is the thesis that society itself is 'crazy'. Conventional standards of 'mental health' are viewed as suffocating and repressive obstacles to the development of a fully human consciousness, as they deny human uniqueness and spontaneity in favour of a sterile and destructive work ethic. Early works by Laing (1970) went so far as to identify the schizophrenic as being 'hypersane', that is as a cultural critic who points out the contradictions between man's innate capacity for joy and the pervasive joylessness of 'normal' society.

Laing's work is largely speculative and his theories remain unsupported by convincing experimental evidence, although he has reawakened interest in the interpersonal aspects of schizophrenia.

Other investigations of family relationships in schizophrenia have suggested possible abnormalities of marital relationships. In 'skewed' relationships there was thought to be a dominant and abnormal parent to whom the other parent yielded. Relationships of this sort were thought to be commoner among parents of male schizophrenics, and the mother was thought to be dominant and the father weakly passive. The dominant mother was then thought to reject her passive partner and direct her emotional energies against her son instead, with destructive consequences (Lidz et al, 1965). In *marital schism* each parent tried to dominate and devaluate the other, each attempting to enlist the child's support in this interpersonal civil war. This background was considered to be commoner in families of female schizophrenics (Lidz et al, 1965).

A study of identical (monozygotic) twins, only one member of which developed schizophrenia despite the fact that they were raised in the same family, revealed that the schizophrenic twin identified more strongly with the parent who was mentally less healthy (Mosker et al, 1971).

Studies of the *'prepsychotic'* or *'premorbid'* personality (personality before the onset of disorder) have suggested that it tends to be marked by seclusiveness, shyness, lack of interest in the environment and a rich fantasy life. This personality type is also referred to as *schizoid* and the presence of these traits may be said to constitute *schizoidia*. Such a personality type does not mean that the development of schizophrenia is inevitable; these traits may, in some cases, bear no relationship to schizophrenia at all. The traits described do, however, occur more frequently in schizophrenics than in their relatives and occur almost 50 times more frequently in the history of schizophrenics than in the population at large (Trethowan and Sims, 1983). This personality type may constitute a *predisposition* to the disorder and is probably determined genetically. *Precipitating* factors (trauma, drug or alcohol abuse, childbirth, metabolic disorder, or sustained family stress) may trigger an outbreak of the disorder proper.

Geneticists refer to the inherent genetic development of the individual as the *genotype*, and the genotype is determined by nothing other than the two genetic memories that have combined to create it. These characteristics are imposed upon by environmental influences to produce the *phenotype*—the egg plus experience.

It is possible that *schizoidia* or a tendency to it is the genotype, and schizophrenia is the phenotype, critical experiences perhaps being included among the biochemical and psychosocial forces discussed.

Features of Schizophrenia

In schizophrenia there seems to be disorder of ego function. Freud defined the Ego as that part of the mind which organizes perception and deals with reality. The Ego regulates awareness of oneself as separate from all external things which are not part of self, thus allowing separation of self from environment.

In schizophrenia ego boundaries become indistinct and may deteriorate, causing diminished awareness of reality. Kurt Schneider, a German psychiatrist, identified a number of symptoms which he considered to be diagnostic of schizophrenia, these being referred to as *'first rank symptoms of schizophrenia'* (Schneider, 1959).

First rank symptons comprise thought disorder (thought insertion, thought withdrawal, thought broadcasting, and primary delusions), feelings of passivity, and auditory hallucinations in the third person.

First rank symptoms of schizophrenia

Passivity experience

This involves thoughts, emotions, impulses or actions experienced by the individual as being under external, alien control. Disturbances of *thought control* are included (thought insertion, thought withdrawal, and thought broadcasting).

Auditory hallucinations in the third person

These are hallucinatory 'voices' maintaining a 'running commentary' on one's actions, or discussing thoughts or behaviour as they occur. The 'voices' are experienced as alien and may be heard discussing or arguing about one in the third person, that is referring to one as 'he' or by name.

Primary delusions

These are delusions arising from perceptions which are in themselves normal.

A diagnosis of schizophrenia may still be made in the absence of first rank symptoms as they may be absent in the very early and acute stages of the disorder. In making the diagnosis of schizophrenia, the following must be excluded: drug or alcohol abuse, affective disorder, or epilepsy. Consciousness must be clear, and memory and orientation intact.

First rank symptoms describe the primary or basic dimensions of schizophrenia, but a wide variety of other disturbances are also often present, many not being peculiar to schizophrenia. They include the following:

1 *Disorder of mood*. Blunting or incongruity of effect—a pervasive apathy may develop.

2 *Disorder of thought*. The first rank experiences of thought control may co-exist with thought blocking, concrete thinking, 'knight's move' thinking or overinclusive thinking and ideas of reference (see Chapter 4).

3 *Delusions*. May be primary or secondary, systematized or unsystematized.

4 *Hallucinations*. May arise in a setting of clear consciousness, usually auditory, but may affect the other senses.

5 *Disorder of volition*. Loss of drive and 'willpower'.

6 *Disorder of expression*. May reflect underlying thought disorders (e.g. neologisms, 'word salads', echolalia).

7 *Withdrawal*. Retreat, seemingly into a distorted inner world of often bizarre fantasies, may take place.

8 *Motor disturbances*. Abnormalities of movement may occur with bizarre grimaces, postures, or gait. In extreme cases flexibilitas cerea or echopraxia may appear. Combinations of the above may interact to produce an overall picture of personality disorganization. This led early psychiatrists to erroneously call schizophrenia 'dementia praecox' (precocious dementia) and this term persisted until 1911 when Bleuler coined the term 'schizophrenia'.

'Whence is this monstrous thing?'—The Experience of Schizophrenia

There are many first person accounts of the experience of schizophrenia which serve to shed some light on the bizarre and often terrifying experience of psychosis. In Book VIII of his Confessions, St Augustine groans under the weight of mental disorder: 'Whence is this Monstrous Thing, and Why is it? The mind commands the body, and it obeys forthwith, the mind commands itself and is resisted . . . For the will commandeth that there be a will, not another, but itself. But it doth not command entirely . . . It is, therefore, no monstrous thing partly to will, partly to be unwilling, but an infirmity of the mind . . .'.

Janet Frame, the New Zealand novelist, describes her experience of the first rank symptom of auditory hallucinations in the third person . . .

'The voices continued their whispering. "We'll give her shock treatment tomorrow", one said. "A worse shock than she's ever had, and she can't escape. You've locked the door securely?"
"Yes", replied the other. "She's down for shock. It will put her in her place I tell you. She needs to be taught a lesson. No breakfast for her tomorrow."
"No breakfast", the other voice repeated. "She's for shock."
My heart beat so fast that I found it hard to breathe. I was overcome by such a feeling of panic that although it seemed like breaking and distorting the only image of the sky that was left to me, I smashed the window with my fist, to get out or get at the glass and destroy myself to prevent the coming of tomorrow . . .'

(*Frame, 1961*).

In *Autobiography of a Schizophrenic Girl*, the author describes experiences indicating disintegration of ego boundaries and a pervasive sense of being controlled by alien forces—'the System':

'Everything was alive, defied me. Outside in the street people were struck mad, moved around without reason, encountered each other and things which had become more real than they.
    At the same time, I received orders from the System. I did not hear the orders as voices; yet they were as imperious as if uttered in a loud voice. While, for example, I was preparing to do some typing, suddenly without any warning, a force which was not an impulse but rather resembled a command, ordered me to burn my right hand or the building in which I was'

(*Sechehye, 1951*).

Mark Vonnegut vividly describes the first visual hallucination of his schizophrenic breakdown:

'. . . out of nowhere came an incredible wrinkled, iridescent face. Starting as a small point infinitely distant, it rushed forward, becoming infinitely huge. My heart had stopped. The moment stretched forever . . . it kept coming and coming 'til I was lost somewhere in some pore in its nose and it still kept coming . . . There was nothing at all unreal about that face. Its concreteness made the Rock of Gibraltar look like so much cotton candy'

(*Vonnegut, 1975*).

In *Living with Schizophrenia* the author describes her voyage into the 'fathomless worlds of unreality' and describes her experience of ideas of reference and thought broadcasting:

'The walk of a stranger on the street could be a "sign" to me which I must interpret. Every face in the windows of a passing streetcar would be engraved on my mind, all of them concentrating on me and trying to pass me some sort of message . . . To feel that the stranger passing on the street knows your innermost soul is disconcerting . . . I had very little ability to sort out the relevant from the irrelevant'

(*McDonald, 1960*).

There are many other accounts of the parallel world of psychosis in which the sufferer may be impelled on strange courses of action by powerful delusional beliefs while 'voices' guide or criticize his actions. Everyday objects and events may assume a mystic or symbolic significance and awareness of reality may ebb and flow as the disorder fluctuates in intensity.

Forms of Schizophrenia

Schizophrenia disorders may assume a variety of forms, though four main types predominate:

1 *Simple schizophrenia* (schizophrenia simplex). Early age of onset (usually during adolescence) with insidious and slowly progressive deterioration of personality. Not a florid or dramatic disorder, and hallucinations and delusions are usually absent. The primary symptoms are emotional blunting and loss of volition, and the patient may simply appear to be rather 'odd' to others. Many cases never reach hospital but drift downwards socially to become vagrants or recluses. Behaviour tends to be eccentric rather than obviously disturbed.

2 *Hebephrenic schizophrenia* (hebephrenia). The early age of onset is reflected in the nature of this disorder (Gk. *hebe* meaning youth); onset is usually in the late teens. The underlying state is one of dullness and apathy, though bizarre hypochondriacal delusions are common. Hallucinations are common and are usually auditory in type. Behaviour may be erratic and unpredictable and odd mannerisms

are common. Mood may be shallow and inappropriate and there may be outbursts of giggling or laughing with an overall suggestion of childishness about the patient's responses. Thought disorder may be marked and the patient may become pre-occupied by pseudoscientific or pseudophilosophical beliefs.

3 *Catatonic schizophrenia.* This form is commoner in females and occurs in the late teens to mid-twenties. It has become increasingly rare in the last 30 years and many catatonic symptoms may have been a response to institutionalization.

The essential feature of this form is psychomotor disturbance, often alternating between the extremes of hyperkinetic excitement and catatonic stupor. Hallucinations, thought blocking and neologisms may occur. Negativism is not uncommon and stereotyped behaviour and posturing may be apparent.

4 *Paranoid schizophrenia.* This form has a later age of onset (30–50 years) and the major symptom is the presence of delusions of persecution with auditory hallucinations. Ideas of reference may be prominent and delusional beliefs may be loosely or well systematized. The patient harbouring delusions of persecution may show enduring attitudes of hostility, suspicion and aggression towards others.

In some cases the delusional beliefs appear to be 'infectious' in that they may eventually be shared by the patient's partner—the so-called *'folie à deux'*.

Uncommon forms

Paraphrenia

This is a schizophrenic reaction occurring in the elderly and, like paranoid schizophrenia, is characterized by persecutory delusions with a relatively intact personality. The delusions are usually systematized and the patient may prove troublesome to neighbours and may plague the police by lodging frequent complaints. It is commoner in elderly people with a degree of hearing impairment.

Paranoia

This is a 'monosymptomatic' psychosis consisting of a rigid delusional belief, often persecutory, without any generalized features of schizophrenic deterioration.

It is uncommon and may manifest itself as an *Othello syndrome*, that is an irrational belief that one's partner is being unfaithful. The flimsiest and most improbable evidence may be cited to support these accusations of infidelity. For example, curtains being parted at a certain angle may be interpreted as a signal to a secret lover.

In *Cap Gras syndrome* the patient develops the strange belief that their partner has been replaced by a 'doppelganger' or double, evidence for this substitution being found in minor errors or slips of the tongue on the part of the replacement.

L'illusion de Fregoli refers to a similar disorder of identification in which the patient believes strangers to be their spouse disguised and may accost strangers in the street firmly persuaded that the hapless person concerned is their spouse or some important person in disguise, perhaps a famous politician or a member of the Royal Family.

In *De Clérambault's syndrome* the patient entertains the delusional belief that some celebrity is in love with them and may bombard this unfortunate person with letters and phone calls.

These 'monosymptomatic psychoses' are rare and the nurse is unlikely to encounter them in the in-patient population of the psychiatric hospital.

Treatment of Schizophrenia

Treatment of schizophrenia remains palliative (directed against symptoms rather than cause) as the cause(s) remain obscure.

Treatments may be divided into three groups: (a) *physical*, (b) *psychological* and (c) *social*, though all three elements are usually involved in any given treatment regime.

Physical treatments

The history of the physical treatment of schizophrenia demonstrates the wide variety of viewpoints which have been generated about the disorder, and the clinical fortress of schizophrenia has been besieged with a strange assortment of therapeutic weapons, with limited success. Due to the often irregular course of the disorder and its tendency to spontaneous remissions, advocates of many physical treatments were able to claim success, though these claims often failed to stand the test of time.

During the eighteenth century schizophrenics

were subjected to burning, cupping, whirling in revolving chairs, starving, immersion in freezing or boiling water, bleeding and binding. These excesses reached such a pitch that a concerned observer (in 1803) commented that 'It is a revolting spectacle to see the brash empiric (physician) cavorting with his mental patient . . . Woe unto the image of God who falls into such hands' (Szasz, 1971).

In 1785 Dr W. Oliver administered large doses of camphor (now used as a chest rub) by mouth to mentally disordered patients and claimed success, saying of one patient: '. . . he became natural, easy and polite . . . and played his game at whist with great accuracy' (Clare, 1976). In 1934 camphor was again used to treat mental disorder. Von Meduna, a Hungarian psychiatrist, made the quite erroneous observation that epilepsy and schizophrenia could not co-exist in the same patient, and induced convulsions in schizophrenic patients, by the intramuscular injection of camphorated oil, in the hope that the convulsions would somehow suppress the schizophrenia. The side-effects (delirium, vomiting and pain) were so unacceptable that camphor was replaced by injections of the cerebral irritant leptazol (Cardiazol), and extravagant claims were made for the success of this treatment. One psychiatrist, recalling Cardiazol treatment, remembers the terror it evoked in even the most psychotic of patients and wryly comments that it was a case of 'first catch your patient' (Rollin, 1980).

In 1937 Cerletti and Bini introduced electroconvulsive therapy (ECT) (having first experimented on pigs in the local slaughterhouse), and ECT became the order of the day for the 'maintenance' of chronic cases of schizophrenia.

It is now recognized that electroplexy should only be administered to those schizophrenics showing marked disturbance of mood or motor activity (e.g. catatonic stupor or excitement) and Berrios (1983) has commented on this group of patients saying: 'Although ECT is rarely necessary in the management of the schizophrenias, it may lead to dramatic improvement in such cases'.

Other physical approaches have included insulin-induced coma, 'malarial therapy' (infection of the patient with a benign form of malaria in the belief that the resultant pyrexia would reduce troublesome symptoms), transplantation of endocrine organs, surgical removal of large parts of the small intestine (Slater and Roth, 1969), removal of septic foci, and renal dialysis (Meyer and Salmon, 1984).

The most consistent relief of schizophrenic symptoms has arisen from the introduction of antipsychotic drugs.

In 1952 a French surgeon noted the ability of the drug chlorpromazine to quieten schizophrenics without stupefying them, and persuaded his psychiatric colleagues to use it in disturbed schizophrenic patients. Chlorpromazine, which belongs to the group of drugs known as *phenothiazines*, proved to be a major advance in the treatment of schizophrenia as it effectively reduced the intensity of tormenting delusions and hallucinations. A whole range of related phenothiazine compounds were synthesized and introduced and proved to be valuable in preventing relapse when used as maintenance treatments after acute episodes had subsided.

The parent drug remains–chlorpromazine (Largactil)–and it may be given orally, intramuscularly or intravenously in doses up to 300 mg daily, though, on occasion, it may be given in doses three times as great. However Davis (1976) has commented that 'megadoses' are 'too often used and produce no better results' (Davis, 1976).

Antipsychotic drugs (sometimes referred to as 'neuroleptics') were initially referred to as 'major tranquillizers', though this term has been rejected as there is evidence of a specific antipsychotic effect (Berrios, 1983). All antipsychotics show an affinity for dopamine receptor sites in the brain and may act by producing a generalized reduction in the level of neurotransmitters in the central nervous system (Weller, 1983).

Sustained release depot injections of antipsychotic drugs (Moditen, Modecate, Depixol) have counteracted the difficulties of non-compliance with oral medication often shown by discharged schizophrenics. These preparations consist of an oily solution of the drug which is given by intramuscular injection forming a 'depot' in the tissues from which the drug is slowly released into the bloodstream, maintaining therapeutic blood levels of the drug for two to four weeks. Thus a single injection, given every two to four weeks, replaced the necessity of swallowing tablets three to four times per day and reduced the risks of overdose as well as non-compliance.

Antipsychotic drugs may be considered in three major groups: the *phenothiazines*, the *thioxanthines*, and the *butyrophenones*. Table 60 lists examples of widely used drugs belonging to each category.

Though antipsychotics reduce the intensity of hallucinations and delusions, they do not effectively reduce emotional blunting or loss of volition (Ingram et al, 1981), and there is, in fact, evidence

Table 60 Some antipsychotic (neuroleptic) drugs used in the treatment of schizophrenia.

Approved name	Proprietary names	Daily dosage (unless specified otherwise)	Comments
Phenothiazines			
Chlorpromazine	Largactil	150–600 mg acute disorder. 100–400 mg for maintenance treatment. Higher doses needed in some cases	The most widely used phenothiazine. Disadvantages include sedative and extrapyramidal effects.
Thioridazine	Melleril	100–500 mg	Less prone to produce extrapyramidal symptoms, though high dosages may lead to retinitis pigmentosa.
Trifluoperazine	Stelazine	15–30 mg	Less sedative in effect and, therefore, more suitable for retarded presentations. More liable to produce extrapyramidal symptoms.
Perphenazine	Fentazin	6–27 mg	
Fluphenazine	Moditen	2.5–15 mg	
Methotrimeprazine	Veractil	10–100 mg	
Fluphenazine enanthate	Moditen enanthate	An injection of 25 mg every 10–14 days	Long acting preparation administered by depot intramuscular injection. Depressive symptoms develop in a proportion of patients.
Fluphenazine decanoate	Modecate	12.5–25 mg every 2–4 weeks	
Thioxanthenes			
Flupenthixol	Depixol	20–40 mg every 1–3 weeks	Long-acting preparation also administered by depot injection. Possibly less likely to produce depression.
Butyrophenones			
Haloperidol	Serenace Haldol		Very potent drugs liable to cause marked extrapyramidal symptoms.
Trifluperidol	Triperidol		
Diphenylbutyl-piperidines			
Pimozine	Orap	2–8 mg	Similar effects to the phenothiazines, but with the advantage that it only needs to be taken once daily and has fewer side-effects.
Flupirelene	Imap	2–6 mg weekly	Administered by intramuscular injection, and has similar effects to pimozine. Used in the maintenance treatment of schizophrenia.

that they may lead to loss of spontaneity, creativity, and initiative (Meyer and Salmon, 1984). Phenothiazines also tend to suppress the gag reflex, and a significant number of deaths due to aspiration asphyxiation have been reported (Weiner, 1979).

Antipsychotic drugs may lead to troublesome side-effects involving the extra-pyramidal system (that part of the nervous system responsible for the fine regulation of muscular movement) and these side-effects are described in Table 61. Most of these side-effects respond well to anti-Parkinsonian drugs.

Other side-effects include retinitis pigmentosa (thioridazine), increased sensitivity to sunlight (chlorpromazine), agranulocytosis, jaundice, postural hypotension, and skin rashes. Agranulocytosis (marked reduction in, or complete absence of, granular white blood cells) is a rare but serious complication which is more common in females and tends to develop rapidly (Slater and Roth, 1969). It presents as a sore throat of sudden onset and the nurse should immediately report such a complaint to the medical staff. In rare cases phenothiazine-induced jaundice may progress to fatal necrosis of the liver (Slater and Roth, 1969) and early signs of jaundice must again be reported immediately.

Increased sensitivity to sunlight means that patients receiving chlorpromazine will rapidly

Table 61 Drug-induced extrapyramidal reactions.

Psychotic patients receiving major neuroleptics may exhibit extrapyramidal reactions. Occasionally such reactions are similar to severe depression, but, if they are recognized as extrapyramidal, respond rapidly to treatment. In many cases these side-effects can be avoided by careful adjustment of dosage. The more serious reactions are briefly described.

Reaction and clinical features	Treatment
Acute dystonic reactions These are characterized by an abrupt onset of retrocollis, torticollis, facial grimacing and distortions, dysarthria, laboured breathing and involuntary muscle movements. Rarely the patients may have an oculogyric crisis. Such an attack begins with a fixed stare for a few moments, the eyes are then rotated upwards, then to the side, and remain fixed in that position. At the same time the head is tilted backwards and laterally, the mouth opened wide and the tongue protruded.	Severe dystonic reactions can be relieved promptly by parenterally administered anti-Parkinsonian agents such as benztropine (Cogentin), procyclidine (Kemadrin), biperiden (Akineton) or orphenadrine (Disipal), the drugs normally taking effect within 10 minutes.
Parkinsonian-like states These include tremor, rigidity and akinesia (difficulty in initiating and stopping voluntary movements). The most obvious effects of these disturbances on the patient are an immobile or wooden facial expression, drooling or saliva due to a disturbance of swallowing, and a shuffling gait without the normal arm swinging. The patient becomes aware of fatigue in a limb used for ordinary, repetitive motor acts such as walking or writing. The slowness of movement and lack of facial mobility often appear similar to severe depression but, unlike the latter, will respond rapidly to the treatment.	Parkinsonian disturbances are usually effectively controlled by oral anti-Parkinsonian drugs such as benztropine, benzhexol (Artane), biperiden, orphenadrine or procyclidine. Apparent depressive states, due to extrapyramidal rigidity and akinesia, can readily be distinguished from true depression by their rapid response to intramuscular or intravenous anti-Parkinsonian agents.
Akathisia Akathisia or motor restlessness is often described as the jitters. The patient feels compelled to pace the floor, or shift his legs or tap his feet when sitting.	It has been reported that diazepam and low dose sedative hypnotics reduce the symptoms of akathisia. Anti-Parkinsonian drugs and antihistamines have proved less effective.
Tardive dyskinesia In contrast to acute dyskinesia, tardive dyskinesia refers to various characteristic involuntary movements which may occur in some patients after prolonged therapy with oral or injectable anti-psychotics may become manifest when dosage is reduced or discontinued. It is characterized by stereotyped, repetitive, involuntary movements of the mouth, lips and tongue and often limbs as well; worm-like rippling of the tongue is sometimes an early sign. Most commonly seen are sucking, smacking movements of the lips, lateral jaw movements and puffing of the cheeks with the tongue thrusting, rolling or making 'fly-catching' movements. Symptoms occur more frequently under emotional stress and disappear during sleep.	Discontinuation of the drug regime has to be balanced against the likelihood of schizophrenic relapse in the individual patient. If the anti-psychotic is withdrawn, the symptoms of tardive dyskinesia may become exacerbated before improvement begins. Anti-Parkinsonian drugs with anti-cholinergic action (e.g. those listed) are not recommended as they may exacerbate the condition. A large number of drugs have been advocated for the treatment of tardive dyskinesia but evidence for their efficacy is conflicting.

develop painful cases of sunburn after minimal exposure to strong sunlight and the nurse should therefore ensure that these patients sit in a shaded area when out-of-doors. Summer trips to the seaside may necessitate the use of ultraviolet screening creams (e.g. Uvistat) and the use of a sunhat is advised.

The antipsychotics are potent drugs, though, as Evans et al (1983) have commented: 'Potency should never be confused with efficacy'. The extreme potency of these drugs creates a risk that patients may become passive and 'easily managed' and thus at risk of institutionalization. Drugs cannot be regarded as an end in themselves, but they do make the patient more receptive to nursing care and other rehabilitative measures. Despite indignant rebuttals of the term 'tranquillizers', there is little doubt that over-zealous use of these preparations may have a crushing effect. Creer and Wing (1974) recount the remark made by a 'tranquillized' patient: 'Medication obviously plays a part but somehow I prefer to be a little "mad" than over-dosed by major tranquillisers'. Wescott (1979) records a similar statement made by a patient maintained on Moditen: 'I think that the richness of my pre-injection days—even with brief outbursts of madness—is preferable to the numbed cabbage I have become'.

Judicious use of antipsychotics need not produce 'numbed cabbages' though the nurse must be aware of the dangers of some patients drifting off into a torpid, drug-induced inertia. Drugs are never a total replacement for effective rehabilitation and nursing care. As Weller (1983) has commented: 'Drugs alone do not help patients to find jobs and accommodation or to adjust to life outside of hospital'. Antipsychotics may dramatically facilitate rehabilitation and may greatly increase the quality of the patient's life by reducing tormenting symptoms and making him/her more socially acceptable to others, thus increasing the likelihood of improved interactions.

Lader (1984) points out that schizophrenics tend to habituate quickly to phenothiazines and suggests that the drugs may start to lose efficacy after 6–12 months. Some clinicians now tend to conserve the drug for relapses and give the patient 'drug holidays' in between, as opposed to the former practice of continuing maintenance medication for several years.

Schizophrenic states coloured by components of anxiety or depression may respond to the administration of an anxiolytic or antidepressant in association with an antipsychotic drug.

Psychological treatments

Insight-directed psychotherapies have proved to be of little value in the treatment of schizophrenia (Stafford-Clark and Smith, 1983), though a variant of psychoanalysis called direct analysis, which holds faulty parenting to be a critical causative element, has claimed some success (Meyer and Salmon, 1984).

Social skills training and selective use of behaviour modification can be useful in counteracting much of the social disengagement of schizophrenia,

and both are related to nursing practice in the next chapter.

The Token Economy Programme

This has proved useful in improving overall social functioning and in restoring self-help skills lost as a result of hospitalization. The token economy is basically a microeconomic system insofar as it reproduces, on a small scale, the system of payment for performance which exists in society.

Behaviours considered important by the therapist (*target behaviours*) are rewarded with tokens which can be exchanged by the patient for goods or privileges. Desirable behaviours are scored and a token value is assigned to them. For example, the dormitory may display signs indicating: Arising by 8 a.m.—10 tokens, Arising by 8.30 a.m.—5 tokens, Arising after 9 a.m.—0 tokens, Acceptable standard at tidiness check—10 tokens. The bathroom may display signs reminding the patients that cleaning teeth is worth 5 tokens, bathing or showering—5 tokens, shaving—3 tokens, cleaning shoes—3 tokens. Acceptable mealtime behaviour may earn 10 tokens, and completing work or therapy assignments will also earn tokens.

The tokens may be exchanged for goods (cigarettes, cosmetics, magazines, sweets, etc.) at a 'token shop' which may consist of a table displaying attractive goods, each with its value indicated in tokens, in a room off the ward. It is important that this 'token shop' contains an imaginative array of goods, attractively displayed, to increase patient motivation.

In the token system, earnings (tokens) must be scrupulously related to performance (response) and it is essential to have a strict policy of NO RESPONSE=NO PAYMENT (TOKEN).

During their stay in the token economy ward, patients must not have access to cash otherwise the efficacy of the programme would be completely destroyed. Likewise visitors must be asked not to bring cigarettes, sweets or similar commodities in for the patient. All goods and privileges must be earned and payed for in tokens for the duration of the patient's stay in the unit (which may be 6–12 months).

Each patient must have a similar earning capacity, and weekly allowances, pensions, etc. may be converted into token equivalents, any unearned balance being lodged as a cash saving for the patient. Each token may be equal to one pence and this may be borne in mind when pricing goods in the token shop. For example a packet of cigarettes which would cost £1.40 in a traditional shop should cost 140 tokens in the token shop.

The token system should make custodial and authoritarian control systems (nagging, scolding, ordering) redundant as patient motivation will increase quickly.

As in all behavioural approaches, reinforcement must be immediate and should be accompanied by warm verbal expressions of approval.

Patients may be allowed to realize the value of tokens on admission to the unit by giving free tokens for a few days before the programme proper starts.

Patients quickly become persuaded of the value of tokens as they have no other means now of gaining access to desired goods and privileges. Privileges may include hours spent watching television or playing preferred games, and eventually patients should be encouraged to save tokens for bigger privileges (trips to the cinema, theatre or pub).

In the beginning everyone is paid *immediately* for making the expected response, but the giving of tokens will gradually be delayed so that the system resembles a normal wages system. Tokens may eventually be given hourly, two hourly, four hourly, twice daily, daily and then weekly, a careful running total of the patient's token earnings being kept so that 'wages' are fair and accurate. Eventually the patient will make the transition from weekly issue of tokens to weekly issue of cash; in other words, he will be placed on the sort of token economy to which we are all subject (banknotes and coins are intrinsically worthless but simply act as tokens).

Gains made by the patient in the areas of improved personal habits, dress and hygiene will quickly produce wider benefits as the patient becomes more acceptable to others and gains in confidence and self-esteem.

Selection of patients for token economy should bear the following principles in mind: (a) no organic psychosis, (b) no patients over the age of 65 years, and (c) every patient should be assured of a place in a halfway house or group home if the programme is completed successfully (there is little point in spending much time and effort in rehabilitating a patient only to return him to a long-stay ward to deteriorate again).

Studies suggest that the token economy will be most beneficial to patients who are low in maturity and efficiency (Meyer and Salmon, 1984). Comparatively independent and intellectually competent patients show more complexity in their behaviours and may adjust to a token economy with difficulty.

The token economy system is discussed in full by Ayllon and Azrin (1968).

Family therapy

This is based on considerations of 'family pathology' and many approaches rely upon the perspectives of Laing and his co-workers. The schizophrenic is regarded as the 'index patient' and attempts are made to encourage the whole unit to confront the disturbed rhythms of the family setting which may have caused, or contributed to, the patient's disorder.

The family of the patient must always be involved in treatment (of whatever sort) as there is strong evidence to show that families can affect the prognosis. Treated schizophrenics do less well in families where there is a high level of expressed emotion (Evans et al, 1983) and may require long-term maintenance therapy.

Social approaches

Schizophrenia is a socially disabling disorder, and care and rehabilitation must be directed towards improving social functioning from the onset. It is perhaps a well-worn cliché that 'rehabilitation starts on the first day of treatment' but this is particularly true of schizophrenia.

Social, occupational, industrial and recreational therapy all have an important part to play in helping the patient to gain confidence and skill in mixing with others and in coping with everyday living. The emphasis should be on promoting maximum independence and autonomy, and the grave dangers of institutionalization must never be overlooked.

The earlier treatment is initiated and the shorter the stay in hospital, the better the prognosis. Some studies suggest that patients should be supported psychologically for several weeks to see if they recover without drugs (Davis, 1976).

Helping the schizophrenic to make an early and smooth transition from the hospital back into the community is critical (Curran et al, 1982).

It is absurd to expend effort and resources on schizophrenic patients while they are in hospital and then to provide ineffective follow-up and community support when they leave.

The author remembers paying a visit to a teenage schizophrenic who had been discharged from hospital three weeks previously, this being the first follow-up visit arranged. The patient's treatment had been regarded as successful (after all, he was discharged from hospital and was thought to be 'relatively symptom free'). When the patient was eventually traced, after hours of inquiry, he was found in a derelict building where he had been squatting since discharge, having left the parental home after a disagreement. He was lying on a pile of dirty rags and was apathetic, dazed, dirty, verminous and malnourished. Immediate readmission was necessary and arranging future discharge was difficult in view of his 'poor performance after last discharge'.

Discharging the schizophrenic without adequate preparation and arrangement of community care is rather like expecting an amputee to compete successfully in a marathon run.

The community psychiatric nursing department and social work department have a vital role to play, and community support should involve more than the monthly administration of a depot phenothiazine injection (which is still unfortunately referred to as 'community care' in many areas). The patient's overall level of social functioning must be comprehensively monitored, and full use should be made of every resource (link clubs, retraining schemes, disablement resettlement officer, sheltered accommodation, day hospital facilities— where applicable), and it must be emphasized that the family will need support as much as the patient and should be actively involved in community care programmes.

Caution must be exercised in selecting accommodation for the discharged patient. Unscrupulous landlords abound and the media frequently report cases of landlords 'specializing' in accommodation for discharged psychiatric patients. Such 'specialist' provision may consist of blatant exploitation. Accommodation may be overcrowded and grossly substandard and there are many reported cases of landlords insisting that patients surrender social security giros to them, the majority being retained as an inflated rent and a small percentage being returned as 'pocket money'. The patients may also spend most of the day aimlessly wandering the streets as they must vacate their rooms by mid-morning and are not allowed to return until mid-evening. Relapse and readmission are almost inevitable under such conditions.

Prognosis

Table 62 indicates some of the positive prognostic indicators in schizophrenia. Catatonic disorders seem to have a better outlook, at least in the short term, than simple or hebephrenic forms, while the paranoid patient may manage to lead a fairly productive existence, even if it is not symptom-free.

Reaction schizophrenia always carries a more favourable prognosis than process schizophrenia in which there is often a tendency to insidious deterioration. Personality deterioration becomes likely if there are repeated relapses, and some degree of lasting impairment is often apparent from the third relapse onwards (Trethowan and Sims, 1983).

Stafford-Clark and Smith (1983) suggest that a quarter of patients remit completely and another quarter do very well. The remaining 50% show varying degrees of progressive deterioration.

The nurse must remember that effective and dynamic nursing care may be one of the most important factors in prognosis.

Table 62 Prognostic indicators for schizophrenia.

Just as there are factors that predict occurrence, several variables (independent of the type of treatment) may predict adequate remission once schizophrenia is diagnosed:

Sexual-marital status: married, or at least a prior history of stable sexual-social adjustment

A family history of affective rather than schizophrenic disorder

Presence of an affective response (elation or depression) in the acute stage of the disorder

Abrupt onset of the disorder: reactive rather than process schizophrenia

Onset later than early childhood

Minor or no paranoid trends in the disorder

Higher socioeconomic status

Adequate pre-morbid vocational adjustment

Pre-morbid competence in interpersonal relationships

Short length of stay in hospital

No history of ECT treatment

Tendency to be stimulation-receptive rather than stimulation-avoidant

Clear precipitating factors at the onset of disturbance

(These variables are correlates, rather than explicit causes in any positive change.)

Key Concepts

1 Schizophrenia is a *relapsing–remitting disorder*, with a tendency to *chronicity*, in which the salient features is *impaired reality testing*.

2 Schizophrenia does not cause splitting of the personality. The personality is not split, but fragmented.

3 Short-lived forms (*reaction schizophrenia*) may arise in response to stress but most are progressive in their course, after an insidious onset (*process schizophrenia*).

4 The disorder tends to develop in adolescence. Persons over the age of 39 have passed the peak risk period, though one form (paranoid schizophrenia) develops in later life.

5 There is much debate about the causes, though it now seems probable that there is a genetic *predisposition* which may or may not be acted upon by *precipitating factors* in the environment to cause the disorder.

6 Research has suggested, but has failed to conclusively establish, faults in cerebral *metabolism* which may be inherited.

7 Studies of *family dynamics* are equally inconclusive but suggest that if some 'pathogenic' families do not actually cause schizophrenia, they may well precipitate and/or maintain schizophrenic responses.

8 'First rank' symptoms of schizophrenia consist of *passivity experiences, auditory hallucinations* in the third person and *primary delusions*.

9 Schizophrenia may take one of four forms: *simple, hebephrenic, catatonic* or *paranoid*.

10 Simple schizophrenia manifests itself in behaviour and ideas which are liable to be regarded by others as being 'odd' or 'eccentric'. Many sufferers exist as recluses or aimless drifters on the fringes of society.

11 Hebephrenic schizophrenia is often florid in its presentation and behaviour and thought processes may be bizarre and *regressive*.

12 Catatonic schizophrenia presents the extreme example of withdrawal and is a rare form in which the patient may withdraw into a *catatonic stupor* which may be succeeded by bouts of *schizophrenic excitement*.

13 Paranoid schizophrenia has a later age of onset (30–50 years) and is characterized by *delusions of persecution* with relatively good perservation of personality. Auditory hallucinations are common.

14 In all schizophrenic disorders there is great loss of self-esteem, and loneliness and isolation may be extreme.

15 Uncommon forms include paraphrenia, paranoia, Othello syndrome, cap gras syndrome, l'illusion de Fregoli, De Clerambault's syndrome, and these forms are often collectively referred to as *monosymptomatic schizophrenic reactions* as each has one prominent symptom, though personality is otherwise well-preserved.

16 Treatment may be physical, psychological or social, though usually a blend of all three approaches is used.

17 Physical treatment mainly consists of *anti-psychotic drugs*, usually given orally or by *depot injection*.

18 Schizophrenic patients are particularly vulnerable to institutionalization (due to their innate tendencies to withdrawal) and drugs may increase this risk if used to produce 'easily managed' patients.

19 *Social skills training* and *behaviour modification* are useful and widely used psychological treatments.

20 Social approaches include occupational, industrial, recreational, and art and music therapy.

21 Discharge must be planned carefully as it is all too easy to inadvertently relegate the passive and withdrawn schizophrenic to an aimless existence on the fringes of society. Regular contact must be maintained.

References

Ayllon, T. & Azrin, N. (1968) *The Token Economy*. New York: Appleton-Century-Crofts.

Berrios, G. (1983) In Berrios, G. & Dowson, J. H. (Eds) *Treatment and Management in Adult Psychiatry*. London: Baillière Tindall.

Clare, A. (1976) *Psychiatry in Dissent*. London: Tavistock Publications.

Creer, C. & Wing, J. K. F. (1974) *Schizophrenia at home*. Sutton: National Schizophrenia Fellowship.

Curran, J., Monti, P. & Corriveau, D. (1982) Treatment of schizophrenia. In Bellack, A. S. et al (Eds) *International Handbook of Behaviour Modification and Therapy*. New York: Plenum Books.

Davis, J. (1976) Recent development in the treatment of schizophrenia. *Psychiatric Annals*, **6**: 33–50.

Evans, L., Eadie, M., Hollister, L. & Tyrer, J. (1983) *Drug Use in Psychiatry*. Maryland: Adis Health Science Press.

Frame, J. (1961) *Faces In The Water*. New York: George Braziller.

Gotesman, I. & Shields, J. (1973) Genetic theorising & schizophrenia. *British Journal of Psychiatry*, **122**: 13–30.

Heston, L. & Denny, D. (1968) Interactions between early life experience & biological factors in schizophrenia. In Rosenthal & Kety (Eds) *Transmission of Schizophrenia*. Oxford: Pergamon Press.

Ingram, I., Timbury, G. & Mowbray, R. (1981) *Notes on Psychiatry, 5th edn*. Edinburgh: Churchill Livingstone.

Lader, M. (1984) In *Inside Out* (Journal of the Glasgow Association for Mental Health), 4.

Laing, R. D. (1970) *The Politics of Experience*. Harmondsworth: Penguin Books.

Laing, R. D. & Esterson, A. (1964) *Sanity, Madness & The Family*. Harmondsworth: Penguin Books.

Lidz, T., Flock, S. & Cornelison, A. (1965) *Schizophrenia & the Family*. New York: International Universities Press.

McDonald, N. (1960) Living with schizophrenia. *Canadian Medical Association Journal*, **82**: 678–681.

Meyer, R. & Salmon, P. (1984) *Abnormal Psychology*. London: Allyn & Bacon.

Mosker, L., Pollin, W. & Stabénau, J. (1971) Families with identical twins discordant for schizophrenia. *British Journal of Psychiatry*, **118**: 29–42.

Rollin, H. (1980) The changing problem of the treatment of schizophrenia. In Rollin (Ed) *Coping with Schizophrenia*. London: Burnett Books.

Schneider, K. (1959) *Clinical Psychopathology, 5th edn*. New York: Grune & Stratton.

Sechehaye, M. (1951) *Autobiography of a Schizophrenic Girl*. New York: Grune & Stratton.

Slater, E. & Roth, M. (1969) *Clinical Psychiatry*. London: Baillière Tindall.

Smith, A. C. (1982) *Schizophrenia & Madness*. London: George Allen & Unwin.

Smythies, J. R. (1975) The biochemical basis of schizophrenia. In Forrest & Affleck, (Eds) *New Perspectives in Schizophrenia*. Edinburgh: Churchill Livingstone.

St Augustine. *The Confessions and Letters of St. Augustine, Vol. 1*. Translated by J. G. Pilkington (1956). Grand Rapids: Erolmans.

Stafford–Clark, A. & Smith, A. (1983) *Psychiatry for Students, 6th edn*. London: George Allen & Unwin.

Szasz, T. (1971) *The Manufacture of Madness*. London: Paladin.

Trethowan, W. & Sims, A. (1983) *Psychiatry, 5th edn*. London: Baillière Tindall.

Tsuang, M. T. (1982) *Schizophrenia. The Facts*. Oxford: Oxford University Press.

Vonnegut, M. (1975) *The Eden Express*. New York: Bantam.

Weiner, M. (1979) Haloperidol, hyperthyroidism and sudden death. *American Journal of Psychiatry*, **136**: 717–718.

Weller, M. (1983) *The Scientific Basis of Psychiatry*. London: Baillière Tindall.

Wescott, P. (1979) One man's schizophrenic illness. *British Medical Journal*. **1**: 989–990.

21

Nursing Care of the Schizophrenic Patient

> The schizophrenic patient is like the sea anemone which puts out frail tendrils in the ocean but withdraws them when the slightest shadow passes over the water.
>
> *Madeline Weiss (1954)*

Nursing the schizophrenic patient may be simultaneously one of the most challenging yet rewarding aspects of psychiatric nursing. Making contact with the schizophrenic patient may be difficult as the patient will often be lonely, frightened, mistrustful and lacking in self-esteem. Withdrawal may be marked and the patient may be difficult to 'reach.' It is almost as though the patient were isolated from reality behind a distorting glass wall through which they see strangely distorted images of reality.

In paranoid forms the patient may be fixated at the level of unsatisfied safety needs, as he sees the world and other people as dangerous and threatening. Feelings of fear and insecurity may be reflected in a hostile or suspicious approach to staff. Movement towards the satisfaction of belongingness and esteem needs will not take place unless nursing staff gently and carefully win the patient's trust so that he begins to feel secure and safe.

In many forms there is marked fixation at the level of unsatisfied belongingness needs as the patient feels unable to affiliate with others, be accepted and belong. Schizophrenics want to be liked and to be like other people, but are so insecure and fearful that they tend to retreat from everyday social situations into a world of fantasy wherein they gain love and approval and avoid threat.

Many patients who appear to be moderately socially competent will also show fixation at the level of unsatisfied esteem needs and are easily hurt by an injudicious word or act which would pass unnoticed by others. Loss of self-esteem may be both pervasive and destructive in schizophrenia and warm, encouraging and supportive attitudes are important on the part of the nursing staff.

Planning Nursing Care

It is difficult to effectively generalize about nursing care of the schizophrenic patient as symptoms may vary enormously between patients and the possible range of symptoms is very wide indeed.

Wing and Creer (1980) list 17 behavioural characteristics observed in a group of 80 schizophrenics and from this list we may isolate commonly occurring characteristics which may become the focus of nursing intervention (see Table 63).

It will be observed that the commonest characteristics are social withdrawal, underactivity and lack of conversation and leisure interests. This highlights the fact that schizophrenics may be the loneliest people in the world.

The nurse must learn to gently penetrate the shell of psychosis, remembering that the schizophrenic may fear interpersonal closeness as much as he fears his extreme loneliness. Mistrust and suspicion of others may be profound in the schizophrenic and he

Table 63 Behavioural characteristics of patients in rank order of frequency

Characteristic	Total (N = 80)	%
1 Social withdrawal	59	74
2 Underactivity	45	56
3 Lack of conversation	43	54
4 Few leisure interests	40	50
5 Slowness	38	48
6 Overactivity	33	41
7 Odd ideas	27	34
8 Depression	27	34
9 Odd behaviour	27	34
10 Neglect of appearance	24	30
11 Odd postures and movements	20	25
12 Threats or violence	18	23
13 Poor mealtime behaviour	10	13
14 Socially embarrassing behaviour	6	8
15 Sexually unusual behaviour	6	8
16 Suicidal attempts	3	4
17 Incontinence	3	4

N.B. Each of these items was rated as occurring to a very, rather, or slightly marked extent or not at all. The numbers given here refer to those rated as occurring to a very marked or rather marked extent.

may develop relationships with the nursing staff slowly and haltingly; any such relationships may be fragile and easily damaged by a thoughtless word or action.

The inner life of the schizophrenic may be characterized by fear and inconsistency and, for this reason, the nursing approach must be warm and consistent. In many ways the nurse may provide reassuring elements of the consistency in which the schizophrenic may be deeply lacking, and her positive attitudes may serve as a 'splint' for deep fractures in the patient's interpersonal functioning.

Self-esteem is often very low in schizophrenia and the nurse may help to bring about improvements in this area by noting and warmly reinforcing positive attributes and achievements. Even in the most extensive forms of the disorder there are recognizable 'fragments' of personality which remain largely unaffected. The perceptive nurse should recognize these when assessing the patient and should use them as 'islands' which may be therapeutically colonized.

By its very nature schizophrenia often makes the patient prone to withdrawal; the risk of institutionalization is therefore great. The schizophrenic patient may be easily 'managed', particularly if maintained on high doses of tranquillizing drugs, and may insidiously slip away into a state of torpid inertia in which 'ward routine' is quietly and unquestioningly adhered to. Such a patient may eventually come to be regarded as a 'chronic deteriorated schizophrenic', and may passively spend his life as a fixture in a back ward of the psychiatric hospital. It is therefore important that the schizophrenic's innate tendencies to alienation and isolation are not intensified by the hospital setting but are instead recognized and dealt with.

Human contact must be consistent and sustained and is the most important factor in nursing care. This contact may be provided in the setting of the industrial, occupational or social therapy department, or may be informally provided as the nurse involves the patient in ward activities.

The patient's perceptions of reality may often be distorted, and the nurse should therefore constantly direct attention to the 'real world' and be a reassuring guide in the patient's often halting or erratic interactions with others.

Elementary social skills may have atrophied and the nurse may play an important re-educative role here, producing improvements in both behaviour and subjective feelings of competence and comfort in social situations. The patient should be encouraged to make 'experiments in living' and progress should be noted and reinforced.

Studies suggest that elementary social skills training can quickly produce positive results in a very short period of time (Trower et al, 1978).

Assessment of the patient's competence in activities of daily living may also reveal loss of basic self-help skills and these may be restored by a simple behaviour modification programme (see Chapter 10).

Delusional verbalizations should not be reinforced by arguing with them, but should be quietly disregarded. The nurse should make it apparent that she is not prepared to spend time with the patient when he is expressing delusional beliefs but should reinforce rational verbalizations and make the patient aware that he is more pleasant to spend time with when speaking rationally.

The nurse must make it clear that she is rejecting the delusion but not the patient and this principle also applies to any other maladaptive characteristics shown by the patient. The patient must not be allowed to delegate responsibility for his life to the nursing staff but should be encouraged to use his initiative, and nothing should be done for the patient which he is capable of doing for himself (acts of friendship excluded). Initially the nurse may have to do things *for* the patient, but she should exchange this approach for doing things *with* the patient as quickly as is feasible.

The emphasis must be on both self-care and self-sufficiency, and the patient should be given as much freedom as is compatible with staff judgement.

The paranoid patient may present particular difficulties as he may be suspicious and resentful of imagined injustices or threats. An attitude of firm, but gentle, consistency is again important and the nurse should be open and truthful and must avoid being drawn into arguments with the patient. This type of patient may be rather 'prickly' and difficult to relate to and the nurse must resist any temptation to avoid him and spend more time with friendlier patients. The paranoid patient should not be forced to take part in group activities, and the nurse should try to recognize his need for reassurance and consistency. It is usually possible to identify and relate to areas untouched by delusional thinking and this should provide the basis for a therapeutic nurse/patient relationship.

In summary, the key points in the nursing approach should be the provision of a therapeutic nurse/patient relationship aimed at promoting trust, confidence and awareness of reality. The grave dangers of institutionalization should be recognized and avoided, while self-sufficiency should be encouraged. Many of the improvements that ensue after hospitalization can be attributed to the nurse-patient relationship.

Assisting the Schizophrenic Patient with Activities of Daily Living

Assessment will have revealed areas of potential difficulty (see Tables 63–73) and planning care now involves establishing *objectives* of care and identifying the necessary *actions* whereby the care plan may be implemented.

1 *Maintaining a safe environment*

The schizophrenic patient may inflict injuries on self or even attempt suicide in response to delusional ideas or hallucinatory 'commands'. Low self-esteem may lead to anxiety or depression, either of which will increase the risk of suicide. Admission to hospital may greatly increase anxiety levels, and careful observation is particularly important for two to three weeks after admission. Many schizophrenics show *anhedonia*, or the inability to experience pleasure, and this will contribute to feelings of

depression. Patients tormented by paranoid beliefs may attempt suicide to escape their imagined persecutors or to avoid the terrible fate they believe to be in store for them. Paranoid verbalizations which are persistent and accompanied by feelings of fear should always alert the nurse to the danger of suicide.

Many suicide attempts by schizophrenics are unpredictable and seem to take place impulsively, without any warning sign being given in the preceding days.

2 *Communication*

The pervasive loss of self-esteem and blurred boundaries of reality may lead to the schizophrenic patient spending much time in a state of passive withdrawal. The patient may seek out quiet corners of the ward and may actively avoid interaction with others. Table 63 reveals that social withdrawal was shown by 74% of the patients studied and lack of conversation by 54%. The nurse should be warmly supportive of the patient, and should share activities, however simple, with him.

Fear and lack of trust may compound the patient's tendency to withdrawal, and the nurse must never forget that schizophrenics learn to trust slowly and cautiously. Carefully established trust may be shattered by a thoughtless word or action by the nurse, so the approach must be consistent. The patient should be gently encouraged to spend time with others and the approach must be graduated

Table 64 Maintaining a safe environment

Problem	Objective	Action
Risk of self-harm or suicide as a result of delusional ideas or impulsive actions	To render the environment safe for the patient	Remove/protect sources of danger Discreet but careful observation

Table 65 Communication

Problem	Objective	Action
Patient withdrawn and uncommunicative	To promote healthy patterns of interaction	Spend time with patient and encourage group activities
Disorder of content of speech	To help the patient communicate effectively with others	Listen attentively to patient and prompt lucid verbalizations
Delusional verbalizations	To reduce the incidence of delusional verbalizations	Define reality of situation. Do not reinforce delusional verbalizations. Reinforce rational verbalizations

carefully. Attempts to enthusiastically and abruptly involve the withdrawn schizophrenic in group settings or demanding social situations may be counterproductive and will simply let the patient retreat further into his schizophrenic 'shell'.

The withdrawn schizophrenic may be gently led into the company of others by simply spending time in the company of a trusted nurse at first, even if this time is largely spent in silence. One or two patients known to the schizophrenic may be introduced into the setting after a day or two, and simple board-games may initiate communications without taxing the patient unduly. The setting, participants and activities should be altered from time to time so that the patient's trust and atrophied social skills are slowly developed.

Communication with the patient should be carefully structured to avoid touching on areas of delusional content, and verbal communications should be supplemented with warm non-verbal communications of the type so important to the timid and perplexed schizophrenic. Warm smiles, eye-to-eye contact and reassuring squeezes of the hand will prevent 'double-blind' situations and will clarify the intent of the communication. Wing (1978) has described the poor eye contact and general lack of use of non-verbal cues which are characteristic of many schizophrenic patients, and there may be a total confusion on the part of the patient as to the significance of such a social interaction. It is therefore important that the nurse models non-verbal communications for the patient and notes and reinforces any returned by the patient.

Underlying thought disorder may be reflected in disordered content of speech, so the nurse must learn to listen attentively to the patient's utterances. Often, seemingly garbled statements contain important cues and statements to which the nurse may respond. Consider the following statements made by a 20-year-old schizophrenic nurse:

'I don't know what it is. You see . . . she says, I don't know, I'm sure. There's Cinderella. There is a much better play than that. I don't know. I said. He is an awful idiot. Oh dear God I'm so stupid . . . I don't like acting the goat at all. A cream sponge sandwich. My memory is so slow, that's all I'm sure. It was caramels then and fruit cakes. Well, well I said, I can't help it, and, well, I don't care. Contrary Mary again, and says Nurse Grant—dogs barking. What's the matter with me anyway? I'm so terribly stupid. I'm fed up with

this place, that's all. Sago pudding. She looks pale and tired often . . . No that won't do. Oh dear God I'm so stupid. I won't see my way—white rabbits. Back home in Tennessee—that's the way it's spelt. Oh I don't know what I'm going to do now. It's all wrong. Dear God I'm so silly. It's killing isn't it? French cakes and meringues. Flies, fleas and butterflies.' (Henderson and Batchelor, 1962).

These statements are reproduced in a textbook of 1962 as an illustration of 'inappropriate emotional manifestations, great incoherence of speech and thought, and apparently absurd ideas'. One is nevertheless tempted to note the overall feelings of distress being conveyed and, in particular, the following despairing appeals:

'Oh dear God I'm so stupid/silly' (repeated four times)
'I don't like acting the goat at all'
'My memory is so slow'
'I can't help it'
'What's the matter with me anyway?'
'I'm fed up with this place, that's all'
'I don't know what I'm going to do now'
'It's all wrong'
'It's killing isn't it?'

The initial impression conveyed by much schizophrenic speech is of a bizarre kaleidoscope of ideas and images, the total strangeness of which may deter the nurse from listening carefully. This tendency should be avoided and the nurse should respond carefully and calmly to the rational fragments often concealed in a 'smoke screen' of words.

Delusional verbalizations must not be reinforced and it is not helpful to attempt to persuade the patient of the falseness of his beliefs (see Chapter 4). The nurse should gently and firmly discontinue the interaction if delusional ideas are intensely expressed, saying: 'I'll come back and talk to you when you want to talk about something else'. It is important that the nurse makes it clear that she is rejecting the delusion, not the patient.

Rational verbalizations should be noted and warmly reinforced, and the nurse may use phrases like: 'What a pleasant change to talk to you when you're feeling relaxed/talking differently' or 'You're much better company when you're talking like this—so much nicer'.

Such an approach will help to decrease the frequency of delusional verbalizations, and such change must be recorded.

3 *Expressing sexuality*

Table 63 indicates that 'sexually unusual behaviour' was a problem in a small minority of the patients studied (8%). Such behaviour may consist of repeated masturbation (sometimes in public) or impulsive sexual gestures or suggestions made to staff or fellow patients. Such behaviour reflects poor ego strength and may be prompted by delusional beliefs or hallucinatory suggestions. The appropriate response is one of firm but gentle dissuasion and the nurse must ensure that inappropriate behaviours of this sort are not inadvertently reinforced by responses of shock, outrage or increased attention. Decrease in the incidence of these behaviours should be warmly and approvingly commented upon. It is important to ensure that other patients do not suffer as a result of sexually inappropriate behaviour and the nurse must also ensure that the patient is not victimized or stigmatized as a result of this behaviour. Content of speech may reveal strange sexual beliefs, often associated with feelings of passivity, paranoid beliefs or somatic delusions, but these beliefs only give rise to troublesome behaviour in a small minority of patients. The innate timidity and insecurity of the schizophrenic usually ensures that negative responses quickly reduce the incidence of inappropriate sexual behaviours.

4 *Working and playing*

Schizophrenics may be afraid of reality, of emotions, and of giving. They want to be liked and accepted, to be like other people and to be part of the group, but tend to be timid and suspicious spectators, rather than participants, in social activities. They are so unsure of themselves that they make blunders, and low self-esteem means that they are very conscious of these blunders. They are often fearful of attracting disapproval or of being laughed at so they tend to retreat into a safe world of fantasy wherein they are the centre of attention, they always appear attractive, they say and do just the right things to gain approval, and they are never without the approval and esteem they want so greatly. Withdrawal may alternate with episodes of childlike attention-seeking behaviour, and everyday social activities may tax the limited resources of the schizophrenic to the extreme. Studies of social learning suggest that social skills are acquired from childhood onwards, partly through *imitation* of others including parents, siblings and peers, partly through *reinforcement* (i.e. encouragement or discouragement on the part of parents and others), partly through the opportunity to *observe* and to *practise* behaviour in a range of settings, partly through the development of *cognitive abilities*, and partly through *innate potential*. Schizophrenia may thus constitute a potent recipe for social inadequacy, and much of the nurse's efforts must be exerted in this direction. Childhood experiences may have been negative in schizophrenia. For example, the child may have been subject to double-bind situations during the formative years or may have developed within a skewed or schismatic family (see Chapter 2). Cognitive ability and innate potential may have been hampered by the erosive effects of the psychosis, and the end result may be extreme social inadequacy. However it has been indicated that the opportunity to *observe* and to *practise* behaviour in a wide range of settings may lead to effective development of social skills. For this reason the hos-

Table 66 Expressing sexuality

Problem	Objective	Action
Inappropriate sexual behaviour	To reduce incidence of such behaviour	Social skills training and behaviour modification

Table 67 Working and playing

Problem	Objective	Action
(a) Withdrawal (b) Underactivity (c) Lack of conversation (d) Few leisure interests (e) Overactivity/underactivity (f) Aggressive behaviour	To promote healthy patterns of interaction and stimulate interest in environment and other people	Social skills training Behaviour modification Provision of therapeutic activities

pital should afford the schizophrenic the opportunity to make 'experiments in living' under the guidance of the staff, and studies suggest that elementary social skills training will quickly produce gains in schizophrenic patients (Trower et al, 1978).

In schizophrenia the patient may seem to have no social goals and the resultant behavioural pattern may seem meaningless or irrational. It is probable, however, that social withdrawal maintains the patient in a sort of negative equilibrium as it reduces feelings of inadequacy and threat and thus enables the patient to cope, after a fashion, with everyday living. If this pattern is allowed to continue uninterrupted, the result may be the chronic schizophrenic who has become 'socially bankrupt' (Longabaugh et al, 1966). Behaviour may be suspended even to the extent of gross neglect of personal hygiene and the appearance of incontinence.

The nurse may provide the elementary social skills training which is so essential in schizophrenia by modelling (demonstrating) appropriate social responses and by encouraging the patient to imitate them. Gutride et al (1974) initiated a form of social skills training which they called structured learning therapy and which consisted of videotaped demonstrations of ways of initiating and sustaining conversation, coaching in important aspects which related to individual difficulties, practice and videotaped feedback, and social reinforcement. The therapy was given in group form and the group met three times a week for four weeks. Ratings of behaviour after therapy showed significant improvements in both acute and chronic patients compared with a no treatment control group, though no follow-up of long-term effects was made (Gutride et al, 1974).

The use of video equipment to demonstrate social skills and to provide feedback is certainly advantageous but is not essential. In the everyday interactions with the patient, the nurse is modelling appropriate social behaviours, and the observational skills of the nurse will reveal areas of individual difficulty with which he/she can assist the patient and on which he/she can provide feedback. Simple roleplay or simulation of everyday activities (mealtime behaviour, shopping, meeting a stranger, asking for directions, initiating and sustaining simple conversations) can prove very helpful and may quickly increase the patient's social competence, adding to confidence and self-esteem in the process.

Social, occupational, industrial and recreational therapy all afford opportunities for developing confidence and social skills, and it is particularly important that such therapies provide activities which are stimulating and rewarding and which lead to personal growth. There is no more sad spectacle than a group of schizophrenics being assigned monotonous and soul-destroying tasks (e.g. sorting out nuts and bolts), this process being referred to as 'industrial therapy'. Such repetitive tasks allow the patient to drift off into withdrawal and fantasy as he automatically carries out these activities in a quiet corner of the 'industrial therapy department'. The damaging effects of monotonous and unstimulating routines on the mentally healthy has been vividly described by sociologists and psychologists; one shudders to think of the effect on the vulnerable and socially incompetent schizophrenic.

Art therapy may provide the perplexed schizophrenic with a means of expressing the confused and vivid images which distort his perceptions of reality and may also provide the nurse with insights into the inner world of her patient, though she should beware of becoming too analytical over the patient's productions.

Acts of aggression may be a response to delusional ideas of hallucinatory 'commands' and the tense and fearful schizophrenic should be approached gently and reassuringly. The tone of the nurse's voice should be calm and she should use non-verbal cues which communicate friendly intent (smiles and a relaxed posture). Do not suddenly approach the tense schizophrenic from behind, and avoid ambiguous communications. The paranoid patient may be quick to misinterpret communications (for example, the nurse leaves the duty room smiling or frowning after a discussion with a colleague and approaches the patient who may imagine that he is being mocked or threatened. Whispered conversations with a colleague may provoke ideas of reference, particularly if one or other nurse should glance in the patient's direction during the discussion. These precautions may be necessary when nursing the acutely disturbed patient but the nurse should beware of becoming over-cautious and thus adding to the patient's feelings of isolation and alienation. A consistently firm, gentle and friendly approach will do much to build a therapeutic nurse/patient relationship and will defuse many of the patient's fears and tensions.

Verbal expressions of aggression should not be reinforced, and calm and relaxed episodes should be strengthened by the potent reinforcers of nursing time and attention. 'Trigger' factors which provoke aggression in the patient should be identified and, where possible, reduced or removed. It is essential that each act of aggression be discussed by the nursing staff afterwards in order to identify precipitating factors. Prevention is much better than cure in this area and a 'post-mortem' on each act of aggression may help prevent any recurrence.

5 Sleeping

The schizophrenic patient may have difficulty in sleeping, especially during the first week or two after admission. A darkened and unfamiliar environment may prove very disturbing to the tense and fearful schizophrenic, and shadows and unfamiliar sounds may provoke illusions or hallucinations. The paranoid patient may lie awake for much of the night fearfully scrutinizing every unfamiliar sound. The creak of a floorboard may signal the approach of an assassin to the delusional patient and the night nurse's smile may be interpreted as having a sinister significance.

The nurse should try to identify those factors which increase or decrease sleep in the case of each individual patient and should be sensitive to the patient's needs for reassurance at this time. A warm milky drink and a quiet well-ventilated room will help, and the night nurse should try to avoid paying too many visits to the patient's bedside during the night. The sight of a shadowy figure looming over the bed may prove terrifying to the patient. If the patient cannot sleep and wishes to sit with the night nurses for a little while, then this should be permitted until the patient feels calmer. It is not helpful to insist that the patient returns to bed immediately as this may simply add to feelings of tension. A night-light may prove reassuring as it will eliminate intimidating patterns of shadow. The patient's bed should not be too near the nurse's station as whispered conversations may be interpreted as evidence of a conspiracy and may provoke auditory hallucinations. At night the schizophrenic's imagination is free to roam unfettered by the distractions of everyday events, and the nurse should be prepared to anticipate episodes of restless or disturbed behaviour.

It is important that the patient does not spend much of the day dozing in a quiet corner of the ward, as in the case of many schizophrenics. Healthy tiredness is much more productive of refreshing sleep than the most effective hypnotic.

6 Eating and drinking

Table 63 indicates that poor mealtime behaviour was a problem in 13% of the patients studied. Behaviour of this sort (eating with fingers, snatching food) should quickly respond to a simple behaviour modification approach as outlined in Chapter 10.

Food may be refused as a consequence of delusional beliefs (for example, the paranoid patient may believe the food to be poisoned). Determined attempts by the nursing staff to demonstrate that the food is unpoisoned may simply reinforce the patient's belief that attempts are being made to poison him (after all, look at the determination to make him eat the stuff!). Food refusal for this reason is actually rare and is usually self-limiting. Hunger will often ensure eating when all the reassurances and admonitions in the world fail. The availability of snacks between meals may help promote the return of food acceptance.

7 Personal cleansing and dressing

Table 63 reveals that neglect of appearance was a problem in 30% of the schizophrenic patients studied. If the patient has distorted perceptions of

Table 68 Sleeping

Problem	Objective	Action
Insomnia	To promote healthy pattern of sleep	Provide restful sleeping environment. Allay fears

Table 69 Eating and drinking

Problem	Objective	Action
Poor mealtime behaviour	Acceptable mealtime behaviour	Behaviour modification
Food refusal	Adequate food and fluid intake	

Table 70 Personal cleansing and dressing

Problem	Objective	Action
Neglect of personal hygiene and dressing	To promote acceptable patterns of cleansing & dressing	Behaviour modification

reality and is preoccupied by delusional beliefs, then the result may be disregard for the conventions of everyday living. In the parallel world of psychosis such activities have low priority. Alternatively, withdrawal may be so marked that there is marked inattention to personal hygiene and dressing.

Simple behaviour modification should quickly restore acceptable standards in these areas, and a rise in self-confidence and self-esteem should also bring about improvements in these areas.

It should be emphasized that attempts to bring about improvements in these areas should respect the adult status of the patient, and the nurse should resist any temptation to treat the patient like a wayward child and must not assume the role of 'Critical Parent'.

If improvements are made in this area the resultant benefits should generalize as the patient becomes more acceptable to his fellow patients and is involved in more social interactions and group activities.

8 Breathing

Problems in this area are unlikely.

9 Elimination

Delusional beliefs about bowel function may be occasionally expressed by schizophrenic patients but should lessen in intensity as overall condition improves. Do not reinforce delusional verbalizations if expressed.

Table 63 indicates that incontinence was a difficulty with a small minority of patients (4%) and may occur in the severely withdrawn or stuporous patient. As awareness of reality improves, this difficulty should disappear. Lasting problems will respond to behaviour modification. Deterioration in eliminatory habits are more likely to be due to institutionalization rather than to schizophrenia.

10 Mobilizing

Table 63 reveals that underactivity and overactivity are common problems in nursing the schizophrenic patient. Fifty six per cent of patients displayed underactivity and 41% displayed overactivity.

The underactive patient will respond to carefully tailored programmes of simple social and group activities, though these must follow a pace suited to the patient's social abilities at first.

David Premack (1959) made the observation that high strength behaviour may be used to reinforce low strength behaviour (*the Premack Principle*). Simply stated, this principle suggests that what a person does a lot of (high strength behaviour) is likely to prove to be an effective reinforcer by which to increase the rate of what he/she does not do very much of (low strength behaviour).

Thus if the nurse wishes to increase the amount of time the underactive patient spends actively partici-

Table 71 Elimination

Problem	Objective	Action
Delusional beliefs about bowel function	To restore rational perceptions of eliminatory function	Behaviour modification
Incontinence	To eradicate incontinence	

Table 72 Mobilizing

Problem	Objective	Action
Overactivity/underactivity	To promote healthy activity levels	Design schedule of daily activities appropriate to healthy activity levels.

pating in group activities (a low strength behaviour) she should identify activities which the patient does a lot of (a high strength behaviour) and make these contingent upon participation in group activities. Thus if the underactive patient spends a lot of time watching television, this high strength behaviour may be selectively used as a reward for spending time with others. Obviously the availability of the reinforcer must be carefully controlled so that it is not randomly available but must be earned, thus constituting an incentive for behavioural change.

It is not enough to simply move the underactive patient in the direction of group activities without carefully assessing the nature of the group activities offered. These activities should be stimulating and rewarding so that participation in them is eventually perceived as being rewarding in itself. Thus the extrinsic reinforcer of television time will gradually be replaced by the intrinsic reinforcers of pleasure and satisfaction gained from activities shared with others.

The overactive patient will also respond to careful use of the Premack Principle, and high strength behaviours (of which there will be many) may be made contingent on an increase in desirable low strength behaviours (quietly chatting with others, quietly playing a board-game or calmly assisting nursing staff with simple tasks). The environment must not be too stimulating for the overactive patient as noise and bustle may increase levels of overactivity by increasing stimulation in the stimulus-sensitive patient.

In the case of both overactive and underactive patients the nursing approach should be consistent and gentle but firm. Any improvements should be noted and warmly commented upon, as nursing approval and attention are probably the most potent reinforcers of all.

11 Controlling body temperature

Problems in this area are unlikely.

12 Dying

The patient tormented by paranoid beliefs may misinterpret both the words and the actions of the nursing staff and may experience intense levels of fear as a result of his belief that he is to die as the result of a conspiracy. This level of fear may be slowly reduced by ensuring that the patient's day is consistently reassuring and non-threatening, thus helping to restore the element of stability which is markedly lacking. Trust and confidence in the nursing staff will reduce these feelings of threat but the nurse must always remember that trust must be earned—it cannot be unconditionally expected. In her attitudes and her actions the nurse should display the stability and consistency which the patient lacks so much.

Delusional verbalizations must not be reinforced, and calmer, more rational verbalizations should be given the reinforcers of nursing approval, time and attention.

Evaluation of the Care Plan

This should take place every time nursing intervention takes place and the care plan should be modified in light of feedback obtained. Rigid adherence to preconceived ideas about nursing care should be avoided. If the care plan is not leading to a reduction in maladaptive behaviours and an increase in adaptive behaviours, then it must be modified. Schizophrenic patients respond well to behaviour modification but this must be weighed against the dangers of allowing care to be delivered in a mechanistic fashion. Selective reinforcement will reduce the level of delusional verbalizations but the nurse must never forget the underlying feelings which gave rise to these verbalizations and must be prepared to work with them. Schizophrenic patients are often very malleable insofar as they will acquiesce with changes in routine and activities suggested by the nursing staff. This may result in a change in the pattern of behaviours as per nursing objectives but the nurse must never lose sight of the *quality* of

Table 73 Dying

Problem	Objective	Action
Unjustified fears of death	To improve patients' perceptions of the situation Reduce feelings of threat	Promote consistency in experience and trust in relationships.

the patient's experiences. Rigidly behavioural approaches may bring about quantitative change in the meek and passive schizophrenic but the effective care plan must never lose sight of the aim of bringing about *qualitative* change in the patient.

Evaluation should be multidisciplinary and should also involve the patient and his family.

Remember that confidence and self-esteem are fragile in schizophrenia and that setbacks may be caused by the nursing approach becoming casual or over-confident.

Preparation for Discharge

Once the patient's level of social competence has improved, and assessment confirms that the patient can cope with activities of daily living, discharge should be considered. It is not helpful to keep schizophrenic patients in hospital any longer than is absolutely necessary, as they are particularly prone to institutionalization and may be rapidly 'desocialized' by institutional living.

Depot phenothiazines will maintain the patient in a state of remission but a measure of social stability must be ensured for the patient before discharge.

The criterion for a successful outcome is no longer simply 'discharged from hospital'. In the not too distant past many schizophrenic patients were discharged to grossly unsuitable accommodation with little attempt being made to monitor progress and provide community support. Sadly, many schizophrenics regressed unnecessarily and were readmitted to embark upon a career as a 'chronic deteriorated schizophrenic' in a back ward of a large mental hospital.

Community care facilities for the discharged patient are still woefully inadequate, but are improving steadily. The patient may now be discharged to a halfway house or to a group home if total independence is not immediately practicable. The community psychiatric nurse and the psychiatric social worker will provide support and guidance, and organizations like the National Schizophrenia Fellowship and The National Association for Mental Health (MIND) will provide support and guidance for patient and relatives alike.

The impact of psychosis on the family unit may be devastating, and relatives will also need support and counselling, both before and after discharge.

With judicious community support there is no reason why the discharged schizophrenic should not resume life in the community and enjoy life to the full extent of his/her capabilities.

Key Concepts

1 The commonest characteristics of the schizophrenic patient are *withdrawal*, *underactivity* and lack of conversation and leisure pursuits.

2 Schizophrenics may be the loneliest people in the world.

3 Self-esteem and confidence are particularly low and there are innate tendencies to *alienation* and *isolation*.

4 Warm and consistent human contact is the most important factor in care.

5 *Social skills training* and *behaviour modification* may dramatically reduce troublesome behaviours, but the nurse must never forget the person behind the behaviour.

6 Schizophrenics are particularly prone to *institutionalization*, and the patient's independence and individuality must be conserved.

7 There may be a risk of aggression, directed towards self or others, and this may occur impulsively.

8 The provision of a safe and non-threatening (but stimulating) environment is therefore important.

9 The nurse should promote healthy patterns of interaction and group activities, paced according to the patient's capabilities, as social skills are often atrophied in schizophrenia.

10 Delusional verbalizations should not be reinforced, but the nurse should make it clear that she is rejecting the delusion and not the patient.

11 Therapeutic activities should be creative and stimulating and should recognize the individuality of the patient. Repetitive and monotonous tasks will allow the patient to drift off into fantasy and withdrawal and are not helpful.

12 Regression may be marked in schizophrenia but the nurse must avoid the role of Critical Parent as this simply fosters dependence and leads to instutionalization.

13 The *Premack Principle* may be used to shape behaviour in a desirable direction, and consists of using a high strength behaviour to reinforce a low strength behaviour.

14 Evaluation of the care plan should consider the quality of the patient's life, and nurses should be aware of the dangers of drifting into a sterile and purely quantitative approach to schizophrenia.

15 Preparation for discharge should involve the primary health care team, and the community psychiatric nurse and social worker have a particularly important role to play.

16 The family should not just be actively involved in care and treatment but should be involved in planning for discharge, as should the patient.

17 If complete independence is not immediately practicable, then discharge to a *halfway house* or *group home* may be indicated.

18 With adequate community support there is no reason why the patient should not enjoy life to the full extent of his/her capabilities.

References

Gutride, M., Goldstein, A. & Hunter, G. (1974) The use of structured learning therapy and transfer training in the treatment of chronic psychiatric pts. *Journal of Clinical Pathology*, **30**: 277–280.

Henderson, D. & Batchelor, I. R. C. (Eds) (1962) *Henderson & Gillespie's Textbook of Psychiatry*. Oxford: Oxford University Press.

Longabaugh, R., Eldred, S. H. & Bell, N. W. (1966) The interactional world of the chronic schizophrenic patient, *Psychiatry*, **29**: 78–99.

Premack, D. (1959) Towards empirical behaviour laws. *Psychology Review*, **66**: 219–233.

Trower, P., Bryant, B. & Argyle, M. (1978) *Social Skills and Mental Health*. London: Methuen.

Wing, J. (1978) *Schizophrenia. Towards a New Synthesis*. London: Academic Press.

Wing, J. & Creer, C. (1980) *Schizophrenia at Home*. London: National Schizophrenia Fellowship.

VI

ALCOHOL AND
DRUG DEPENDENCE

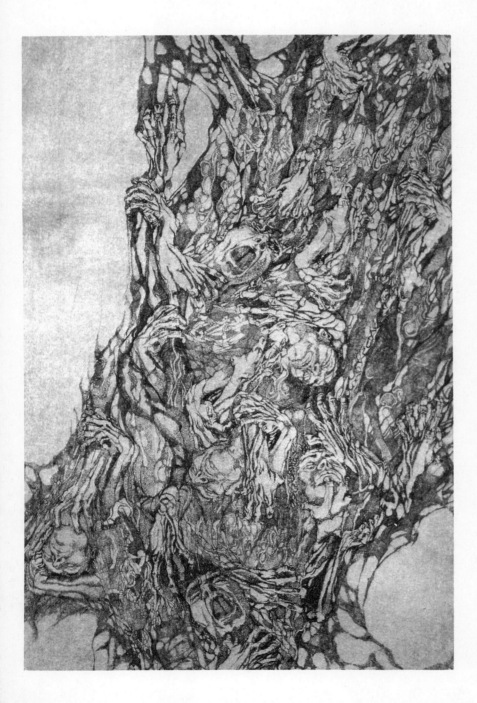

22
Drug Dependence

If you drink very much from a bottle marked
'poison' it is almost certain to disagree with you
sooner or later.

Lewis Carrol: Alice in Wonderland

From the dawn of recorded history man has used a variety of substances to induce intoxication. Neolithic farmers in Mesopotamia cultivated the opium poppy, and clay tablets more than 6000 years old refer to opium as the 'plant' of joy. Coca leaves, the source of cocaine, were chewed by the Aztecs and are still used by at least four million Indians in Peru and Bolivia (Van Dyke, 1981). The Aztecs also used the peyotl cactus (a potent source of the hallucinogen mescaline) as an integral part of religious ceremonies, and this cactus (the 'mescal button') still forms part of the ritual of the Peyotl Society or Native American Church in the Southern USA today (Birdwood, 1971).

A Chinese pharmacological text, dated 2737 BC, describes hemp extract (cannabis) as the 'delight giver' and Meyer and Salmon (1984) describe cannabis as currently forming 'an important part of American culture'.

Opium (from the Greek *opion*, meaning poppy juice) was enthusiastically advocated by Hippocrates and Galen and, in 1680, Thomas Sydenham commented that 'among the remedies which it has pleased Almighty God to give to man to relieve his sufferings, none is so universal and so efficacious as opium'. In China the poppy was largely grown as an ornamental plant until the seventeenth century, when opium smoking was introduced from India (via Turkey), despite the popular belief that China is the ancestral home of the 'opium den'. Opium use was prohibited by the Ching dynasty emperors in the late eighteenth century but opium continued to be smuggled extensively into China with the help of the British East India Company which grew opium in Bengal, and which deliberately fostered the vastly profitable opium trade. British attempts to pursue the trade and preserve their business interests led to the first Opium War of 1839–1842 and resulted in the opium trade continuing for the rest of the nineteenth century.

Tincture of opium (laudanum) and other opiates were freely available in Victorian Britain, being sold from grocers as well as from pharmacists, and were as casually used as aspirin is today.

By the early 1900s there were in the USA more than 50 000 over-the-counter medicines containing addictive drugs—including Kohler's One Night Cough Cure—a mixture of morphine, cannabis and chloroform which, as Freemantle (1985) comments: 'was enough to cure anything in one night'.

In Britain feeble attempts at control were incorporated in the Poisons and Pharmacy Act of 1908 but, in practice, anyone could obtain large amounts of opium, heroin or cocaine by simply signing the poisons register—no prescription being required—and the first restrictive Act was only passed in 1920.

Until the first Dangerous Drugs Act (1920) casual and widespread use of substances, now regarded with misgivings, was rife. In 1886 Dr J. C. Pemberton blended caramel, cola nuts and coca leaves into a 'brain tonic' to cure 'headaches and melancholy' and called it Coca-Cola. Coke (containing coca—the source of cocaine) was 'The Real Thing' until 1903 when the use of coca in its manufacture was discontinued.

In the mid 1880s another cocaine-based elixir, named Mariani Wine after its inventor, was introduced and became a huge success. The Tsar and Tsarina of Russia used it, as did Queen Victoria, US President William McKinley, Alexandre Dumas, Emile Zola and Jules Verne. In 1898 Pope Leo XIII awarded Mariani a gold medal as a 'benefactor to humanity' (Freemantle, 1985).

Morphine (named after Morpheus, the god of dreams) was isolated from opium in 1803 and diacetylmorphine (heroin), a semi-synthetic derivative of morphine, was first produced at St Mary's Hospital, London, in 1874. In 1898 heroin first came onto the market. It was sold as a remedy for coughs.

In the mid 1850s the hypodermic syringe was introduced and led to an increase in the medical use of morphine. The opiates, formerly regarded as harmless sedatives and analgesics, were finding their way from the grocers' counters into the hospitals.

In the 1870s concern was expressed in the medical press about an epidemic of morphine abuse which was nevertheless regarded as a moral failing similar to drunkenness. Excess was regarded as a failing but use was not.

Morphine was freely used to control pain arising from combat wounds, and the resultant wave of morphine addiction after the American Civil War led to morphine addiction becoming known as the 'soldiers' disease'. The doctors of the time decided that cocaine was best used to reduce morphine addiction, and a second addiction became commonplace in armies. In 1916 Britain had to prohibit the gift or sale of cocaine to soldiers except on prescription, but there was no restriction on sale to civilians.

Opiate use was attracting increasing legislative attention—from the casual view of the cheap working class self-medication of Victorian times, opiates were becoming increasingly regarded as a dangerous substance of abuse, leading to moral decay and vice. In the first two decades of the twentieth century most addicts had been introduced to opiates (opium, morphine and heroin) in the course of medical treatment, or had occupations that gave easy access to supplies (doctors, nurses and pharmacists). An increasing number of people were, however, beginning to seek opiates for purely 'recreational' reasons.

In 1926 the Rolleston Committee firmly defined addiction as a 'disease' and as a legitimate target for medical treatment. In 1926 addiction was still relatively rare and, if anything, seemed to be diminishing. Cocaine was less commonly used and the problem largely consisted of a small number of morphine and diamorphine (heroin) addicts who, it was suggested by Rolleston, could be treated by medically prescribed opiates with the aim of maintenance, thus stabilizing the lifestyle and reducing criminality, or gradually reducing the dose and thus weaning the user from the drug.

Rolleston formed the basis of the 'British system' which was to continue largely unaltered for half a century. Drug abuse did not become a major problem in Britain until the late 1950s when the 'British system' began to break down. In the 1950s drug abuse slowly began to escalate, almost imperceptibly at first, and the growth seemed to have the London area as its nucleus.

Cannabis appeared on the streets in ever-increasing amounts and was thought to have been largely introduced by seamen. Recreational use of the drugs was now increasing steadily and seemed to be largely confined to young people living in the larger cities. Heroin use was still rare (it was only in 1954 that the Home Office began to record heroin abusers as a separate category—57 were known to them in 1954, rising to 94 by 1960) (Stimson and Oppenheimer, 1982).

Synthetic analgesics and stimulants were now being produced by pharmaceutical companies and were finding their way onto the illicit market—the increase in drug abuse was becoming qualitative as well as quantitative.

The first Brain Committee (1961) concluded that the majority of addicts were respectable citizens addicted in the course of medical treatment or were themselves members of the medical professions. Illicit drug use is only mentioned in passing and the Rolleston proposals remain unchanged.

Amphetamines (powerful synthetic stimulants) and the potent hallucinogen LSD (lysergic acid diethylamide) were now figuring larger in seizures of illicit drugs (until 1956 amphetamines could be obtained without prescription), and cannabis convictions rose steadily each year. An increasing number of young people were being prescribed heroin by unscrupulous doctors (often with cocaine), and a sizeable heroin market began to develop in London.

The second Brain Committee reported in 1965 and brought about the creation of drug dependence units ('drug clinics') which were to largely replace the prescription of opiates by private doctors. The clinics would continue to prescribe opiates, and addicts were to be notified to the Home Office as they were seen to be suffering from a 'socially infectious' condition.

The USA had steadfastly refused to emulate the 'British system' and had recorded its opposition to any plan for drug clinics. American legislation was Draconian and adopted a punitive attitude towards the entire issue of drug abuse. Harry J. Anslinger (1959), chairman of the Federal Narcotics Bureau, and a man not noted for his balanced view of the problem, recorded his opposition thus:

'Following the line of thinking of the "clinic plan" advocates to a logical position, there would be no objection to the state setting aside a building where on the first floor there would be a bar for alcoholics, on the second floor licensed prostitutes, with the third floor set aside for sexual deviates and, crowning them all, on the top floor a drug dispensing station for addicts'.

This equation of drug abuse with 'prostitution, alcoholism and sexual deviance' was a theme that was to be enthusiastically developed by the press who popularized terms like 'junkie' and 'drug fiend' to the extent whereby impartial assessment of the problem by the layman became increasingly difficult.

Methadone (Physeptone), a synthetic substance with some opiate-like qualities, was introduced in the hope of weaning heroin users from their drug of choice. Methadone substitution therapy aims to gradually reduce the craving for heroin as its effects are more protracted and hopefully 'block' the desire for heroin. Initially, methadone was prescribed by the clinics in injectable form, but now tends to be supplied in linctus form. Once the user is stabilized on methadone it is then possible (in theory) to gradually withdraw the drug until the user is drug-free, though some researchers consider that supplying methadone simply changes one addiction for another.

Some clinics are now using Librium (chlordiazepoxide)—a benzodiazepine anxiolytic—instead of methadone and claim some success with this regime, though benzodiazepines are also an integral part of the drug abuse scene.

Pharmaceutical advances have led to the introduction of a wide range of psychotropic and potent analgesic drugs, many of which have become drugs of abuse and some of which have created many 'therapeutic' addicts (one study estimated that a quarter of a million people in the UK are dependent on tranquillizers prescribed by doctors) (Lacey and Woodward, 1985).

Currently there is a wide spectrum of drug abuse—from problem users of 'hard' drugs (opiates and cocaine) to problem users of LSD (and other hallucinogens), barbiturates and amphetamines, and to the so-called 'soft' drugs (cannabis and 'over-the-counter' analgesics).

Attitudes towards the 'drug addict' are often ones of distaste and revulsion, the addict being viewed as an undesirable and potentially poisonous weed in the social undergrowth. Yet we live in a drug-orientated society. Many of you reading this book will be under the influence of a drug (nicotine, caffeine, alcohol or a medically prescribed 'tranquillizer'). Very few people set out to become dependent on drugs. Drugs are an integral part of the western way of life and acceptance of them is often conditioned in childhood. Children may be given an aspirin for every minor headache, and vitamin tablets are bestsellers in most chemists—many mothers in the USA include vitamin tablets in their children's lunch packs, (Barrymore, 1975). General practitioners may prescribe antibiotics for every minor sore throat; indeed, the patient who emerges from a consultation with a general practitioner without a prescription may feel cheated. Emotional difficulties are liable to provoke a prescription for a 'tranquillizer'. One study revealed that most patients who were prescribed tranquillizers saw their doctor for less than 10 minutes on the first visit when the drug was prescribed, and half of the patients were not even told that the drug was a tranquillizer (Lacey and Woodward, 1985). Overworked and hard-pressed general practitioners may tend to over-prescribe tranquillizers (five million people in Britain are thought to be currently taking medically prescribed tranquillizers) (Lacey and Woodward, 1985) and may not always be aware of the risk of dependence. Benzodiazepine tranquillizers are now amongst the most commonly prescribed drugs in the western world; in fact they are becoming as widely used as laudanum was in Victorian England.

Our attitudes towards problem drug use should not only be coloured by awareness of the fact that western society freely uses addictive drugs for accepted recreational purposes (alcohol, nicotine) but should also take account of the fact that drugs regarded with horror by many Westerners (cannabis, cocaine, opium) are accepted recreational drugs in other societies (many of which view our use of alcohol with horror). Use of cannabis is widespread in the West Indies and is related to the Rastafarian religion, and South American peasants have chewed coca leaves (the source of cocaine) from the start of recorded history. Some North American Indian tribes regarded tobacco as a hallucinogen—to be smoked during religious ceremonies by shamans who would then 'see' into the world of spirits. It is misleading to regard the 'drug user' as being an alien, and essentially inferior, being.

Routes into Dependence

There are many routes into dependence, some obvious, some less so. In the main, people use drugs because they make them feel better, the effect of the drug is being used to create feelings which are desired for their own sake or which block previously obtaining troublesome feelings. Think of reasons for use of accepted recreational drugs, like alcohol—a gin and tonic may induce feelings of relaxation (intrinsic effect) and block feelings of tension after 'a hard day in the office' (blockade of troublesome feelings). Alcohol consumption tends to be a social practice; it usually takes place in the company of others, and there is often also a strong social element in the use of illicit drugs.

As *tolerance* to a drug develops, higher doses are required to obtain the desired effect. Many chronic drug abusers continue to take drugs largely to prevent the appearance of withdrawal effects (e.g. opiate use), the early pleasurable effects having disappeared as tolerance develops. In this case self-medication with illicit drugs has become a form of maintenance therapy, physical, psychological and social equilibrium now being dependent on continuing use of the drug.

Three factors often combine to produce problem drug use. These are *availability*, coupled with predisposing *social pressures*, and *positive attitudes* towards drug use, the latter perhaps forming part of a youth or ethnic subculture.

Availability

History provides many examples of the simple axiom that people cannot become dependent on substances they have never experienced. Opium was imposed upon a reluctant Chinese people by the East India Company, supported by a British government which was prepared to go to war to establish profitable opium markets, and opium use became not only firmly established in China but was exported to North America by Chinese workers during the latter part of the nineteenth century. In South America the coca leaf became the monopoly of the conquering Spaniards during the sixteenth century and was used as a form of payment to slaves employed in the silver mines, (Willis, 1974).

At the present time heroin is (relatively) cheaper than ever before and is easier to obtain. Overprescribing by a small group of unscrupulous or careless doctors released large amounts of pharmaceutical heroin onto the London black market in the 1960s. One private practitioner (Lady Isabella Frankau) prescribed up to 1800 mg of heroin per patient per day (the therapeutic dose is 5–10 mg) and introduced many others to cocaine. Stimson and Oppenheimer (1982) comment that: 'it was her prescribing that resulted in heroin and cocaine being relatively easily available on the black market . . . many addicts were selling their surplus'. Freemantle (1985) adds that

'Lady Frankau didn't create the heroin outbreak in Britain . . . but she fuelled it . . . she stands accused—rightly—in the history of British drug addiction as the person who re-introduced into England a cocaine culture that had flourished in London briefly before and then between the two world wars but which was otherwise virtually unknown after 1945. And a heroin culture as well'.

It is probable that Lady Frankau over-prescribed so carelessly as a result of naïvety rather than a desire for personal gain. This was not so in the case of some other notorious 'drug doctors'. Dr James Petro indiscriminately prescribed heroin and cocaine to London drug users. He initially issued prescriptions at the buffet at Baker Street underground station. Evicted from there he used a room at the Winton Hotel, was fined £1700 for failing to keep a drugs register, and went on to issuing prescriptions from a former cinema. Again evicted he wrote prescriptions from a Vauxhall Viva car parked in Victoria Street and was struck off the medical register in 1968. Pending his appeal he switched to prescribing amphetamines (24 906 ampoules to 110 'patients' during one month), finally lost his appeal and was struck off in October 1968.

Amphetamines expanded the 'needle culture' and now barbiturates like Tuinal and Nembutal were being crushed and injected.

Advances in pharmaceutical research coupled with ineffective safeguards against careless prescribing led to a wide range of potent new hypnotics, stimulants and psychotropics finding their way on to a complex and steadily expanding black market in drugs.

In the early sixties Canadian and American drug users were coming to the UK to benefit from the 'British system'. One American 'drug refugee' wrote of the 'British system':

'Over here it's beautiful. Over here I can stand up and walk around like a man. Over here I am a man. I can walk straight and live decently . . . I don't have to steal or rob anybody. I don't have to wake up sick and wonder where my next fix is coming from—But, Jesus! The United States! . . . All those junkies . . . those poor dogs lying in the Tombs (cells) . . . throwing up over each other' (an American addict, 1970).

Cannabis was increasingly smuggled into the UK by seamen (largely Asian or African), largely for their own use, and found its way onto the streets and into 'youth culture' in the late fifties and early sixties.

By the late seventies the main source of heroin was Iran and it was thought by police sources that middle class Iranians used heroin as a means of transferring their wealth from a politically troubled Iran.

As the drug dependence units (drug clinics') moved towards a policy of prescribing methadone linctus, the resultant deficit in supply seems to have been largely filled by Iranian heroin, though there have been significant seizures of heroin from Hong Kong, Pakistan and Afghanistan. Availability of a wide variety of drugs, particularly of cheap heroin, has increased, but availability does not in itself account for the steady rise in the incidence of drug dependence.

Social Pressures

These must be added to the recipe for dependence.

Finigarette and Hasse (1978) describe the new problem drug user as 'young, poor, disadvantaged, occupationally unskilled, socially uprooted and psychologically immature'. Burr (1984) describes the illicit drugs scene in Kensington Market and indicates that 36% of the buyers (of illicit drugs) were aged 22 years or under, adding that British buyers over the age of 25 years tended to be long-term drug users mainly from working and lower middle class backgrounds. The study indicated that 23% of the buyers were female (aged 17–30 years).

The same reseacher (Burr, 1983) has described the illicit drugs scene in Piccadilly, a notorious haunt of drug users and a focus for the illicit market in hard drugs since the sixties. More than 90% of the Piccadilly buyers were of working or lower middle class origin and about 40% of them stated that they had had no fixed address in the last six weeks. The 'over-25s' made up the vast majority of drug users in Piccadilly and the drugs that changed hands were very largely manufactured pharmaceutical substances rather than illicitly imported or manufactured drugs.

It is still often stated that problem drug use is associated with major personality disorder (Willis, 1974) but this position becomes less convincing when one takes into account the fact that the great majority of the studies supporting this conclusion are based on groups of institutionalized drug abusers. Finigarette and Hasse (1978) point to the existence of a population of drug users who do not become dependent, and the individuals involved in the hospital studies may represent a relatively small percentage of the drug-abusing population.

Jamieson et al (1984) summarize that 'opinions differ between those who see the addict's problems as in some sense an individual inadequacy and who therefore set out to make radical changes in their personality, and those who prefer to stress the social causes of addiction, that in a drug-taking society there are cultural pressures encouraging drug taking, and vested interests, commercial, professional and criminal exacerbate these'.

Some basic dimensions of the sociopathic personality (impulsiveness, thrill-seeking, resentment of convention) lead to vulnerability to drug and alcohol abuse. This personality type is heavily represented in most hospital studies, and probably also forms a major component of the indigenous population of chronic misusers of hard drugs.

Social pressures must firstly create a situation conducive to experimentation with drugs; the final push into drug misuse may be provided by *curiosity*, *rebellion* against parents or other authority figures, *imitation*, *peer pressure* or the wish to escape from chronic *stress* or *inertia* (e.g. young unemployed persons). Mann (1983) comments that 'drug taking became an attempt to accomplish style in a symbolically impoverished world'.

Routes into drug misuse may vary as much as patterns of misuse. The middle class user of psychedelics (LSD, cannabis) in the sixties differs dramatically from the 'glue sniffer' of the eighties. 'Glue sniffing' (solvent abuse) has become endemic in deprived urban areas and misuse of solvents may form an integral part of the street 'subculture' in such settings. (A subculture is an alternative set of beliefs and attitudes embedded in the broader culture which are nevertheless at variance with social norms in some respects.)

Cohen's classic theory of '*status frustration*' may partially explain some forms of 'low status' drug misuse (e.g. solvents, barbiturates). This theory suggests that the school system nurtures ambitions among working class boys which the social structure cannot accommodate. The solution to the resultant feelings of anomie and alienation is to 'hit back' at the system which has stigmatized them as failures and to acquire status in the terms of 'expressive' oppositional values which they can more readily meet (solvent abuse and delinquency) (Cohen, 1956). In this sense drug taking may represent an act of communion—an entrance ritual into a subculture which provides alternatives to the values of a society which are perceived as being spurious or irrelevant. The rejecting culture has in turn been rejected.

The youth subculture of the sixties and the early seventies revolved around the explosion of popular music taking place at that time. Disillusionment with traditional values was high. The Vietnam War led to much discontent amongst American students, and the literature of the new discontent began to form a '*counter culture*' which found expression in the writings of 'acid poets' like Timothy Leary and Allan Ginsberg. Leary, the self-acclaimed high priest of the underground counter culture extolled the use of LSD as an illuminating experience which opened caged areas of the mind:

'And their minds did indeed open like zooz (sic) with all the cages open—and this became the metaphor of our journey. *Open the cage doors*! Let the wild animals be free! When the domesticated discover their wild nature the result is chaos only to the zoo-keeper jailor with his brass ring of keys. When the cage doors open nature rules' (Leary, 1970).

The steadily emerging counter culture was attractive to many young people; it was opposed to war, nuclear weapons and all forms of institutionalized violence and coercion. It was politically radical (though this element was often implicit rather than explicit) and it valued love, peace and compassion. Above all it suggested that the traditional social arena in which many young people had failed was an absurd circus. Internationally this message found expression in the lyrics of famous rock bands, and the 'establishment' and its values seemed distinctly tattered in the conflict. (The mood of the era is encapsulated in the cover illustration of a book by Norman Mailer—*Armies of the Night*—which shows a smiling young woman placing a flower in the barrel of a bayoneted rifle held by a glowering national guardsman at an anti-Vietnam War protest.)

Rock music continued to elaborate the message (Bob Dylan warned that 'the times, they are changing, your sons and daughters are beyond your command'). Drugs formed an integral part of the counter culture; drugs were no longer the province of sordid 'junkies' and 'drug fiends' but were part of a sophisticated and glamorous alternative lifestyle. The Beatles sang of *Lucy in the Sky with Diamonds* (LSD), and The Rolling Stones of *Brown Sugar* (heroin)—the press abounded with accounts of drug arrests and casualties among the heroes of the young. The casualties of drug misuse among rock stars began to constitute an alarming roll-call—Janis Joplin, Brian Jones, Keith Moon (The Who's drummer who died of a drug overdose in the same apartment as Cass Elliott, co-founder of The Mamas and the Papas), Elvis Presley (whose autopsy confirmed a long-term pattern of polydrug abuse), Brian Epstein, the Beatles' manager—another drug victim—had his suits tailored with 'pill pockets' inside the jacket (Freemantle, 1985) and Keith Richard, the heroin-addicted lead guitarist of the Rolling Stones, was sentenced by a Toronto court to play a public charity concert. John Lennon used every drug, including heroin, and was sometimes 'so stoned' that he had to record lying on the studio floor (Stimson and Oppenheimer, 1982).

The supply increased to meet the demand. Psychedelics, such as LSD and cannabis, figured largely in drug seizures during the 'swinging sixties' and were openly on sale at rock festivals. Positive attitudes towards illicit drugs were here to stay and young people often hesitated to condemn drug misuse out of hand for fear of being regarded as 'square' (reactionary).

From the late sixties onwards drug misusers became less respectable as the death toll among the famous rose, and harder drugs (cocaine and heroin) began to figure larger in the drug scene. Despite this the sixties left a residue of liberal attitudes towards drug misuse which has become a part of youth culture (if a less overt part).

Some of the factors discussed interact ominously—young, unemployed persons, suffering from anomie and alienation (social pressures) may have little else to do but embrace 'rock culture', many exponents of which are still involved in drugs (positive attitudes), and hard drugs have never been cheaper or easier to acquire (increased availability).

Drug abuse is not simply going to go away—it is probably here to stay.

The Substances Abused

Five categories of drug may be identified:
1 Sedatives and narcotics
2 Minor tranquillizers
3 Stimulants
4 Hallucinogens (psychedelics)
5 Solvents

Sedatives and narcotics

These are substances which dull consciousness and often produce states of euphoria or increased well-being. Many are powerful analgesics and some have a hypnotic action (i.e. they induce sleep). This category includes the opiates and the barbiturates.

The opiates (opioids)

These are alkaloid substances derived from the opium poppy, *Papaver somniferum* (e.g. morphine and heroin), and this category also includes powerful synthetic analgesics with similar effects. Soon after the opium poppy flowers, slits are made in the unripe seed capsules which then exude a milky sap which dries in the air to become a dark sticky substance—raw opium—used as an analgesic and as a recreational drug for thousands of years (the nepenthe mentioned in Homer's *Iliad* as the drug of sleep given to warriors wounded in the Trojan War was probably opium). Crude *opium* is usually smoked or eaten but the practice is now uncommon in the UK and is restricted mainly to Chinese nationals.

One hundred and fifty years ago *morphine* was isolated from opium; it is ten times more potent than the crude opium base. *Diacetylmorphine* (heroin or diamorphine) was introduced in 1898 when it was claimed not only to be non-addictive but also to be a useful substance to use in the treatment of morphine withdrawal. *Codeine* is also related to the opiates but does not (by itself) have the addictive properties of morphine or heroin. A number of synthetic opiates have been introduced as analgesics and have found their way on to the illicit market; these include *pethidine*, *dipipanone* (Diconal) and *methadone* (Physeptone).

Opiate powders can be swallowed or dissolved in water and injected either intravenously ('mainlining') or subcutaneously ('skin popping'), though it is probable that most users now sniff or smoke the powder. Smoking heroin is a practice known as 'chasing the dragon', the heroin is heated on a piece of tin foil and the thin column of heavy acrid smoke is then inhaled, often using the plastic tube which forms the outer casing of cheap ballpoint pens. (A popular song of the sixties was called *Puff the Magic Dragon*.)

Heroin is sold on the illicit drugs market as pink, grey or brown bricks and as pills, ampoules or more usually in small paper packets caled 'bags' which contain a white or brown crystalline powder. Illicit heroin is often heavily adulterated or 'cut' before sale, using talc, glucose, flour or powdered baby food. (Occasionally more alarming substances are used to 'cut' heroin—Harpic in one recent case.) A 'bag' usually contains around a quarter of a gram and the street price (in 1986) is £10–15 per 'bag'. A regular user will probably use one 'bag' per day, a habit thus costing £70–105 per week.

The practice of 'cutting' creates hazards. A heavy habitual user may buy from a new source and unwittingly obtain heroin which is much purer than that to which he has been accustomed. Use of the same volume may then lead to death from overdose.

Tolerance to opiates develops readily; more of the drug has to be taken to obtain the desired effect. One heroin user was noted to be using 1140 mg of heroin each day; 10 mg has been known to lead to respiratory failure in a non-tolerant individual (Stimson and Oppenheimer, 1982). Habituation to the euphoriant 'flash' which occurs after immediate use in the early stages occurs quickly, and the pleasurable effects may soon vanish completely, the user continuing with the habit to avoid withdrawal symptoms.

'Speedballing' is another way of using heroin; it means using a mixture of cocaine (which gives a 'high') and heroin (which gives a 'low') and is a practice which has been responsible for a high number of fatalities.

Contrary to popular belief heroin is not instantly addictive and it is possible to use morphine or heroin regularly without becoming physically dependent [Institute for the Study of Drug Dependence (ISDD), 1982]. 'Casual users' of opiates are uncovered in most research studies (Burr, 1983), though the risk of intractable dependence is always present. The myth of instant addiction is so widespread that terminally ill patients in some countries are refused diamorphine lest they become addicted (Trebach, 1982) which is, to say the least, unfortunate, as diamorphine is a potent analgesic which does not cloud consciousness.

The effects of opiates are to induce a feeling of warmth, well-being and contentment—a state of dreamy detachment which is often accompanied by episodes of dreamy contemplation ('gouching'). Some users report an initial 'kick' or 'flash' of almost orgasmic proportions, associated with intravenous use. Some first-time users simply become violently nauseated and avoid the drug in future.

Intravenous use is accompanied by many hazards [hepatitis B, acquired immune deficiency syndrome (AIDS), septicaemia, gangrene, nerve damage] largely due to insterile injection technique or communal use of a syringe and needle. Heavy habitual users may spit into a syringe to 'clean' it, and public lavatories are favourite place for self-injection, water from the lavatory bowl often being used to make up the heroin solution.

Regular use of heroin reduces appetite and sex drive, lowers general health, causes intractable constipation and interrupts the menstrual cycle. There can also be fatal reactions to injected adulterants due to the uncertain composition and purity of street heroin. Given the dangers of street heroin, many users prefer it to pharmaceutical heroin as it may be cut with caffeine or strychnine and thus is less sedating than 'medical' heroin.

Withdrawal. After as little as several weeks on high doses, sudden withdrawal results in a variable degree of discomfort generally comparable to a severe bout of influenza. The effects appear 8–24 hours after the last 'fix' and may be mild, moderate or severe.

Willis (1974) describes the effects of opiate withdrawal as follows:

1 *Mild symptoms*:
yawning
rhinorrhoea (runny nose)
tears
sweating
anorexia

2 *Moderate symptoms*:
trembling
'gooseflesh'

abdominal cramps
insomnia

3 *Severe symptoms*:
vomiting
diarrhoea
restlessness
weight loss

Craving for the drug may be marked during withdrawal, and the combination of gooseflesh and shivers led to the nickname 'cold turkey' for the effects of abrupt withdrawal. Involuntary muscle jerks may occur during withdrawal, often involving involuntary kicking movements of the legs—hence 'kicking the habit'.

Withdrawal symptoms reach their peak about 48 hours after the last dose of opiate and remain at this height for 72 hours. They then gradually subside during the next 5–10 days (Kolb and Brodie, 1982). Withdrawal may be unpleasant but does not remotely resemble the tortured ravings invented by the media. The problem is not so much that of withdrawal, which can be relatively easily accomplished, but of staying off.

The user may have invested heavily in the lifestyle of the illicit drugs user and may feel alienated from 'normal' society. There may also be deep-seated fears about the quality of life without drugs. Stimson and Oppenheimer (1982) comment that

'sooner or later people talked less about getting buzzes and more about using heroin to "keep me straight", "to keep me normal", "to stop me being sick", "to be able to talk and do normal things that people do without thought". By this stage, continued use less often brings pleasure, but rather alleviates discomfort' (Stimson and Oppenheimer, 1982).

Chronic heavy use will eventually create the risk of personal and social deterioration. Theft (usually shoplifting) or prostitution may be resorted to in order to pay for an increasingly expensive habit. Heavy use is not often compatible with continued employment, and unemployment benefit is not enough to pay for an opiate habit. Crime or dealing in drugs may seem to be the only answer to the user. One heavy user described to the author (1985) how she received £28 per week in benefits but spent £90 per week on heroin. Her bedsit cost £15 per week and she spent 'around £5' per week on food. Her life now revolved around making good the £82 weekly deficit. She shoplifted from city centre stores (mainly clothes and electrical appliances) and occasionally dealt in small amounts of heroin when she made a big 'score'. 'Life is just a big hassle now—the only thing that makes it bearable is smack (heroin)'. She was introduced to heroin by a boyfriend (now in prison as a result of drug offences) and for the first year or so smoked heroin at weekends only. After this period (which she bitterly described in retrospect as the 'honeymoon period') she graduated to subcutaneous injections of heroin (occasionally supplemented with cocaine).

> 'You lose interest in sex and all sorts of things you used to like . . . everyday life gets . . . out of focus . . . becomes unreal and irrelevant . . . you don't think you will ever become a junkie . . . you think you can handle it . . . but you can't . . . people I used to know walk past me in the street now.'

She was pale and emaciated and both ankles were spotted with dried blood from recent injections.

Barbiturates

Barbituric acid and its homologues—the hypnotics—have effects which are similar to alcohol and, in general, opposite to the stimulants. This group of drugs is often known as the *hypnosedatives* as some have a sedative (calming) effect, while others have a hypnotic effect (induce sleep). Many have a sedative action if given in low doses but induce sleep if given in higher ones. Those with a medium duration of action, and used as sleeping pills, are the ones most often abused for their intoxicating effects. They include Sodium Amytal, Tuinal, Seconal and Nembutal. Mandrax ('Mandies') is a hypnotic combining methaqualone (a hypnosedative) with an antihistamine and is no longer manufactured in the UK due to its widespread abuse, but is still occasionally illegally imported.

In 1979 there were thought to be 15 000 persons dependent on barbiturates in the UK (ISDD, 1982), though the level of barbiturate abuse is thought to be declining.

Burr (1983) revealed that drugs on sale around the Piccadilly area still included many hypnosedatives (Tuinal, Nembutal, Seconal, Amytal and Doriden).

Barbiturates and other hypnosedatives are produced in the form of tablets, capsules, ampoules, solutions and suppositories and may be taken by mouth (sometimes with alcohol), or capsules may be opened, or tablets crushed and the resultant powder made into a solution and injected. Use of injected sedatives is possibly the most dangerous form of drug misuse—large doses produce unconsciousness, respiratory failure and death. Heavy users are also liable to pneumonia (the cough reflex is depressed and hypothermia (normal responses to cold are suppressed) and the dependence produced is both physical and psychological. Barbiturate dependence causes rapid psychosocial deterioration, and 'barb freaks' are often regarded with contempt by users of other illicit drugs. The user who is 'barbed up' is likely to be incoherent and aggressive: 'you don't know what you are doing', 'you just start fighting people'. The user frequently wakes up in hospital 'with stitches around my eyes' and will not be able to 'remember a thing about it' other than 'fighting with ambulance drivers'—'when you're stoned you don't know what you're doing, you go out and get more and take them without realizing' (Stimson and Oppenheimer, 1982). The lethal dose may be only three to four times the therapeutic dose, or less if combined with alcohol—10 Tuinal capsules can be enough.

Withdrawal effects set in within 24 hours and reach a peak on the second or third day. Delirium, convulsions and transient psychotic states may occur and there is a risk of brain damage or death. Of all withdrawal states, the barbiturates present the most serious physical problems (Willis, 1974).

Minor tranquillizers

This group includes the benzodiazepines (anti-anxiety drugs including Librium and Valium). The majority of problem users are women who have been prescribed these drugs by their general practitioner and who have insidiously developed dependence. Some tranquillizers find their way onto the illicit market where they are known as 'tranx' and are used as 'downers'. In 1982 Valium and Librium were being illicitly sold at about £1 for four 5 mg tablets or capsules (ISSD, 1982).

The British National Formulary (BNF) contains a warning about benzodiazepines, indicating that they should only be used for

> 'patients whose anxiety is clearly handicapping . . . treatment should be limited to short periods because tolerance to its effects develops within four months of continuous use and because of the insidious development of dependence and subsequent difficulty in withdrawing the drug' (Lacey and Woodward, 1985).

This viewpoint was again emphasized in an article in the British Medical Journal (Einarson, 1980) which acknowledges withdrawal effects and points out that these drugs lose effectiveness after four months. This report recommends that these drugs should be prescribed for 3–14 days for sleeping problems and for up to four months for anxiety; yet a survey of more than 2000 people who were prescribed benzodiazepines revealed that 62% had been taking them for longer than five years and 40% had been taking them for longer than ten years (Lacey and Woodward, 1985). Benzodiazepines are among the most commonly prescribed drugs in the Western world (40 million prescriptions in 1980) (Lacey and Woodward, 1985) and are twice as likely to be prescribed for women than for men.

Perry (1979) writes of this sex discrepancy in benzodiazepine prescription and comments that

'modern medicine has incorporated stereotypes of women as emotional, sensitive, introverted and physically and psychologically weak, with interpretations of Freud ascribing these deficiencies to biological factors'.

Once having had a benzodiazepine prescription, women are also more likely than men to be given further prescriptions.

Attempts to give up benzodiazepines are likely to lead to withdrawal symptoms (insomnia, anxiety, perceptual distortions, tremor, nausea vomiting and, after high doses, convulsions and confusion). These withdrawal effects are liable to result in the agitated patient paying a return visit to the doctor who is likely to prescribe more of the drug, being now convinced that the patient needs it to control his/her anxiety. The state of chronic dependency thus fostered is undesirable for reasons other than the effect on the patient:

'If Mum reaches for the Valium every time she's depressed or has a problem it's hardly surprising if her teenage children look for chemical solutions to their problems too' (Perry, 1979).

Stimulants

As the name suggests, these stimulate the nervous system, banish fatigue and produce feelings of alertness and confidence in the user. The street name for this category of drugs is 'uppers'. The compounds most widely misused are amphetamines ('speed') and cocaine ('coke').

Amphetamines were used to increase the effectiveness of troops in the Second World War and the Vietnam War (ISDD, 1982) and enjoyed a vogue on the illicit market during the sixties when they were known as 'pep pills'. The best known amphetamine was a combination of amphetamine and barbiturate called Drinamyl (known as 'purple hearts' because of their distinctive shape and colour). Others misused included amphetamine itself (Benzedrine), methylamphetamine (Methedrine and phenmetrazine (Preludin or 'Prellies), dexamphetamine (Dexedrine or 'Dexies') and methylphenidate (Ritalin). Street amphetamines today are largely illicitly manufactured amphetamine sulphate powder (ISDD, 1982). Much illicit 'amphetamine' is actually diethylpropion hydrochloride—the active ingredient of Tenuate Dospan, an appetite-reducing drug prescribed widely in the treatment of obesity.

Amphetamines, now most commonly known as 'speed', may be taken by mouth, injected or smoked, though the most common method is to sniff the powder up the nose. Use does not cancel fatigue and hunger but merely postpones them; when the user wakes the next day he/she is liable to feel deeply depressed (the 'speed blues'), lethargic and ravenously hungry.

'I stayed up all night in the club taking these pills every hour or so and I'd never enjoyed myself so much in my life, I felt on top of the world, as though I could go on dancing and talking and laughing for ever and ever, just listening to records on the juke box and drinking coffee, but next morning . . . oh, you feel shocking, terrible, I can't describe it. All I wanted to do was to go to bed and sleep and sleep and sleep' (Parker, 1965).

Amphetamines do not cause addiction insofar as physical dependence does not occur, but psychological dependence may be intense and prolonged use leads to debility and decreased resistance to infection. There is also a risk of heart failure due to the hypertension produced by amphetamine intoxication. Regular users are liable to develop feelings of paranoia accompanied by delusions and hallucinations, these symptoms sometimes developing into a psychotic state (amphetamine psychosis) which may take several months to abate. There is no generally recognized withdrawal syndrome.

Cocaine ('coke', 'snow') is a white powder derived from the leaves of the coca bush which is a powerful stimulant and is much more expensive than its poorer relatives—the amphetamines. Its effects are similar to those of the amphetamines but are more intense and short-lived (a dose of amphetamines lasts for 3–4 hours but a dose of cocaine may have to be repeated every 20 minutes to maintain the desired effect). A sequence of quickly repeated doses (a 'run') may lead to violent or erratic behaviour, sometimes accompanied by hallucinations and, as with amphetamines, there is a risk of heart failure or residual psychosis (Willis, 1974).

Cocaine is usually sniffed ('snorted') but is sometimes mixed with heroin and injected (the dangerous 'speed ball'). Repeated sniffing may cause necrosis (and eventual destruction) of the nasal septum, and paranoid feelings are sometimes accompanied by an unpleasant sensation as though insects were crawling under the skin (the 'cocaine bug').

Neither tolerance nor significant withdrawal symptoms occur, but psychological dependence may be intense and depression following heavy use may reinforce the temptation to repeat the dose.

'Freebasing' is a method of ingesting a purer form of cocaine by holding an extraction pipe over a flame to burn away the hydrochloride salt. 'Freebasing' is hazardous as the ether or alcohol used as a solvent is liable to ignite explosively. (Richard Pryor, the American comedian, almost burned himself to death when 'freebasing'.) (Freemantle, 1985).

'Angel dust' (phencyclidine) is a potent stimulant which may be sniffed, swallowed or injected, though it is popularly ingested by smoking it in a cigarette made from either parsley or marihuana. It can provoke berserk states of homicidal violence, hallucinations, coma and sometimes death. Originally introduced as a veterinary anaesthetic, its illicit use reached a peak in the USA during 1981 and 1982, though its popularity seems to be tapering off. Phencyclidine did not reach the UK illicit market in significant amounts.

Caffeine is perhaps the most widely used stimulant being found in coffee, tea, soft drinks and over-the-counter analgesics and headache pills (one cup of coffee may contain caffeine equivalent to the minimal stimulant dose). Soft drinks usually contain less caffeine than coffee but because of their lower body weight, children consuming a full can could ingest the caffeine equivalent of four cups of coffee (ISDD, 1982).

Fencamfamin (Reactivan) and pemoline (Kethamed) are mild stimulants with effects similar to those of caffeine.

The pharmacologically active stimulant dose of caffeine is 200 mg (a cup of brewed coffee contains 100–150 mg, a cup of instant coffee about 70 mg, tea 50–75 mg and a can of soft drink 35–55 mg).

Caffeine is a powerful central nervous system stimulant and, in moderate doses, allays fatigue and postpones the onset of sleep. Performance on simple or well-learnt motor skills is improved, and blood pressure, heart rate and secretion of urine is increased. More than 1 gram taken as a single dose may induce restlessness, excitement and delirium. Death from overdose is rare (it would take the equivalent of more than 100 cups of coffee) but there is a well-established withdrawal syndrome (fatigue, headache and irritability).

Needless to say, caffeine ingestion in the form of strong tea or coffee should be discouraged in the patient who is tense, anxious or suffering from insomnia.

Hallucinogens

From the dawn of recorded history mankind has used substances which distort perceptual processes and alter awareness, the resultant 'mind-expanding' experience often being an integral part of religious ceremonies. The substances used are extremely diverse and include the seeds of the piptadena tree (Haiti), fly agaric mushrooms (Siberia), the eating of 'dream fish' (east coast of America), morning glory seeds, and the peyotl cactus (Mexico), 'Kava' roots (New Zealand and Polynesia) and nutmeg (Great Britain), (Birdwood, 1971), but the best known drugs in this category are powerful synthetic hallucinogens such as LSD 25 (lysergic acid diethylamide). The English hop plant is a type of morning glory, of which two varieties contain powerful hallucinogens, so it is not impossible that ordinary British beer has traces of hallucinogens (Laurie, 1971).

Besides LSD, modern chemistry has produced a number of potent synthetic hallucinogens [for example, the tryptamine group—dimethyltryptamine, diethyltryptamine, dipropyltryptamine, Serotonin (5-hydroxytryptamine), Psilocybin and Bufotenine (the latter occurring naturally in the skin secretions of many species of toad and perhaps explaining their frequent inclusion in the 'witches brews' of folklore)]. Illicit use of synthetic hallucinogens other than LSD is rare in the UK. Phencyclidine (or 'angel dust') has both stimulant and hallucinogenic effects and is again rare in the UK.

LSD is the most powerful mind-affecting chemical known, being effective in doses of millionths of a gram.

In 1938 the Swiss chemist, Albert Hoffman, synthesized LSD by adding diethylamide to lysergic acid, a naturally occurring substance found in morning glory seeds and the ergot fungus (and a hallucinogen in its own right). Five years later he accidentally ingested a small amount (20 micrograms, or 20 millionths of a gram, are enough to have a detectable effect) and described the results as follows:

> 'I was seized by a peculiar sense of vertigo and restlessness . . . in a dream-like state I left for home . . . and fell into a peculiar state . . . characterized by exaggerated imagination. With my eyes closed, fantastic pictures of extraordinary plasticity and intensive colour seemed to surge towards me—space and time seemed more and more disorganized . . . I was overcome by a fear that I was going out of my mind.' Hoffman awoke the next morning 'feeling tired but otherwise perfectly well' (Hoffman, 1980).

Laurie (1971) summarized the effects of the drug by saying that

> 'the drug dissolves the crust that separates us both from the sensually experienced world and our own unconscious. 'The effect on civilized man is often that he discovers—to his surprise—as large and strange a world inside his head as there is outside' (Laurie, 1971).

An LSD-induced 'trip' begins about half an hour to an hour after taking LSD, peaks after 2–6 hours and fades out after about 12 hours (depending on the dose), and the drug is usually taken absorbed on small pieces of paper ('micro-dots') or sugar cubes. The resultant 'trip' may be 'good' or 'bad', and a 'bad trip' may be associated with overwhelming feelings of terror and episodes of disturbed behaviour. Short-lived vivid re-experiences of part of a previous trip ('acid flashes') may occur:

> 'the next day we felt cold and remote, but got through a lot of work. Driving the children to school I nearly crashed when a coloured girl came out of a grey house wearing day-glo orange trousers: they went off on my retina like a bomb in a free-church assembly' (Laurie, 1971).

LSD was used in research into the psychoses as it was thought to have a *psychotomimetic* (or 'madness-mimicking') effect, though the effects of LSD differ from those of psychosis. In the sixties the use of 'acid' was widely advocated by the 'hippy culture' (which was opposed to the use of 'needle drugs') as a sort of 'mental vitamin' which enhanced awareness and provided experiences which transcended the world of everyday reality (transcendental experiences). LSD was used at this time with a wide range of psychedelic (mind-altering) drugs—some powerfully hallucinogenic, others only feebly so (e.g. cannabis).

LSD also enjoyed a brief vogue as an adjunct to psychotherapy due to its ability to open up areas of the unconscious quickly and so to penetrate into buried experiences and emotions from very early childhood.

Suicides or deaths due to 'bad trips' are rare but much publicized, though there is a risk that the drug may quickly precipitate latent psychosis. Some users have 'gotten lost in inner space' and have never come back (Leech, 1983).

Use of LSD is uncommon overall, but recent reports suggests that its availability has increased since the seventies and that its use has spread to a wider range of youth subcultures (ISDD, 1982). LSD does not induce physical dependence.

Hallucinogenic mushrooms

A dozen or so species of hallucinogenic fungi grow in the British Isles (notably *Amanita muscaria*—'fly agaric'—and *Psilocybe semilanceata*—the 'liberty cap'). These fungi contain psilocybin and psilocin, both of which have a hallucinogenic effect, though 20–30 mushrooms may be required (ISDD, 1982). The mushrooms may be eaten fresh, cooked or brewed into a tea, though boiling or crushing makes possession illegal as it constitutes making 'a preparation or other product'.

The effects include euphoria and hilarity (unlike LSD) and there is the risk of a 'bad trip' or 'flashes'. Physical dependence does not develop, though tolerance rapidly increases, but the greatest risk arises from the possibility that poisonous *Amanita* species (e.g. *Amanita bhuroides*—the Death Cap) may be picked by mistake. Few users possess the necessary knowledge of fungal taxonomy to enable them to select mushrooms with confidence. Eating of hallucinogenic mushrooms has been reported as a common event in urban conurbations in Great Britain (ISDD, 1982), though accurate assessment of the hazards is not yet possible due to a lack of comprehensive studies.

Cannabis is conventionally included among the hallucinogens, rather inappropriately as it is only hallucinogenic in very high doses, being used to induce euphoria and relaxation, though a degree of perceptual distortion may occur.

Cannabis is derived from *Cannabis sativa*, a plant rather resembling a tall and ungainly nettle which grows wild in most parts of the world and is easily cultivated in Britain. The active ingredient is delta-g-trans tetrahydrocannabinol (THC) and the resin exuded by the flowering heads of the female plant is rubbed from the plants and compressed to form blocks of 'hash' (hashish), the commonest form of cannabis in the UK. Hash may be brown, black or golden in colour depending on the country of origin (e.g. 'Paki black' or 'Moroccan gold'). The dried plant material is shredded, dried and sold as 'grass' ('marihuana' in the USA). Grass is much less potent than hash, but the strongest preparations of all are 'hash oil' (made by percolating a solvent through cannabis resin) and synthetic THC (both uncommon in the UK).

In Britain cannabis was widely used until this century. Culpepper's Herbal (1652) claimed that it was 'so well known to every good housewife in the country that I shall not need to write any description of it' (Leech, 1983).

Cannabis use is widespread—it is known as 'bhang' in India, 'kif' in Morocco, 'dagga' in South Africa, 'ganja' in the West Indies and 'marihuana' in the USA. As bhang it is brewed into a sort of tea and consumed during religious ceremonies. West Indians associate use of ganja with the Rastafarian religion and claim that use of it enables them to work harder in the fields. In many societies it is an accepted recreational drug, viewed much as we view tobacco or alcohol. In Britain cannabis was available on prescription until 1973 (ISDD, 1982), though not much used, and illicit use began to escalate in the fifties until it became the most widely used illicit drug—cannabis features in 80–90% of all drug seizures and convictions and 'it's generally accepted that cannabis smoking is now established in the leisure activity of large sections of the population' (ISDD, 1982), and a survey in 1973 suggested that 3.8 million people in the UK had used cannabis (ISDD, 1982).

In the late sixties the popularity of cannabis became so great that those unable to obtain, or afford any, resorted to substitutes. 'Mellow yellow' consisted of a preparation of the dried lining of banana skins which had been baked in an oven. It was claimed to have mild effects similar to cannabis but, unfortunately, caused abrupt episodes of explosive diarrhoea (which tended to disrupt the desired state of relaxed meditation in no small way).

Cannabis may be smoked (usually rolled into a cigarette in combination with tobacco to produce a 'joint'), eaten, brewed into a drink, added to food or smoked in a pipe (usually a water-pipe, or 'hookah', which cools the hot irritant smoke). The drug induces a fatuous euphoria (it isn't called 'dope' for nothing), relaxation, and heightened appreciation of sex, music and colour. In higher doses distortion of perceptions may occur, though florid hallucinatory experiences are unlikely.

There is no conclusive evidence to show that long-term use causes damage to physical or mental health and cannabis use does not induce physical dependence (ISDD, 1982), though the smoke is as carcinogenic as tobacco smoke. Heavy use is hazardous for persons with pulmonary or cardiovascular disorder and may precipitate underlying mental disorder. There is little evidence that cannabis use leads to misuse of 'harder' drugs. Most (but not all) heroin users have used cannabis and various pills in the past, but a progression on to harder drugs takes place only in a minority of cases (and these probably include those with personality disorder who would be more likely to escalate any drug habit). Recreational use of cannabis is endemic in the West Indies where there is not only no evidence of progression into harder drugs but often marked disapproval of 'hard' drug use.

Leech (1983) comments that some heroin users have at some point used cannabis but

'it is also probably true that most methylated spirits drinkers have at some point drunk beer . . . the point is that most beer drinkers do *not* become methylated spirits' addicts or alcoholics of any kind. Similarly most cannabis users . . . do *not* become heroin addicts or addicts of any kind. If they did we would have millions of drug addicts in Britain today.

There is considerable controversy as to whether or not cannabis use should be partially or completely legalized. The constabularies of Merseyside, Northumbria, South Yorkshire and Suffolk have adopted policies of caution rather than prosecution for persons found with small amounts of the drug for personal use (Freemantle, 1985) and a spokesman for the Police Federation has stated in January, 1984, that 'the law on (cannabis) possession is fairly unenforceable and it points to a growing lack of conviction that it is a sensible law' (Freemantle, 1985).

The decriminalization of cannabis may mean that much of its appeal would be lost. In 1983 the Netherlands made cannabis available from controlled distribution centres, and the percentage of the population (aged 13–25 years) using cannabis dropped from the 1976 level of 15% to between 1–2% (Freemantle, 1985).

There are dangers in unrestrained arguments in favour of legalization. The 'legalise grass' camp tend to portray cannabis as a healthier alternative to tobacco or alcohol but no-one is seriously suggesting that alcohol or tobacco be *replaced* by cannabis; the suggestion is that another intoxicant be made available to a society which cannot cope with the health problems created by the two major intoxicants already in accepted recreational use (tobacco and alcohol). Perhaps a more balanced approach would consist, not of open legalization, but of decriminalization of possession of small amounts for personal use, thus freeing police manpower to concentrate on the growing market in 'hard' drugs.

Table 74 Drugs and the law.

The Medicines Act (1968) prohibits sale of barbiturates without a prescription. Possession of barbiturates is not an offence.

The Misuse of Drugs Act (1971) divides controlled drugs into three categories:
Class A includes heroin, morphine, methadone and a number of synthetic opiates, cocaine, LSD, PCP, synthetic hallucinogens and amphetamines prepared for injection.

Class B includes cannabis, codeine, DF 118, amphetamine, Preludin and Ritalin.

Class C includes methaqualone (Mandrax) and some stimulants.

Maximum penalties under the Act:

	Possession	Possession with intent to supply, and supply
Class A	7 years or unlimited fine	14 years or unlimited fine
Class B	5 years or unlimited fine	5 years or unlimited fine
Class C	2 years or unlimited fine	5 years or unlimited fine

Most of the drugs used are subject to minimal controls (alcohol, barbiturates) or no controls at all (solvents, tobacco, caffeine, 'over-the-counter' analgesics).

Certain sectors of the press have behaved irresponsibly by luridly overstating the case against cannabis. Young people who have used cannabis may recognize 'dope fiend' headlines for the nonsense they are, and mistakenly assume that the polemic argument directed against 'hard' drugs is equally unfounded. Health educators may have suffered inestimable loss of credibility due to the excesses of irresponsible and ill-informed journalists. A typical example of counter-productive polemic is provided by the Northants newspaper which announced: 'Thirty registered LSD addicts in Northampton' (Leech, 1983)—LSD is not addictive and there is not, and never has been, any system of registration of its users.

In Canada the report of the Le Dain Commission (Non-Medical Use of Drugs, 1973) proposed that the prohibition against the simple possession of cannabis be repealed, and in the USA, the report of the Shafer Commission (First Report of the National Commission on Marihuana and Drug Abuse, 1973) recommended that possession of small amounts of cannabis in private should not be regarded as an offence. In Britain the Wootton Committee (1968) recommended that penalties for cannabis possession be reduced and that the association of cannabis with heroin and other opiates was inappropriate and should be changed (Logan, 1974).

These reports simply recognize that cannabis is readily available in urban areas (much British cannabis is now home-grown) and that a large number of people will continue to use it despite legal sanctions. No-one is suggesting that packets of '20 hash-tipped' be made available at the corner shop.

Solvent abuse

The practice of seeking intoxication by inhaling vapours or gases is, like most patterns of drug misuse, very ancient indeed. The Pythia, a young priestess in Ancient Greece, experienced visions after inhaling vapours escaping from fissures in the rocks (probably carbone dioxide vapour) and in the Bible lands, vapours from aromatic gums and burning spices were inhaled as part of the ritual of worship in Judaic culture. During the Renaissance the French essayist, Montaigne, noted the pleasant mind-changing effects of some odours and wrote: 'Incense and perfumes raise our spirits and excite and purify our senses' (Essais I, LV) (O'Connor, 1983).

In the mid and late nineteenth century nitrous oxide ('laughing gas') was used recreationally for its euphoriant effect (Coleridge, Southey and Wedgewood used it) and public demonstrations were arranged where 'the gas will only be administered to highly respectable men' (Black, 1982). In the nineteenth century inhalation of the fumes of ether or chloroform was practised and 'ether frolics' enjoyed some popularity. In 1855 an outbreak of ether sniffing occurred at Draperstown in Northern Ireland where it was used as a substitute for alcohol following a successful temperance movement (O'Connor, 1983), predicting the 20th century practice of 'glue sniffing' as a cheap alternative intoxicant to alcohol. During the First World War (1914–1918) there were accounts of allied troops sniffing fumes from the metal polish used for their equipment (O'Connor, 1983), and during prohibition in the USA soft drinks were often 'spiked' with ether, but widespread problems arising from inhalation of intoxicant vapours first became apparent in the USA during the fifties. Solvent abuse has been known in Britain since 1962 but concern has only become apparent since the mid seventies.

Substances used are diverse and include glues (notably Evo-Stik), nail varnish remover, dry cleaning fluids, petrol, butane lighter fuel and propellant gases from aerosols or fire extinguishers.

Inhaled vapours pass rapidly from the lungs into the bloodstream. Given the large surface area of the lungs available for absorption the effect is as rapid as an intravenous injection, and most of the volatile substances are fat soluble (e.g. toluene—a common constituent of adhesives and solvents) and are concentrated in the brain and spinal cord. Most of the absorbed solvent is metabolized in the liver and excreted in the urine, though considerable amounts are excreted unchanged through the lungs (hence the strong smell of solvents from the breath which is apparent for some time after sniffing). Urine tests carried out within 24 hours can identify the type of solvent which has been abused.

Sniffers often attempt to heighten the effect by sniffing from a plastic bag (or crisp packet) in which a quantity of glue or solvent has been placed. The bag is placed over the nose and mouth and the vapours are inhaled to cause rapid and gross intoxication. Sometimes the vapours are concentrated by placing the volatile substance in a wide-necked bottle or jar (milk bottles are widely used) from which the vapours can be inhaled. In some cases

Steradent tablets are added to the solution or the substances are warmed to speed up release of the fumes (Rogers, 1982). Sometimes a blob of Evo-Stik is placed on top of a ball point pen which is then inserted into the nostril, or the plastic outer casing of such a pen is filled with glue and used as a 'sniffing stick'. There have been reports of children inhaling petrol fumes directly from the petrol tanks of cars or even inhaling car exhaust fumes (Rogers, 1982), the latter practice creating a risk of brain damage from carbon monoxide poisoning. The abuse of the anaesthetic gas Trilene (especially by anaesthetists) has been reported and even the vapours from burning ping-pong balls have been used (Wilson, 1981).

The effects of solvent abuse are similar to alcohol intoxication, and the sniffer will develop a sense of euphoria and may develop blurred vision, drowsiness, slurred speech, discoordination and an unsteady gait. One study found that 42% of those interviewed experienced hallucinations (mainly visual) (Scott, 1982), and Steradent tablets added to solvents are thought to increase the probability of hallucinatory experiences (and are added for this reason). The effects come on quickly and disappear within a few minutes to half an hour if sniffing is stopped, though the sniffer will experience a hangover (headache, lethargy, impaired concentration) for about a day afterwards.

The hazards are many. 'Sniffing' practices (actually a misnomer as vapours are inhaled deeply, not sniffed) may be hazardous in themselves, especially when plastic bags are placed over the head or when sniffing occurs in a confined space. The practice of spraying aerosols (particularly of butane) directly into the mouth may freeze the larynx and cause death by asphyxiation. Vomiting may occur at any stage, with a risk of inhalation asphyxia. Toxic effects on the central nervous system, kidneys, liver and heart have been described and several cases of solvent encephalopathy (presenting with coma, ataxia, convulsions, diplopia or hallucinations) have also been described (King et al, 1981), as have isolated cases of severe uncontrolled status epilepticus (Allister et al, 1981).

Solvent abusers tend to be adolescents from low socioeconomic backgrounds, disrupted families and poor neighbourhoods (Lowenstein, 1982) and there is also the likelihood that they are abusing, or will abuse, other forms of drugs. Other factors identified are general boredom, lack of interesting pursuits in the home area, lack of money to purchase alcohol, depression, and high availability. Males are more likely to 'sniff' regularly than are females; the ratio of male sniffers to female sniffers was found to be 3:1 in one study (Ives, 1981).

Solvent abuse is a widespread problem and is regarded as having reached 'serious' levels in the USA, UK, Canada, Mexico, Sweden, West Germany, Hungary, Israel, Japan, Australia, Eire and parts of Africa (O'Connor, 1983). A study in Dallas found that 29% of high school pupils had inhaled solvents at least once (Ives, 1981) and it is thought that a significant proportion of adolescents in the UK experiment with volatile substances. The trend in Scottish returns seems to indicate that solvent abuse is progressively affecting younger age groups each year. The age range has been reported as between 8 and 17 years with an average age of 12 or 13 years, but there are alarming reports from Strathclyde and Ayrshire of solvent abusers as young as 5 or 6 years of age (O'Connor, 1983).

Between 1970 and 1981, 117 deaths from solvent abuse were reported in the UK, the commonest causes of death being heart failure or laryngeal spasm. The same study reported a disproportionately high number of deaths among males (9 males per female), the median age for death being nearly 16 years (Scottish Health Education Group, 1983).

Polydrug Abuse

This refers to concomitant use of a variety of drugs (often including some prescribed drugs). Lethally dangerous 'cocktails' of drugs may be consumed with disastrous results.

Elvis Presley died from an apparent heart attack in 1977 and autopsy confirmed a reported pattern of long-term polydrug abuse. Most of the drugs had been obtained by prescription, and blood and tissue samples were found to contain toxic levels of methaqualone (Mandrax), 10 times more codeine than would be needed for any therapeutic purpose and residual amounts of at least 10 other drugs including Valium, barbiturates and various stimulants and opiates (Meyer and Salmon, 1984). For the last few years of his life Presley (aged 42 at death) was

'grotesquely bloated, incomprehensible in speech and song, and wearing a nappy because of the incontinence caused by his addiction to amphetamines and sedatives—his doctor admitted

that in the twenty months prior to the singer's death he had prescribed 10 000 pills' (Freemantle, 1985).

Most polydrug abusers are young (many are adolescents) and are more psychologically disturbed than other types of drug misusers. Continuing polydrug abuse carries a grave prognosis, particularly if the drug misuser is not even aware of the identity of all the drugs consumed (as is often the case).

'Over the Counter' Misuse

Many drug misusers drift into a pattern of dependence by over-use of drugs available from any chemist without prescription (many polydrug misusers include 'over the counter' drugs in their 'menu'). Analgesic preparations (particularly combinations of aspirin and codeine), expectorants and 'pick-me-ups' may be used. Aspirin is the most widely used drug in the world (35 000 tons of it are used each year) (Breckon, 1978), and though not addictive, may be widely misused. Over-use may lead to mental disturbances—the 'salicylate jag'—of a psychotic nature, and delirium, convulsions and coma may occur. The early signs of aspirin intoxication include tinnitus (ringing in the ears), deafness and drowsiness. Compound pain killers are widely abused; there are persons dependent on Askit powders who take up to 25 a day and it has been estimated that there are 250 000 aspirin abusers in the UK (Breckon, 1978).

Other drugs abused include Feminax (sold for the relief of period pains), Solpadeine (and other preparations often containing aspirin, codeine and caffeine), paracetamol and Benylin Expectorant (the latter often being used in combination with alcohol). Some codeine abusers take up to 50 tablets a day.

Recognizing the Signs of Drug Misuse

The following are indications that certain categories of drug may have been misused. Remember that many of these signs may have alternative causes and try not to jump to conclusions by identifying behaviour as 'odd' and therefore as an indicator of drug abuse.

Opiates

Changes associated with a recent 'fix':
'Pin-point' pupils
Dreamy and detached manner and responses
Anorexia
Slow and slurred speech
Poor concentration
Rubbing of eyes, chin and nose and scratching of arms and legs
Resentment at being disturbed and of noise and bright lights
Wakefulness interrupted by drowsing ('gouching')
Relaxed posture
Frequent visits to the lavatory
Eyes wide open but glazed

There may be fresh injection marks and constant examining of arms. The injection site used by chronic heavy users is usually the antecubital area but almost any area may be used as veins collapse or sclerose with over-use. Heroin users have been known to inject into the nose, penis, scalp and breasts. A favourite site for subcutaneous injections ('skin popping') is the ankles.

Changes associated with a 'come down':
Irritability
Restlessness and fidgeting
Rhinorrhoea
Perspiration
Yawning
Heavy smoking

Changes in 'lifestyle' associated with chronic use:
Loss of interest in personal appearance
Loss of weight and anorexia
Pallor
Sleeping out and frequent unexpected absences from home
Increased number of telephone calls and new visitors at home, with evasive explanations for these
Loss of efficiency
Blood spots on clothing
Fully burnt matches, blackened pieces of tinfoil and litter in rooms and pockets.
(After Leech 1983)

Amphetamines ('Speed')

Changes associated with recent use:
Euphoria
Restlessness and overactivity
Inexplicable laughter
Dilated pupils (often so dilated that no iris can be seen)
Lips and tongue dry and crusted with dried saliva
Tremor
Picking of the skin around the fingernails and on the face (especially associated with intravenous use)
The user has a 'bright eyed' look coupled with lack of tact
A tendency to stay out all night

Changes associated with 'come down':
Lethargy
Irritability
Depression
Photophobia (dark glasses often worn)
Paranoid mood (there may be angry accusation made against others for the most trivial of reasons)
A tendency to sleep late and over-react to disturbance

Cannabis ('Hash', 'Pot', 'Grass')

Changes associated with recent use:
Fatuous euphoria
Dreamy expression
Glazed eyes
Slow, slurred speech
Episodes of excitability (the user may over-react to auditory and visual stimuli, especially to music and bright colours)
Relaxed but unsteady gait
Inane laughter

Changes associated with habitual heavy use:
Poor memory and concentration
Passivity
Reddened eyes
Odour of 'burnt grass' from clothing and breath
Dry cough
Preference for sweet foods and drinks

Hallucinogens

Changes associated with recent use:
Dreamy, glazed expression
Over-reaction to auditory and visual stimuli
Preoccupation with examination of everyday objects (inspected as though never seen before)
Inappropriate laughter or comments
Sudden mood changes

After-effects:
Emotional flatness
Risk of 'acid flashes'
Sometimes anxiety feelings of depersonalization

Solvents

Indications of recent use:
Redness and watering of the eyes
A hacking cough
Excessive nasal discharge
Spots, rash or a ring around the mouth
Stomach pains and nausea
Smell of solvents from clothing or breath
Signs of glue on clothing
Episodes of erratic, uncharacteristic or disturbed
behaviour
Complaints of numbness or tingling feelings in the
hands or feet
'Hangover behaviour' with lethargy and irritability,
often with headache

Barbiturates

Indications of recent use:
Gross intoxication
Staggering gait
Slurred speech
High risk of episodes of disturbed or violent
behaviour
Drowsiness/stupor
Possible incontinence

After effects:
Risk of delirium, coma or convulsions—remember
severe withdrawal syndrome

Treatment

Treatment consists of:
1 Detoxification (where appropriate)
2 Stabilization of physical state, if this is reduced
3 Stabilization of any critical difficulties in life circumstances arising from drug misuse
4 Reaching agreement with patient about treatment
objectives and preparing a contract of treatment
5 Aiding patient to break ties with the drug subculture (this is critical)
6 Arranging continuing support by referral to
appropriate agency

Detoxification consists of guiding patient through
any withdrawal effects until he/she is drug-free.
Withdrawal effects may be mild, moderate or severe
depending on the type and amount of drug(s) used.
Many patients will be referred to the psychiatric
hospital from the general hospital where they
will have received treatment for a drugs overdose
(which may have been deliberate or accidental).
Corrected for age the suicide rate for persons misusing hard drugs is around 50 times that of non-users
(McCullogh and Philip, 1972) and a significant rise
in drug abuser deaths has been reported (Spear,
1983).

The patient who is transferred after overdose is
still likely to be very debilitated (physically and
mentally) and will require careful observation and
treatment until stable. Barbiturate abusers present
the greatest difficulties during withdrawal (the
biggest hazard being of withdrawal fits) and require
careful monitoring until stable. Heroin abusers
experiencing 'cold turkey' (withdrawal unsupported by substitute drugs) will not experience the tortured ravings fondly depicted by the media but will
require careful nursing attention for 7–10 days.

Some units still offer methadone (Physeptone)
during withdrawal but opinions differ about the
validity of this practice, as many consider that this
simply replaces one addiction with another. A
survey of 190 American heroin users being maintained on methadone revealed that 78% felt that
methadone takes away the craving for heroin, but
88% felt that methadone had simply replaced one
addiction with another; 61% felt that 'it's better
being abstinent than taking methadone' (Brown et
al, 1975).

In Glasgow (1986) the heroin user may be offered
methadone, chlordiazepoxide or 'cold turkey',
depending on the treatment centre to which he/she
is referred.

A controversial book by Arnold Trebach has
argued that the 'British system' of the Rolleston era
whereby heroin may be prescribed by private
doctors is the correct solution to the problem, as it
would destroy the black market, decriminalize and
enable effective treatment and control (Trebach,
1982) a view endorsed by a report suggesting
responses to the rapid increase of heroin addiction in
Glasgow (Ditton and Speirits, 1981).

Ghodse (1983) has expressed the opposite view.
He feels that the black market will always be endemic and will be supplied in part by an overspill of
legally prescribed drugs. Frugal prescription of

methadone linctus is recommended to keep such overspill to a minimum.

Though the debates about maintenance and substitution continue, there is no debate about the fact that current provision of treatment facilities is less than adequate. Voluntary agencies have struggled heroically to fill the gaps in the provision of care and treatment but the current rise in 'hard' drug abuse threatens to completely overwhelm them.

Stabilization of physical state may be difficult to accomplish on an out-patient basis as the problems may be both multiple and severe.

Needle users may present with injection abscesses, lymphadenitis, septicaemia, hepatitis B, pneumonia, AIDS, venereal disease or malnutrition. Some heroin users add vinegar or lemon juice to heroin before injecting (to heighten the 'buzz') and major abscesses are common in association with this practice.

Life circumstances may be chaotic and psychosocial damage may be as great as physical damage. Benzodiazepines may be used (in the short term) to combat anxiety, and formal psychotherapy and counselling has been found to benefit the majority of drug misusers (Woody et al, 1983). The social worker may be enlisted to assess social background and suggest ways of reducing social problems created by drugs misuse.

A 'contract' agreeing to the conditions applying to treatment is usually signed by the patient and usually incorporates the following provisos:

1 You are expected to use *no drugs* other than those prescribed by the hospital staff.
2 Visitors must be discussed with the staff. Nobody other than those agreed upon will be allowed to visit.
3 The staff reserve the right to inspect parcels.
4 You will be expected to remain dressed in pyjamas and dressing gown while in the hospital.
5 You must remain on the ward throughout your stay in hospital.
6 You must attend the daily ward group and should participate constructively in it.

Once withdrawal has been accomplished and the physical condition stabilized, the patient may be placed in contact with one of the agencies specializing in offering support to the drug misuser who is attempting to break his/her habit (see Appendix 5).

Treatment is most effectively provided in the setting of a specialized unit, most of which are organized on therapeutic community principles, and a stay of 12 months in such a unit may be required to break ties with the drug subculture and to reorganize life around activities which do not involve drugs. Therapeutic communities demand total abstinence and the emphasis is on dismantling allegiance to the drug misusing way of life, building motivation, strengthening coping resources and planning a drug-free future.

The clinics (drug dependence units/centres) continue to play a major part in treatment but the picture is not encouraging of late. Stimson et al (1978), in a follow-up study of young heroin misusers attending London clinics, found that seven years later 48% were still using drugs, 12% were dead, and only 32% were abstinent.

Out-patient treatment of solvent abusers is beginning to have a major impact on the problem. An example of such a unit is Acorn Street Day Hospital, Glasgow, which commenced a solvent abuse clinic in 1980 and has received more than 440 referrals during 1980–1985. Of these, 63% have stopped abusing solvents in response to counselling.

Prevention

Prevention must involve sober assessment of the drug industry and of prescribing practices. Despite the (justified) concern about the illicit market in illegally imported opiates, the fact remains that most drugs which are misused are manufactured by reputable companies, prescribed by doctors and dispensed by chemists. So long as drug companies continue to produce an ever-increasing range of addictive substances and doctors continue to routinely prescribe them, there will be a steady increase in the number of 'therapeutic addicts' with overspill of the prescribed drugs onto the black market. Leech (1983) has commented that 'some drug companies have exploited personal and social problems and have often been dishonest about their claims and about the effects of their products'. The benzodiazepines provide an alarming example. Concern about diazepam and other benzodiazepines became so great in the USA that patients prescribed these substances had, by law, to be given a leaflet stating: 'You can become dependent on Valium. Dependence is a craving for the drug, or an inability to function normally without it . . . if you have been taking Valium for a month or more your doctor should reassess your condition and your continued use of the drug'. This regulation has now been rescinded by the Reagan administration due to pressure from the drug industry (Lacey and Woodward, 1985).

There is debate about the form health education about drug misuse should take. Television campaigns may simply heighten drug awareness and make images of misuse part of the young person's everyday repertoire. Continual reminders of availability are not a good idea. Ditton and Speirits (1981) suggest that there are three possible approaches to the problem:

1 Throw more policemen at the problem (increased criminalization)—unlikely to be successful—as the American experience shows. Furthermore, prisons do not cure but create drug awareness.

2 Throw more money at the problem—there is an urgent need for more realistically supported recovery programmes. Glasgow has an alarmingly escalating heroin problem but the nearest therapeutic community for drug misusers is in Oxford.

3 Throw more NHS heroin at the problem—a return to Rolleston—confining the fire in a therapeutic hearth rather than letting it rampage through the streets. This policy would erode the black market, decriminalize and reduce the death and disability rate among needle users. This option would also be the cheapest.

Lastly, the role of the media must be examined. Irresponsible and lurid reporting has already been mentioned; the effects may be devastating.

In 1972 the Consumer's Union published an article called *How to start a nationwide drug menace* which discussed early press coverage of solvent abuse. A Denver newspaper investigated reports of a few incidents of glue-sniffing in Arizona and Colorado and printed lurid headlines combined with illustrations of 'how to do it'. The reports were emulated elsewhere. Within a few years a minor problem had been manufactured into a national epidemic with mass panic reactions (Leech, 1983). Overstated, distorted or simply untrue press statements about drug misuse also foster attitudes of contempt and cynicism in young people and undermine valid exercises in health education. Headlines about 'junkies', 'addicts', 'drug freaks' or 'glue-sniffers' also foster attitudes of hostility towards the drug misuser and reinforce negative stereotypes which compound an already deteriorating situation.

Every 'drug misuser' has a unique personality of his/her own, has a unique pattern of psychosocial difficulties and has individual hopes, wishes and aspirations for the future. Treatment and nursing care must recognize and accept the individual behind the label if any progress is to be made.

Table 75 A short glossary of drug slang.

Acid—LSD
Acid head—LSD user
Amp—ampoule (usually methadone)
Bag—quantity of heroin
Barbs—barbiturates
Bread—money
Breadhead—non-user dealer—involved in drugs only for money
Bust—police arrest
Buzz—immediate pleasant effects of drug
Coke—cocaine
Cold turkey—coming off heroin without supportive medication
Come down—to lose the drug effect as it wears off
Crash out/crash—to pass out, go to sleep, after drug use
Deal—drug transaction
Dikies—Diconal
Dope—drugs in general (often used to describe cannabis in particular)
DS—Drug Squad
Fix—to inject a drug
Flash—short, strong sensation occurring immediately after injection of opiates and lasting about 20 seconds (see Rush)
Gouching—drowsing off after using heroin
Grass—herbal cannabis
H—heroin
Hash—cannabis resin
Hep—Hepatitis B
Hit—an injected dose of drugs
Hit it up—injecting drugs
Hot shot—bag of drugs contaminated with poison (e.g. heroin cut with strychnine)
Jack up—inject heroin or other drug
Joint—cannabis cigarette
Junk—heroin or other opiate
Junkie—user of heroin or other injectables
Kick—stop taking drugs
OD—overdose
Pillhead—amphetamine user
Pinkies—Diconal
Popping—injecting subcutaneously
Pusher—drug dealer
Rip off—to con, steal, obtain by deceit, take advantage of
Rush—see Flash
Score—obtain drugs
Script—prescription
Shot—a dose of drugs
Shit—cannabis resin (hash)
Shoot—inject
Sleeper—sleeping pill (e.g. barbiturates)
Smack—heroin
Snort—to sniff or inhale a drug (e.g. cocaine)

Speed—amphetamines
Speed ball—combination of stimulants and depressants,
  prepared for injection (e.g. heroin and cocaine or diconal
  and ritalin)
Spike—hypodermic needle
Stoned—drugged, 'high'
Strung out—in bad shape, suffering from withdrawal
Trip—experience with LSD or other hallucinogen.
  Sometimes used loosely to describe any drug experience.
Turn on—to smoke cannabis: to introduce someone to
  drugs
Turn over—to steal
Weed—cannabis
Works—the equipment used for injecting drugs (e.g. needle
  and syringe)

Key Concepts

1 Recreational use of drugs is as old as recorded
history, and drugs regarded with distaste in the
West are often socially accepted elsewhere (e.g.
cannabis, coca leaves).

2 The opiates were constituents of everyday
household medicines for almost half a century
(e.g. laudanum, paregoric).

3 Heroin was first marketed as a cough
suppressant and as a harmless remedy for
morphine dependence.

4 In 1926 the *Rolleston Committee* defined drug
dependence as a 'disease' and provided for the
prescription of opiates by doctors to stabilize
misusers' lifestyles and to (hopefully) eventually
wean most of them from the drug.

5 In 1961 the first *Brain Committee* reviewed the
situation, recorded that drug abuse was rare and
did not amend the Rolleston proposals.

6 In 1965 the second *Brain Committee* established
drug dependence units to replace the prescription
of opiates by private doctors. 'Addicts' were to be
notified to the Home Office.

7 *Methadone* (Physeptone) was introduced in 1964
and gradually began to replace opiates as the
prescribed drug at drug dependence units,
initially being supplied in injectable form and,
more recently, in linctus form.

8 *Tolerance* develops to many drugs (e.g. opiates);
higher and higher doses are then required to
create the desired effect.

9 *Availability* coupled with *social pressures* and
positive attitudes towards drugs and drug users is
thought to be a major causative factor.

10 Some chronic heavy users of drugs have overt
personality disorder but the majority of misusers
do not.

11 *Status frustration* may lead to misuse of drugs
(especially solvents and opiates) in the young,
disadvantaged urban poor.

12 The substances abused fall into five main
categories: sedatives and narcotics, minor
tranquillizers, stimulants, hallucinogens and
solvents.

13 Substances abused are so diverse (tobacco,
analgesics, opiates, Steradent tablets, mushrooms,
ping-pong balls, Askit powders, caffeine,
tranquillizers, alcohol, petrol, plant seeds) that
some writers despairingly write of *substance abuse*.

14 The opiates are not instantly addictive but are
dangerously habit-forming, and a heavy habit is so
expensive that many users resort to crime to
obtain money for drugs.

15 *Barbiturates* produce gross and unstable effects
and, of all withdrawal states, barbiturates present
the most serious problems. Sudden withdrawal
from barbiturates can be fatal.

16 Minor tranquillizers, notably the
benzodiazepines (e.g. Valium and Librium) have
produced vast numbers of 'therapeutic addicts'.

17 Stimulants ('uppers') mainly consist of
cocaine and amphetamines and may be ingested,
sniffed or injected.

18 Heavy amphetamine use creates the risk of
residual *amphetamine psychosis*.

19 *Hallucinogens* induce perceptual distortions
resembling transient psychosis; the most widely
abused are LSD and hallucinogenic fungi.

20 *Cannabis* (active ingredient THC) induces
relaxation and euphoria and, in heavy doses, may
induce hallucinations.

21 Amphetamines, LSD, cocaine and cannabis
do not cause physical dependence ('addiction'),
but variable degrees of psychological dependence
may develop.

22 *Solvent abuse* consists of the inhalation of
vapours from a variety of volatile substances in
order to induce intoxication.

23 Young people from deprived urban areas seem
to constitute the majority of solvent abusers.

24 The risks associated with solvent abuse are
high but the practice is not illegal.

25 *Polydrug abuse* consists of the concomitant use
of a variety of drugs (usually pills) and is a
particularly hazardous form of drug misuse.

26 Treatment objectives include *detoxification* and
stabilization of physical and psychosocial
problems.

27 Therapeutic community care seems most
effective and requires a stay of 12–24 months.

This approach requires total abstinence from drugs.
28 Many voluntary organizations in the community claim high success rates for programmes based on teaching self-help skills.

References

Allister, C. et al (1981) Status epilepticus caused by solvent abuse. *British Medical Journal*, **283**(6300): 1156.

An American addict living in England (1970) In Trebach, A. (1982) *The Heroin Solution*. London: Yale University Press.

Anslinger, H. J. (1959) In Trebach, A. (1982) *The Heroin Solution*. London: Yale University Press.

Barrymore, R. (1975) *Drugs*. London: Wolfe Publishing.

Birdwood, G. (1971) *The Willing Victim*. London: Martin Secker and Warburg.

Black, D. (1982) Misuse of solvents. *Health Trends*, **14**: 27–28.

Breckon, W. (1978) *Your Everyday Drugs*. London: BBC Publications.

Brown, B. S. et al (1975) Methadone maintenance: some client opinions. *American Journal of Psychiatry*, **132**(6): 623–626.

Burr, A. (1983) The Piccadilly drug scene. *British Journal of Addiction*, **78**: 5–19.

Burr, A. (1984) The illicit non-pharmaceutical heroin market and drug scene in Kensington market. *British Journal of Addiction*, **79**: 337–343.

Cohen, A. (1956) *Delinquent Boys*. Harmondsworth: Penguin Books.

Ditton, J. & Speirits, K. (1981) The rapid increase of heroin addiction in Glasgow during 1981. *Background Paper No. 2, Dept. of Sociology*. University of Glasgow.

Einarson, T. R. (1980) Systematic Review of the Benzodiazepines. *British Medical Journal*, **11**: 1009.

Finigarette, H. & Hasse, A. (1978) *Mental Disabilities and Criminal Responsibility*. London: University of California Press.

Freemantle, B. (1985) *The Fix*. London: Michael Joseph.

Ghodse, A. (1983) Treatment of drug addiction in London. *Lancet*, **i**(8325): 636–639.

Hoffman, A. (1980) *LSD. My Problem Child*. Maidenhead: McGraw-Hill Book Co.

ISDD (Institute for the Study of Drug Dependence (1982), *Drug Abuse Briefing*.

Ives, R. (1981) *Solvent Abuse*: A Review of Research. National Children's Bureau (Highlight No. 43).

Jamieson, A., Glanz, A. & McGregor, S. (1984) *Dealing with Drug Misuse. Crisis Intervention in the City*. London: Tavistock Publications.

King et al (1981) Solvent encephalopathy. *British Medical Journal*, **283**: 663–664.

Kolb, L. & Brodie, H. (1982) *Modern Clinical Psychiatry*, 10th edn. Philadelphia: W. B. Saunders.

Lacey, R. & Woodward, S. (1985) *Survey on Tranquillisers*. London: BBC Publications.

Laurie, P. (1971) *Drugs. Medical, Psychological and Social Facts*. Harmondsworth: Pelican.

Leary, T. (1970) *Jail Notes*. US: Douglas.

Leech, K. (1983) *What Everyone Should Know About Drugs*. London: Sheldon Press.

Logan (Ed.) (1974) *Cannabis—Options for Control—Report of a Study Group—ISDD*. Quartermaine House.

Lowenstein, L. (1982) Glue sniffing. Background features and treatment by aversion methods and group therapy. *Practitioner*, **226**: 1113–1116.

Mann, M. (1983) *Student Encyclopaedia of Sociology*. London: Macmillan.

McCulloch, J. & Philip, A. (1972) *Suicidal Behaviour*. Oxford: Pergamon Press.

Meyer, R. & Salmon, P. (1984) *Abnormal Psychology*. Herts: Allyn & Bacon.

O'Connor, D. (1983) *Glue Sniffing and Volatile Substance Abuse*. Hants: Gower Publications.

Parker, T. (1965) *Five Women*. London: Hutchinson Books.

Perry, L. (1979) *Women and Drug Use: An Unfeminine Dependency*. London: Institute for the Study of Drug Dependence.

Rogers, H. (1982) Glue sniffing among schoolchildren. *Health Visitor*, **55**: 236–239.

Scott, J. (1982) Solvent abuse—a growing problem. *Occupational Health*, **34**: 405–407.

Scottish Health Education Group (1983) *Solvent Abuse*. (1983) *A Report for Professionals Working in Scotland*. Scottish Health Education Group: Intermediate Treatment Resource Centre.

Spear, H. (1983) Drug abuser deaths. *British Journal of Addiction*, **78**: 173–178.

Stimson, G. & Oppenheimer, E. (1982) *Heroin Addiction*. London: Tavistock Publications.

Stimson, G., Oppenheimer, E. & Thorley, A. (1978) Seven years follow up of heroin addicts: drug use and outcome. *British Medical Journal*, **i**(6121): 1191–1192.

Trebach, A. (1982) *The Heroin Solution*. London: Yale University Press.

Van Dyke, C. (1981) Cocaine. In Lowinson & Ruiz. *Substance Abuse*. Baltimore: Williams and Wilkins.

Willis, J. (1974) *Drug Dependence*. London: Faber and Faber.

Wilson, C. (1981) Glue Sniffing. *Health Visitor*, **16**: 6–8.

Woody, G. et al (1983) Psychotherapy for opiate addicts. *Archives of General Psychiatry*, **40**: 639–645.

23

Nursing the Drug-Dependent Patient

'. . . his sense of happiness . . . was now nothing more than a thin cover beneath which anguish and the obsession of death were awakening'.

Andre Malraux

Getting someone off drugs (or alcohol) is not difficult. Getting someone to *stay* off drugs (or alcohol) may be very difficult.

Simply admitting the drug-dependent person to hospital, detoxifying and then discharging will rapidly lead to re-establishment of problem patterns of drug abuse, this time with diminished faith in the efficacy of helping agencies and reduced inclination to seek help in the future. The drug-dependent person should leave hospital with increased awareness of faulty lifestyles and equipped with self-help strategies which will reduce the chances of relapse. There is no magical solution to the problem; it will require high levels of determination and support from others before progress is made.

The largely passive approach which was implicit in substitution therapies (doctor and his methadone will make me better) must be replaced by an active and critical approach (*Why* do I need drugs? *How* did I come to lose control when others didn't? *Which* factors maintain my habit? *How* do I sabotage myself?).

Before progress of any sort can be made it will be necessary to treat withdrawal states and any troublesome complications apparent at initial assessment.

Assessment

The complications of drug abuse may be physical, psychological or social and, commonly, all three will be present and will interact.

Physical complications

These are often particularly apparent in the case of needle users, irrespective of what has been injected. Complications may be local or systemic.

Local complications are associated with the use of unsterile needles and include injection abscesses, lymphangitis (inflamed lymph vessels showing as red, angry streaks around injection sites) lymphadenitis (inflamed lymph glands, usually in the axilla or groin), nerve damage (manifesting itself as areas of paralysis and/or paraesthesia) and, occasionally, gangrene. Over-use of vessels (usually in the forearm) may lead to the formation of sclerosed and scarred vessels, readily visible and known as 'track marks' by drug abusers.

Systemic infections which are possible include *hepatitis B* (serum hepatitis) which is usually spread parenterally (communal use of contaminated needles) but may also be spread orally or by direct contact. The incubation period is long (45–180 days—60 days average), onset is insidious (seldom febrile) and mortality is high (50%). Recovery provides immunity.

AIDS

AIDS (acquired immune deficiency syndrome) is another blood-borne disease which may affect needle users; 38% of drug abusers were estimated as having the disease in a survey carried out in Edinburgh (90% of the sample also had hepatitis B) and the European incidence of AIDS in drug users has been reported to vary from 1.5–6.4% in England, 6% in West Germany, 20–22.5% in Italy, 32–42% in Switzerland and 44–48% in Austria and Spain (Peutherer et al, 1985). These figures reveal that AIDS is more common in drug users than in any other group (including homosexuals), while American studies revealed a seropositivity of 64% amongst parenteral drug users and suggested that this group was the bridge to other potential risk groups (73% of heterosexuals with AIDS have had sexual contact with an intravenous drug user and 51% of children with AIDS have at least one parent who used intravenous drugs (Bennett, 1985). AIDS is caused by a virus which leads to severe and irreversible damage of the immune system of the body. The disease is incurable; no-one who has contracted AIDS has lived for more than four years after diagnosis, and the average time from diagnosis to death ranges from 8 to 18 months.'

Death usually occurs as a result of *opportunistic infections* (arising as microorganisms seize the 'opportunity' offered by deficient immune responses) or *Kaposi's sarcoma*, a cancer of skin and connective tissue usually first noticed as small purplish blotches on the skin.

Symptoms of AIDS include persistent diarrhoea, night sweats, unexplained weight loss and lymphadenopathy (swollen lymph glands, mainly in the neck, axilla and groin). AIDS may occur among homosexuals (the virus is blood-borne and anal intercourse is often associated with minor bleeding as the rectal wall is much thinner than that of the vagina), haemophiliacs (who have inadvertently been given contaminated blood products) and drug abusers who use contaminated needles (often shared with other users). The incubation period is long (up to four years) but the presence of the virus is no guarantee that the person will develop AIDS; over a period of two years between 1% and 10% of infected persons have gone on to develop the disease.

The virus is present in semen, saliva, blood and phlegm and it need hardly be said that great care should be exercised in disposing of excreta from infected persons. Even greater care should be exercised when giving injections. At least one British health worker has died after accidentally pricking his finger with a needle that had been used to inject an AIDS patient, and a British nurse has been found to be harbouring the virus after a similar incident (Fisher, 1985).

There is now strong evidence that AIDS is being transmitted heterosexually and the Royal College of Nursing has pointed out (1985) that the present rate of increase could lead to more than a million cases in this country by 1991 (Fisher, 1985).

It has been suggested that the public response to AIDS is amounting to a 'plague mentality' redolent of panic, superstition and bigotry, and it is hoped that the nursing response would not fuel this undesirable state of affairs. On the other hand, realistic and balanced awareness of risk is essential for the nurse. If a patient is suspected or known to have AIDS (or hepatitis B), the following precautions should be observed:

1 Do not bend needles after use but place them promptly in a puncture-resistant container for disposal. Do not reinsert needles into their original sheaths before discarding as this is a common cause of needle injury.

2 Wear gloves when handling blood specimens, blood-soiled items, body fluids, excretions and secretions, as well as when handling surfaces, materials and objects exposed to the same.

3 Wear a gown when clothing may be soiled with body fluids, blood or excretions.

4 Wash hands thoroughly, using a bactericidal solution, after removing gown and gloves and before leaving the patient's room.

5 Label blood and other specimens prominently with a warning (e.g. AIDS: PRECAUTION).

6 Place blood or excreta-soiled articles from an AIDS patient in an impervious bag, labelled (prominently) AIDS: PRECAUTION, before sending them for re-processing or disposal.

7 A single room is most appropriate for known or suspected sufferers.

8 Should mouth-to-mouth resuscitation be necessary, the use of a Brook's airway is advised.

Though realistic precautions should be taken, it should be remembered that direct contact with the body fluids of an infected person is required to spread the disease. No-one has yet caught AIDS from a toilet seat or a drinking glass or by breathing the same air as a person with the disease. Infection with the virus is stressful enough in itself—being treated like a leper will only ravage the well-being of the sufferer further.

Long-term abuse of opiates depresses respiratory function and increases the likelihood of *chest infections*, and *malnutrition* may develop as diet is neglected. Some chronic heavy users of opiates resort to prostitution to raise money for drugs, where the risk of *venereal disease* is greatly increased. Male users may resort to homosexual prostitution and will then be doubly at risk of AIDS (infected needles + frequent homosexual contacts).

It should be clearly recognized, however, that only a small minority of illicit drug users will develop a chaotic lifestyle and descend the steep slope into intractable addiction. The gaunt, needle-scarred drug abuser who leads a life punctuated by episodes of criminality and promiscuity does exist, but exists as a small minority. It is a myth that drug abuse inevitably leads to physical and psychosocial degeneration followed by early death, and this myth has been propagated in no small way by the irresponsible journalism of some of the tabloid news-papers, some of which seem to exercise an almost planetary influence on the tides of public super-stition and prejudice.

Plant (1977) points out that the majority of drug misusers are not physically dependent on the substances they take and that there is a sizeable population who pass through a phase of recreational drug use without coming to any evident harm.

The nursing approach to drug dependence should show realistic awareness of the dangers involved in some types and patterns of drug misuse but should be free of the alarmist global exaggerations of the problem so frequently encountered. Remember that drug abusers encountered in hospital tend not to be typical of the drug-abusing population as a whole.

Psychosocial complications

These may include mounting anxiety or depression associated with loss of control. Fear of withdrawal reactions may be marked and the heavy user may have experienced a marked level of psychosocial deterioration tinged by fear of punishment by the police and/or complete rejection by family. As dependence increases the drug misuser may lose employment, well-being and any semblance of social stability, and will often lead an anxiety-ridden existence on the fringes of society. A process of disengagement tends to occur whereby the user feels more and more alienated from the non-user society and only feels safe in the company of fellow users. There may be little faith in the ability of non-users to understand the problem. Repeated relapses may lead to feelings of hopelessness and great loss of self-esteem. Drug misuse may become the most impor-tant part of life and the demands of daily living may evoke feelings of impatience or irritation. As drugs are more and more valued, so the non-user society is devalued in the eyes of many users.

Treatment must involve help in stabilizing unsta-ble lifestyles and there must be realistic attempts to help fill the vacuum which will be created when drug misuse is stopped or reduced. Getting off may be largely a hospital or clinic-based exercise; staying off involves recognition of sociocultural pressures and restructuring of lifestyle.

Withdrawal states

Withdrawal states will develop in most heavy habi-tual users after admission but only if the drug causes physical dependence. The severity of these states varies with the drug of abuse but most have been grossly exaggerated in their intensity by the film industry, writers of popular fiction and the tabloid press.

Severe withdrawal states (delirium, convulsions, possible coma or brain damage) may occur in mis-users of *barbiturates* and in some types of *polydrug abuse*. In this case the patient requires careful obser-vation and full nursing care which does not differ in essence from that employed in the DT's of alcohol withdrawal. In the event of a patient with a history of barbiturate abuse being admitted, careful obser-vation and monitoring of vital signs is essential from the outset.

Benzodiazepine withdrawal produces unpleasant effects:

> 'I couldn't go anywhere; in fact my wife had to force me to go out. I'd have anxiety attacks, palpitations, sweating. I'd be walking along and it's as if the road itself was coming up to meet you'
>
> (*Melville, 1984*).

Benzodiazepine withdrawal has effects which may mimic the initial anxiety responses which led to pre-scription in the first place—anxiety may reach panic levels in the patient who is unaware of withdrawal effects.

The unfortunate response of many general prac-titioners confronted by a patient who has tried to come off benzodiazepines is to wrongly diagnose a relapse of the original anxiety state and to re-prescribe benzodiazepines (sometimes increasing the dose). Not all general practitioners are aware of the effects of prolonged benzodiazepine use. One woman who complained (to her general practitioner) that she was addicted was tersely told 'You women read too much rubbish' (Melville, 1984), while another woman experiencing withdrawal was told by her child 'Oh, Mummy, you need a tablet' (Mel-ville 1984). Sadly, some children seem to be more aware than some general practitioners of the nature of the benzodiazepine problem. Anxiety and associ-ated unpleasant autonomic responses associated with benzodiazepine withdrawal will take 2–4 weeks to subside (Peterson and Lader, 1981), and the patient will benefit from relaxation exercises (see Chapter 17) and will need much support and reassur-ance. In essence, nursing care is that appropriate to care of the patient suffering from an anxiety state, with the addition of informative interventions aimed at increasing the patient's awareness of the effects of benzodiazepine withdrawal. Teaching the patient self-help skills which will enable him/her to handle future anxiety without drugs (see Chapter 17) will also reduce anxiety and increase confidence and self-esteem.

Opiate withdrawal produces symptoms resembling a bout of gastric 'flu; these are unpleasant but manageable. The symptoms (sweating, shivering, abdominal cramps and insomnia) appear a day or two after withdrawal and will be marked for 3–5 days thereafter. After this period they decrease steadily, though insomnia and restlessness may persist for some weeks. Bed rest and copious oral fluids will help when withdrawal is at a peak and frequent warm baths will promote relaxation. Anorexia is common when abdominal cramps are present; milky drinks of the Complan type may then be used.

The effects of opiate withdrawal have been greatly exaggerated by the media (which may have discouraged attempts to come off by many users) and the nurse should maintain a positive, reassuring and cheerful attitude. Opiate withdrawal is considerably less dangerous than withdrawal from alcohol or barbiturates.

Cocaine does not produce significant withdrawal effects but the user may feel fatigued, sleepy and depressed after withdrawal.

Amphetamine ('speed') withdrawal will also produce feelings of fatigue and depression—greater than those caused by cocaine withdrawal—and there may also be strong paranoid feelings. Prolonged amphetamine use may lead to hypertension and decreased resistance to infection; blood pressure, temperature, pulse and respirations should therefore be monitored during withdrawal.

LSD, hallucinogenic fungi and cannabis do not cause physical dependence, so there are no physical withdrawal symptoms.

Some drug misusers will be admitted while still under the influence of drugs and there is a risk of disturbed or aggressive behaviour (greatest in the case of polydrug abuse or abuse of barbiturates, solvents or amphetamines). The disturbed abuser should be 'talked down' slowly and firmly in a quiet, distraction-free room. Remember to exercise caution when checking and storing the clothing of drug abusers—pockets may contain unprotected contaminated needles or needles may be stored behind the lapels of jackets. Incautious approaches may lead to needlestick injuries.

Opiate abuse during pregnancy

Opiates readily cross the placenta and can induce physical dependence in the foetus. After birth the baby is suddenly cut off from opiates circulating in the maternal bloodstream, and withdrawal effects (coarse, floppy tremor, muscular rigidity, vomiting, diarrhoea, sneezing and yawning) may occur. Treatment is that appropriate to neonatal irritability (phenobarbitone or chlorpromazine). If it is suspected that the mother has been resorting to prostitution in order to maintain her habit, then the baby requires examination for syphilis and gonorrhoea. Early identification of opiate abuse during pregnancy is important and the mother should be weaned off drugs to prevent neonatal withdrawal syndrome.

Potential Nursing Problems

Once assessment is complete, potential (and actual) nursing problems will emerge. These include the following:

Maintaining a safe environment

Observation must be continuous during major withdrawal states associated with serious physical hazard (e.g. barbiturates). Any lowering of vital functions should be reported to medical staff immediately. A quiet, well-ventilated room is the most appropriate setting. Temperature, pulse, respiration, blood pressure and fluid balance should be charted at 1 hourly intervals (or more frequently if so prescribed). Confusion may be marked during some withdrawal states (barbiturates, polydrug abuse) and the risk of injury may be high. Suicide risk is greatly increased and the appropriate precautions should be taken. Disturbed or aggressive behaviour (directed against staff or fellow patients) may occur.

Amphetamine withdrawal often causes paranoid depression and may even lead to a residual psychosis. The paranoid and irritable amphetamine abuser

Table 76 Maintaining a safe environment.

Problem	Objective	Action
Physical hazards associated with withdrawal/complications	Maintain physical integrity	Careful observation/monitoring
Increased suicide risk	Render environment safe	Remove/protect sources of danger

may misinterpret sudden movements by staff (or fellow patients) and may lash out. Do not approach such patients from behind or startle them in any way. Remember that there is a very high probability that visitors will attempt to supply the patient with drugs. Many units bar visitors completely during withdrawal for this reason. Medicine trolleys and drug cupboards should be protected with even greater than usual vigilance.

Communication

The drug-using subculture tends to place great emphasis on being 'street-wise', 'cool' and 'hip' and often views non-users with suspicion. The resultant communication gap may be considerable. Nursing staff may be viewed as authority figures and the patient may be over-sensitive to anything which may be interpreted as criticism. The patient will tend to be initially defensive of his/her way of life and will freely employ the argot of the drug user in conversation, often in an attempt to romanticize an unstable and dangerous way of life which can be as debilitating psychologically as it is physically. There are dangers in unrestricted use of drug slang by the nurse as this may simply reinforce maladaptive subcultheral values. In the early stages some use of drug slang may foster good communications but this should be gradually and gently replaced by firm reminders of an often unpalatable reality. For example, the patient may say 'I was really strung out

(suffering from withdrawal) one morning so I went round to the East End and dug out this guy and managed to score some smack (obtain some heroin). I fixed the stuff in his flat and felt really great—it was so good—we were laughing and joking'. A suitable response might be: 'How did you feel when you were suffering from withdrawal, before you injected the heroin?' or 'How did you get the money? Was this at the time when you had major financial problems?' Do not be deceived by the exterior show of bravado displayed by many drug misusers. Loss of confidence and self-esteem is often colossal and the need for support and reassurance is great. Try to avoid letting conversations degenerate into boastful and distorted accounts of drug misuse; gently steer the conversation back to the here and now and encourage attempts at problem identification and solving. Discussion should have educative themes (hazards and complications of drug misuse) and should promote insight: 'Why do you think you need drugs? Why do you worry about facing life without drugs? Can you tell me how you lost control when others didn't? What are your greatest fears for the future?'

Expressing sexuality

Some young drug abusers may attempt to elicit sympathy or preferential treatment by manipulative professions of admiration for staff members: 'I feel

Table 77 Communication.

Problem	Objective	Action
Value systems and social norms of staff and patient likely to be at variance	To promote effective communication	Active listening; non-judgemental stance; supportive approach

Table 78 Expressing sexuality.

Problem	Objective	Action
Possible attempts to manipulate staff	To prevent same	Limit setting; confrontation

very attracted to you—you understand me so well'. Gently and firmly confront the patient with this behaviour and set limits to it while keeping the therapeutic dimensions of the relationship open.

Working and playing

The preoccupied and morose drug misuser may irritably reject attempts to involve him/her in group activities, and gentle persistence may be necessary. Elements of the therapeutic community approach are helpful here: 'You are responsible for your actions and your behaviour and should be prepared to discuss their effects with your fellow patients as they should with you'. Informal group discussion provides a forum for ventilation of troublesome feelings and enables learning to take place. Time weighs heavy on the hospitalized drug misuser, and the provision of opportunities for confidence-building and inertia-dispelling activities is important. Much aggression and tension has been worked off on an exercise cycle or during a game of table tennis or badminton. Try to ensure that group activities do not become the occasion of boastful exercises in 'symptom swopping' or mutual reinforcement of undesirable subcultural values. Remember that a group of drug misusers will have few topics of conversation other than drugs.

Sleeping

Marked insomnia is common during withdrawal from opiates, barbiturates and stimulants (amphetamines and cocaine). A quiet, well-ventilated room is essential and frequent warm baths will promote relaxation. Once withdrawal is over, relaxation exercises and meditational techniques may be usefully taught.

Eating and drinking

Personal cleansing and dressing

Elimination

Constipation (often intractable) may occur in long-standing opiate or stimulant misuse. Reduced dietary intake and lack of exercise are common causes and some opiate misusers will have been self-medicating against withdrawal by consuming a bottle of codeine phosphate syrup a day. Codeine phosphate slows peristalsis (it is used in the treatment of diarrhoea) and regular ingestion will cause intractable constipation. It also depresses the cough reflex (increasing likelihood of respiratory infections), may cause liver and kidney damage and is itself addictive.

Mobilizing

Introspective brooding is fostered by inactivity and gentle exercise—even a walk in the fresh air is to be encouraged. Exercise will also reduce tension and contribute to overall feelings of well-being.

Controlling body temperature

Dying

Suicidal feelings have already been mentioned and should not be dismissed but should be listened to carefully with a view to assessing the degree of suicidal risk and allowing ventilation of tensions.

The drug subculture is one haunted by awareness of the risks of death or disability (hepatitis B, overdose, septicaemia) despite exterior displays of bra-

Table 79 Working and playing.

Problem	Objective	Action
Loss of interest and efficiency due to preoccupation with drugs	To restore interest and efficiency	Group discussion and activities; provision of stimulating activities

Table 80 Sleeping.

Problem	Objective	Action
Insomnia	To reduce same	Provide suitable sleeping environment; promote relaxation

Table 81 Eating and drinking.

Problem	Objective	Action
Anorexia/food intolerance	To correct same	Light, nourishing diet
Poor nutritional status		Cater (where possible) to dietary likes and dislikes

Table 82 Personal cleansing and dressing.

Problem	Objective	Action
Poor personal hygiene; loss of interest in personal hygiene	To restore adequate standard of personal hygiene and restore interest in personal appearance	Prompt and reinforce appropriate cleansing behaviour; ask visitors to bring in patient's personal clothing

Table 83 Elimination.

Problem	Objective	Action
Constipation common	To reduce same	Copious fluids, dietary fibre and exercise

Table 84 Mobilizing.

Problem	Objective	Action
Inertia due to apathy and withdrawal	To promote healthy patterns of activity	Provide opportunities for exercise and encourage same

Table 85 Controlling body temperature.

Problem	Objective	Action
Shivering and goose flesh ('cold turkey') during opiate withdrawal	To reduce associated discomfort	Provide electric blanket and encourage oral fluids and frequent warm baths

Table 86 Dying.

Problem	Objective	Action
Suicidal feelings and/or fears of drug-related death	To reduce these	Active listening; educative interventions

vado or nonchalance. The fear of AIDS is now currently casting a shadow over the drug-misusing population. The patient should be reminded that one of the advantages of hospitalization is the opportunity for effective screening for drug-related disease and should be encouraged to approach the medical staff for advice.

Assessment and identification of problems should help to provide some perspective on the possible difficulties on admission and during the initial period of adjustment to hospitalization. The pervasive degree of psychosocial disorganization often encountered is perhaps best described in the words of a 26-year-old heroin abuser interviewed by the author (November, 1985).

Pete describes the processes of 'starting' and

'stopping' and the period of limbo in between. He is a tall, thin, dark haired young man, long haired and unshaven, who gesticulates nervously as he speaks. His clothing is untidy, in need of repair, but clean. During conversation he speaks slowly, hesitates frequently, and smiles rarely. He listens intently but drops eye-to-eye contact when speaking. Pete is both intelligent and articulate and his statements about heroin abuse are, in the main, carefully considered. On occasion he is defensive and he still rationalizes about some aspects of his heroin abuse. Overall he gives the impression of being depressed and is patently low in self-esteem and confidence. At the time of interview he had discontinued his moderate to heavy heroin habit for 14 months, with one or two relapses. The social vacuum created by stopping the habit was proving troublesome and he was making insightful efforts to occupy himself constructively and to cultivate friends outside the drug subculture. He lost his job due to his drug habit 18 months ago. His account is as follows:

'I started about three years ago. I used to use a fair amount of hash and speed before then but was always rather contemptuous of "junkies". You used to see some real junkies in a couple of pubs I used to go to—they were real oddballs—screwed up people—and the crazy thing was they thought they were "the beautiful people". They were so dirty and nervous-looking—always had one eye open for the DS (drug squad) and another for the dealer. Once a junkie sat beside me in a pub—he was well known locally—right into smack—used to fix in the pub toilet—he could be a violent bastard, too, and he stank. He had been inside (in prison) a few times and was really paranoid—what an advert for smack: I mean this guy was a freak and he looked the part. He never offered me any—this "pusher" business is a myth—if you want junk you better go looking for it—no-one's going to come looking for you. This "free bag" business—to get you started—is nonsense—any I ever got I had to go to a lot of hassle to obtain and I never heard of anyone being given free smack to hook them. The papers are so full of . . . they haven't the faintest idea what the real situation is—they just don't live in the real world. Right—how did I get into smack? I met this girl—she was really attractive—bright, too—a bit middle class though. She used to chase the dragon (smoke heroin) now and then—had been doing it occasionally for years. I mean she was very different from the local junkies—she had no time for junkies either. We both liked music and I

really respected her—though I wouldn't admit that to her. I don't know why—maybe she made me feel a bit inferior—though she never put me down. Anyway I chased the dragon with her a few times—and it was so good! I felt really terrific! So confident—I mean I could have lectured to the Royal Philosophical Society without hesitating—it's impossible to tell you what it's like—it just makes a grey world seem technicolour for a while—nothing could bother you when you're like that.

We used to use a bag every Friday—sometimes Saturday, too—some of our friends tried it, too—I mean good people—not junkies—and eventually about six of us were using it. Those were the good days—before all the hassle started.

I tried fixing once—it made me sick—but the feeling was indescribable. Soon we fixed regularly—then it was every day. We used to fix about nine o'clock at night so we would be okay for work in the morning. We would still chase the dragon occasionally—burnt tin foil everywhere. Then the hassle about money started—I mean it costs a fortune—I thought nothing of spending £100 on smack—nothing. You start to think of money in terms of the smack it will buy: £10 = 1 bag; a ten pound note is just a voucher for a bag. I don't think I was a junkie even then—I think I could probably have stopped then, but why should I?

About then I used to get really "strung out" in the mornings. You get this headache—it's hard to describe—it's sort of above and behind your eyes and it buzzes. At work I used to be sweating and yawning—my nose was streaming and I was covered in goose flesh. You get a bit paranoid about other people when you're like that—you imagine things—but the relief when you make a hit—oh! the feeling is glorious. Suddenly you feel confident and alive again—and it happens so fast—only two or three minutes—the contrast is incredible.

I split with that girl then—we argued a lot about money—she became a real breadhead. About then I got a lot of hassle from the dealer—half the stuff he was selling me was just brickdust. I felt really hurt and angry—he got so much money from me. Around then I had to jump on a train and go up to the city to score—my life revolved around scoring—so much hassle. I just used to get bored and go get that smack—why not?

Yes, it was affecting me physically then. I lost two stone and only had a bath about every six weeks or so—I used to really smell. Then I got the Hep (hepatitis B). That was a bad period that I don't much want to remember. I didn't go into hospital though and I was alright—more or less.

Then I said "Pete—you're a junkie"; and I thought—so what? Did you know that the Victorians were all junkies? They were into opium, laudanum, paregoric and stuff like that. You could just buy it in shops for a few coppers—nobody bothered then. What worried me then was sort of sliding down the social scale—there is this sort of pecking order among junkies. You get the occasional smoker—you know—very controlled just chasing the dragon now and then; then you get fixers—I used to look down on them—then, at the bottom, the hopeless cases—the real junkies—VD and prison and things like that.

Round about then I spent a lot of time begging money from people; my parents got really pissed off with me. I stole some of their stuff—sold my own long ago—did a bit of dealing and a bit of shoplifting. Lost my job—it was like a kind of death wish. I could see it coming. I was heading for the sack for a long time. Used to feel suicidal then—still do sometimes—spent most of my life really strung out and chasing a fix. The things you do—it's unreal.

Losing my job finally made me try to get off. I felt so angry—rejected as a hopeless junkie—I wanted to show them. I started to taper off and I drank a lot of codeine phosphate; it wasn't so bad. The big problem is carving out a drug-free way of life. You don't know what the hell to do with yourself—just a day at a time till you get your confidence back—that's how to do it. Self-help—that works. My GP wanted me to go into hospital but I conned him into giving me a prescription for 100 DF118—I mean—imagine giving 100 DFs to a junkie! Hospital wouldn't help me—shuffling around for a few weeks in a dressing gown and pyjamas—what's that going to do for anyone? I got involved with a self-help group. You need so much reassurance. You need people to tell you that you're doing well. You have to be told that continually. Eventually your motivation reaches a sort of critical mass—but you need help—a lot of help and support to keep that going. I started fishing again—I do a lot of that now.

For the last year I've been drinking a bottle of codeine phosphate syrup every day—I know I've changed one addiction for another but I can handle this one. I worry about kidney damage though—that and AIDS. Now money means something to me—five pounds is a lot of money now. Three months ago I got really fed up and made a hit. It was really disappointing. If you're not strung out when you make a hit, it's nothing—rubbish.

I don't want to go back to the way I was though, but I might have some smack now and again—never regularly though.'

Relapses—the Problems of 'Staying Off'

Relapse has been defined as 'any situation where a person has made a resolution to change their behaviour and fails (even for a short time) in that resolution' (Allsop, 1984). Medical model explanations of relapse have largely emphasized 'craving' and 'loss of control' as factors critical to relapse (in the case of drugs *or* alcohol). These concepts have been described as having 'little explanatory value' (Allsop, 1984) and laboratory studies have produced results that were inconsistent with 'craving' and 'loss of control' (Mello and Mendelson, 1965).

It has been suggested that clients may have relapses for two reasons: (a) inability to cope in high-risk situations, or (b) the client's decision not to employ coping strategies—the 'planned relapse'—'having appropriate skills is not the same as deciding to use them' (Allsop, 1984).

It is certainly essential to teach clients *coping skills* which may be used to deal with high-risk situations, and *behavioural rehearsal* will help to build confidence and increase commitment to change. For example, 'OK you're sitting in your local pub and I (your best friend) come in and tell you that I have just bought a bag of heroin and offer to share it with you. How are you going to handle the situation? Let's practise being assertive until you feel comfortable with your responses'. This approach—essentially social skills training—does not differ in essence from similar exercises (described in Chapter 25) for the alcohol-dependent patient.

The behavioural approach, in itself, may be dangerously simplistic. Fulton (1983) has indicated that coping skills alone are not enough; increased motivation is also required as many clients 'decide to have a relapse' . . . 'it appears that some individuals relapse because they choose not to exercise coping skills . . . and not because of deficient coping skills in high risk situations'.

Wikler (1972) identifies powerful reinforcing processes in opiate dependency. Sources of reinforcements include the need to belong, boredom, anomie and hostility to the establishment, and the reinforcement of events includes acceptance by, and increased status within, the deviant subculture culminating in drug-taking in accordance with rituals and affirmation of cultist beliefs.

The nurse should help the client to develop increased awareness of reinforcing situations and should clearly identify these as dangerous situations, and should also identify tendencies towards self-sabotage. Discussions may also profitably explore the function served by drugs in the client's life.

The Blenheim Project (1983) encourages a self-help approach to drug dependence and suggests that clients ask themselves two questions:
1 Why has your drug abuse become a problem? Many people who use drugs do so on a casual basis without ever running into problems or becoming addicted. Why have you?
2 How will you cope with your problems when you stop using? Drugs can be used as short-term solutions to otherwise unsolved troubles. They kill pain, relieve anxiety, give you that 'little bit extra' when you feel you need it, or ease inhibitions. Whatever your drug does for you (and the same drug can do different things for different people) you must be aware that when you stop using it you will need to find other ways of dealing with these things.

The author (October, 1985) interviewed 14 persons who had had moderate/heavy opiate habits (age range: 18–32 years; 11 males and 3 females, period of abuse ranging from 2–11 years, mean duration of period of abuse 3 years) and asked them to identify those psychosocial changes which had filled the post-dependence vacuum and which had sustained motivation. The results were as follows:
(a) Voluntary work with drug misusers, 9
(b) Marriage/lasting relationship, 7
(c) Gaining employment, 7
(d) Developing hobbies/interests, 6
(e) 'Geographical escape', 3
(f) Embarking upon university/college course, 2
(Factors a+b were jointly identified by 6 persons; a+b+c by 5; a+c by 6 and e+f by 2.)

Placing the patient in contact with a self-help group (many of which are conducted along similar lines to AA) will help to ensure community support and will bolster determination. The heavily dependent drug misuser who has developed a chaotic lifestyle may benefit from a drug-free community which offers a visibly helpful alternative lifestyle. One of the best known is the Phoenix House Movement which offers a programme based on three premises (Warren Holland, 1976):
1 An individual's reliance on chemical substances prevents him from reaching solutions to his real problems; therefore total withdrawal is a necessary prelude to problem solving.
2 Most addicts are emotionally immature, as characterized by 'irresponsible and demanding attitudes, avoidance of unpleasant reality and inability to communicate effectively'. To counteract this the community fosters emotional growth and the development of a sense of responsibility, and an ability to communicate and come to terms with reality.
3 Addicts are helpless, incapable people who must be made to assume responsibility for their lives.

Some helping agencies recognize that (as in alcohol dependence) total abstinence may not be a practical goal for some individuals (Blenheim Project, 1983) and that controlled use may be aimed for by some clients. Many clients will turn to alcohol as a form of substitution therapy, so the dangers of replacing one form of dependence with another should be warned against. Above all, clients should be advised that the occasional relapse does not mean failure but offers the opportunity to learn more about dangerous situations and factors adversely affecting motivation. Relapses should not become an excuse for abandoning attempts to come off drugs.

In summary, staying off involves:
1 Improving *assertive skills* which may be used to deal with high risk situations
2 Increasing the client's *confidence, self-esteem* and *motivation* by supportive client-centred discussion of flawed lifestyle and associated emotional difficulties
3 Ensuring contact with *helping agencies* in the community
4 Emphasizing that a relapse does not equal failure and encouraging discussion of causes of relapse, emphasizing that many are not accidental but are carefully planned

Family Therapy in Drug Dependence

Drug abuse does not simply affect the abusing member of the family; parental distress is likely to be considerable and one or both parents may develop troublesome anxiety or depression as the problem continues. Initial parental responses tend to be of shock and disbelief, even if long-standing suspicions have finally been confirmed. In the early stages most parents are supportive, though episodes of anger may punctuate this support. In the long-term, weary resignation and rejection are common, fuelling feelings of anomie on the client's part. The drug-abusing client will also provide an undesirable role model for younger siblings and the total stresses on the family unit will be great. Recriminations and accusations may be exchanged between parents ('if only you had spent more time with him when he was younger!') and marriage guidance counselling may be necessary.

Parental distress may be unnecessarily high in the early stages when abuse may not yet have led to dependence. Tabloid images of heroin as the 'white death' may persuade parents that their son or daughter is beyond redemption and it must be emphasized that, while drug abuse is always to be regarded seriously, many young people go through a phase of recreational experimentation with drugs without coming to any lasting physical or psychosocial harm. Discovering that a son or daughter is abusing drugs is not an occasion for panic or moral outrage. It certainly is the occasion for much calm and serious dialogue aimed at open and honest discussion of the problem, and early involvement of helping agencies should be considered. Referring a son or daughter who occasionally smokes heroin to a self-help group for heavy parenteral users is not a good idea, and careful advice should be taken to ensure that referral is appropriate. In the case of intermittent drug abuse or early dependence it may be more appropriate for the client to see a counsellor from one of the many voluntary agencies involved in this field, initially on a one-to-one basis and then with parents. Many drug counsellors will advise a self-help approach to getting off and will offer supportive and educative interventions to client and parents.

Kaufman and Kaufman (1979) identify certain features which they claim to be common within families with a drug-abusing member:

1 The drug abuser is the symptom carrier of the family dysfunction.

2 The drug abuser helps to maintain family homeostasis (equilibrium).

3 The abusing member reinforces the parental need to control and continue parenting, yet he finds such parenting inadequate for his needs.

4 The abuser provides a displaced battlefield so that implicit and explicit parental strife can continue to be denied.

5 Parental drug and alcohol abuse is common and is directly transmitted to the abuser or results in inadequate parenting.

6 The abuser forms cross-generational alliances which separate parents from one another.

7 Frequently the crisis created by the drug-abusing member is the only way in which the family gets together and attempts problem solving, or is the only opportunity for a 'dead' family to experience emotions.

The family therapy approach assumes that the problem is not simply the drug abuse but the problem of a family and young person disengaging from one another, and assumes that 'if the family organisation does not change the young person will continue to fail, year after year, despite therapy efforts' (Stanton and Todd, 1979).

Therapy involves bringing the client back into contact with the family (even in the case of married clients), requiring the family to take charge and focus on the problem behaviour, emphasizing the 'here and now'. 'The past and past causes of the problem are ignored and not explored. The focus is what to do now' (Stanton and Todd, 1979). 'Normalization' commences immediately (normal work or school should be expected immediately, not later). This approach emphasizes intense involvement and a rapid disengagement as independence re-emerges. Total involvement usually occurs within three to five months.

The stability conferred by family therapy is helpful as identification with quasi-parenting older abusers, peers and siblings is common (Kaufman and Kaufman, 1979) and re-engagement with the family will reduce feelings of anomie and alienation and will help to sustain motivation.

The theme of the 'index patient' as scapegoat and the associated theme of the family as battleground, with the index patient a casualty of emotional crossfire, will help provide clearer perspectives on *some* family units. Remember, though, that it may be difficult to separate cause from effect—Is John abusing heroin as a retaliation against his mother's authoritarian and demanding attitudes? Or does mother show these attitudes as a result of John's drug abuse? Or, are both perspectives partially true?

Family therapy should studiously avoid any

implications of blame, whatever the circumstances. Remember that parents are likely to be traumatized and vulnerable. Haw (1985) describes the effects on parents of discovering that a son or daughter is abusing drugs: 'The current tendency to present opiate users as helpless, hopeless victims probably serves to heighten the panic, fear and anxiety that accompanies the discovery of the problem'. The same researcher describes a range of parental reactions including fear, confusion, anger, guilt and, especially, the painful feeling of total loss of trust between the parents and the drug-abusing child. Many parents felt too stigmatized to discuss the problem openly and nursing staff should be sensitive to the parents' need to discuss the problem.

Nurses should also critically review their own attitudes towards drug abuse. Critical, authoritarian, moralistic or judgemental stances are not helpful—the nurse will simply begin to play the part of Critical Parent, thus fostering a Rebellious Child stance in the client. Interactions should be Adult to Adult and should be undistorted by the nurse's personal value system.

In conclusion, the nursing approach should seek to replace hostility with trust, confusion with increased understanding, and fear with balanced optimism and increased awareness of alternative ways of being.

Key Concepts

1 Getting someone off drugs is not difficult; helping them to stay off will require more effort.
2 Drugs may come to progressively displace more and more activities until they dominate lifestyle and consciousness.
3 Coming off drugs leaves a vacuum which must be filled by helping the patient to restructure lifestyle—if this is not done relapse is almost inevitable.
4 The first step is assessment. Physical, psychological and social problems are likely to be present and to interact with each other.
5 Monitoring of physical state is essential for the first week after admission due to the risk of withdrawal states or serious systemic infections.
6 Teaching *coping skills* and encouraging identification of high-risk situations will help but must be accompanied by attempts to motivate the patient to use these skills where appropriate.

7 The emphasis throughout is on promoting an active *self-help* approach and discouraging passive adoption of the 'sick role'.
8 Underlying emotional problems (be they cause or effect of the problem) require supportive psychotherapy.
9 Family therapy recognizes and responds to the stresses on the family unit and on the client and aims to promote re-engagement with the family, without any suggestion of apportioning blame either to client or family.

References

Allsop, S. (1984) Relapse—the failure of resolution. *Scottish Council on Alcoholism (Edinburgh) 10th Annual Report*.

Bennett, J. (1985) *AIDS Epidemiology Update*. AJN.

The Blenheim Project (1983) *How to Stop—a Do it Yourself Guide to Opiate Withdrawal*. The Blenheim Project: 7 Thorpe Close, London W10.

Fisher, R. (1985) AIDS and a plague mentality. *New Society*, 71(1157): 322–325.

Fulton, A. (1983) Relapse fantasies. *Post-Graduate Diploma in Alcohol Studies Dissertation*. Alcohol Studies Centre, Paisley College of Technology, Paisley.

Haw, S. (October 1985) *Drugs Problems in Greater Glasgow. Report of the SCODA (Standing Conference on Drug Abuse) Fieldwork Survey in Greater Glasgow Health Board*. London: Chameleon Press.

Kaufman, E. & Kaufman, P. (1979) From a psychodynamic orientation to a structural family therapy approach in the treatment of drug dependency. In Kaufman, E. & Kaufman, P. (Eds) *Family Therapy of Drug and Alcohol Abuse*. New York: Gardner Press Inc.

Mello, N. & Mendelson, J. (1965) Operant analysis of drinking habits of chronic alcoholics. *Nature*, 206: 43–46.

Melville, J. (1984) *The Tranquilliser Trap—and How to Get Out of It*. London: Fontana Paperbacks.

Petursson, H. & Lader, M. (1981) Withdrawal reaction from Clobazam treatment. *British Medical Journal*, 282: 1931–1932.

Peutherer, J. et al (1985) HTLV-III antibody in Edinburgh drug addicts. *Lancet*, November 16.

Plant, M. (1977) *Drug Takers in an English Town*. London: Tavistock Publications.

Stanton, M. & Todd, T. (1979) Structural family therapy with drug addicts. In Kaufman, E. & Kaufman, P. (Eds) *Family Therapy of Drug and Alcohol Abuse*. New York: Gardner Press Inc.

Warren Holland, D. (1976) *The Featherstone Lodge Project*. In Madden Walker Kenyon (Ed) *Alcoholism and Drug Dependence*. London: Plenum Press.

Wikler, A. (1972) Sources of reinforcement for drug using behaviour. In Cochin, J. (Ed) *Pharmacology and the Future of Man. Proceedings of the 5th International Congress on Pharmacology, 1972, Vol. I*. Basle, Switzerland: Karger.

24

Alcohol Dependence

'He drank, not as an epicure, but barbarously, with a speed and dispatch altogether American, as if he were performing a homicidal function, as if he had to kill something inside himself—a worm that would not die'—*Baudelaire* (*writing about Edgar Allan Poe*)

The World Health Organization defines alcoholics as 'those excessive drinkers whose dependence on alcohol has attained such a degree that it causes a noticeable mental disturbance or an interference with their bodily and mental health, their interpersonal relations and their smooth social and economic functioning'.

The images of physical, psychological and social impairment incorporated in this definition may generate a vision of the 'Skid Row' alcoholic for many people—a pitiable creature alienated from normal social relations by virtue of a suicidal overconsumption which seems difficult to understand. Alcohol addiction, however, is not the problem of an unfortunate and eccentric few but is firmly rooted in 'normal' social patterns of alcohol use. The 'typical' alcoholic does not exist (any more than the 'typical' drug addict exists). Alcoholics are to be found in all social classes, all environments and come from all walks of life.

For most people alcohol is a social lubricant equated with relaxing and pleasurable social occasions and, indeed, small amounts of alcohol not only do no harm but may even do some good. Recognition of this fact should, however, be coupled with recognition of the fact that regular alcohol use may lead to alcohol abuse and eventually to dependence. The door to alcoholism is not forced open by a determined and suicidal few but lies open and may be inadvertently entered by any social drinker. Not all 'problem drinkers' progress to fully established alcoholism and there seems to be considerable migration in and out of the 'problem drinking' pool (Goodwin, 1981).

Social and Anti-social Drinking

Archaeological evidence suggests that alcohol has been used since the Stone Age, and alcoholism was recognized in Ancient Egypt and Babylonia.

The basis of all commercially marketed alcoholic preparations is ethyl alcohol (ethanol) which is a waste product excreted by yeasts as they grow in sugar solutions.

Ethyl alcohol mixes freely with water so that, once in the body, it is rapidly dispersed throughout all the tissue fluids and thus has ready access to all organs. It is also soluble in fat and thus readily infiltrates the fat-rich cells of the central nervous system, exerting rapid effects on thinking, feeling and behaviour.

Alcohol is said to affect a person in four ways: first he becomes jocose, then bellicose, then lachrymose, and finally, comatose. Initially alcohol loosens inhibitions and may induce mild feelings of relaxation.

Alcohol acts as a *depressant* of the central nervous system (despite the widely held belief that it is a stimulant). The functions of higher centres in the brain seem to be inhibited first, and continuing rise in blood alcohol levels will soon lead to emotional lability and impaired judgement with an increase in the likelihood of impulsive or anti-social behaviour. As intoxication progresses, loss of coordination, unsteadiness, slurred speech and drowsiness will rapidly ensue.

The ingestion of even small amounts of alcohol dramatically increases the risk of accidents of any kind. One in three of the drivers killed in road accidents have levels of alcohol which are over the legal limit, and the risk of occupational accidents involving dangerous machinery is greatly increased by even minimal amounts of alcohol. The risk of anti-social behaviour is also greatly increased by alcohol consumption. Intoxication may cause the individual to become quarrelsome or aggressive, and even 'social drinking' may have widespread effects on social relationships. Hayman (1967) criticizes the 'myth of social drinking' as follows: 'We cannot say that all who drink are alcoholics, but can we say that they are "social drinkers" who, because of drinking, have hurt others by hostile criticism, made unwelcome passes at other men's wives, had unreasonable fights, given their children a model of drunkenness, squandered time needed for constructive pursuits, driven while in a drunken state, had accidents coming home from a cocktail party, impatiently punished their children, or sat detached from wife and children in front of the television set evening after evening in a semi-stuporous state, following several "social" drinks before dinner? We need another category "anti-social drinking" to replace much of what we call "social drinking".'

Anti-social drinking is characterized by *abuse*, rather than use, of alcohol. Alcohol abuse is a general term applied to the misuse of alcohol resulting in one or more problems for the drinker and does not necessarily involve alcoholism, though it is often a prelude to it. The act of getting drunk is in itself a form of alcohol abuse.

The person who regularly abuses alcohol will become a *problem drinker* as they create personal, social or professional problems arising from alcohol abuse. The distinction between problem drinking and alcoholism is largely a matter of degree and depends on both the number of difficulties exhibited and the tolerance of the social 'audience'. Attitudes towards alcohol abuse vary widely from culture to culture and there may be much variation within any given culture. Heavy drinking may be regarded as 'manly' or 'sophisticated' in some cultures (Scotland, Ireland, Australia, West Germany, Russia) while it may evoke responses of distaste and censure in others (Israel, Islamic societies, China). In general terms it seems that the farther we go from the Equator, or the nearer we get to the Poles, the higher the prevalence of alcoholism tends to be.

At What Point does Social Drinking Create the Risk of Dependence?

Considerations of alcohol intake levels are usually based on the *standard unit* of alcohol. One standard unit is equal to a half pint of beer, a single measure of spirits (whisky, gin, rum, vodka), a glass of wine, a glass of sherry or a measure of vermouth (see Figure 12 and Table 87). For men, a sensible limit is 4–6 standard units (or 'standard drinks') two or three times a week. For women, a sensible limit is two or three standard units, two or three times a week. The limit is lower for women as females are more readily affected by alcohol than are males. In men, 55–65% of body weight consists of water, whereas 45–55% of women's body weight consists of water. Alcohol is distributed throughout the body fluids so, in men, the alcohol is more 'diluted' than it is in women. Women also tend to weigh less than men so that the same amount of alcohol will produce much higher blood concentrations than in a man drinking an equivalent amount. Women are also more susceptible than men to alcoholic cirrhosis of the liver, and there may be an interaction between menopausal hormonal status and the susceptibility of the liver to the toxic effects of alcohol (O'Brien and Chafetz, 1982). You may wish to consider keeping a record of your alcohol intake for one week, calculating the total number of standard units consumed, and comparing the total to the table of thresholds shown in Table 88. Twelve to eighteen units spread over a week may do no harm to the average healthy male but if this intake is concentrated into one 'binge', serious impairment of judgement will ensue and there is a very real risk of problems arising.

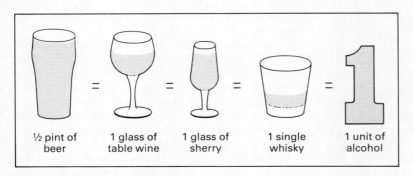

½ pint of beer = 1 glass of table wine = 1 glass of sherry = 1 single whisky = 1 unit of alcohol

Figure 12 The standard unit of alcohol.

Table 87 Alcohol intake levels based on the standard unit of alcohol.

	Standard drinks
Beers and lagers	
Ordinary strength beer or lager	
½ pint	1
1 pint	2
1 can	1½
Export beer	
1 pint	2½
1 can	2
Strong ale or lager	
½ pint	2
1 pint	4
1 can	3
Extra strength beer or lager	
½ pint	2½
1 pint	5
1 can	4
Ciders	
Average cider	
½ pint	1½
1 pint	3
quart bottle	6
Strong cider	
½ pint	2
1 pint	4
quart bottle	8
Spirits	
1 standard single measure in most of England and Wales (⅙ gill)	1
1 standard single measure in Northern Ireland (¼ gill)	1½
⅕ gill measure	1¼
¼ gill measure served in some parts of Scotland	1½
1 bottle	30
Table wine (*including cider wine and barley wine*)	
1 standard glass	1
1 bottle	7
1 litre bottle	10
Sherry and fortified wine	
1 standard small measure	1
1 bottle	12

These figures are approximate

Table 88 Interpretation of alcohol intake levels.

Weekly totals standard units Men	Women	Interpretation
up to 20	up to 13	Drinking at this level carries no long-term risk.
21–36	14–24	If spread throughout the week unlikely to cause any long-term damage but if concentrated into say 2 hours, increases the risk of accident.
51–95	36–63	May already be doing some harm—liver and stomach may both be affected—high risk of social/legal problems (drinking/driving)—this level of drinking should be reduced.
96 and more	64 and more	It is rare for anyone drinking as much as this to escape unscathed! Physical and mental health will be deteriorating and there is now a high risk of damage to liver, nervous system or heart. Personal/social problems are now inevitable.

Source: *That's the Limit—A guide to sensible drinking* (Scottish Health Education Unit)

The Development of Dependence

Meyer and Salmon (1984) describe the progression towards chronic alcoholism that typically takes place. Three stages are identified:

1 *Pre-alcoholic phase* (a) Social drinking and an occasional weekend drink are the major symptoms, (b) both tolerance and frequency of drinking increase, usually slowly, (c) alcohol serves primarily as an escape from anxiety, mild depression or boredom.

2 *Initial alcoholism* (a) Tolerance, frequency and abuse increase, (b) more is drunk per swallow; often there is a shift to more potent drinks, (c) depression increases along with loss of self-esteem over drinking patterns, (d) occasional blackouts occur.

3 *Chronic stage* (a) True loss-of-control patterns, such as drinking throughout the day and using any source of alcohol, predominate, (b) inadequate nutrition affects functioning and physical health, (c) signs of impaired thinking and hallucinations and tremors emerge.

As tolerance increases, the problem drinker will find that intake has to be increased to achieve the desired state of intoxication, and surreptitious drinking may take place with a feeling of urgency attached to consuming the first drink of the day. As alcohol is abused steadily, memory blackouts (*palimpsests*) will occur and the problem drinker will make excuses and produce rationalizations in an attempt to justify escalating consumption levels and increasing frequency of problems associated with drinking.

Attitudes tend to be very defensive at this stage (despite attacks of guilt) and the problem drinker will often indignantly insist that his/her consumption is no greater than that of friends. These comparisons, however, tend to be based on underestimation of personal consumption and overestimation of that of others. The problem drinker will often refuse to realistically discuss his/her drinking pattern at this stage and may become surly and resentful if criticized.

Initial episodes of alcohol abuse will be replaced by a discernible pattern of problem drinking which is the basis of the pre-alcoholic phase.

As dependence increases, efforts at control will be attempted repeatedly without lasting success and, as initial alcoholism asserts itself, psychological and social deterioration will become apparent. Family and friends will be avoided as the company of fellow 'hard drinkers' is cultivated and willpower fails. As alcoholism becomes chronic, complete defeat is likely to be admitted as alcohol becomes the central factor in the person's life.

What Causes Alcoholism?

A variety of factors may interact to cause alcoholism, though any one of these single factors may emerge as the dominant influence in any given case. Surveys of the aetiology of alcoholism have considered possible physical, psychological and social causes.

Physical explanations

Physical or biological hypotheses are organized around the 'illness' or 'disease' model of alcoholism which emphasizes the physiological effects of alcohol abuse. The inference here is that an underlying physiological malfunction leads to dependence and that this metabolic defect is probably hereditary.

Studies indicate that a small minority of alcoholics have a genetic predisposition for alcohol abuse insofar as adopted children, raised apart from their alcoholic parents, show an increased incidence of alcohol abuse (Goodwin et al, 1973), though these persons may have inherited depressive tendencies rather than a metabolic defect.

Another study indicates that heavy drinkers eventually begin to metabolize alcohol in the liver differently (Seixas, 1981), though this may be simply the *effect* rather than the *cause* of problem drinking.

The 'illness model' has been criticized on two grounds. First, the supportive physiological evidence is flimsy as most symptoms are effects rather than causes. Second, in describing alcoholism as an 'illness' we may be encouraging problem drinkers to assume the passive 'patient role' at the expense of more productive exploration of areas of psychosocial difficulty which may be crucial to the continuation of the person's alcohol abuse.

Psychological explanations

The psychoanalytical explanation is that alcoholics are fixated at the oral stage (most alcoholics are also heavy smokers), though there is little supportive evidence for this theory. There have been many other attempts to relate personality type to alcohol abuse in an attempt to isolate vulnerable types, and a frequent conclusion is that alcohol serves as a potent self-administered tranquillizer for highly anxious individuals (Grant and Gwinner, 1979); that is, alcohol is used for the purpose of *self-medication*. Despite the frequency of this finding there is little evidence that anxiety is more prevalent among alcoholics than among other groups of individuals for whom alcohol has become an important method of coping, though many alcoholics do identify the tranquillizing effects of alcohol as one of their motivations for drinking.

Jones (1971) found that male alcoholics were likely to be impulsive and rebellious while female alcoholics were likely to be passive and socially avoidant. Another view is that alcoholics are individuals who suffer from pervasive feelings of inferiority which result in an enhanced need for power in the face of inadequate personality resources. Consequently they drink to achieve this power, relieve tension and bolster self-esteem.

The behaviourist explanation is simply that problem drinking behaviour is caused and maintained by the association of drinking with rewarding experiences. Alcoholism is regarded as a conditioned behavioural response that can be 'unlearned' by the modification of environmental stimuli and reinforcement situations, though these 'unlearning' strategies have not had the dramatic success one would anticipate were this explanation to be comprehensive.

Steiner (1969) has used the language of transactional analysis to identify three 'games' frequently played by alcoholics. There is the 'aggressive' game where the alcoholic invites disapproval and allows those who disapprove to appear virtuous and blameless ('you're good, I'm bad, try and stop me'). The basic objective of this game is to make persecuting parental figures so angry that they lose control of the situation and display their impotence and foolishness. Secondly, there is the *self-damaging game* usually played with a partner who has difficulty in providing emotional or sexual support. By continuing to abuse alcohol, the drinker diverts attention from the partner's inadequacies. The third game, based on tissue destruction, centres around the alcoholic obtaining satisfaction (or 'strokes' as transactional analysts call them) by making himself physically ill. The 'pay-off' in this game is the provision of medical care and treatment, nursing attention and all the associated rewards of the 'sick role'.

Almost any type of mental disorder may contribute to the development of alcohol dependence, notably depressive disorders and anxiety states, and chronic alcohol abuse may *result* in mental disorder where none was discernible in the early stages of increasing dependence. It is difficult to assign a percentage to the number of alcoholics suffering from mental disorder, be it cause or effect of alcohol abuse, and it must be stressed that not all alcoholics suffer from mental disorder other than the profound disturbances of psychosocial integrity associated with chronic alcohol abuse.

Sociocultural explanations

The prevalence of alcoholism varies widely from culture to culture and this serves to underline the importance of cultural attitudes towards alcohol abuse. France and Italy are easily the leaders in annual per capita consumption (6.56 and 4.0 gallons respectively) (Meyer and Salmon, 1984), yet Italy has a very low prevalence of alcoholism. In Italy permissive attitudes towards alcohol consumption are coupled with strong and consistent social sanctions

against drunkenness or loss of control, and Spain and Portugal provide similar examples of this combination of factors. France couples permissive attitudes towards alcohol with indulgent views of insobriety and has a much higher rate of alcohol-related problems than Italy, Spain or Portugal. Jews have lower rates of alcoholism than other ethnic groups, though 95% of the Jewish people use alcohol (O'Brien and Chafetz, 1982). Jewish cultural practices include the introduction of alcohol to children at an early age, coupled with the use of alcohol at religious ceremonies and social gatherings, yet intoxication and drunken behaviour are not tolerated. There appears to be a correlation between a move away from Jewish orthodoxy and an increase in the incidence of alcoholism (O'Brien and Chafetz, 1982).

Muslims and Mormons reject social use of alcohol as being incompatible with their religious beliefs and have very low rates of alcoholism, though an increase in incidence among the Bedouin of Kuwait has been reported (Kinney and Leaton, 1983).

Drinking patterns within the United Kingdom vary considerably with a far higher incidence of alcohol abuse in Scotland and Northern Ireland than in England and Wales. Admissions for alcoholism in Scotland have increased sixfold in the last 20 years (Ingram et al, 1981) and there are thought to be four to five times as many alcoholics in Scotland as in England and Wales (Plant, 1975).

Ireland has a large, but declining, percentage of non-drinkers (43% in 1974) but the drinking population spends a larger proportion of their income on alcohol than in any other country (O'Brien and Chafetz, 1982), their closest competitors being the Finns and the British. The result seems to be that the rising rate of alcoholism in Ireland results from the problem-drinking of a smaller pool of the population than elsewhere in Europe. The number of admissions to mental hospitals for the treatment of alcoholism rose by more than 300% from 1965 to 1977 in Ireland, though overall prevalence remains lower than in many other countries (e.g. the USA).

Irish-Americans have a rate of problem-drinking three times as high as that of other ethnic groups (O'Brien and Chafetz, 1982).

Sociocultural attitudes towards alcohol abuse seem to be of critical importance in determining the incidence of alcohol-related problems.

In many working class European and North-American cultures, alcohol abuse may be regarded as a sign of 'toughness' or 'manliness' while females from these backgrounds may see heavy alcohol consumption as a sign of 'sophistication'. Permissive attitudes towards insobriety seem to open the door wide to alcoholism.

The acquisition of attitudes which positively value heavy alcohol use may start in the home; children of alcoholics have two to three times the risk of developing alcoholism than that of the general population and identification with an adolescent subculture which views insobriety indulgently increases the risk further.

Unemployment also augments the risk of alcoholism (as it does of suicide) and an analysis of the records of New York City revealed that the rate of alcoholism rose sharply during times of high unemployment (Mangen, 1982).

People working in certain occupations are known to run a much higher risk of becoming alcoholics (see Table 89) and these occupations often share the common factors of the availability of free or cheap alcohol, relative freedom from direct supervision, and greater than average separation from the stabilizing influence of the home.

Advertising which attempts to portray alcohol use as 'glamorous' or 'sophisticated' has been considered as a possible factor contributing to the alarming rise in the incidence of alcoholism in Britain. While such distorted presentations can in no way be considered desirable, the fact remains that some countries, (e.g. the Soviet Union and Sweden) which ban *any* advertising of alcohol, have a high incidence of alcohol-related problems.

Considerations of the causes of alcoholism reveal that many factors may be involved and that the interaction of several factors is often involved in any given case, though the importance of sociocultural factors is not to be underestimated.

Table 89 Deaths from cirrhosis in different occupations in England and Wales.

	Standard mortality ratio
Company directors	2200
Publicans	773
Actors and entertainers	550
Hotel keepers	450
Armed forces	350
Medical practitioners	350
Barmen	200
Commercial travellers	150
Total male population of England and Wales	100

Source: Understanding Alcohol & Alcoholism in Scotland. (Scottish Health Education Group—HMSO)

Prevalence

This is difficult to estimate as many drinkers may move in and out of the problem-drinking pool undetected. Overall prevalence is thought to be about 1% in Britain (Ingram et al, 1981) and rising, though 2% of the population over 15 years of age are likely to have significant drinking problems (HMSO, 1981). In Scotland alone, alcoholism accounts for 20% of all admissions to psychiatric hospitals (HMSO, 1981), and this admission rate has been rising steadily since the mid-1950s.

Male alcoholics outnumber females by roughly five to one, though drinking problems are on the increase among women, as they are among teenagers.

Clinical Features of Alcoholism

These are physical, psychological and social and are characterized by an increase in dependence, initially in psychological dependence and eventually in physical dependence.

Physical effects of alcohol abuse

These may be varied and widespread and range from the irritating to the potentially fatal. Widespread organ damage is likely to occur in association with chronic alcohol abuse, and physical health will deteriorate steadily and dangerously. In the early stages (initial alcoholism) there will be loss of appetite as alcohol is a rich source of calories (one pint of beer contains 180 kCal), and vitamin deficiency and anaemia may herald the onset of malnutrition. Thereafter, a number of target organs will register the destructive effects of alcohol abuse. These are as follows:

The stomach

Gastritis, nausea and heartburn are the responses of a stomach which is raw and inflamed from heavy drinking, and peptic ulceration may eventually result. Gastric symptoms are the commonest in alcoholism.

The liver

Cirrhosis of the liver is a chronic inflammatory disease in which functioning liver cells are gradually replaced by scar tissue; it will be developed by roughly 10% of alcoholics. No effective treatment for cirrhosis has been devised and 60% of alcoholics who continue to drink after a diagnosis of cirrhosis has been made will die (O'Brien and Chafetz, 1982). Cirrhosis is the final stage of liver injury and occurs as the liver unsuccessfully attempts to detoxify large amounts of ethyl alcohol over a period of years. Cirrhosis is usually preceded by *fatty liver* or *alcoholic hepatitis* as the liver enlarges and becomes inflamed. As cirrhosis progresses, the liver shrinks and nodules of scar tissue develop until the liver eventually becomes incapable of sustaining life.

Blood flow through the liver almost comes to a halt in cirrhosis as capillaries and venules are replaced by scar tissue. The result is that back-pressure develops in the portal system (portal hypertension) as veins unsuccessfully attempt to feed blood into a shrunken and scarred liver which can no longer handle it. The paper-thin veins of the oesophagus will dilate and become varicosed due to this back-pressure, forming *oesophageal varices*, which may rupture causing a fatal haemorrhage. The type of cirrhosis developed by alcoholics is called *portal cirrhosis* (or Laënnecs' cirrhosis) and female alcoholics are more liable to develop it than males. Jaundice may be an early sign of cirrhosis, and suppression of female sex hormones by the liver soon fails in men, causing atrophy of the testicles, enlargement of the breasts (gynaecomastia), loss of body hair and increase in the pitch of the voice.

Brain and peripheral nerves

There is little direct evidence that alcohol alone causes brain damage but a small minority of chronic alcohol abusers suffer brain damage due to deficiency of *thiamine* (vitamin B_1, also called aneurine). Chronic deficiency of thiamine is associated with the malnutrition common in many alcoholics who fail to eat an adequate diet, as calorie needs are satisfied by energy-rich alcohol.

Severe and sustained deficiency of thiamine leads to degeneration of certain well-demarcated areas of the brain causing devastating impairment of cerebral functioning.

Wernickes' encephalopathy is characterized by confusion, unsteadiness and memory impairment. These symptoms are often accompanied by *alcoholic neuritis* in which a peripheral form of neuritis associated with degeneration of long peripheral nerves manifests itself in wrist and foot drop, weakness and wasting of the leg and hand muscles, and loss of sensation. Peripheral neuritis may arise in the absence of cerebral involvement but it should be regarded as an ominous sign of generalized insult to nervous tissue.

Wernickes' encephalopathy may progress to *Korsakoff's psychosis* which is characterized by a grossly defective short-term memory, the patient often being unable to remember events which happened only a few minutes before. The patient tends to attempt to conceal these memory 'blanks' by *confabulation*, that is by inventing imaginary events. Memory impairment is the most prominent feature of Korsakoff's psychosis (hence the fact that it is sometimes called the *dysmnesic syndrome*) but variable degrees of confusion, disorientation in time, emotional apathy and loss of insight are usually present. Patients are often moderately cheerful and non-comprehending and the condition is usually irreversible, the patient requiring hospital care for the rest of his life, unlike Wernicke's syndrome which is often reversible if large doses of thiamine are given early. It may be difficult to distinguish late Wernicke's encephalopathy from early Korsakoff's syndrome and, for this reason, the generic term of *Wernicke–Korsakoff syndrome* is often used.

Degenerative disease of the cerebellum (also associated with vitamin deficiency) may also develop causing ataxia (unsteady gait). Fortunately most alcoholics show little or no signs of mental impairment after many years of heavy drinking (Goodwin, 1981) and although computed tomography scanning shows ventricular enlargement in a proportion of chronic alcoholics, this is not necessarily associated with clinical impairment and may be reversible should the alcoholic decide to mend his ways (Trethowan and Sims, 1983).

Subdural haematoma occurs with increased frequency in alcoholics and is associated with heavy falls, and major epileptiform seizures may occur during withdrawal (seizure threshold rises with alcohol ingestion but falls below normal as blood alcohol levels drop).

Other physical effects of alcohol

Alcohol abuse includes a variety of physical effects.

Table 90 Drugs which commonly interact with alcohol.
(interactions of major or moderate significance)

Central Nervous System Depressants
Hypnotics (e.g. barbiturates, chloralhydrate,
chlormethiazole, nitrazepam).
Tranquillizers (e.g. benzodiazepines, dichloralphenazone,
glutethimide).
Phenothiazines (e.g. chlorpromazine, haloperidol).
Anti emetics (e.g. hyoscine, cyclizine, promethazine).
Pethidine.
Additive effects may be seen with concomitant use of
ethanol and CNS depressants.

Hypoglycaemic Agents (e.g. tolazamide, tolbutamide, insulin)
Accentuate hypoglycaemia due to hypoglycaemic effect of
alcohol.
With metformin there is an increased risk of lactic acidosis.
Chlorpropamide may cause flushing with alcohol in
susceptible patients.

Oral Anticoagulants
Coumarins (dicoumarol, warfarin) and indamediones
(diphenadione, phenindione)
Alcohol tends to enhance the effect of oral anticoagulants.
Increased warfarin metabolism in heavy drinkers is
probably due to alcohol induced stimulation of hepatic
microsomal enzymes.

Tricyclic Antidepressants (amitriptyline, imipramine,
desipramine)
Tricyclics and alcohol have combined effects on the CNS,
giving a potentiated sedative effect.

Tetrachloroethylene
CNS depression caused by tetrachloroethylene is additive
with that caused by alcohol. Alcohol also increases
absorption of the drug and hence the risk of liver damage.

Diphenylhydantoin
Alcohol induces production of hepatic microsomal enzymes
resulting in enhanced diphenylhydantoin metabolism.

Antihypertensives
Ethanol produces vasodilatation which may enhance
orthostatic hypotension.

Nitroglycerin
Hypotension may occur following combined use of alcohol
and Nitroglycerin. Probably due to vasodilation which both
agents produce.

Salicylates (e.g. Aspirin)
Ethanol appears to increase gastrointestinal bleeding
produced by salicylates.

Metronidazole
Acts in a similar manner to disulfiram by inhibiting
aldehyde dehydrogenase, hence may get an 'Antabuse
reaction' if alcohol is taken.

MAOI (e.g. phenelzine)
Many alcoholic beverages contain tyramine. In presence of
MAOI, there is an enhanced pressor response to tyramine.

Anaesthetics
Many anaesthetics are less effective at a given dose because
chronic excessive alcohol consumption results in enhanced
metabolism due to prior induction of microsomal enzymes.

With kind permission of the publisher, The Medical Council on
Alcoholism.

Pancreatitis (acute, relapsing and chronic)

This may be caused by heavy drinking; a study in
Glasgow found a quarter of cases of pancreatitis to
be associated with alcohol abuse (Imrie et al, 1977).
Pancreatitis is commonest in young male bout
drinkers and presents with epigastric pain, radiating
through to the back, abdominal tenderness and
tachycardia. Heart disease (alcoholic cardiomyopathy), hypertension, muscle disease, anaemia
and some forms of cancer all show an increase in
incidence associated with heavy drinking.

Foetal alcohol syndrome (FAS)

When a pregnant woman drinks, alcohol passes
freely across the placental barrier to cause concentrations in the baby's bloodstream at least as high as
those in mother—if mother gets drunk the baby
does too. The undeveloped liver of the foetus burns
up alcohol at less than half the rate of the adult liver
so that alcohol remains in the foetal system for a
longer period than in the adult system. The foetus is
not equipped to handle alcohol. The resultant dangers to the unborn baby have long been recognized.
(The Ancient Greeks noted that alcohol abuse by
pregnant women often resulted in harmful effects to
their unborn children and the Talmud contains
warnings against drinking during pregnancy for this
reason.)

Alcohol abuse during pregnancy may result in
FAS which is a combination of physical and mental
defects. The baby has a small head, short nose, thin
upper lip, an absent or indistinct philtrum (the
groove in the midline of the upper lip), small eye
openings and flat cheeks. These facial features are
considered characteristic of FAS and usually occur
in association with low birth weight, mental retardation, heart murmurs, hernias and retarded growth
as an infant and child.

Studies have suggested that 30–50% of women who

Table 91 Some physical complications of alcoholism.

Liver
Fatty liver
Alcoholic hepatitis
Jaundice
Cirrhosis

Pancreas
Pancreatitis
Cancer of pancreas (often a complication of chronic
   pancreatitis)

Gastrointestinal tract
Atrophy of mucosa of mouth, pharynx and oesophagus and
   larynx
Smooth tongue
Cancer of pharynx and oesophagus
Acute gastritis
Peptic ulcer
High incidence of gastrectomy

Heart
Cardiomyopathy

Hypertension

Disturbance of fat metabolism
Hyperlipaemia
Hyper-triglyceridaemia

Blood
Thrombocytopenia
Leucopenia
Anaemia, haemolytic
Macrocytic

Vitamin deficiency
B1, B2, B6 [e.g. wet Beri Beri (B1 deficiency)],
   Wernicke–Korsakoff (B complex deficiency, esp. B)

Endocrines
Cushing syndrome
(?) Thyroid
Pituitary
Hypoglycaemia

Respiratory system
Lowered resistance to intermittent infection
Cancer of larynx (especially supraglottic growth)

Skeletal muscle
Acute myopathy
Chronic myopathy

Skin
Hyperaemia
Telangiectasias—(groups of dilated capillaries)
Rhinophyma—(bulbous enlargement of nose)
Erythema of palms and feet
Spider naevi—(small red areas surrounded by dilated
   capillaries)

Genital system
Testicular atrophy
Gynaecomastia
Impotence

Dupuytren's contractures

Neurogenic oesteoarthropathy

Perinatal
Foetal alcohol syndrome
Spontaneous abortion

Nervous system
Cerebral atrophy (widened sulci and Sylvian fissure,
   dilatation of ventricles)
Wernicke–Korsakoff syndrome
Cerebellar cortical atrophy
Polyneuropathy
Alcoholic tremor
Marchiafava–Bignami syndrome
Alcoholic myelopathy
Retrobulbar neuritis
Epileptiform attacks
Subdural haematoma

drink 'heavily' during pregnancy have infants with
one or more of these defects (Goodwin, 1981) while
other studies have failed to find FAS in *any* of the
offspring of 'heavy drinking' mothers (Goodwin,
1981). Gordis and Kreek (1977) summarize the
research by stating that 'it was not possible to state
with confidence' whether alcohol caused birth
defects in man but, until the issue is resolved, these
authors felt the wisest recommendation to be total
abstinence during pregnancy.

The risk of *spontaneous* abortion increases with
alcohol intake and studies suggest that it may result
from even *moderate* drinking (Glatt, 1982).

Psychological effects of alcohol abuse

Preoccupation with alcohol. Drinking dominates the
alcoholic's thinking from morning until night and
craving for alcohol becomes intense as psychological
dependence increases.

Self-deception and rationalization. The alcoholic not
only lies to others—he lies to himself and excuses for
continuing drinking become more and more flimsy.
The alcoholic at this stage is still refusing to admit
that he has a problem (I could stop drinking
anytime. I don't drink any more than my friends.
What a fuss about nothing).

Guilt. As loss of control becomes more pronounced and behaviour more erratic, self-deceit begins to fail and guilt begins to punctuate episodes of drinking. The alcoholic is liable to suppress these feelings of guilt by simply drinking more.

Anxiety. This occurs as physical symptoms and social deterioration can no longer be ignored and the future seems more threatening. Like guilt, it is unfortunately likely to be suppressed by drinking more.

Depression. This begins to assert itself, particularly during the 'morning after', and is often associated with irritability. Again, it tends to be alleviated by more alcohol but may assert itself even when the problem drinker is intoxicated.

Amnesia. Memory lapses will become more frequent as problem-drinking continues; these 'blanks' may be due to unconscious feelings of guilt.

Persistent remorse. This may give rise to wild promises and 'crocodile tears', and sweeping guarantees of sobriety will be offered to family and friends. These are most unlikely to be kept, and broken promises increase feelings of guilt and remorse and may become the excuse for more episodes of abuse in an attempt to blot out these troublesome feelings. Thus drinking bouts may assume a circular quality—alcohol abuse causes troublesome feelings of guilt, shame and remorse, and these troublesome feelings provoke further alcohol abuse as the alcoholic 'drinks to forget'. This produces more of the troublesome feelings which leads to more drinking, etc.

Grandiose, aggressive and uncontrolled behaviour. This is likely to occur frequently. The Super-Ego is highly soluble in alcohol. Alcohol intoxication leads to loss of inhibitions and 'releases' sexual desire, though it impairs sexual performance. Drunken men have difficulty in achieving an erection or ejaculating, and orgasmic potential is reduced in women:

> 'Lechery, sir, it provokes and unprovokes;
> it provokes the desire,
> but it takes away the performance'
>
> (*Macbeth—Act II, Scene 3*).

Pathological jealousy. Impotence may persist long into sobriety and may contribute to the well-known syndrome of *alcoholic conjugal paranoia* in which husbands convince themselves that their wives are unfaithful and persecute them endlessly with accusations based on the most improbable of 'evidence' (Why did you take 20 minutes longer with the shopping today?—Are you meeting a man? I can smell after-shave from your blouse!).

Eventually the overall picture becomes one of failing efficiency, distorted thinking, behavioural excesses, emotional lability and psychological defeat.

Social effects of alcohol abuse

Neglect. Neglect of family, friends, occupation and previous interests becomes marked. The alcoholic will cultivate the company of social inferiors, that is anyone unlikely to criticize him and likely to join him in alcohol abuse.

The casualties of his heavy drinking will increase in number—spouse, children, relatives, employer, fellow workers, pedestrians, hapless victims of uncontrolled behaviour, police and bar staff.

Alcoholics are three times more likely to be divorced than non-alcoholics, and the average policeman in the USA spends half of his time dealing with alcohol-related offences (Goodwin, 1981).

Absenteeism from work will increase and efficiency at work will decrease until loss of employment takes place in a large majority of cases.

Suicide. The suicide rate in alcoholics has been estimated at 50 times that of the general population (Glatt, 1982) and alcohol abuse dramatically increases the risk of criminal behaviour, though the full extent to which alcohol is responsible for crime is not known. Studies suggest alcohol involvement in 13–50% of rape offenders and in 6–31% of rape victims, and also indicate that alcohol was involved in 28–86% of assault offenders and in 14–87% of the victims of assault (O'Brien and Chafetz, 1982).

Child abuse and neglect (including incest). This shows an increased incidence in relation to alcohol abuse, and a climate of family violence is not uncommon in this respect.

Driving offences. These are common in association with heavy drinking and may involve death or injury of others. Fifteen drivers per hundred involved in driving offences in Britain were over the legal blood alcohol level (80 mg per 100 ml of blood) and the corresponding figure for Australia is 50% (Swinson and Eaves, 1978) (the Australian limit is 100 mg/100 ml).

Moral deterioration. This is common in both male and females who are chronic alcohol abusers, and a pattern of casual promiscuity may be adopted, increasing the risk of venereal disease.

Effects of Alcohol Withdrawal

The most common effect of alcohol withdrawal is *tremulousness* which may be so marked that the alcoholic has difficulty in lifting a cup to his mouth without spilling the contents. Tremors may prompt the alcoholic to have a morning or midday drink as the alcoholic who is used to drinking heavily in the evenings will eventually feel himself shaky the next morning. As heavy drinking continues, the alcoholic may find that further boosts of alcohol are necessary during the day to maintain a blood alcohol level sufficient to prevent the shakes.

The physically dependent alcoholic will also find that withdrawal leads to a state of restless apprehension (the 'jitters') associated with tremor which, (like tremor), is reduced by having a drink.

Acute and chronic *alcoholic hallucinosis* occurs in some 25% of persons withdrawing from alcohol (Kinney and Leaton, 1983) and this syndrome includes alarming auditory and visual hallucinations, though auditory hallucinations predominate. The patient is *not* delirious and may only mention the 'voices' if sympathetically questioned. Alcoholic hallucinosis may persist for weeks or months and is not always associated with withdrawal as the patient may experience persistent hallucinations while drinking. The 'voices' often offer a running commentary on the patient's actions and may be friendly or accusatory and threatening. Alcoholic hallucinosis may resemble paranoid schizophrenia or an amphetamine psychosis, and differential diagnosis is important.

Recovery may be abrupt or the 'voices' may fade away slowly, though one attack of alcoholic hallucinosis means that the risk of recurrence once drinking starts again is often high. In most cases hallucinosis does not indicate an underlying psychiatric disorder but is simply the response of the central nervous system to alcohol withdrawal, though a small percentage of patients with chronic hallucinosis will go on to develop mental disorder resembling schizophrenia.

Convulsive seizures ('rum fits') develop in response to withdrawal in a minority of alcoholics and these reflect the fact that seizure threshold drops with blood alcohol levels. The seizures are major epileptiform seizures, of the grand mal type, and an uncommon but serious complication is the development of *status epilepticus* in which seizures follow one another with virtually no intervening periods of consciousness. Seizures are most likely to occur from 12 to 41 hours after stopping drinking but they can occur up to one week after the last drink.

The most serious form of alcohol withdrawal syndrome is *delirium tremens* (DT's), which literally translates as 'trembling delirium'. Not all patients experiencing DT's will develop a state of delirium as some will simply experience tremor and hallucinatory experiences. The presence of delirium is a serious sign as mortality rates of 15–20% have been reported (Kinney and Leaton, 1983).

Edwards (1982) lists nine classical features of delirium tremens. These are as follows:

1 *Delirium.* The patient has clouded consciousness and grasp of reality fluctuates. There is often disorientation for time, place and person. Delirium may remit briefly, only to reassert itself.

2 *Hallucinations.* These may affect any of the five senses and are usually vivid and bizarre. The patient may 'see' visions of animals (snakes, rats, insects) and hallucinations are often horrifying or threatening. Hallucinations may be triggered off by illusory misperceptions—the pattern on the wallpaper may be mistaken for snakes (illusion) and the snakes may leave the wall and crawl towards the patient (hallucination). *Lilliputian hallucinations* may occur (hallucinations of objects or people reduced in size, e.g. small animals or men dancing around the room).

3 *Tremor.* At worst the patient may be shaking so badly that the bed is rattling or, at the other extreme, the tremor may not be discernible unless the patient is asked to stretch out his hands. Tremor, in extreme cases, may affect the facial muscles so that teeth chatter and speech becomes indistinct. The tongue may even flutter uncontrollably.

4 *Fear*. There is often a prevailing mood of terror ('the horrors') in response to hallucinatory experiences and for illusory misperceptions, though some patients appear to be quite unperturbed.

5 *Paranoid delusions*. Contribute to feelings of terror, particularly if coupled with paranoid *mood*. The patient suspects that some nameless conspiracy is afoot and that assassins lurk behind every corner.

6 *Occupational delusions or hallucinations*. These are common and the patient acts out activities associated with his occupation. The barman pours out imaginary drinks or the bricklayer builds an imaginary wall.

7 *Restlessness and agitation*. This is partly a consequence of the fearfulness of the hallucinatory experiences and the patient may jump out of bed and attempt to flee from imaginary enemies or may startle at any sound. The risk of falls and accidents is high.

8 *Heightened suggestibility*. The patient will deal from an imaginary pack of cards or drink from an empty glass if these are offered to him. This may serve to confirm suspicions of DT's in the early stages.

9 *Physical disturbances*. These include tachycardia, low grade pyrexia, sweating, dehydration, hypertension and exhaustion. There is a risk of a sudden and disastrously steep rise in temperature followed by collapse, so careful nursing observation must be coupled with careful monitoring of vital signs.

The condition tends to last for 3–5 days with the occasional case continuing for some weeks (Edwards, 1982) and there is always the risk of intercurrent chest infection or pneumonia, causing serious risk. In 80% of cases DT's subside within three days, the patient then falling into a deep sleep and awakening feeling better with little memory of what has happened.

Personal accounts of the experience of DT's abound in literature and a recent graphic account has been given by a senior nurse who describes 'The day the strangers came' (Anon, 1984):

'As I went about my business, weird bangs had suddenly materialized from God knows where, very sonorous deep and menacing. They frightened the life out of me but I put it down to atmospherics, leaky gas and so on. Then there were voices. Not too loud, not persistent, but whispers in passing, subtle giggles or a firm intonation from just outside the window. Again, this puzzled me but did not unduly worry me as they always went away very quickly. I tried to talk back once or twice, I remember, but no-one replied. I put it all down to rich imagination. So, the voices and I formed an uneasy alliance, companions in a sinister precursor to the nightmare which was to follow.' (As withdrawal progresses, alcoholic hallucinosis is replaced by DT's—Ed.) 'I first noticed my two little sons hugging each other in terror, huddled together on a chair. Their eyes burned into me and silently accused me of being anything but a father . . . all around the room little furry animals were hopping and running . . . my body was now becoming wracked with convulsions . . . then the insects arrived, but insects of a nature I had never seen before. Large, multi-coloured masses moved and crawled over the walls; vicious heads and tentacles lashed from them. They moved towards me then disappeared. I couldn't understand this behaviour and felt an awesome curiosity . . . (the convulsions worsened and then the 'voices' reappeared—Ed.) . . . male voices of a coarse nature. "Get him, the bastard" I heard them say quite plainly. They were hatching some vile plot to get me and I could not understand why! (At this stage, the patient's wife drove him to hospital at his request and he was admitted—Ed.). 'Faces appeared, floated in space for a while, and then disappeared. And all the time around me the haunting, taunting voices, plotting, planning and conniving . . . I can remember drinking my own urine . . . that example is all I can give . . .'

The patient fortunately made a good recovery and was discharged home to his family.

This account describes how alcoholic hallucinosis may progress into DT's which is heralded by major epileptiform seizures. This progression is not inevitable and may be arrested by prompt treatment.

Not all cases of DT's or hallucinosis are associated with withdrawal. Sometimes these syndromes arise while the patient is still drinking and may be associated with intercurrent illness or physiological upset.

Chronic Brain Failure

There is some dispute about alcoholism as a course of chronic brain failure (alcoholic dementia) per se (Trethowan and Sims, 1983), though it has been suggested that cerebral atrophy can occur in alcoholics in their fifties and sixties (Kinney and Leaton,

1983)—the so-called 'wet brain'. Korsakoff's syndrome, though severely incapacitating, should not be considered as a form of dementia (Trethowan and Sims, 1983) although it may mimic it.

Residual defects of memory and perception may be the result of years of alcohol abuse, though these defects may only be apparent at psychometric testing (Meyer and Salmon, 1984). Residual disability of this sort is most likely in females.

The Treatment of Alcoholism

Treatment must be directed against the physical, psychological and social problems exhibited by the alcoholic and a first step is usually *detoxification* ('drying out'), sedation usually being required to cover withdrawal symptoms. Chlormethiazole (Heminevrin) is useful as it has sedative, anticonvulsant and muscle-relaxant qualities, and phenothiazines or benzodiazepines may also be used (the latter group also possessing muscle-relaxant properties). Anticonvulsants and hypnotics may also be necessary but major attention must be paid to the patient's general health and nutritional status, both of which are often poor.

High dosage vitamin preparations are given parenterally at first (Parentrovite) and then orally (Orovite) in order to correct deficiencies and reverse any tendencies towards Wernicke–Korsakoff syndrome or delirium tremens. Detoxification and stabilization of general health and nutritional status are usually adopted as virtually first-aid measures.

Fear of withdrawal effects may be high on admission and much psychological support will be needed.

Intervention aimed at psychological problems may commence after detoxification and a variety of approaches have been tried. *Behavioural techniques* may be based on classical or operant conditioning and aim to break down the maladaptive drinking behaviour shown by the alcoholic. *Aversion therapy* involves establishing an association between the drinking of alcohol (or the thought of it) and an unpleasant stimulus such as nausea and vomiting (resulting from the administration of an emetic) or pain (resulting from electroshock).

Therapeutic gains have been modest and of short duration (Berrios and Dowson, 1983) and the use of emetics carries considerable risk (of inhalation of vomitus or cardiovascular complications). Aversion

therapy may also be interpreted as punitive by the patient and may thus militate against the formation of therapeutic relationships.

Other behavioural approaches, for which some success has been claimed, include filming the patient when he is intoxicated and subsequently showing him the film when he is sober (filming of drunken comportment) and giving electroshock in response to inappropriate drinking behaviour (e.g. drinking too fast). Environmental control of drinking (similar to environmental control of obesity) has also been used and encourages the patient to identify environmental 'triggers' which lead to problem drinking and devise strategies for their modification or avoidance.

Biofeedback may be used to provide problem drinkers with information about their blood alcohol levels. As obese individuals are often unaware of how much and how fast they eat, alcoholics are often surprisingly less competent than 'normal' drinkers in judging their blood alcohol level (Meyer and Salmon, 1984).

Psychotherapy may be offered formally or informally. Formal approaches have included rational emotive therapy, family and/or marital therapy and insight-directed psychotherapy. Studies suggest that persons receiving formal psychotherapy had higher recovery rates than those only receiving standard care, though they tended to relapse at 12-month follow-up (Brandsma, 1979).

Controlled drinking may be offered as an alternative to total abstinence but is only suitable for carefully selected groups of alcohol abusers. Davies (1962) reported a group of seven former chronic alcoholics who were all drinking in a moderate, controlled manner for periods ranging from 7 to 11 years after treatment. None had been intoxicated during the follow-up period and none had received extensive psychotherapy or continuous follow-up assistance. These findings initiated controlled drinking programmes which aim to return the patient to a pattern of 'normal' social drinking which will not interfere with physical, psychological or social well-being, though there is a danger that even small quantities of alcohol may continue to have harmful effects on already established cerebral or hepatic disease.

Controlled drinking is only suitable for highly motivated problem drinkers who have a stable personality and who enjoy social support (e.g. have a job and/or family and supportive friends). Cerebral or hepatic pathology are contraindications and these

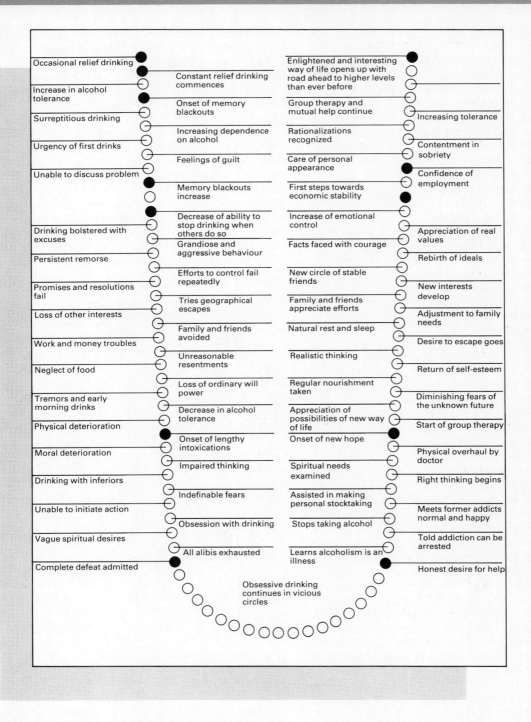

Figure 13 A chart of alcohol addiction and recovery. (From Glatt, M. M. with kind permission of the author and editor of *The British Journal of Addiction*.)

programmes are also unsuitable for the 'derelict' or insightless alcoholic.

Complete abstinence may be regarded as the most appropriate objective for many problem drinkers. This is the philosophy of Alcoholics Anonymous for example ('one drink, one drunk').

Aversive drugs may be used to promote abstinence. These are drugs which arrest the metabolism of alcohol at the level of *acetaldehyde*, a toxic degradation product of alcohol, causing unpleasant physiological reactions.

Disulfiram (Antabuse) is one such drug. It causes a range of aversive responses associated with a rise in acetaldehyde levels together with a relative deficiency of noradrenaline. The reaction starts 10–25 minutes after ingestion of alcohol, and is characterized by palpitations, profuse sweating, skin flushing, nausea (sometimes followed by vomiting), severe headache and general malaise. A severe reaction could include a fall in blood pressure followed by cardiovascular shock which might prove fatal (Berrios and Dowson, 1983).

Disulfiram should not be given until the patient has been administered a *test dose* to induce a controlled reaction in hospital. The patient is given disulfiram (400 mg orally) for at least four days, followed by 600 mg on the day of the controlled reaction. An hour after the 600 mg dose, 50 ml of ethanol is given and the patient is observed closely while vital signs (blood pressure and pulse) are recorded at 10-minute intervals. If no reaction occurs, the same dose of ethanol is repeated at 15-minute intervals up to a maximum of 150–200 ml. In the case of hypotensive shock, 10 mg of intravenous noradrenaline may be administered and the administration of alcohol is discontinued. This induced reaction not only ensures that the patient is fit to be maintained on the drug but also reinforces the deterrent effect of the drug. The daily maintenance dose of disulfiram is 200 mg and side-effects include headache, nausea, fatigue or impotence and an unpleasant taste in the mouth. Severe side-effects may require the discontinuation of disulfiram and its substitution by *calcium carbamide* (*Abstem*), which has fewer side-effects, at a daily dose of 100 mg.

Both disulfiram and calcium carbamide can be taken for an indefinite period, though occasional psychotic states and basal ganglia disturbances have been described in association with prolonged use of disulfiram (Berrios and Dowson, 1983).

Compliance may be low and abdominal wall

implants have been tried in patients who defaulted on drug regimes or lacked the determination to take it by mouth. Implants frequently do not produce plasma levels required for a reaction to take place and, overall, the use of aversive drugs has not made major inroads into the problem of alcohol abuse (Meyer and Salmon, 1984).

Social difficulties may be widespread in alcoholism and treatment of psychological problems may generalize to produce gains in social functioning. Social support may be provided by *Alcoholics Anonymous* (AA), a self-help organization founded in 1935 by two recovered alcoholics. AA clearly accepts the disease model of alcoholism but, paradoxically, has tried to urge the patient to reject the 'sick role' (Brandsma, 1979). The objective of AA is total *abstinence* and the approach incorporates

Table 92 AA members' alcohol-related problems 1976 and 1964.

Problems	Men 1976 %	Men (1964) (%)	Women 1976 %	Women (1964) (%)	Total 1976 N	Total %
Physical						
Blackouts	88.9	(95.0)	83.9	(91.0)	149	87.1
Too drunk to stand	85.2		87.1		147	85.9
Severe morning shakes	79.6	(84.0)	76.2	(72.0)	131	77.1
'Seeing things'	44.4		41.9		75	43.5
DTs	38.0		37.1		65	35.3
'Heard voices'	38.9	(48.0)	29.0	(38.0)	61	33.6
Mental						
Deep shame	89.8		96.8		158	92.4
Extremely depressed	90.7		91.9		156	91.2
Extremely frightened	82.4		83.9		141	82.9
Uncontrollable anger	67.6		67.7		115	67.6
Unable to trust anyone	62.0		59.7		104	61.2
Attempted suicide	34.3	(26.0)	48.8	(47.0)	68	39.4
Social						
Neglected the family	72.8		70.5		124	71.7
Severe money problems	66.7		37.7		98	56.0
Trouble with police	62.9		26.2		87	49.4
Lost a job	58.1	(63.0)	31.1	(43.0)	85	48.2
Broken marriage	38.1	(35.0)	44.3	(28.0)	72	40.4
Been in fights	38.1	(40.0)	21.3	(19.0)	58	31.9

From Robinson (1979) with kind permission of the publisher, Croom Helm.

four elements: (a) the requirement that they clearly admit that they need help, (b) the informal group-therapy type format of AA meetings, (c) the availability of support at times of crisis, and (d) the chance for broad-spectrum social contacts with non-drinkers. AA has proved successful in the treatment of many problem drinkers but accurate assessment of the efficacy of their approach is difficult as anonymity is conferred on those who attend. When the alcoholic has been coerced into attending, AA is less effective than other approaches (Trethowan and Sims, 1983), and some patients find AA's evangelical approach overpowering (Jahoda and Cramond, 1972).

Al-Anon is an offshoot of AA and offers support and counselling to the spouses and families of alcoholics and to teenagers with an alcoholic parent.

Prevention of Alcohol Abuse

Many of the problems resulting from alcohol abuse are the result of the distorted attitudes which society holds towards alcohol. Jahoda (1972) indicates that children seem to form their attitudes towards alcohol at a very early age, and health education units suggest that health education during the first few years of primary school would be more effective than the common practice of delaying it until the final years of secondary schooling when drinking patterns are already established.

Alcohol education for the young is generally known as *primary prevention* and has as its aim 'the communication of a realistic and unambiguous set of values related to drinking'. Health education measures aimed at the general population are known as *secondary prevention*, and measures aimed at those known to be damaging themselves by problem drinking are known as *tertiary prevention*. The aim of preventive programmes should be to destroy the myths that heavy drinking may be evidence of 'sophistication' or 'manliness' and to indicate clearly the levels at which 'social drinking' becomes dangerous. Identification of the physical, social and psychological hazards of alcohol abuse is usually incorporated into these programmes as awareness of these dangers is often low.

Meyer and Salmon (1984) suggest the following steps in any prevention effort:

1 If children are to be allowed to drink alcohol at all, introduce them to it early and in moderation.
2 Associate use of alcohol with food and initially allow its use only on special occasions.
3 Provide a consistent model of low to moderate drinking, and use beverages such as beer and wine that have low alcohol content.
4 Never associate drinking behaviour with evidence of attainment of adulthood or other identity accomplishments.
5 Label excess drinking as stupid and in bad taste rather than as stylish or sophisticated.
6 Label help-seeking behaviour in people who have an alcohol problem as evidence of strength rather than weakness.
7 Encourage alcoholism education programmes in the community and public health measures such as a restriction on the use of alcohol in certain settings and age groups.

Clearly the nurse has a major role to play as health educator in this respect and may provide valuable informal and formal inputs to health education programmes.

Key Concepts

1 Alcoholism is a disorder in which dependence upon alcohol is causing interference with *physical*, *psychological* and *social* well-being.
2 Alcoholism may develop through the following progression: social use of alcohol → episodic abuse of alcohol → problem drinking → initial alcoholism → chronic alcoholism.
3 A sensible limit is 4–6 standard units two or three times a week for men and 2–3 units two or three times a week for women.
4 Women are more vulnerable than men to the risks of problem drinking, though there are fewer women alcoholics than men.
5 Suggested causes include genetic predisposition, metabolic defect, oral fixation, learned maladaptive drinking patterns, self-medication against anxiety, depression or low self-esteem and sociocultural pressures.
6 In any given case, a blend of these factors may interact to initiate and sustain heavy drinking.
7 Sociocultural norms seem to play a major part in determining international differences in incidence insofar as cultural attitudes may predispose to, or militate against, alcohol abuse.

8 Physical effects of chronic alcohol abuse may include widespread organ damage, and gastrointestinal, hepatic and cerebral symptoms are particularly serious complications.

9 Chronic alcohol abuse will cause the liver initially to become enlarged, then inflamed and finally to become cirrhosed.

10 *Alcoholic cirrhosis* (Laennec's cirrhosis) is a serious complication to which women are more prone.

11 Many physical complications are serious and some (e.g. cirrhosis) are potentially fatal.

12 *Wernicke–Korsakoff's syndrome* arises from cerebral deterioration associated with the vitamin deficiency common in chronic alcoholism.

13 Wernicke's syndrome is reversible but may progress on to the chronic, dysmnesic state of Wernicke–Korsakoff's syndrome.

14 *Foetal alcohol syndrome* places the unborn children of alcohol abusers at risk and consists of characteristic facial abnormalities usually combined with mental handicap.

15 Psychological effects are diverse and include craving, anxiety, depression, loss of efficiency and low self-esteem.

16 Social deterioration occurs as the alcoholic's lifestyle is adjusted to centre around alcohol at the expense of the family, friends and occupation.

17 Physical dependence is marked by withdrawal effects (tremor, seizures, hallucinosis and delirium tremens) which occur as the blood alcohol levels fall.

18 In *alcoholic hallucinosis* consciousness is unclouded, while there is variable clouding of consciousness in *delirium tremens*.

19 Delirium tremens (trembling delirium) is characterized by tremor delirium and hallucinations.

20 Delirium tremens does not always arise in response to withdrawal and not all patients show market tremor and delirium.

21 Treatment of alcoholism commences with *detoxification* coupled with correction of malnutrition and stabilization of general health.

22 Multi-vitamin preparations (Parentrovite) and anxiolytics/sedatives are used to prevent/suppress unpleasant effects of withdrawal.

23 Treatment may include *behavioural techniques* (aversion therapy, operant conditioning of drinking behaviour, biofeedback), psychotherapy, controlled drinking programmes, the use of aversive drugs (Antabuse or Abstem) and the teaching/reinforcement of coping skills.

24 Social stabilization may be assisted by attendance at Alcoholics Anonymous, while Al-Anon and Al-Ateen offer support to the spouses and teenage children of alcoholics.

25 Prevention programmes may be *primary* (aimed at young non-drinkers), *secondary* (aimed at the general population) or *tertiary* (aimed at those known to be damaging themselves by abuse of alcohol).

26 The major aim of prevention programmes is to create realistic and adaptive perceptions of the use of alcohol and to highlight the risks of abuse.

References

Anon (1984) The day the strangers came. *Nursing Times*, **80**(26): 51–54.

Berrios, G. & Dowson, J. (1983) *Treatment and Management in Adult Psychiatry*. London: Baillière Tindall.

Brandsma, J. (1979) *Outpatient Treatment of Alcoholism*. London: University Park Press.

Davies, D. (1962) Normal drinking in recovered alcohol addicts. *Quarterly Journal of Studies on Alcohol*, **23**: 94–104.

Edwards, G. (1982) *The Treatment of Drinking Problems*. Oxford: Grant McIntyre.

Glatt, M. (1982) *Alcoholism*. Kent: Hodder & Stoughton.

Goodwin, D. (1981) *Alcoholism—The Facts*. Oxford: Oxford University Press.

Goodwin, D., Schulsinger, F. & Hermansen, L. (1973) Alcohol problems in adoptees raised apart from alcoholic biologic parents. *Archives of General Psychiatry*, **28**: 243–289.

Gordis, E. & Kreek, M. (1977) *Current Problems in Obstetrics and Gynecology*, **1**(3): 27–30.

Grant, M. & Gwinner, P. (1979) *Alcoholism in Perspective*. Kent: Croom Helm.

Hayman, F. (1967) The myth of social drinking. *Psychiatric Spectator*, **8**.

HMSO (1981) *Understanding Alcohol and Alcoholism in Scotland*. Scottish Health Education Group.

Imrie, C. et al (1977) In Grant & Grant (Eds) *Alcoholism—New Knowledge and New Responses*. Kent: Croom Helm.

Ingram, I., Timbury, G. & Mowbray, R. (1981) *Notes on Psychiatry*. Edinburgh: Churchill Livingstone.

Jahoda, G. & Cramond, J. (1972) *Children and Alcohol*. London: HMSO.

Jones, M. (1971) Personality antecedents and correlates of drinking patterns in women. *Journal of Consulting and Clinical Psychology*, **36**: 61–70.

Kinney, J. & Leaton, G. (1983) *Loosening the Grip—A Handbook of Alcohol Information*. Oxford: C. V. Mosby.

Mangen, S. (1982) *Sociology and Mental Health*. Edinburgh: Churchill Livingstone.

Meyer, R. G. & Salmon, P. (1984) *Abnormal Psychology*. Herts: Allyn and Bacon.

O'Brien, R. & Chafetz, M. (1982) *The Encyclopaedia of Alcoholism*. London: Library Association.

Plant, M. (1975) Alcoholism in Scotland. *New Psychiatry*, Dec 4th.

Seixas, F. (1981) Alcohol. In *Substance Abuse*. Bristol: Williams and Wilkins.

Steiner, C. (1969) The alcoholic game. *Quarterly Journal of Studies on Alcohol*, **30**: 920–938.

Swinson, R. & Eaves, D. (1978) *Alcoholism and Addiction*. London: Macdonald & Evans.

Trethowan, W. & Sims, A. (1983) *Psychiatry, 5th edn*. London: Baillière Tindall.

25

Nursing the
Alcohol-Dependent Patient

In my judgement such of us who have never fallen
victims (to alcoholism) have been spared more by
the absence of appetite than from any mental or
moral superiority over those who have. Indeed, I
believe if we take habitual drunkards as a class,
their heads and their hearts will bear an
advantageous comparison with those of any other
class.

Abraham Lincoln

Alcohol-dependent persons may be unpopular
patients. Psychiatrists rate them as the least rewarding of psychiatric patients despite the evidence that
most improve with treatment (Manson and Ritson,
1984) and nurses should carefully consider their own
attitudes towards alcohol abuse before working with
this client group. Stereotyped beliefs about alcohol
abuse may give rise to critical judgemental or unrealistic attitudes which will create major obstacles
towards progress as they will be quickly detected by
patients. It may be helpful for the nurse to discuss
her attitudes with other staff members if there is a
tendency to regard the alcohol-dependent person
from the viewpoint of the 'Critical Parent'.

On admission, the alcohol-dependent patient is
likely to present a multiplicity of physical, psychological and social problems and may lack faith in
his/her own ability to restore balance to life. For this
reason hope and optimism, reflected in positive nursing attitudes, are essential. Lasting improvement
requires commitment—not just from the patient—
but from all members of the care team.

Nursing Assessment of the
Alcohol-Dependent Patient

Physical difficulties may present nursing
problems—for example, withdrawal syndrome,
poor nutritional status, food intolerance and
insomnia—and careful observation and charting of

vital signs may be required for the first 72 hours.

Psychological problems may include failure to
recognize and accept alcohol dependence,
resentment, lack of cooperation, and disruptive attitudes and behaviour.

Social problems may include marital/domestic
friction, impaired employment prospects, financial
difficulties, and criminal charges pending, and all
will be worsened by any reluctance on the patient's
part to break ties with the 'alcoholic subculture'.
Family and relatives will have much need of
support, and the social worker may help to restore
some order to the chaos alcohol abuse may have
caused.

Planning nursing care falls into three phases:

1 Guiding the patient through *detoxification* and
possibly the *withdrawal syndrome*
2 Assisting the patient to formulate realistic strategies for *coping* with life without alcohol, and
completing unfinished psychological 'business'
associated with the period of abuse
3 Helping to arrange continuing *support* for the
patient and his family in association with other
members of the care team

Throughout all three phases the patient may also
require assistance with problems related to activities
of daily living.

Implementing Nursing Care

Detoxification/withdrawal

Bed rest for the first 72 hours will promote the physical and mental rest that most patients will need and
will enable accurate nursing observations to be
made. During withdrawal most patients are anxious
and fearful as they have very real fears of the withdrawal syndrome. In consequence some patients
may be uncooperative or even aggressive and much
reassurance will be needed. The nurse should show
that she recognizes the problem drinker as an individual confronting a difficult task and should

explain withdrawal symptoms, emphasizing that they will pass.

The patient should be nursed in a quiet, well-ventilated room with adequate lighting (day and night). Fluid balance should be charted and oral fluids encouraged. Excessive quantities of tea, coffee or cigarettes should be avoided as these have a stimulant effect. Large quantities of fruit juice are preferable and intramuscular vitamins (Parentrovite) are usually given daily for the first week, while oral vitamins are given for four weeks thereafter. Temperature, pulse and respiration rates should be charted at 4-hourly intervals, as a rising pulse or temperature are common warnings of severe withdrawal effects. Appetite will be poor for most of the first week and a light diet, rich in protein, is desirable. Dyspepsia and nausea may be marked and food supplements (of the Complan variety) may then be used.

The nurse should discreetly observe for signs of the withdrawal syndrome and should report these immediately. Withdrawal responses may be mild, moderate or severe and always necessitate increased nursing support and observation. Mild withdrawal responses will include tremor, nausea and vomiting (even attempts to use a toothbrush may cause retching), tachycardia and sweating. Moderate withdrawal responses include agitation, restlessness, marked tremor, convulsions, hallucinations and disorientation. Severe responses consist of fully blown delirium tremens, usually accompanied by pyrexia. Ataxia and/or paralysis of the eye muscles indicate the onset of Wernicke's encephalopathy and necessitate urgent treatment with intravenous thiamine.

During withdrawal the patient may be prone to illusional misinterpretation of sensory stimuli—shadows seem like threatening monsters and the pattern on the counterpane may seem like snakes. For this reason a quiet, well-lit room and quietness in manner and speech are essential. Sudden and abrupt approaches to the patient should be avoided.

Detoxification is not an end in itself but merely enables the patient to consider lasting solutions. The patient who is discharged after detoxification is simply fit enough to start drinking heavily again.

Assisting the alcohol-dependent person with activities in living

The alcohol-dependent person may require assistance with many activities in living during the first week or two of hospitalization.

1 Maintaining a safe environment

The patient who is experiencing delirium tremens is liable to be confused and restless. Falls and other accidents are likely unless careful and discreet observation is maintained. Cot sides are not a good idea as the bars may trigger illusional misinterpretation and heighten restlessness. Risk of suicide or parasuicide may be high. Many problem drinkers accrue enormous debts, and loss of employment, status, self-esteem and loss of stable family relationships may have taken place. Feelings of guilt and depression may be high and should be noted. Early involvement of the community psychiatric nurse and the social workers' department may help to repair some of the damage caused, and stresses should be identified (rates/rent arrears, building society threatening to foreclose on mortgage, gas/electricity disconnected due to failure to pay bills, spouse/children experiencing hardship, children taken into care). In cases like this the maxim that 'the whole is more than equal to the sum of its parts' is certainly true and the client must be encouraged to rationally sort out jumbled and overwhelming areas of threat so that they may be addressed in order of priority, and appropriate assistance enlisted.

Suicidal verbalization or plans should be reported and the feelings giving rise to them should be calmly and supportively discussed by the nurse who may

Table 93 Maintaining a safe environment.

Problem	Objective	Action
Risk of accidental injury during withdrawal	To ensure patient's safety at all times	Careful observation
Risk of suicide/parasuicide		Supportive and empathetic identification and discussion of problems

provide a valuable 'safety valve' for pent-up tensions by simply active listening.

2 *Communication*

Robinson (1979) comments that 'before a problem can be shared it has to be defined'. Communication will not be effective unless the problem drinker feels enough trust in the nurse to be able to make a thorough personal inventory without evoking unrealistic or judgemental responses from the nurse. Such self-examination may be prompted by the nurse briefly discussing the physical, psychological and social hazards of uncontrolled drinking and by inviting the client to briefly sketch out the history of his/her own alcohol problems. Factual understanding of the problem is essential and educative work must be free from any suggestions of censure on the nurse's part.

Feelings of shame and guilt are likely to be particularly high in the case of female problem drinkers and attitudes of acceptance and unconditional positive regard on the part of the nurse will do much to reduce these feelings.

Self-esteem will often be very low and it is often helpful for the nurse to emphasize positive achievements and to convey feelings of optimism and commitment. The problem drinker may initially find it difficult to trust the nurse; one survey revealed that 62% of male and 60% of female AA members felt 'unable to trust anyone' (Robinson, 1979) (Table 92). Trust cannot be demanded but must be earned and should develop against a background of openness, warmth and consistency on the part of the nurse.

3 *Expressing sexuality*

Many alcohol abusers develop deeply ingrained suspicions that their spouse has been unfaithful. These feelings range from mild but lingering suspicions to a deeply held delusional conviction that the sexual partner is being unfaithful (the *Othello syndrome*). Men are affected three times as often as women and states of morbid jealousy may lead to physical violence being directed against the partner, usually on the flimsiest or most improbable 'evidence' of infidelity.

Impotence may result from chronic alcohol abuse and this may be mediated, at least in part, physiologically (remember hypogonadism associated with an increase in circulating female hormones). The spouse may have rejected the partner completely as a steadily failing and stressful relationship, punctuated by neglect and physical or emotional violence, hardly makes for positive interpersonal attitudes. The client may benefit from 'talking out' tensions to the nurse, and the spouse may be involved in these sessions at which much unfinished psychological business may emerge.

In the case of profound or intractable difficulties, assistance may be sought from the psychology department and/or a marriage counsellor.

4 *Working and playing*

The client should be encouraged to realistically review employment prospects and to consider alternative options. The person in a high-risk occupation (e.g. bar staff) should consider seeking alternative employment.

Table 94 Communication.

Problem	Objective	Action
Low recognition of the problems of dependence; reluctance to confront difficulties	To improve awareness of and insight into the nature of dependence	Development of a nurse/patient relationship which educates, supports, guides and also facilitates self-awareness

Table 95 Expressing sexuality.

Problem	Objective	Action
Jealousy, sexual dysfunction, rejection by spouse	To help restore stable patterns of sexual functioning	Supportive discussion with referral to specialist counselling where necessary

Table 96 Working and playing.

Problem	Objective	Action
Loss or risk of loss of employment and friends	To stabilize employment prospects	Counselling with referral to social work department
Atrophy of previous patterns of recreational activities	Re-establish awareness of constructive social activities	Provide patterns of recreational activity

Many clients will attempt to make some reparation to friends who have suffered from the results of the client's uncontrolled drinking. The nurse may help here by ensuring that the client has ready access to the telephone and writing requisites, and by ensuring that visiting policy is informal and flexible.

Discussion of previously enjoyed hobbies, interests and recreational pursuits may help provide outlets and there should be provision of recreational outlets in hospital.

5 Sleeping

Provision of a quiet, evenly lit and well-ventilated room will reduce insomnia and will also reduce the likelihood of illusional misinterpretation (most frequent at night). Stimulants (tea, coffee) should be avoided before bedtime and the doctor may prescribe a hypnotic.

6 Eating and drinking

Malnutrition is commonly observed in the recently admitted problem drinker. Alcohol will have been providing the majority of the client's dietary calories and will also have created gastrointestinal problems leading to food intolerance. A light diet, rich in protein, should be provided and the patient's likes and dislikes should be respected (where possible). Vitamin supplements (Parentrovite followed by Orovite) are likely to be routinely prescribed. Fluid balance should be charted for the first week and the client should be weighed weekly.

7 Cleansing and dressing

If self-esteem is low there is often loss of interest in personal hygiene and appearance. The nurse should gently prompt the patient to attend to personal

Table 97 Sleeping.

Problem	Objective	Action
Insomnia	To ensure adequate sleep and rest	Provide suitable sleeping environment. Reduce factors worsening insomnia

Table 98 Eating and drinking.

Problem	Objective	Action
Risk of inadequate dietary intake	To restore nutritional status	Provide balanced diet with vitamin supplements, and monitor nutritional status

Table 99 Cleansing and dressing.

Problem	Objective	Action
Risk of loss of interest in personal hygiene and dress	To restore same	Prompt, shape and reinforce

hygiene and visitors may be asked to bring in some of the client's favourite clothes or toilet requisites. Improvements should be noted and warmly reinforced.

8, 9 and 10 *Breathing/elimination/mobilizing*

No specific problems are likely, though care must be taken to observe for any signs of peripheral neuritis (mobilizing).

11 *Controlling body temperature*

Temperature, pulse and respiration rate should be recorded at 4-hourly intervals for the first week, and any pyrexia reported.

12 *Dying*

Risk of suicide should be taken into account (highest in female problem drinkers).

Coming to terms with dependence

The alcohol-dependent person must accept that his/her drinking pattern is dangerous to his/her continuing physical, psychological and social well-being and must seriously consider ways of coping without alcohol. Critical or moralistic nursing attitudes will simply foster rationalization and denial of the problem, whereas a supportive and positive interpersonal climate will foster self-examination and the motivation to break the drinking pattern.

Self-esteem and self-confidence will often be low and agitation or depression may ensue as the patient now has time to survey his/her recent past from a standpoint of sobriety. Feelings of guilt about harm caused to others during the period of lost control may be strong and the nurse should be prepared to sympathetically act as 'confessor' on occasion. Need to make some form of reparation may be strong and the nurse should try to dissuade the patient from making impulsive or extravagant gestures in this respect (one patient wanted to sell his house so that he could make financial reparation to a large number of 'victims' of his drinking). There may be much 'unfinished business' in the form of feelings of resentment, guilt, jealousy or anger and the nurse may promote constructive consideration of these feelings so that the patient may approach the task of considering sobriety unburdened by excessive tensions.

Setting of goals with the patient should be realistic

and should emphasize the 'here and now'. Alcoholics Anonymous recognizes the dangers of sweeping or over-ambitious goal setting in their suggestion that the alcohol-dependent person should approach life 'one day at a time'. Living in the 'here and now' should be coupled with commitment towards not only eradicating problem drinking patterns but towards considering the future activities which will replace problem drinking.

The alcohol-dependent person will have spent most of his/her recent past either drinking, recovering from drinking, thinking about alcohol or confronting difficulties arising from problem drinking. Life will have revolved around drinking and the removal of alcohol will leave an enormous void which must be filled with constructive patterns of activity. Hospitalization and detoxification will temporarily stabilize the life circumstances of the problem drinker and will provide a vantage point from which the future can be realistically considered. If detoxification is simply followed by discharge in a cloud of well-meaning promises, the chance of rapid relapse is very high. The problem drinker must be encouraged to consider ways of restoring stability to life, of restoring some order to the social ruins often created by problem drinking. This task may present seemingly insurmountable obstacles to the patient, so support, guidance, reassurance and education from the nurse is essential.

The problem drinker may have to consider repairing damaged relationships (with spouse, children, parents, friends and employers) and movement in this direction will help to create the social support which is so important if gains are to be maintained after discharge.

The problem drinker must also be encouraged to consider how he/she may constructively fill the 'empty hours' which will be created by the removal of uncontrolled drinking behaviour. Hobbies, interests and recreational activities formerly enjoyed may be discussed and encouraged in an attempt to lend some structure to the future.

It is not enough for the patient to verbalize commitment. This commitment must find expression in the formulation of a set of realistically structured goals—a plan for facing the future without alcohol abuse. Discussions aimed at identifying and reinforcing a stable lifestyle may identify abstinence or controlled drinking as the foundation of future strategies. Those with a long history of fully developed alcohol dependence and those who lack social support or who suffer from alcohol-induced physical problems are unlikely to achieve stable or safe patterns of controlled drinking; abstinence is then the only realistic goal.

Unthinking adherence to a philosophy of total abstinence will narrow the horizons of the health care professional if consideration of controlled drinking as a realistic and practical option for many clients does not take place. Edwards (1982) comments that the goal of abstinence may involve a change in lifestyle which is too difficult for many clients and 'the decision to advise the patient to aim for total abstinence may sometimes be ill-advised and result in the patient alternating sobriety with explosive relapses'.

Controlled drinking programmes aim at restoring 'normal' patterns of drinking by reducing the quantity and frequency of intake. A programme of this sort may resemble the following:

1 Buy a newspaper before entering pub.
2 On entering pub buy a pint of beer.
3 *Do not* begin to drink this first pint immediately but read newspaper for 5 minutes before commencing drinking.
4 Start pint but *do not gulp* and take at least 10 minutes over pint, replacing it on the table between mouthfuls and reading paper.
5 On finishing first pint wait for at least 5 minutes before ordering a second.
6 Take at least 10 minutes over second pint, again resisting the urge to gulp.
7 Wait for 5 minutes before ordering third (and final) pint.
8 Take 15 minutes over last pint—again—*no gulping*.
9 On finishing last pint wait for 5 minutes before leaving pub.
10 Make no more than 2–3 similar visits to the pub in a week—no drinking at home.

The client may be advised to choose times when the pub is likely to be quiet; Friday and Saturday night crowds should be avoided. Speed of drinking should be gradually reduced and the aim should be to eventually make a pint of beer last for 25–30 minutes.

'Competing activities' should be identified. For example, the client may discover that a game of darts, chess, draughts or pool may divert attention away from drinking by providing substitute channels of activity. The lonely housewife who has identified afternoons as a peak risk period for heavy drinking should decide upon suitable competing activities for this time (e.g. shopping, visiting a friend).

Initially the nurse may accompany the patient to the pub to prompt, support and perhaps to provide a model of controlled drinking (if only of fruit juice). The spouse is the person with whom controlled drinking may most safely be attempted and thus should be involved in such a programme from its inception.

Intense craving for alcohol does not build up until it becomes intolerable, but passes after an hour or so, during which time support and competing activities are important. The fact that craving will reduce after reaching a peak should be emphasized to the problem drinker and competing activities should be decided upon.

Arranging continuing support

Continuing support should involve the family, who should be involved in discussing the programme from the outset. It is important to ensure that the family (a) understands the facts about alcohol dependence, and (b) is motivated to help. Marriage guidance counselling may help the couple to re-establish mutual trust and the nurse may promote constructive and sympathetic discussion of any residual tensions or resentments which may militate against progress after discharge.

The client should be encouraged to practise saying '*no*'; simple role-play will help develop confidence in this direction. The nurse may ask the client 'What will you say when you meet an old friend in the street and are promptly invited into the pub? How will you respond when well-meaning friends try to force a drink upon you? (for example, "go on—one won't hurt you—don't be a wet blanket") What will you say when friends arrive at your door with a bottle/cans? How are you going to handle Christmas, New Year, holidays?'

The client must consider these risk situations in advance. It will be too late to try to 'ad lib' in an unprepared way once the situation has developed.

The nurse may role-play the part of the insistent but well-meaning friend who is outraged at the refusal of a drink. Make it realistic—make the dialogue as taxing as it may be in real life—and keep it up until the client feels confident about his/her ability to say '*no*' in a variety of situations. Then get another staff member or patient to play the part of the insistent friend and continue until the response pattern becomes one that the client is comfortable with. Some clients prefer to say 'I have a liver problem and the doctor has told me that even small amounts of alcohol could be dangerous for me'. Others prefer to say bluntly 'I have had a drink problem and I would appreciate it if you could help by not offering me alcohol'.

Situations creating high risk of relapse should be identified. It is not a good idea for the recovering problem drinker to go on holiday with friends to a Mediterranean resort where alcohol is liable to be both cheap and almost constantly available. The office party, pub lunches with colleagues, weddings, and attending a football match are all danger areas that must be identified, and the client must either decide that, realistically, some are best avoided altogether or that ways of coping should be carefully worked out *before* the event.

Job interviews may be highly anxiety-evoking for the recovering problem drinker and, again, the client must be prepared for these. Previous work record may have been poor due to uncontrolled drinking, and absenteeism may have been high. Employers may have found it necessary to adopt disciplinary action and the client may have been dismissed from one or more previous posts.

The client may feel stigmatized and discredited—social identity has been 'spoiled'. It is helpful for the client to consider his/her feelings in this respect and the nurse should facilitate discussion of troublesome feelings in an attempt to enable the client to come to terms with them. The client must recognize that others may well have negative feelings about the problem drinker but must be cautioned against accepting as his own the negative attitudes that others may display. What other people think of us may, to a large extent, determine what we think of ourselves. Self-image is influenced by the overt and covert judgements of others, and persistent negative feedback may lead the problem drinker to wearily accept the negative role assigned to him by others.

Goffman (1963) warns against the resignation which may set in 'whereby the stigmatized person ingratiatingly acts out before normals the full dance of bad qualities imputed to his kind, thereby consolidating a life situation into a clownish role'. A combination of relapses and rejection (the relapses often triggered by rejection) may sap commitment and self-esteem and may lead the problem drinker to embark upon a new 'career' as a hopeless 'drunk'.

Optimism may be high before discharge as self-confidence returns with sobreity, and this is both desirable and helpful. Feelings of confidence must not become dangerously unrealistic, however, as incautious or over-confident attitudes simply pave the way to relapse and despair.

Job interviews highlight the importance of comfortable and confident 'presentation of self', Many clients find it best to simply say to prospective employers: 'yes, I have had a drink problem but have obtained help and have been abstinent/controlled for some time now. I realize that this may cause you to immediately regard me as being unsuitable but I would appreciate it if you would give me a trial for three months'. Prospective employers are just as liable to respond positively to honesty as they are to respond negatively to lies or evasions.

Alcoholics Anonymous has been claimed to be responsible 'for the sobriety of more alcoholics than any other therapy' (Robinson, 1983), though it is difficult to assess the veracity of statements like this due to the lack of comprehensive studies.

Alcoholics Anonymous (AA) has 1500 groups in the UK and an estimated world membership of upwards of one million (Edwards, 1982). The nurse should be willing to discover how AA works and the best way of doing this is to attend an open meeting (one open to all comers)—the telephone number is in the directory. The nurse should have all the facts available concerning an agency before suggesting attendance by a client.

Once the nurse has made personal contact with AA it is thereafter possible to refer clients to members of AA who are now known personally to the nurse, rather than impersonally supplying a telephone number or address. AA members will visit the client before discharge and may provide a valuable source of social support and increased motivation. AA meetings are informal and only first names are used. Each meeting starts when the chairman (who will introduce himself by his first name only and acknowledge that he is an alcoholic) reads the AA preamble:

'Alcoholics Anonymous is a fellowship of men and women who share their experience, strength and hope with each other that they may solve their common problem and help others to recover from alcoholism. The only requirement for membership is a desire to stop drinking. There are no dues or fees for membership; we are self-supporting through our own contributions. AA is not allied with any sect, denomination, politics, organisation or institution, does not wish to engage in any controversy, neither endorses nor opposes any causes. Our primary purpose is to stay sober and help other alcoholics to achieve sobriety.'

As the meeting goes on, one or two speakers will each give a short autobiographical account of how alcohol abuse created problems for them and led to dependence, and how AA promoted sobriety and stability. The tenor of these accounts is open and honest and the speaker often emphasizes the deceit (of self and others), evasions and rationalizations which, for a long time, prevented him/her from confronting the problem of uncontrolled drinking. The 'Twelve Steps' which encapsulate the basic philosophy of AA are usually referred to during the meeting. They are as follows:

1 We admitted we were powerless over alcohol—that our lives had become unmanageable

2 Came to believe that a Power greater than ourselves could restore us to sanity

3 Made a decision to turn our will and our lives over to the care of God as we understood him

4 Made a searching and fearless moral inventory of ourselves

5 Admitted to God, to ourselves and to another human being the exact nature of our wrongs

6 Were entirely ready to have God remove all these defects of character

7 Humbly asked Him to remove our shortcomings

8 Made a list of all persons we had harmed and became willing to make amends to them all

9 Made direct amends to such people wherever possible, except when to do so would injure them or others

10 Continued to take personal inventory and, when we were wrong, promptly admitted it

11 Sought through prayer and meditation to improve our conscious contact with God as we understood Him, praying only for knowledge of His will for us, and the power to carry that out

12 Having had a spiritual awakening as the result of these steps, we tried to carry this message to alcoholics and to practise these principles in all our affairs.

The meeting ends with informal discussion over tea or coffee and the new member will meet regular attenders and perhaps find a 'sponsor' who will offer personal advice and will also provide his telephone number so that he may be contacted informally at any time.

Edwards (1982) identifies four dimensions of AA

through which the organization operates. These are:

1 Coherent flexible ideas

2 An action programme (e.g. the 'Twelve Steps')

3 Rewards of sobriety

4 Possibility of recovery

Remember that AA describes alcohol dependence as an incurable 'disease' and has only one approach—lifetime abstinence ('one drink, one drunk').

Manson and Ritson (1984) point out that 'the character of AA meetings varies enormously and it is worth encouraging the patient to shop around until they find a congenial setting'. Edwards (1982) points out that AA 'has much to teach the therapist about the processes which aid and influence recovery. There is wisdom to be borrowed from AA'.

The spouse of the problem drinker may benefit from contact with Al-Anon, an allied organization for 'anyone who loves an alcoholic', and the teenage children of problem drinkers may benefit from contact with Al-Ateen.

Councils on alcoholism also exist in most cities throughout the UK and will provide voluntary counselling and advice to problem drinkers and their families. Again, numbers are readily obtained in the directory.

The homeless problem drinker may be placed in a hostel/detoxification/rehabilitation centre where drinking is not allowed, thus promoting the development of social stability, without which sobriety is unlikely.

Relapses may often occur after discharge and should be regarded as positive learning experiences and not as evidence of the client's constitutional inability to make progress. Regular attendance at out-patient clinics is important and the client may admit to a relapse at such a return visit. The nurse should ask:

Where were you when the relapse occurred?
What were you doing when the relapse occurred?
How were you feeling when the relapse occurred?
Which factors can you identify which contributed to loss of control and commitment?
Who were you with?

Exercise of this kind may enable the client to develop greater awareness of 'trigger' factors and thus to develop strategies for coping with these.

Repeated relapses should lead to re-evaluation of the treatment programme and consideration of alternative approaches. The client should never be allowed to identify relapses as evidence of the fact that he/she is a 'hopeless case' and thereby rationalize further drinking. The 'hopeless case' does not exist.

Key Concepts

1 Alcohol-dependent patients are often unpopular and the nurse should critically assess her attitudes towards this client group.

2 Assessment may reveal multiple problems associated with reduced physical state.

3 Assessment of psychological factors should consider *motivation* and the patient's ability to recognize and deal with *high risk situations* in which relapse is likely.

4 Assessment of social difficulties may reveal multiple problems associated with disorganized lifestyle, domestic friction, employment and financial difficulties.

5 Planning care involves preparing to support the patient through *detoxification* and possibly *withdrawal*, helping the patient to formulate realistic strategies and arranging community support.

6 Much assistance with activities of daily living is often necessary during detoxification/withdrawal and the nurse should be alert to early signs of nervous system involvement.

7 *Psychotherapy* will help the patient to confront and resolve troublesome feelings (shame, depression, anger, resentment and lost self-esteem) generated during the period of problem drinking.

8 Goal setting should be realistic and should emphasize the skills of recognizing and dealing with high-risk situations (*coping skills*).

9 Coping skills may be developed and strengthened during the stay in hospital but must be accompanied by an increase in motivation—otherwise the patient may decide not to use these newly acquired skills.

10 *Abstinence* is most appropriate for patients with organ damage or who lack social support or minimal levels of motivation and control.

11 *Controlled drinking programmes* will benefit many problem drinkers who do not have alcohol-related organ damage and who do possess social support and reasonable levels of motivation.

12 Behavioural rehearsal will help clients to practise coping skills before discharge, and may take the form of simple role-play.

13 *Alcoholics Anonymous* will fulfil valuable educative, therapeutic and supportive functions for many clients, and contact should be made before discharge.

References

Edwards, G. (1982) *The Treatment of Drinking Problems*. Oxford: Grant McIntyre.

Goffman, E. (1963) *Stigma. Notes on the Management of Spoiled Identity*. Harmondsworth: Pelican.

Manson, L. & Ritson, E. (1984) *Alcohol and Health*. London: Medical Council on Alcoholism.

Robinson, D. (1979) *Talking out of Alcoholism*. Kent: Croom Helm.

Robinson, L. (1983) *Psychiatric Nursing as a Human Experience, 3rd edn*. Philadelphia: W. B. Saunders.

VII

MOTHERHOOD, PSYCHOSEXUAL DISORDERS, ANOREXIA AND SUICIDE

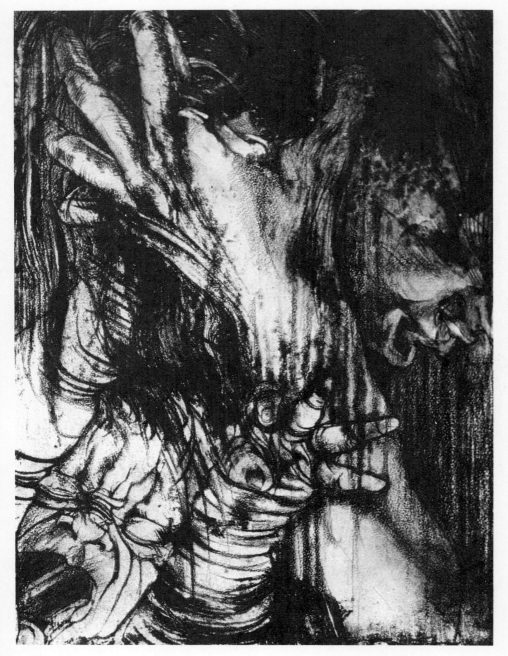

26

Motherhood and Mental Disorder

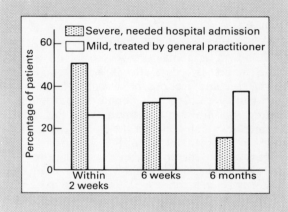

Figure 14 Time of onset of postnatal depression in 413 patients. From Dalton (1980), with kind permission of the publisher, OUP.

The 'happy event' of childbirth may be associated with an increased incidence of depressive disorders, ranging from the mild and transitory 'baby blues' to episodes of psychotic depression which may be of a schizophrenic nature.

Pitt (1982) identifies three conditions associated with childbirth: (a) the *'baby blues'*, (b) *neurotic (reactive) depressions*, and (c) *psychotic reactions*. He suggests that these disorders may lie along a continuum, the person's place on which is determined by constitution and stress.

Incidence

The incidence of post-partum psychosis is generally quoted as one admission per 1000 births, though it has been suggested that only a minority are admitted to psychiatric hospitals and that the true incidence may be of the order of one in 200 births (Pitt, 1982). In the first three months post-partum, women experience a four to five-fold increase in the risk of emotional disorder, particularly of psychosis (Melges, 1968).

Kumar (1984) estimates that a degree of neurotic depression may arise in as many as one in 10 recently delivered mothers, while the mild and transitory 'baby blues' is difficult to assess in terms of incidence as it has not often been deemed worthy of serious study (Yalom et al, 1968) though it has been estimated as arising in 50–66% of recently delivered women (Nott et al, 1976).

The Baby Blues (or 'post-partum blues syndrome')

This is a transient self-limiting state of emotional lability, sometimes called the 'three, four, or five day blues' after the usual time of onset, and sometimes called the 'ten day blues' after the usual duration of this state of emotional upheaval.

Weeping is the most characteristic symptom and may arise for relatively minor reasons. Weeping may alternate with rapid mood changes—for example, to hearty laughter—and the patient is usually apologetic for her displays of sadness. The patient will also show increased sensitivity to minor rebuffs and there may be feelings of helplessness, fatigue and poor concentration.

The episodic bouts of weeping seem to have a 'contagious' nature, and one writer comments that 'The nurses in the postnatal ward know that if they happen to drop a cup or saucer the whole ward will be crying in unison within a few minutes of the crash' (Dalton, 1980).

During the nineteenth century the 'baby blues' was known as 'milk fever' as it occurred during those days when milk was appearing in the breasts in quantity, and there is a possibility of endocrine causes (perhaps progesterone withdrawal). The contribution of social/psychological factors cannot be ignored as the recently delivered mother has undergone an abrupt change in body image and social status and is recovering from an experience which is as psychologically taxing as it is physically demanding. The euphoria of late pregnancy may be succeeded by feelings of 'flatness' as the new arrival now becomes the focus of attention.

Childbirth is a major psychosocial crisis and, while the first two days after delivery bring relief, satisfaction and feelings of accomplishment, the third and succeeding days herald the beginning of feeding, washing and changing. As Pitt (1982) comments: 'a baby outside the womb can be a lot more trouble than one within!'

Pressure on maternity beds often means that mother is discharged on the third or fourth day, and the abrupt increase in responsibilities, coupled with an equally abrupt withdrawal of the support of the hospital environment, may also play a part.

The importance of psychosocial factors (as opposed to endocrine factors) is supported by the findings of several studies which indicate that adoptive mothers have exhibited symptoms of depression typical of the psychological reactions often observed in post-partum mothers (Howell, 1981).

Reactive Depression following Childbirth

This does not differ significantly from reactive depression due to other causes, though the content is coloured by the recent event of childbirth.

The depression varies from day to day (with more bad days than good), and *irritability* is usually a marked feature. Women suffering from post-natal depression may have a yearning for sleep and can never get enough (Dalton, 1980) though there may be a degree of initial insomnia.

The mother may become preoccupied by the baby's health and crying—regurgitation of foods, rashes and snuffles may cause the greatest alarm. It has been suggested that the 'ailing' infant may be the presenting sign of post-natal depression (Carne, 1966).

Feelings of resentment and helplessness may result in 'baby battering', though post-natal depression accounts for only a very small minority of non-accidentally injured babies (Pitt, 1982).

Reactive depression is most likely in women suffering from work overload and isolation, particularly if there is lack of support from the partner.

It has been suggested that the extended family provided support and supplementary care for mother and infant of a nature unavailable to the now prevalent nuclear family. Accounts of cultures where the extended family is still prevalent describe little evidence of post-natal depression (Rossi, 1968), and the transition to parenthood may extract a high price in terms of social deprivation. Professional women who give up their work tend to be vulnerable to severe post-natal depression (Howell, 1981), and women returning to inadequate housing have an increased risk also (Pitt, 1982).

Mothers may be reluctant to admit to depression at a time traditionally regarded as a happy one, and many cases of reactive depression may therefore be undetected.

Post-natal Psychosis

Psychotic reactions to childbirth were, at one time, of a toxic, delirious nature, though these are now fortunately rare due to modern aseptic delivery practices.

The type of psychotic reaction most often observed now is of an *affective* nature (occasionally of *schizo-affective* nature), and these psychoses do not differ from those arising from causes unrelated to childbirth. The concept of a psychosis peculiar to childbirth ('puerperal psychosis') has waxed and waned in popularity, though consensus seems to be that 'the concept of a specific puerperal psychosis has long been discredited' (Pitt, 1982).

A nineteenth century observer commented that measles arising during the puerperium are not known as 'puerperal measles' (Brockington et al, 1982), though the risk of psychotic breakdown in the post-natal period is well-established, and the content of the disorder will be coloured by the recent crisis of childbirth.

Onset is usually acute after a night or two of restlessness, and symptoms usually appear a week or so after delivery.

The psychotic reaction is florid—persecutory delusions and auditory hallucinations are common, and there may be marked disorder of thought. Mothers sometimes express the belief that they or their babies are possessed, or even that the baby is dead or strangely altered in some unnatural way, only apparent to the mother.

One mother was noticed hammering the head of her baby: 'It's the wrong shape. It's too long', she explained (Dalton, 1980).

Depersonalization and derealization experiences may be marked: 'The day after the Caesarean operation I woke up and the world looked different and smelled different. Horrible. I was swearing at everyone. Everyone was laughing at me and shouting obscenities' (Brockington et al, 1982).

One patient explained that she had not given her baby a name because she thought she was a frog— she no longer believes this. 'It was a silly idea wasn't it?' She explained that the baby had been born in a ward named the Faraday Ward. 'He was the man who measured electricity in frogs' nerves wasn't he?' She remembered the doctors attaching wires to the baby's scalp during delivery (Kumar, 1984).

Suicidal impulses, and/or impulses to harm the baby, necessitate close observation: 'It was when baby Hugh looked up at me when I was breast-feeding. Those big blue eyes seemed to hypnotize me. I had a mad urge to stick a pin into those dark, black circular pupils—I loved the baby, yet felt absolutely murderous towards him (Dalton, 1980).

Despite the dangers of these impulses, actual injury to the baby occurs in only a small minority of cases and one study revealed that only three out of 93 mothers affected by psychosis during the post-natal period made any form of attack on the baby (Brockington et al, 1982).

Women suffering from any form of mental disorder form a minority of those who kill their babies under six months, being outnumbered by impulsively battering mothers, and comprising only 27% of a series admitted to Holloway prison (D'Orban, 1979).

Fortunately, the prognosis is excellent, and most mothers make a good recovery in 6–10 weeks, though there is often a tendency towards recurrence after future births (Brockington et al, 1982).

Risk is highest in women with a previous history of mental disorder and the incidence doubles amongst primiparae (women giving birth for the first time).

Treatment

Treatment is non-specific. 'Baby blues' is usually self-limiting and the only intervention required is increased support from family and nursing staff.

Reactive depressions respond to antidepressants and supportive psychotherapy, and many women benefit from attending a self-help group for depressed mothers.

Psychotic reactions to childbirth almost invariably require hospitalization as it is difficult to provide the careful observation required in the home setting—a moment's inattention could have catastrophic consequences. Electroplexy, antidepressants and antipsychotic drugs may be used, and marital and/or group therapy is beneficial. Hormone therapy (progesterone, thyroid extracts) have been tried without evidence of success (Pitt, 1982). The spouse and family should be involved and social support strengthened, and the patient should spend weekends at home as soon as this is feasible. Baby and mother are admitted together so that 'bonding' is not impaired and mother/child relationships are not disrupted unnecessarily.

Identification of the 'High-Risk' Mother

Gordon et al (1965) developed a list of 14 stress factors predictive of post-natal difficulties. These were as follows:
1 Primipara
2 No relatives to help with the baby
3 Complications of pregnancy in family history
4 Husband's father dead
5 Wife's mother dead
6 Wife ill during pregnancy
7 Wife ill, apart from pregnancy
8 Wife's education higher than that of her parents
9 Husband's education higher than that of his parents
10 Wife's education incomplete
11 Husband's occupation higher than that of his parents
12 Husband's occupation higher than that of his wife's parents
13 Husband often away from home
14 Wife has had no previous experience with babies

Forty per cent of women with scores above five (i.e. five of the 14 factors) experienced post-natal emotional difficulties, while only 6% of women with scores under four experienced these difficulties (Gordon et al, 1965).

To this list one may add poor housing, professional status of mother, family history of mental disorder, previous history of mental disorder and unsupportive attitudes of spouse. Post-natal difficulties do not seem to bear any relationship to social class.

Mental Disorder during Pregnancy

Psychotic reactions during pregnancy are rare, though there is a minor increase in neurotic (reactive) depressions during the first trimester (the first three months). High anxiety during the last trimester may forecast depression during the post-natal period.

Suicide during pregnancy is now extremely rare.

Mental Disorder Following Abortion

Psychosis after abortion is only a fifth as common as psychosis after childbirth while depressive and guilt reactions are neither common nor severe (Clark et al, 1968).

Repeat aborters tend to be in poorer health, have less favourable personality structures, have more sexual partners and have tried more types of birth control (Jacobsson et al, 1976).

Abortion during the second trimester carries increased risk of emotional difficulties, and supportive counselling is essential. Kahn-Edrington (1981) comments that 'the counsellor must have worked out his or her own feelings regarding abortion and birth. A belief in the client's right and responsibility to make her own decision is essential'.

The nurse may hold negative views on abortion and these should not colour nurse/patient interactions as they may then precipitate or exacerbate adverse psychological reactions. The bedside of an emotionally and physically traumatized woman is no place for displays of moral or religious bias.

Prevention of Post-Natal Depression

Primary prevention consists of identifying high-risk patients and ensuring that support and counselling are available, both during pregnancy and in the post-natal period.

Secondary prevention consists of rapid identification of those women showing adverse reactions to either pregnancy or childbirth and ensuring that prompt intervention is made.

Tertiary prevention involves effective treatment of established cases of mental disorder associated with childbirth in order to reduce both the severity and duration of emotional distress experienced by the mother.

The Short Report (Social Services Committee, 1980) was critical of the prevalent indifference in antenatal clinics and post-natal wards to women's emotional and social needs, and discussion of these aspects of care has taken place within the profession of midwifery. Ball and Stanley (1984) comment that ward 'routine' had three main effects in maternity hospitals: (a) it gave a false sense of security, (b) the lack of flexibility militated against patient-centred care, and (c) it sapped initiative and critical appraisal of practice among midwives. The authors go on to comment that 'Midwives seemed to be valued for "getting the work done in the morning", rather than for giving personalised care'.

Improved education about the psychosocial stresses associated with childbirth should not only be directed towards mothers (and their spouses) but should include all care givers.

Gordon et al (1965) showed that systematic education of expectant mothers reduced psychiatric morbidity in the post-natal period, and best results were obtained when husbands attended with their wives. Robson and Powell (1982) suggest that 'it would seem appropriate to forewarn mothers routinely about the possibilities of feeling detached from their infant after childbirth'.

It would be appropriate to indicate to primiparae that they must not expect a sudden gush of 'maternal instincts' as women are *not* automatically 'programmed' to love and effectively care for newly born babies. The appropriate skills and responses are *learned* ones, and supportive and insightful nursing staff can facilitate the development of a positive mother/child relationship.

Nursing Care

Nursing care is non-specific insofar as the nurses' interventions are the standard ones, directed against the difficulties experienced by the person suffering from depression (or mood elevation).

It should be emphasized that supportive psycho-therapy is the major nursing contribution and can produce rapid and lasting gains. Hayman (1962) points out that particularly rapid progress can be made in post-natal psychotherapy with achievements being made within months which, under different circumstances, may take years.

'Baby blues' is self-resolving and usually merely requires additional support during the period of emotional liability, from both nursing staff and spouse.

Reactive depressions tend to respond particularly well to supportive psychotherapy (as indicated), and psychotherapy is also usually productive of good results in psychotic reactions to childbirth.

Maintaining a safe environment is particularly important in severe depressions and in psychotic reactions as the safety of both mother and baby may be at risk.

Careful, but discreet, observation is essential, and the nurse should note any expression of aggressive feelings (whether directed against baby or self) by the mother. A moment's inattention could be catastrophic if the mother is harbouring marked delusional ideas or is expressing destructive impulses.

Communication with the depressed mother should encourage discussion of her emotional responses and should promote identification of difficulties in the 'here and now', while encouraging the formulation and strengthening of coping responses.

The patient may have problems in expressing sexuality due to loss of libido or hidden feelings of anger for her husband. The patient should be reassured that loss of libido after childbirth is both common and self-limiting and that it has no organic cause.

Feelings of hostility towards the spouse are an indication for involving him in discussion of the woman's emotional state, and the nurse may facilitate and coordinate such discussion, usually with the involvement of a psychiatrist and/or a psychologist.

Difficulties in 'waking and playing' are common due to loss of drive, low self-esteem and feelings of helplessness. Informal group activities, particularly those involving women with similar difficulties, will help to restore confidence and drive.

Insomnia may be a difficulty and relaxation therapy is helpful here, most women having acquired the basic skills at antenatal classes.

Self-neglect and poor personal hygiene will be exacerbated if the patient adopts the 'sick role' and becomes withdrawn and passive. Frequent visiting should be encouraged and weekend visits home arranged as soon as possible to improve motivation in this direction.

Before discharge the patient may benefit from arranging contact with one of the many informal self-help groups for depressed mothers, and the community psychiatric nurse and social worker will monitor progress.

Key Concepts

1 Depressive responses after childbirth are relatively common and may take the form of 'baby blues', reactive depression or psychotic depression of a schizophrenic nature.
2 *Baby blues* is a transient and self-limiting state of emotional lability which usually appears on the third day post-partum and resolves by the tenth day.
3 *Reactive depression* may appear and is characterized by irritability and lethargy, coupled by feelings of helplessness and resentment.
4 *Postnatal psychosis* is usually of an affective nature (occasionally schizo-affective) and produces florid symptoms, though the prognosis is usually good, most cases resolving in 6–10 weeks. However, the risk of recurrence after future births is high.
5 The risk of non-accidental injury to the baby is always present in affective disturbances following childbirth.
6 Treatment is non-specific and group or marital therapy is often helpful.
7 Major affective responses are less common during pregnancy and after abortion.
8 The nursing approach should involve major elements of supportive psychotherapy and counselling of the spouse is often helpful.

References

Ball, J. & Stanley, J. (1984) Stress and the mother. *Midwives Chronicle and Nursing Notes*, **97**(1162): 28–32.
Brewer, C. (1978) Post-abortion psychosis. In Sandler (Ed) *Mental Illness in Pregnancy and the Puerperium*. Oxford: OUP.

Brockington, I., Winokur, G. & Dean, C. (1982) *Motherhood and Mental Illness*. London: Academic Press.

Carne, S. (1966) The influence of the mother's health on her child. *Proceedings of The Royal Society of Medicine*, **59**: 1013.

Clark, M. et al (1968) Sequels of unwanted pregnancy. *Lancet*, **ii**: 501.

Dalton, K. (1980) *Depression After Childbirth*. Oxford: Oxford University Press.

D'Orban (1979) Women who kill their children. *British Journal of Psychiatry*, **134**: 560.

Gordon, R. et al (1965) Factors in postpartum emotional adjustment. *Obstetrics and Gynecology*, **25**: 158–166.

Hayman, A. (1962) Some aspects of regression in non-psychotic puerperal mental breakdown. *British Journal of Medical Psychology*, **35**: 135.

Howell, E. (1981) Psychological reactions of postpartum women. In Howell & Bayes (Eds) *Women and Mental Health*. London: Basic Books.

Jacobsson, et al (1976) Repeat aborters. *Social Psychiatry*, **11**: 75–86.

Kahn-Edrington, (1981) Abortion counselling. In Howell & Bayes (Eds) *Women and Mental Health*. London: Basic Books.

Kumar, R. (1984) Motherhood and mental illness. *Midwives Chronicle and Nursing Notes*, **97**(1154): 70–73.

Melges, F. (1968) Postpartum psychiatric syndromes. *Psychosomatic Medicine*, **30**: 95–108.

Nott, et al (1976) Hormonal changes and mood in the puerperium. *British Journal of Psychiatry*, **128**: 379.

Pitt, B. (1982) Depression and childbirth. In Paykel (Ed) *Handbook of Affective Disorders*. Edinburgh: Churchill Livingstone.

Robson, K. & Powell, E. (1982) *Early Maternal Attachment in Motherhood and Mental Illness*. London: Academic Press.

Rossi, A. (1968) Transition to parenthood. *Journal of Marriage and the Family*, **30**: 26–39.

Social Services Committee (1980) '*Short Report*'. *Perinatal and Neonatal Mortality*, Vol. 1. London: HMSO.

Yalom, et al (1968) Postpartum blues syndrome. *Archives of General Psychiatry*, **18**: 16–27.

27

Psychosexual Disorders

> 'One half of the world cannot understand the pleasures of the other.'
>
> *Jane Austen*

Psychosexual disorders are disorders of sexual functioning arising from psychological causes. These disorders cause much unhappiness and impaired psychosocial functioning in themselves and are often the cause of related psychiatric disorder (e.g. depression, anxiety).

It is extremely difficult to identify sexual behaviours which may be regarded as 'normal' . . .

> 'There is no form of sexual activity, even including heterosexual intercourse, which has not at some time or other been condemned. Likewise there are possibly no sexual practices (even including incest) which, however occasionally, have not been approved and encouraged' (Trethowan and Sims, 1983).

One cross-cultural study of sexual behaviour found such wide variance that no one society could be considered truly representative of normative human sexual behaviour. Some cultures encouraged sexual exploration by their children but imposed severe restrictions on adults; others repressed female sexuality while condoning variation for males— others did the opposite. Some cultures followed their stated codes of sexual mores, others did not (Ford and Beach, 1951).

The conflict between powerful biological urges and the need to channel these in the interests of social stability has led to many formulations and re-formulations of sexual codes, most religious and some secular. The accusation that much of psychiatry is simply morality translated illegitimately into the language of medicine acquires particular cogency when the societal response to sexuality is considered. Throughout history, attitudes towards sexuality reveal a pattern of incredible diversity and contradiction.

In Ancient Greece, attitudes towards sexuality were both positive and permissive.

> 'Two tendencies in Greek life helped to further a sane and healthy approach to sexuality. One was the emphasis on beauty. This led to the idealisation of the naked body and to its glorification in the plastic arts. The second factor was the robust sexuality they ascribed to their gods' (Ellis and Arbanel, 1961).

Homosexuality was widely practised, the sexual initiation of young boys by older men was accepted and nudity in public places was common. The individual was regarded as being bisexual but Greek marriage was monogamous and virginity was expected of the wife before marriage, as was fidelity afterwards. Men were not precluded from extra-marital sexual relations as long as these did not involve the wife of another man. Divorce was simple and easy to obtain.

Ancient Rome developed a sexual morality profoundly different from the Greeks. If a man and woman lived together for a year they were considered to be married and this became the commonest form of marriage in later times as it emancipated the wife from the authority of her husband. Divorce was almost impossible to obtain and it is said that for 500 years after the foundation of Rome there was no instance of divorce and no process by which it could be obtained (Ellis and Arbanel, 1961). Virginity was esteemed and adultery (by women) punishable by death or banishment. Double standards prevailed insofar as men were accorded much greater sexual freedom than women. Homosexuality was accepted as a natural and inevitable part of man's sexual life.

With the emergence of the Judaeo-Christian ethic, concern about sexuality became widespread and institutionalized. Sex was now believed to be a form of satanic temptation and those who yielded to sexual impulses were considered to be weak and sinful (Meyer and Salmon, 1984). Pleasure was now regarded as a secondary by-product of procreative sex. Masturbation, which the Greeks regarded not as a vice but as a harmless safety valve, was regarded by the Hebrews as a major sin. Kinsey (1948) noted that 'in orthodox Jewish codes masturbation constitutes a major sin and, at times in Jewish history, a sin which was penalized with death' (Kinsey et al, 1948). St Thomas Aquinas was later to regard masturbation as more sinful than fornication (Meyer and Salmon, 1984).

Catholicism was later to assert that 'a rightful sense of shame is proper and should not be abolished through faulty sex education' (Ellis and Arbanel, 1961) and also resisted divorce; 'Whosoever shall put away his wife . . . and shall marry another committeth adultery' (Matthew 19,9). Procreational sex was now heavily emphasized: 'having supernatural purposes, sex must ever be used so as to be an act of justice, charity, chastity and religion' (Ellis and Arbanel, 1961).

Celibacy was now advocated for clergy. Moore (1959) writes:

'From the times of St Paul on, there was a body of celibates, men and women in the Church of whom the Church was proud. Those who had decided to lead a celibate life . . . soon attained a special position in the Church'.

The equation of sexuality with sin and of celibacy with righteousness had some startling results. Matthew (19, 12) says: 'and there be eunuchs which have made themselves eunuchs for the Kingdom of Heaven's sake', and as recently as 1759 a religious sect in Russia (the Skopsti) believed that it was necessary to atone for the sexuality of Adam and Eve by mass castration, and in Eastern Russia whole communities embraced this idea (Kushner, 1973).

The first penalty and result of the Fall of Adam and Eve was, according to Catholic theologians, concupiscence, the ravages of lust . . . 'This malady is by no means confined to man's sexual life, it pervades his entire existence' (Ellis and Arbanel, 1961). This view of sexual instincts as a 'malady' was by no means confined to the Catholic Church. John Calvin agreed that the sexual life of man contains 'an irregularity, which I allow, is beyond others violent and next to brutish' but had a remedy for this 'vice and baseness'—marriage—by means of which 'the fault is covered over so that it no longer appears in the sight of God' (Ellis and Arbanel, 1961).

The theologically sophisticated may protest that these are simplifications which have evoked much corrective theological dialogue. The mass of people, be they active religious practitioners or not, are not theologically sophisticated and the collective uncon-

scious of Judaeo-Christian man probably contains archetypal anxieties about sexuality which have their origin in primitive Hebraic codes. These anxieties, together with the suppression of Id instincts demanded by civilized societies, may extort a heavy interpersonal and emotional price. Fromm (1957) comments that:

'If we speak about love in contemporary Western culture we mean to ask whether the social structure of Western civilisation and the spirit resulting from it are conducive to the development of love. To raise the question is to answer it in the negative. No objective observer of our Western life can doubt that love—brotherly love, motherly love and erotic love—is a relatively rare phenomenon, and that its place is taken by a number of forms of pseudo-love which are in reality so many forms of the disintegration of love'.

Freud (1908) also viewed with concern the effects of the suppression of instincts inherent in 'civilized' sexual morality: 'We must view all factors which impair sexual life, suppress its activity or distort its aims as being pathogenic factors in the psychoneuroses'.

Max Weber, one of the founding fathers of sociology, suggested that the *Protestant ethic* was one of the factors giving rise to the rigid and sterile social organization of capitalist societies as it overvalued hard work, diligence, prudence and acquisition: 'the acquisition of more and more money, combined with the strict avoidance of all spontaneous enjoyment . . . is thought of . . . as an end in itself' (Weber, 1958). Giddens (1971) has pointed out that 'the movement to Protestantism involved acceptance of a much higher degree of regulation of behaviour than that which was demanded by Catholicism . . . Protestantism adopts a resolutely stringent attitude towards relaxation and enjoyment—a phenomenon which is particularly pronounced in Calvinism'.

Critiques of the destructive effects of capitalist society on the emotional life of the individual reached a new level of vehemence in the writings of *Wilhelm Reich* (1897–1957), a psychoanalyst who developed Marx's claim that capitalism 'fatally corrodes all human relationships' (Marx, 1956) into a radical criticism of the sexual and economic dependence of women, the family and human relationships in general under capitalism. For Reich, sexuality is the answer, society the mistake; the family is identified as suppressing the sexuality of individuals and enforced monogamy as being destructive of sexual happiness (Mitchell, 1975). Reich is sometimes accused of wishing to destroy the family, but this is an inaccuracy:

'What we want to destroy is not the family but the hatred which the family creates; the coercion, though it may take on the outward appearance of love . . . No sensible person will talk of love when a man cohabits with a woman who is bound hand and foot. No half-way decent man will be proud of the love of a woman whom he buys by supporting her or by power. No decent man will take love which is not given freely' (Reich, 1969).

Thus the broad theme often evoked suggests that the Graeco-Roman sexual ethic was a healthy and liberating one associated with positive religious views of sexuality, while the Judaeo-Christian sexual ethic is seen as basically repressive and evocative of guilt and anxiety associated with negative religious views of sexuality. An additional theme is the suggestion that the drive repression associated with the latter ethic was sublimated into the spirit of capitalism which perpetuates emotional and interpersonal stagnation and defeat. Philosophical observations supported this viewpoint, Sartre (1960) suggesting that

'Shortly after semi-automatic machines were introduced investigations showed that female skilled workers would allow themselves to lapse while working into a sexual kind of daydream . . . but it was the machine in her which was dreaming of caresses',

and Marcuse (1964) suggesting that

'The machine process in the technological universe breaks the innermost privacy of freedom and joins sexuality and labour in one unconscious, rhythmic automatism'.

The view of man as being innately wracked by quite inevitable sexual conflicts is to a great extent part of psychoanalytical orthodoxy and, to some extent, diverted attention away from broader social structures. Anthropological studies cast doubt on this thesis as they accumulated evidence to the effect that the 'difficulties' of childhood and adolescence are not the inevitable outcome of conflict between psychic forces but are a reaction to the constraints put upon us by civilization. The anthropologist, *Margaret Mead*, commented (in 1928):

'One by one, aspects of behaviour which we had been accustomed to consider invariable complements of our humanity were found to be merely a result of civilisation, present in the inhabitants of one country, absent in another country' (Mead, 1943).

The myth of the sexually emancipated 'noble savage', which saw primitive people living in a state of sexual and emotional freedom and innocence (in ethnic 'Gardens of Eden' interrupted by the arrival of missionaries who were seen to import Western notions of shame and guilt, and who to that extent played the role of the serpent in the Garden), was also modified by anthropological investigation. Mead described societies in which sexual awareness and honesty were so apparent that the rigid and joyless sexuality of Western civilization seemed to suffer in comparison. She also described 'puritanical' attitudes to sex in New Guinea coupled with negative attitudes to intercourse: 'every woman, however, successfully conveys to her growing daughters her own affective reaction to the wearisome abomination which is sex' (Mead, 1943).

In Samoa 'husbands and wives never walk side by side through the village for the husband, particularly, would be "ashamed"' (Mead, 1943). Nevertheless, sex was not seen as being 'wrong'; 'the adult attitude towards all the details of sex is characterized by this view that they are unseemly, not that they are wrong' (Mead, 1943).

The view of sexuality as a social rather than biological product, and its reflection of religious and ethical codes incorporated in the socialization process (rather than inexorable psychic conflict), adds weight to the criticism of arbitrary division of sexual practices and attitudes into the categories of 'normal' and 'abnormal'.

Suggestions that civilization leads to sexual repression often evoke irate responses which take the form of criticisms of the 'permissive' society: 'What of failing moral codes and the rising tide of pornography?' say such critics. Many replies would suggest that some moral codes fail because they are biologically and psychologically untenable and unnatural and that the use of pornography (which is as old as mankind itself, for example, the instructional 'pillow books' given to Japanese brides) is not always 'unhealthy'. There is a fine dividing line between pornography and erotic art; one can hardly legitimately classify Goya's 'Nude Maja' or Michelangelo's 'David' with hard core pornography which often degrades and debases. The theme of debased pornography as a product of strict sexual codes has evoked much debate, and pornography has been said to hold attractions for those 'who find their sexual needs in conflict with the moral and religious values of society from which they have not been able to fully emancipate themselves' (Ellis and Arbanel, 1961).

Whatever the causes, sexual conflict and anxiety are social realities that cause much psychosocial disorganization and elicit varying social responses. 'How can the Church at one time stand for stern moral codes and accept those who violate the codes? Roman Catholicism manages it with the anonymity of the sacrament of penance which provides both personal protection and sacramental power. The Protestant pharmacopoeia possesses no such balm and therefore loses its wounded to the secular priesthood, the psychiatrist and the psychoanalyst.' (Ellis and Arbanel, 1961)

This secular priesthood has historically produced some strange medical demonologies to explain 'abnormal' sexuality and has resorted to even stranger methods of exorcizing unruly or disordered sexual impulses. Women in particular have suffered as a result of the medicalization of sexuality . . . 'the (alleged) psychic vulnerability of women provides an unbroken thread in the medical literature' (Skultans, 1979). Medical misogyny (hatred of women) has ancient antecedents. St John Chrysostom in the fourth century AD advised a friend who had fallen in love: 'The groundwork of her bodily beauty is phlegm and blood and yellow bile and black bile, and the fluid of masticated food' (Meyer and Salmon, 1984), while the Roman philosopher, Boethius, advised that 'woman is a temple built upon a sewer' (Meyer and Salmon, 1984).

In his morning prayer the Orthodox Jew says 'Blessed be God . . . that he did not make me a woman' (Szasz, 1973). St Paul advised that 'It is well for a man not to touch a woman', with the grudging concession: 'It is better to marry than to burn' (I Corinthians, 7). St Augustine enlarged on the theme: 'The act of generation is sin itself and determines the transmission of the sin to the new creature' (Ellis and Arbanel, 1961). Aristotle taught that the sexual urge was a source of shame (Ellis and Arbanel, 1961) and Calvin asserted that 'the immodest desires with which persons burn is a fault arising from the corruption of nature' (Ellis and Arbanel, 1961).

Physicians were soon to legitimize misogyny:

Burton (1621) in *The Anatomy of Melancholy* wrote of woman: 'That other madness is a woman . . . pleasant at first she is, that fair plant to the eye, but poison to the taste . . . her house is the way to hell, and goes down to the chambers of death'. Thomas Sydenham, in 1848, asserted that females were physiologically prone to hysteria: 'there is hardly one who is wholly free from them' (hysterical complaints) (Skultans, 1979) and the 'vulnerabilities' of the 'weaker sex' were enthusiastically charted in Victorian times.

Szasz (1973) writes of 'the abysmal devaluation of women in the ethics of ancient Judaism' and adds that 'the Christian ethic did not raise the worth of female life much above the Jewish; nor did the clinical ethic raise it much above the clerical'.

Masturbation was regarded as both an illness and the cause of further illnesses (Freud called it the 'primal addiction') (Szasz, 1973). The term 'masturbatory insanity' was widely used and hysteria (believed to have a sexual origin) was treated by brutal and mutilating surgery—clitoridectomy, removal of the ovaries and cauterization of the clitoris (Szasz, 1973). Concern over masturbation persisted well into the twentieth century and Henderson and Batchelor (1962) say of it: 'this is the most frequent sexual habit which the family doctor and psychiatrist may be consulted about', while Slater and Roth (1969) say it may 'strictly be regarded as a perversion which may arise when the child is "seduced" by older children or an irresponsible nanny'. As more than 90% of males and 65% of females will have masturbated at some time (Kinsey et al, 1948), this 'perversion' is remarkably widespread (there must be a remarkable number of 'irresponsible nannies' around). Far from regarding masturbation as a problem, Kaplan (1979) regards the absence of masturbation in adolescent males as carrying 'clinical significance of severe sexual repression'.

Old ideas often die hard, however, and needless anxieties about masturbation still surface in the form of distressed letters to the 'problem pages' of popular periodicals. Fortunately sexual myths are now regarded with increasing cynicism, and Meyer and Salmon (1984) suggest that 'our more permissive culture of today is somewhat closer in spirit to that of Ancient Greece'.

It should be emphasized that 'permissive' writers on sexuality are not advocating sexual anarchy. They are simply advocating healthy awareness of sexual needs and behaviour in order that these may be expressed without inappropriate guilt and anxiety. Weinberg (1982) also suggests that 'a necessary prerequisite to helping others is the ability to talk openly and non-judgementally about sex'.

We have discussed the difficulties of distorted views of sexuality and their historical roots. What then is 'normal' sexuality? Trethowan and Sims (1983) offer an admirably succinct definition:

> 'A definition of normal sexuality which might at the present time fit Western culture could therefore well comprise any explicitly sexual act between two people which is acceptable to, and enjoyed by, both and which damages neither, physically or emotionally'.

The Sexual Response Cycle

The sexual response cycle is divided into four phases:
1 Excitement
2 Plateau
3 Orgasm
4 Resolution

The excitement (or arousal) phase is the longest and is accompanied by vasoconstriction leading to engorgement of penis, clitoris and nipples. Myotonia (increase in muscle tension) accompanies the vasoconstriction and vaginal lubrication takes place. The plateau phase precedes orgasm and is accompanied by increase in vasoconstriction, myotonia, heart rate, blood pressure and respirations. This phase is sometimes called the pre-orgasmic phase.

Orgasm involves rhythmic contraction of genital muscles accompanied in the male by emission of 2–5 ml of seminal fluid in a series of squirts. In the female orgasm there is no emission, but rhythmic contractions of the vaginal muscles occur at the rate of 8 per second. Women tend to have greater variation in the length and intensity of the orgasmic responses than do men. Following orgasm the resolution phase sets in which is an involuntary period of tension loss. Women have been found to have the potential for multiple orgasm and can return to an orgasmic state from any point in the arousal cycle, including the resolution phase. Men undergo a *refractory period* during the resolution phase during which effective restimulation is not possible. The refractory phase lasts for 20–30 minutes. Even thereafter the physiological ability of the male to respond to restimulation is less than the female. Men reach plateau much more quickly than women and effective foreplay is necessary if both partners are to reach plateau together.

Sexual Difficulties

There are large numbers of persons who have difficulties arising from their sexual behaviour, attitudes or orientation and these difficulties may be assigned to three broad categories:
1 Sexual dysfunction
2 Sexual deviation
3 Disorders of gender identity
Sexual dysfunctions largely involve individuals who complain of inadequate sexual performance or feelings within a sexual relationship, while sexual deviations consist of departures from accepted sexual codes or practices that cause problems for the person concerned or for others.

Sexual dysfunction

Organic disorder must be excluded and a careful history is necessary before the diagnosis of sexual dysfunction is made. Sexual dysfunction is extremely common. One study examined the incidence of it in several societies and concluded that the greater the sexual restrictiveness of the society, the higher the incidence of dysfunction (Welch and Kartub, 1978). Common sexual dysfunctions in the male are:
Impotence
Premature ejaculation
Retarded ejaculation

In the female, common dysfunctions are:
Lack of libido
Orgasmic dysfunction
Vaginismus

All of these dysfunctions have a similar aetiology. Kaplan (1979) comments that 'on one level the sexual dysfunctions as well as the sexual phobias are caused by a single factor: anxiety'.

Impotence

This may be defined as the inability to achieve or sustain an erection that is sufficient for vaginal penetration. It is extremely common. In 1912 Freud commented that 'if a practising psychoanalyst asks himself on account of what disorder people most often come to him for help he is bound to reply, disregarding the many forms of anxiety, that it is physical impotence'. Impotence may be drug induced (alcohol, phenothiazines – especially thioridazine – steroids, spironolactone, haloperidol, tricyclic antidepressants, monoamine oxidase inhibitors, antihypertensive drugs and opiates) or there may be neurological causes, but the vast majority of cases have simple psychological causes. It has been estimated that more than half of all males have experienced transient episodes of impotence (Meyer and Salmon, 1984).

Emotional tensions in a relationship may give rise to sexually disruptive anxiety, and these are often heightened by simple communication failures. The belief that sexual dysfunction may be ascribed specifically to serious unconscious conflict (Oedipal conflicts and castration anxiety in the male and penis envy in females) is no longer uncritically accepted.

Masters and Johnson (and others) have shown that mild or superficial anxiety can also produce dysfunction (Masters and Johnson, 1970) and Kaplan (1979) comments that 'clinical experience with patients who complain of sexual disorders does not support the specificity hypothesis' and 'the immediate causes of sexual dysfunctions operate in the here and now' (Kaplan, 1974). Anxieties operating in the here and now are a common cause of impotence. '*Performance anxiety*' in which unrealistic expectations about performance generate fears of not meeting these standards is common and may result in 'spectatoring' in which the person detaches from natural and spontaneous sexuality and instead focusses on the outcome (Masters et al, 1982) like a nervous referee. Apprehension is incompatible with natural sexuality. Performance anxiety sometimes arises out of the partner's attitudes towards sex.

Meyer and Salmon (1984) reject the concept of castration anxiety: 'few substantive empirical data exist to support this view', but point out that one partner (male or female) may perform a symbolically castrating role by being critical, demeaning and hard to please, creating a cycle of failure—self-blame—heightened anxiety—avoidance behaviour and repeated failure.

Treatment is both simple and effective. Sensate focus exercises encourage the couple to get in touch with their feelings by initially practising coital abstinence in favour of relaxed caresses. Both partners caress and are caressed and give verbal feedback; initially the genitals and nipples are avoided until sensitivity and awareness are increased. Second level sensate focus exercises move on to non-demanding genital stimulation in which orgasm is avoided. Once optimism and relief have appeared and sensitivity has increased, the couple may move on to the final level of intercourse (Masters et al, 1982). Sensate focus exercises encourage a degree of 'selfishness'; some men neglect their own needs for arousal because they concentrate exclusively on the needs of their partner (Dowson, 1983).

Communication must also be improved. Fromm (1957) comments that

> 'if a sexually inhibited person can emerge from fear or hate, and hence become capable of loving, his or her sexual problems are solved. If not, no amount of knowledge about sexual techniques will help'.

In the case of deeply rooted hostilities, psychotherapy may be required before sensate focus is used.

Premature ejaculation

This is usually cited in the literature as the most common of the male sexual dysfunctions (Kaplan, 1974) and consists of loss of control over the ejaculatory reflex so that ejaculation occurs before penetration can take place or immediately after it has happened. It is only defined as a clinical problem if it occurs 50% of the time (Masters and Johnson, 1970) and is commonest in young males. Treatment may consist of prescribing masturbation before intercourse. After ejaculation, the male experiences a refractory period during which the sexual organ is unable to function and after which ejaculatory sensitivity is decreased. 'Stop-start' techniques may also be used whereby the male signals impending orgasm so that the female may discontinue stimulation (which may be manual or oral) until the pre-ejaculatory phase has subsided, whereafter stimulation may be recommenced. The '*squeeze technique*' may be coupled with this approach (the female applies a quick, moderately hard squeeze just below the glans penis (head of the penis) which interrupts the pre-ejaculatory phase).

Once control has been learned in these situations, stop-start technique is transferred to intercourse (Kaplan, 1974).

Retarded ejaculation

This consists of the inability to ejaculate even though erection and penetration have been achieved. Intercourse is usually prolonged and unsatisfactory and the female partner may become concerned about being unable to become pregnant (Dowson, 1983). Mild forms of this disorder seem to be highly prevalent (Kaplan, 1974), despite the belief that it is uncommon.

Underlying conflicts about parenthood must be discussed and psychotherapy may be necessary. This disorder may have phobic dimensions and in this case systematic desensitization (in vivo) is encouraged. The partner helps the male to reach the pre-ejaculatory stage by any manner and then allows insertion and ejaculation to occur. Many males who have ejaculatory difficulties at intercourse climax easily at masturbation or in response to manual or oral stimulation.

Lack of libido

This is a term often used to describe loss or reduction of sexual desire. The term may be somewhat of a misnomer as libido is often suppressed rather than absent. Fear of a close and intimate attachment may be a cause. 'Sometimes it seems that people in our culture are more afraid of intimacy than they are of sex' (Kaplan, 1979). Fear of pregnancy may also be a cause, as may simple ignorance of sexuality. Ignorance simply requires counselling of the couple and information that more clitoral stimulation is required (Masters et al, 1982).

Many men believe that the vagina is the seat of female sexual sensation and think that rhythmic, vigorous thrusting is the only route to female orgasm. The vagina is a tough, elastic organ, designed to cope with the physical stresses of childbirth, and many couples will benefit if attention is directed towards the clitoris. Some couples feel that clitoral orgasm is 'immature' or 'not proper—not the real thing' and 'clitoral guilt' must be overcome by counselling. Masturbatory exercises may be prescribed for the female and are particularly helpful in the presence of an approving partner (Kaplan, 1979), while a vibrator will help condition and strengthen orgasmic responses. Once clitoral responses are strongly established, 'clitoral assistance' is offered by the partner during intercourse. The male, female or both may manually stimulate the clitoris during intercourse, discontinuing stimulation once orgasm is imminent.

Sexual guilt may militate against relaxed and natural intercourse, some women feeling that sexual images and fantasies aroused during foreplay are 'dirty' or 'not proper'. Sexual imagery should be encouraged in this case and erotic stimulation in the form of books or videos may be employed (Kaplan, 1979). Kaplan (1974) has commented that 'it may be said that sex is composed of friction and fantasy'. Sensate focus exercises will also be helpful and the couple should be encouraged to openly and frankly discuss their sexual needs and attitudes.

The media have implanted many unfortunate images of sexuality which may lead to impotence in males and orgasmic difficulties in females. Cinematic sex tends to occur with carefully orchestrated and unrealistic precision and predictability: the young couple embrace on the beach—the camera pans away discreetly to the rhythmic movements of the surf—the music reaches a climax (as presumably do the young couple) and some months later they are fondly gazing at an engaging and flawless baby (who often becomes an eminent brain surgeon). Real life does not consist of happy clichés, and the young female who has been weaned on a diet of cinematic clichés and pulp romantic novels (peopled by sun-bronzed young ship's doctors and blushing Anglo-Saxon maidens) may find 'real' sex disappointing, uncomfortable or frightening, thus developing a conditioned aversion to sex which may cause much psychosocial difficulty. Her Sir Galahad who will 'make the earth move for her' probably does not exist and she may embark upon a quest for a sexual Holy Grail which will be frustrating and damaging of self-esteem.

Orgasmic dysfunction

This consists of impaired ability to experience orgasm during intercourse. In this case libido is not lacking as most females concerned can easily orgasm at masturbation. Orgasmic sensations may be transferred to intercourse by clitoral assistance during coitus and this assistance may be provided by the female, her partner or both.

Clumsy or ill-informed attempts at intercourse by the partner may be responsible and educative counselling will benefit both partners. A variable period of foreplay of up to, and sometimes beyond, half an hour is often necessary if the female is to reach orgasm (Dowson, 1983) and males should be advised of the 'erogenous zones': breasts, nipples, inner aspect of thighs and arms, ear lobes, the perianal area, buttocks, clitoris, labia, mouth and lips. Interpersonal difficulties must be assessed and explored in a productive manner.

Vaginismus

This is involuntary sustained contraction of the muscles surrounding the entrance of the vagina which renders sexual intercourse impossible or painful. The result is often dyspareunia (painful or difficult sexual intercourse). Vaginismus is not necessarily associated with sexual inhibition or orgasmic difficulties as many women with this condition enjoy sex and have a strong desire for it.

Anatomically the genitalia of vaginismic women are normal, but attempts at penetration provoke painful spasm with the result that the woman may become phobic of intercourse. The general consensus is that this condition is relatively rare (Kaplan, 1974). Factors identified as playing a causative role include strict religious upbringing, sexual guilt, the husband's impotence or prior experiences with molestation, assault or rape (Masters and Johnson, 1970).

The impact of rape on later sexual functioning has given rise to another cliché—that of the man-hating woman unable to tolerate sex as a result of her experience. Research findings do not confirm this picture. Studies reveal that most women (correctly) identified the act of rape as an act of violence rather than sexuality. 'Having sex again didn't bother me. That was one thing I could separate out . . . I never equated that rape was sex, so I never had trouble in my sex life.' (Wolbert-Burgess and Lyttle-Holmstrom, 1981) One study of 63 sexually active women who had been victims of rape reported that 16 experienced a degree of vaginismus for some time afterwards, though 26 (41%) reported lasting orgasmic difficulties (Wolbert-Burgess and Lyttle-Holmstrom, 1981).

Vaginismus may have a devastating impact both on the woman's self-esteem and on the quality of her relationships. Repeated 'failures' may give rise to deeply seated feelings of sexual inadequacy, and husbands may develop secondary impotence as a reaction to their wives' disorder.

In the past, vaginismus was treated surgically by dividing the perineal muscles but this procedure often compounded the trauma felt by the highly frightened woman (Kaplan, 1974). Treatment aims at modifying the conditioned response of vaginal spasm by in vivo deconditioning. One widely used method is to insert successively larger catheters into the vagina, starting with one as thin as a pencil and eventually finishing with one as large as an erect penis (Tollison and Adams, 1979).

Masters and Johnson (1970) recommend that the partner participates in the insertion of the graduated catheters and report a success rate of almost 100%. Intercourse is not attempted until the patient can tolerate insertion of the largest catheter without discomfort (usually after 4–10 dilatation experiences). When intercourse is attempted, the husband should refrain from thrusting and the female superior position (lying, kneeling or squatting) will reduce the woman's feelings of being 'overpowered' or 'losing control'.

Kaplan (1974) points out that intercourse should not be discontinued at the first sensations of discomfort: 'The therapeutic manoeuvre which has proven most useful in treating vaginismic patients is the advice and encouragement to "stay with your unpleasant feelings"'. By 'staying with' unpleasant sensations and attempting to relax, most women overcome these feelings in time.

Sexual deviation

There is no clear demarcation between 'normal' and 'abnormal' sexual behaviour as many of the sexual deviations differ only quantitatively from normal sexual behaviour (Braude, 1983). What one society may regard as unacceptable deviation may be regarded as a normal sexual practice in another. Two groups of sexual deviations are usually described: disorders of sexual preference and disorders of sexual behaviour.

Disorders of sexual preference

include:
  Homosexuality
  Paedophilia
  Transvestism
  Fetishism
  Bestiality

Homosexuality. Homosexuality provides a rich illustration of Simmons' (1969) claim that 'deviants do not exist in nature but are man-made categories' . . .

'this does not mean that there is really no such thing as deviance or that the deviant is an innocent bystander. It means that society is an active partner in producing the phenomenon called deviance and that we must look at the work of both partners if we want to understand'.

Becker (1963) comments that 'social groups create deviance by making the rules whose infraction constitutes deviance'.

Historically, attitudes towards homosexuality have fluctuated, through regarding it as an accepted practice in Graeco-Roman times, to the hatred of homosexuality incorporated in Judaism (which regarded it as a sin punishable by death), to the ambivalent attitudes of the Middle Ages. During the Middle Ages homosexuality was practised by monks, archbishops and saints and St Ethelred prescribed that his monks be allowed to hold hands in public (Boswell, 1980).

By Victorian times social organization was more rigid and many eminent Victorians were both persecuted and prosecuted because of their homosexuality which was now regarded as a sin by the Church and an offence by the law. Psychiatrists were soon to add a third stigmatizing label to homosexual behaviour—that of 'disease' (Szasz, 1973).

Szasz writes of '*homophobia*': 'our secular society dreads homosexuality in the same way and with the same intensity as the theological societies of our ancestors dreaded heresy' (Szasz, 1973). Despite the medicalization of this form of sexual heresy, Freud (1959) wrote that

'homosexuality is assuredly no advantage but it is nothing to be ashamed of, no vice, no degradation. It cannot be classified as an illness . . . it is a great injustice to persecute homosexuality as a crime and it is cruelty, too'.

For the first half of the twentieth century, psychiatrists attempted to justify the (often involuntary) treatment of this 'disease' by investigating hormone levels, body build and chromosomes in homosexuality in an (unsuccessful) effort to find a biological basis for the 'disease'. The 'disease' has now been largely 'demedicalized'; this is exemplified by Braude's (1983) comment that 'homosexuality per se should not be regarded as a clinical problem'. The 'rules', whose infraction constitutes deviance, have largely been redrawn, though the current rise in the incidence of acquired immune deficiency syndrome (AIDS) already shows signs of provoking a rebirth of homophobia.

It should be mentioned that the word 'homosexual' does not mean a man who sexually desires other men. The word is not derived from the Latin *homo* meaning 'man' but from the Greek *homos* meaning 'the same as' and describes those persons (male or female) who emotionally, sexually and socially are drawn to their own sex, often to the exclusion of the other.

One cross-cultural study found that 64% of the 76 societies studied considered homosexuality normal (Ford and Beach, 1951) and it has been estimated that about 4% of adult men and a much lower proportion of women have been exclusively homosexual all their lives, while about 25% of men and about 15% of women enter upon frankly homosexual relationships at one time or another (Stafford-Clark and Smith, 1983).

A small percentage of homosexuals wish to change their sexual preference and may embark upon psychotherapy, though research revealed that homosexual men and women attending a clinic were as well adjusted as 'normals' (Siegalman, 1972).

Paedophilia. This refers to a strong desire for sexual contact with pre- or early pubertal children of either sex (the word literally means 'love of children'). Aggression is an important component and there is a major risk of serious injury or homicidal assault on the victim.

Paedophilia is rare in females and paedophiliacs are mostly heterosexual, many being impotent or sexually inadequate. Treatment has included aversion therapy, psychosurgery and treatment with female hormones. Success rates are low.

Transvestism. This refers to the wearing of clothes of the opposite sex (usually female) as a source of sexual arousal (cross-dressing). Should this behaviour be causing problems, it usually responds well to aversive conditioning techniques, coupled with psychotherapy.

Fetishism. This refers to the use of inanimate objects (usually articles of female clothing) to attain sexual arousal. Most subjects are male and use the object as a masturbatory stimulus or as an adjunct to intercourse. Most cases are harmless but troublesome instances respond to aversive conditioning.

Bestiality (zoophilia). This refers to sexual intercourse with animals and is a rare condition usually associated with males of limited intelligence who live in rural areas.

Disorders of sexual behaviour

These include:
    Exhibitionism
    Voyeurism
    Sadomasochism

Exhibitionism. This refers to intentional display of the genitals, almost invariably by a man, to adults or children of the opposite sex, though paedophiliacs may display this behaviour towards either sex. Exhibitionists constitute about one-third of all sex offenders and show the highest rate of relapse—about 25% (Meyer and Salmon, 1984). Most are impulsive or inadequate and are not dangerous, but some aggressive types may attempt sexual assault. Primarily the action is an attempt to shock by a sexually inadequate individual and the responses of shock and outrage are often sexually stimulating to him.

Obscene telephone calls are a variation on the same theme, though in this case there may be underlying feelings of hostility towards women. Neither behaviour should be reinforced by producing the desired responses of shock and outrage. Aversion therapy has been tried but the results are poor.

Voyeurism. This refers to the seeking of sexual arousal by secretly observing unclothed or undressing individuals or persons engaged in sexual activity. We live in a voyeuristic society where sexual images are used in advertising and are commonplace in newspapers, television and cinema.

The voyeur (or 'peeping Tom') differs from the institutionalized voyeurism condoned by society in that he often uses this behaviour as his sole sexual outlet, risking imprisonment (and assault). Most are harmless and timid and aversion therapy is moderately successful.

Sadomasochism. This refers to the practice of deriving sexual pleasure by giving (*sadism*) or receiving (*masochism*) pain during sexual activity. Both elements are often combined (sadomasochism). This practice provides another example of the blurred boundaries between what is perceived as 'normal' or 'abnormal'. There is a fine margin between pleasure and pain (e.g. the practice of giving 'love-bites') and much sadomasochistic behaviour takes place within the confines of 'normal' marriages, while many prostitutes cater for variations of this sort.

Some masochists enjoy 'bondage'—being tightly tied up during sex so that he/she feels a helpless 'victim'—and many males of this sort are thought to be displaying a regression to guilty infantile sexuality which also manifests itself in aggressive or dismissive attitudes towards women.

Disorders of gender identity

Gender differences are those socially constructed attributes of 'femininity' and 'masculinity' as opposed to sex differences which are anatomical and physiological. Each society has constructed some form of gender differentiation based on its view of what should be regarded as typical of the male and female roles. 'Typical' roles have been found to vary widely from society to society. Women's role in one society may be the men's role in another, a finding which contradicts the once widely held viewpoint that men and women behave differently for innate biological reasons. The assumption that women are 'naturally' programmed to assume the roles of wife and mother is a somewhat tattered one rooted in the nineteenth century view of women as weak and passive creatures totally controlled by their ovaries and the rhythms of the menstrual cycle.

To assume the role of man or woman is to act out a script which is not written genetically but socially, and this script changes dramatically across cultures and throughout history.

The 'gender disorders' involve a basic conflict between the gender identity ascribed by society and a deeply felt conviction that this identity is in some way inappropriate at the personal level.

Transsexualism

This is a gender disorder affecting individuals who have a firm conviction of belonging to the opposite sex, despite normal genitalia (Braude, 1983). Transsexuals are persons who believe that their mind is trapped in a body of the wrong sex and they often wish to have their bodies altered by any means possible. Male transsexuals want to live as women and female transsexuals want to live as men. Transsexuals should not be confused with transvestites who simply wish to derive sexual satisfaction from wearing the clothing of the opposite sex (cross-dressing) and who do not show distaste for their genitalia. Transsexuals feel and react like the opposite sex and feel trapped in a body of the wrong sex . . . 'it is not the dubious "masculinity" and "femininity" which bothers them, but a sense of belonging to the opposite sex' (Wolff, 1977).

Many transsexuals seek escape from the body they regard as being inappropriate by surgery, which is usually preceded by hormonal treatment. Surgery is not agreed to lightly and is usually the third of three stages. Stage one involves asking the individual to dress and live as a member of the opposite sex and to develop modes of behaviour and social skills appropriate to the opposite gender role. Those individuals who do not select themselves out after this stage go on to the second stage which involves the administration of hormones. Oestrogens are prescribed for males and androgens for females and will reduce secondary sexual characteristics (men experience a degree of breast enlargement and women experience suppression of menstruation, increased growth of facial hair and lowering of the pitch of the voice). Should the individual respond favourably the final stage, that of surgery, is reached.

Masculinizing surgery includes mastectomy, hysterectomy and the construction of an artificial penis from a flap of abdominal skin, plastic testicles being inserted into the constructed scrotum and a rigid penile prosthesis sometimes being included.

Feminizing surgery includes removal of the penis, breast augmentation (silicon implants are often used) and construction of a simulated vaginal cavity.

One study revealed that only 10% of transsexuals requesting surgery eventually received it (Laub and Fisk, 1974). Client satisfaction levels after 'sex-change' surgery are often low. Feminizing surgery cannot lead to menstruation or childbirth, and artificially constructed vaginas often cannot cope effectively with intercourse, which is often painful. Masculinizing surgery has an even lower reported client satisfaction level (about 50%) (Meyer and Salmon, 1984).

Factors which have been suggested to play an important part in the aetiology of transsexualism include (a) confusion in gender-role modelling, and (b) prolonged reinforcement of opposite gender-role behaviours in childhood (Money and Weideking, 1980), though hormonal imbalances have been suggested.

Approximately 75% of males who cross-dress do so before age four and the average age of onset for females is only slightly later (Meyer and Salmon, 1984), though concern is only warranted when this behaviour persists for several months, as most children occasionally manifest aspects of this behaviour.

Bisexuality

This reflects a bi-gender identity which may or may not lead to bisexual orientation.

The bisexual nature of human beings is an ancient theme. Greek mythology describes Hermaphroditos, the son of Hermes and Aphrodite, a beautiful youth who was half-male, half-female. The hermaphroditic image is a recurring motif in Greek sculpture and literature. Jung incorporated the hermaphroditic legend into the psychological literature by writing of the *anima* and *animus*. The anima is the female aspect of a man and the animus the male aspect of a woman. According to Jung it is the man's anima which drives him to search for a love partner who corresponds to the female part of himself and a woman's animus seeks her own maleness in the person she loves. The anima in a man may express itself in moodiness, sentimentality and tenderness, and the animus in a woman in aggression and opinionated behaviour, according to Jung.

Freud also subscribed to the view of the basic bisexuality of humans: 'in every sexual act four persons are involved' (Freud, 1949).

The clinical use of the term bisexuality does not refer to subtle nuances of psychic energy but to sexual behaviour. 'Bisexuals are individuals who respond sexually . . . to a variety of people, regardless of their sex' (Weinberg, 1982).

These individuals often define themselves as being unwilling to deny themselves the opportunities for sexual exchange which exist and which are stifled by highly restrictive cultural pressures, though many homosexuals consider professions of bisexuality to be a 'cop-out' by other homosexuals who are unable, or unwilling, to confess to attraction to members of the same sex.

Another viewpoint considers the bisexual to be someone who is on the way to a homosexual orientation but is, as yet, unready to totally abandon the security of heterosexual relationships.

Key Concepts

1 Psychosexual disorders are disorders of sexual function which do not have a physical basis.
2 The concepts of 'normality' and 'abnormality' become particularly elusive if applied to sexual behaviour.
3 Historically and culturally there is tremendous variation in patterns of 'acceptable' sexual behaviour.
4 Three potentially problematic areas may be identified: *sexual dysfunction*, *sexual deviation* and *disorders of gender identity*.
5 Common male dysfunctions include *impotence*, *premature ejaculation* and *retarded ejaculation*.
6 Common female dysfunctions include *lack of libido*, *orgasmic dysfunction* and *vaginismus*.
7 *Anxiety* is the commonest shared component of sexual dysfunctions.
8 Increased knowledge about sexual techniques must be coupled with improved *communications* between partners if tensions are to be resolved and dysfunctions reduced.
9 Sexual deviations include disorders of *sexual behaviour* and disorders of *sexual preference*.
10 Disorders of sexual behaviour include *exhibitionism*, *voyeurism* and *sadomasochism*.
11 Disorders of sexual preference include *homosexuality*, *paedophilia*, *transvestism*, *fetishism* and *bestiality*.
12 Disorders of gender identity include *transsexualism* and *bisexuality*, though the latter category is a contentious one.

References

Becker, H. (1963) *Outsiders*. New York: Free Press.
Boswell, J. (1980) *Christianity, Social Tolerance and Homosexuality*. London: University of Chicago Press.
Braude, W. (1983) Management of sexual deviation. In Berrios and Dowson (Eds) *Treatment and Management in Adult Psychiatry*. London: Baillière Tindall.
Dowson, J. H. (1983) Management of disorders of sexual function. In Berrios, G. & Dowson, J. (Eds) *Treatment and Management in Adult Psychiatry*. London: Baillière Tindall.
Ellis, A. & Arbanel, A. (Eds) (1961) *The Encyclopaedia of Sexual Behaviour, Vol. 1*. London: The Corsano Co.
Ford, C. & Beach, F. (1951) *Patterns of Sexual Behaviour*. New York: Harper.

Freud, S. (1908) 'Civilised' sexual morality and modern nervous illness. In *The Standard Edition of the Complete Psychological Works of Sigmund Freud, Vol. 9*. London: Hogarth Press.
Freud, S. (1912) In Strachey, J. (Ed.) *Standard Edition of Complete Works, Vol. 10*. London: Hogarth Press.
Freud, S. (1949) *Collected Papers Vol. II Letters to Fliess*. London: Hogarth Press.
Freud, S. Letter quoted in Friedman, M. & Rosenman, R. (1959) Association of specific overt behaviour patterns with blood and cardiovascular findings. *Journal of the American Medical Association*, **169**: 1289.
Fromm, E. (1957) *The Art of Loving*. London: George Allen & Unwin.
Giddens, A. (1971) *Capitalism and Modern Social Theory*. Cambridge: Cambridge University Press.
Henderson, D. & Batchelor, I. (1962) *Henderson and Gillespie's Textbook of Psychiatry, 9th edn*. Oxford: Oxford University Press.
Kaplan, H. (1974) *The New Sex Therapy, Vol. 1*. New York: Brunner Mazel.
Kaplan, H. (1979) *Disorders of Sexual Desire*. London: Baillière Tindall (Volume II of *The New Sex Therapy, Vol. 1*. New York: Brunner Mazel).
Kinsey, A., Pomeroy, W. & Martin, C. (1948) *Sexual Behaviour in the Human Male*. Philadelphia: W. B. Saunders.
Kushner, A. (1973) Two cases of auto-castration due to religious delusions. In Brown, L. (Ed.) *Psychology and Religion*. Harmondsworth: Penguin Books.
Laub, D. & Fisk, N. (1974) A rehabilitation programme for gender dysphasia syndrome by surgical sex change. *Plastic and Reconstructive Surgery*, **53**: 388.
Marcuse, H. (1964) *One Dimensional Man*. London: Routledge & Kegan Paul.
Marx, K. The communist manifesto. In Bottomore, T. & Rubel, M. (Eds) (1956) *Karl Marx, Selected Writings in Sociology and Social Philosophy*. Harmondsworth: Pelican.
Masters, W. & Johnson, V. (1970) *Human Sexual Inadequacy*. Boston: Little Brown.
Masters, W., Johnson, V. & Kolodny, R. (1982) *Human Sexuality*. Boston: Little Brown.
Mead, M. (1942) *Growing Up in New Guinea*. Harmondsworth: Pelican (first published 1930).
Mead, M. (1943) *Coming of Age in Samoa*. Harmondsworth: Pelican (first published 1928).
Meyer, R. & Salmon, P. (1984) *Abnormal Psychology*. Herts: Allyn & Bacon.
Mitchell, J. (1975) *Psychoanalysis and Feminism*. Harmondsworth: Pelican.
Money, J. & Weideking, C. (1980) Gender identity/role normal differentiation and its transpositions. In (Wolman, B. (Ed.) *Handbook of Human Sexuality*. New Jersey: Prentice-Hall.
Moore, T. V. (1959) *Heroic Sanity and Insanity*. London: Grune and Stratton.

Reich, W. (1969) *The Sexual Revolution*. New York: Glencoe.

Sartre, J. P. (1960) Tome, I. (Ed.) *Critique de la raison, dialectique*. Paris: Gallimard.

Siegalman, M. (1972) Adjustment of homosexual and heterosexual women. *British Journal of Psychiatry*, **120**: 477.

Simmons, J. (1969) *Deviants*. New York: Glendessary Press.

Skultans, V. (1979) *English Madness—Ideas on Insanity 1580–1890*. London: Routledge & Kegan Paul.

Slater, E. & Roth, M. (1969) *Clinical Psychiatry*, 3rd edn. London: Baillière Tindall.

Stafford-Clark, D. & Smith, A. (1983) *Psychiatry for Students*, 6th edn. London: George Allen & Unwin.

Szasz, T. (1973) *The Manufacture of Madness*. London: Paladin.

Tollison, C. & Adams, H. (1979) *Sexual Disorders*. New York: Gardner Press.

Trethowan, W. & Sims, A. (1983) *Psychiatry*, 5th edn. London: Baillière Tindall.

Weber, M. (1958) *The Protestant Ethic and the Spirit of Capitalism*. New York: Glencoe.

Weinberg, J. (1982) *Sexuality—Human Needs and Nursing Practice*. Philadelphia: W. B. Saunders.

Welch, M. & Kartub, P. (1978) Socio-cultural correlates of incidence of impotence: a cross-cultural study. *Journal of Sex Research*, **14**: 218–230.

Wolbert-Burgess, A. & Lyttle-Holmstrom, L. (1981) Rape: sexual disruption and recovery. In Howell, E. & Bayes, M. (Eds) *Women and Mental Health*. New York: Basic Books.

Wolff, C. (1977) *Bisexuality—A Study*. London: Quartet Books.

28

Anorexia Nervosa and Obesity

Appetite comes with eating.

Rabelais

Food is a subject of great interest to most people, often to a degree which cannot be simply explained by the biological necessity of eating. To eat may be pleasurable indulgence but to refuse food, and thus arouse guilt, may be equally rewarding.

In this section we explore the worlds of the fat and the thin, the obese and the anorexic, both of whom are liable to be encountered in both general and psychiatric hospitals and certainly amongst our acquaintances.

Anorexia Nervosa

In 1689, in his 'Treatise of Consumptions', Dr Richard Morton described the case of Miss Duke, aged eighteen, who suffered from 'an ill and morbid state of the spirits'. Her appearance was 'like a skeleton, only clad in skin', and she was given to self-starvation and continual studying. Miss Duke refused any treatment and died.

We now recognize that she was suffering from the condition named 'anorexia nervosa' by Gull in 1874.

The term is somewhat misleading as anorexia means loss of appetite and the sufferer from anorexia nervosa does not refuse food because of simple loss of appetite but embarks upon a fanatical course of fasting which may terminate in death. Follow-up studies have revealed a mortality of 21.5% (Halmi, 1975) and, although the condition is uncommon, an increasing incidence has been noted (Bruch, 1970).

We have already stated that mental disorder is often difficult to separate from its social context, and this becomes particularly apparent in considerations of anorexia nervosa— the 'slimmer's disease'.

The media continually remind us that 'slim is beautiful'. Adverts for calorie-reduced breads, biscuits, soups, crackers and soft drinks abound. Women's magazines contain much advice for the dedicated dieter, and there are magazines aimed solely at a target audience of slimmers. The calorie conscious may even join a slimmers' club. Slim actresses and models stare at us haughtily from the pages of newspapers and magazines and from the television and cinema screens. Official health propaganda reminds us that fat is unhealthy and that overeating is the cause of it.

The slim person is presented as attractive, controlled, healthy and desirable, while the fat person is liable to be regarded as unattractive, sloppy, unhealthy and undesirable. This potent message may have particular impact during the vulnerable years of adolescence when self-image is readily influenced by social pressures.

In some people, usually sensitive adolescent girls, there develops a compulsive desire to pursue thinness by continuing to lose weight far beyond the bounds of sensible or reasonable dietary adjustment. Fasting may be pursued to the point of death. This is anorexia nervosa.

Features of anorexia nervosa

The patient is invariably thin and has sometimes lost so much weight that the skin seems to be lying loosely over bones only just beneath the surface. Loss of weight down to 30 kg (approximately five stones), or even less, is common.

The skin itself is dry and papery, without normal suppleness and elasticity, and it may show a prominent growth of downy hair (*lanugo*) on the extremities and trunk.

The basal metabolic rate is greatly reduced, blood pressure is low, and the circulation in the extremities is poor. Hands and feet are cold and may be cyanosed. The patient feels the cold bitterly and may wear several layers of woollens (which have the added advantage of disguising the weight loss).

There is amenorrhoea, which has usually been

present from early in the illness, and which sometimes precedes the most obvious signs of reduced dietary intake.

Obstinate constipation is often present, probably due to the low fluid and food intake.

Most foods, especially the most nutritious, are regarded with revulsion, and the strongest resistance is made to taking an adequate diet, even to taking food at all.

The patient will often readily promise to eat, but all efforts are made in the opposite direction.

Much cunning is shown in disposing of food by ways other than eating it. Hiding places will be found where food can be concealed until it is disposed of down the lavatory.

If anything is taken voluntarily it will be something without nutritive value such as sips of water and fruit or salads. The diet may become a bizarre one of nuts and pickles, radishes or carrots.

An orange/yellow pigmentation may appear on the palms and soles, around the nose and on the axillary folds. This is due to elevated blood levels of carotene (*carotenaemia*) and may persist for years, even when weight returns to normal.

The face is pallid, though gross anaemia is often absent, and some patients attempt to disguise this by use of make-up so that they look like rather garish painted dolls. Muscular weakness and shrinkage appear and growth eventually ceases.

Head hair becomes thin, dry, brittle and lifeless and may fall out, though pubic and axillary hair are normal.

Bradycardia usually accompanies the low blood pressure of emaciation, though tachycardia may occur in the terminal stages, when it is a grave sign. Tachycardia also develops when the patient is treated with chlorpromazine (Dally and Gomez, 1979).

There may be an increased incidence of epileptiform seizures amongst patients with anorexia nervosa. One study revealed that 10% of patients had one or more fits, often after heavy drinking of alcohol, vomiting, purging or during treatment with chlorpromazine (Dally and Gomez, 1979).

Some patients have episodes of *bulimia* (compulsive over-eating) as self-control of appetite weakens. Some writers refer to variants of anorexia nervosa in which eating binges are prominent as 'bulimia nervosa'. These episodes are often followed by feelings of disgust leading to self-induced vomiting caused by tickling the back of the throat with a finger or spoon. Some girls learn to induce vomiting by drinking large volumes of water. Persistent vomiting may lead to erosion of dental enamel by acidic stomach contents.

Dependence upon laxatives may develop, particularly after bulimic 'binges'. One girl took 100 Senokot tablets at a time whenever she had an eating binge, which was sometimes several times a week. Electrolyte imbalance may develop as a result of persistent vomiting and purging.

Despite fanatical fasting, the patient may be preoccupied by food and may take pleasure in cooking for others and may avidly read about food and become very knowledgeable about calorific values.

Hunger is very intense in many patients but gradually diminishes with time and may disappear altogether. As control over hunger is established, the patient's sense of triumph may mount in proportion.

Libido wanes with weight loss although it may have been normal before the onset of the disorder, but sexual intercourse has occurred for the first time in only 1% of patients who are still thin and unrecovered after five years (Dally and Gomez, 1979).

Body image is often distorted and patients may strenuously deny that they are thin even when they have begun to resemble walking skeletons.

Many patients spend long periods of time studying themselves in the mirror and seem to derive satisfaction from the sight of the emaciated body which is visible evidence of the success of their grim dietary campaign. Prolonged mirror gazing (an hour or more a day) is thought to indicate a poor prognosis (Dally and Gomez, 1979).

Stealing may occur, particularly during overeating phases and when weight is beginning to return. This stealing is of a compulsive nature and may take the form of shoplifting of jewellery, perfume, clothing and other symbols of femininity, these being used to enhance a basically unsure femininity. Food may be stolen during bulimic binges.

Despite her physically reduced state the patient nearly always shows a remarkable degree of energy, alertness and initiative. Up to the time of admission she will frequently have been engaged in usual social activities, even dancing, swimming and playing tennis (Slater and Roth, 1969).

In many cases she does not feel ill, and her anorexia is not so much a symptom to her as the guiding principle of her life.

Diagnosis of anorexia nervosa

The following are the criteria used to make the diagnosis of anorexia nervosa, as distinct from anorexia due to other causes (Halmi et al, 1975):

1 Onset before 25 years of age
2 Food rejection or restriction, with weight loss of at least 25% of body weight
3 A distorted implacable attitude towards food, eating or weight, that overrides hunger, admonitions, reassurance and threats. For example:

Denial of illness, with a failure to recognize nutritional needs
Apparent enjoyment in losing weight, with overt manifestation that food refusal is pleasurable indulgence
A desired body image of extreme thinness, with overt evidence that it is rewarding to the patient to achieve and maintain this state
Unusual hoarding or handling of food

4 No known medical illness that could account for the weight loss
5 No other known psychiatric disorder, with particular reference to primary affective disorders, schizophrenia, obsessive-compulsive or phobic neurosis.
6 At least two of the following manifestations:

Amenorrhoea
Lanugo
Bradycardia
Periods of overactivity
Episodes of bulimia
Vomiting (often self-induced)

Secondary anorexia nervosa

The term secondary anorexia nervosa is used to describe a different type of anorexic disorder arising in older girls, often in the late teens or early twenties. It differs from true or primary anorexia nervosa in some important respects.

In secondary anorexia nervosa, thinness is not pursued for its own sake but rather for the effect it will have on others, usually people close to the patient. Secondary cases may be precipitated by relationship difficulties or an unsatisfactory sexual experience, and there may be unconscious fear of pregnancy.

Weight loss will lead to a lowering of libido and this may come as a relief to the psychosexually immature girl who may be confused and distressed by her sexuality. The personality type may be char-acterized by immaturity, dependence, obsession-ality and sometimes hysterical traits, though the precipitating factor is almost always sexual.

Lanugo, cyanosis of the extremities and caro-tenaemia are unlikely in secondary types, and amen-orrhoea is unlikely to develop for six months or more after marked weight loss. Menstruation tends to resume promptly with weight gain in secondary types, whereas primary anorexics may wait for up to a year or more for menstruation to resume after weight has been gained.

In contrast to the drive and energy of the primary anorectic, secondary cases may complain of fatigue.

Loss of weight may be as extreme as in the primary form and loss of appetite may be genuine. There may be associated anxiety and depression, coupled with marked insecurity about sexuality and relationships. Relationships are often viewed in a very idealistic way and, should reality fail to match the patient's exaggerated expectations, high levels of anxiety and insecurity may result.

Male anorexia nervosa

Anorexia nervosa may, less commonly, develop in males and may be of a primary or secondary type. The incidence has been variously estimated at one male per 10 females (Slater and Roth, 1969) and one male per 15 or 20 females (Dally and Gomez, 1980). Male cases may be inhibited and unassertive and may show both severe weight loss and marked obsessional features.

Anorexia nervosa of late onset (tardive anorexia nervosa)

Anorexia nervosa may also less commonly develop in older women, often over the age of forty, who have a long history of minor illnesses and may show a resentful dependence on her daughter, coupled with thinly veiled disdain for her husband.

Depression and sleep disturbance may accompany this form and the patient may both identify and compete with her daughter. Egocentricity and immaturity may be prominent.

Causes of anorexia nervosa

Anorexia nervosa is probably due to a complex of interacting factors, and research has tended to concentrate on the primary form.

Studies of primary anorexia have commented that

it often appears with the secondary sexual changes of puberty. Menstruation signals the arrival of womanhood with all its attendant demands and responsibilities, and the adolescent girl may be highly conscious of the pressures of her new feminine role and may have high levels of sexual and social anxiety. Her family may also have high academic expectations of her and this adds to the difficulties of adjusting to new sexual and social expectations.

Fasting may represent an attempt to 'turn the clock back', to return to the safer world of childhood. As weight is progressively lost, menstruation ceases—the persistent reminder of her new status has been eradicated. As more weight is lost, the female curves which develop at puberty fade with progressive loss of subcutaneous fat and the patient once again assumes the angular contours of childhood. To this extent anorexia nervosa may be regarded as a flight from femininity.

This theory of faulty sexual development is perhaps given added weight by the finding that many anorexic girls fail to get married, and, of those who do, many complain of frigidity (Evans, 1982).

Fasting may also be used as a potent weapon of protest against real or imagined injustices, for example the political prisoner who embarks upon a hunger strike or the Chinese custom of sitting upon a debtor's doorstep and visibly starving to shame him into payment.

This may well be an important factor in anorexia nervosa.

The protest of fasting may not just be against the female role, and all that it embodies, but may also incorporate elements of protest against parental expectations and family dynamics.

The dynamic situation within the family is nearly always found to be out of the ordinary, most typically with an overprotective mother who tends to be dominant and obsessionally rigid and who is driven into extremes of anxiety by her daughter's behaviour (Barcai, 1971).

A history of feeding difficulties in childhood is relatively common (Barcai, 1971), though a proportion of patients are obese in the pre-anorexic period and may have a strong interest in food (Slater and Roth, 1969).

There may be a family history of neurosis and there may have been signs in earlier years of hysterical or obsessional traits (Barcai, 1971).

Minor psychological abnormalities are relatively common around puberty, some patients being con-

spiciously tomboyish, and others showing prudishness or disgust with matters relating to sex, including the development of their secondary sexual characteristics.

Siblings may become upset by the patient's refusal to eat and may themselves refuse to eat. By the time referral is made, the family unit may have been stressed by the patient's behaviour for some time and may be touchy and oversensitive in discussions concerning their daughter's difficulties. This may make it difficult to obtain a clear impression of what family functioning was like before the food refusal began.

Discussion with the patient may reveal marked levels of psychosexual anxieties; the anorexia nervosa may then seem a long, slow form of suicide provoked by the prospect of assuming the role of woman.

Precipitating factors

The disorder may be triggered by one or more of a variety of factors, any one of which may serve to precipitate underlying tensions and unhappiness about the patient's life circumstances.

Significant factors which may emerge include anxiety over examinations, disappointment over a job, an engagement to marry which the patient secretly does not feel willing to carry out, or loss of friendship or affection (Sim, 1974).

At this stage the patient may successfully divert attention onto their prominent physical symptoms, thus concealing both the underlying conflicts and the reduced food intake.

Treatment and nursing care

A variety of treatments have been tried including hypnosis, psychoanalysis, electroplexy, anabolic steroids and prefrontal leucotomy, all with a failure to produce consistent results (Halmi et al, 1975).

Large numbers of cases were misdiagnosed as suffering from hypopituitarism (Simmonds' disease) and were treated accordingly, not infrequently with fatal results. It has been estimated that, between 1914 and the 1940s, only one in six patients diagnosed as having Simmonds' disease actually had it; the rest had anorexia nervosa (Dally and Gomez, 1979).

Tube feeding was once widely used but this is fortunately now uncommon as it is hazardous and barbaric and does not in any way serve to restore normal eating patterns. Tube feeding also tended to engender feelings of animosity towards medical and nursing staff which were not conducive to the creation of a climate wherein the underlying conflicts could be satisfactorily explored.

Traditional treatment consisted of exhortations to eat (largely from the nursing staff) coupled with a strictly supervised high protein diet and, often, large doses of chlorpromazine or imipramine. There is a risk that such a regime may simply recreate the family scenario of admonitory and anxious parent figures pressuring the reluctant patient to eat.

The most consistent published results of successful treatment have described a behaviour modification approach, with or without concomitant use of drugs. This approach has resulted in substantial weight gain while hospitalized, and this gain has been maintained on discharge, as evidenced by follow-up studies (Halmi et al, 1975).

The basic principles of behaviour modification are applied, that is the desired behaviour (eating, with associated weight gain) is reinforced, while the undesired behaviour of food refusal is stripped of reinforcers. Positive reinforcements of social activities, increased physical activities and visiting privileges are made contingent on weight gain.

Nursing considerations

Girls suffering from primary anorexia nervosa are usually attractive and of above average intelligence, and, by the time hospitalization occurs, may be accomplished interpersonal manipulators.

The nursing approach should be consistent, and firm but gentle, and awareness of the ruses employed by the anorectic is essential.

Food may be concealed or disposed of in a variety of ways and unobtrusive observation should be maintained at meal-times. Food may be flushed down the lavatory, perhaps being transported there in pockets, sponge bag or wrapped in a towel or newspaper. Fellow patients may be persuaded to eat or conceal food, and food may even be thrown out of windows. The author recalls an incident when an anorectic girl disposed of a plate of custard by tipping it out of a second storey window to land over a passing visitor who gazed skyward, apparently under the impression that he had been dive-bombed by an unusually large pigeon. Food may be pushed down the waste pipes of sinks or down wash hand basins.

The nurse should also be alert to the possibility of self-induced vomiting, perhaps caused by drinking large volumes of water.

The immediate priority is weight gain and this takes precedence over attempts to explore underlying conflicts.

Weight gain should be monitored by weighing under standardized conditions; that is, the patient should be weighed each morning in her nightdress, after passing urine, but having had nothing to drink. The nurse should be aware of the fact that the patient may try to give the false impression of weight gain by drinking large volumes of water before weighing, or by concealing heavy objects (e.g. collections of coins) about her person.

The patient who is mutinously starting to eat again may attempt to burn up calories by relentlessly exercising in her room or by spending hours walking up and down corridors.

The nurse may make a valuable contribution to treatment by actively participating in a behaviour modification programme of the type outlined below.

Behaviour modification programme for anorexia nervosa

The patient is stripped of social privileges (visitors, phone calls, mail, television, mixing with staff and fellow patients) and these are gradually returned contingent on satisfactory weight gain. A target weight (appropriate to patient's height and age) is established and identified to the patient.

Initially the patient is isolated and restricted to a single room, devoid of the social privileges mentioned above. This regime may seem unduly harsh but it has a high success rate and can literally be life saving, and may be experienced as less harrowing than an authoritarian regime of tube feeding.

For the first three weeks the patient is given a formula feed (prepared from Complan or Sustagen or the like) diluted to one kcal/ml, since too rapid a weight gain can have serious medical complications.

For the first week the patient receives 125% of the basal requirement, that is the ideal requirement for her height and age, plus 25%. During the second week, 150% of the basal requirement is given and this is increased to 200% during the third week.

During the fourth week the patient is given three meals of a regular diet, including a morning, afternoon and evening snack. These meals are given in the ward dining area, the patient being given 30 minutes to finish each meal. The patient must record all food returned to the kitchen.

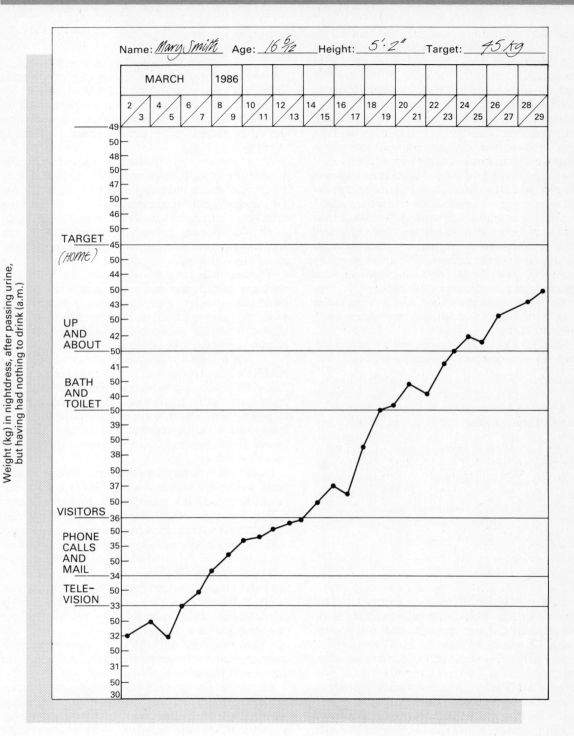

Figure 15 Chart of weight gain and targets.

Thereafter the patient is required to gain 0.5 kg per 5-day period, with the exception of the first 5-day period when she is required only to maintain her weight.

Staff, relatives and visitors are instructed not to discuss food and weight with the patient.

Thereafter privileges are gradually returned with increasing weight (see Figure 15) and the patient can begin to receive re-educative therapy, with particular emphasis on her interactions with others.

The average length of hospitalization necessary is 6–8 weeks, and after discharge, the patient is maintained on the behaviour modification programme.

The programme must be explained to the family and their cooperation is important. Individualized positive reinforcements (e.g. new clothes, records and books) and special activities may be arranged by the family for a weight gain of 0.5 kg per week until the patient reaches normal weight range.

If the patient loses more than 1 kg at any follow-up visit, arrangements are made for readmission.

Treatment of secondary anorexia nervosa

In secondary forms treatment must be directed against the underlying cause, and psychotherapy is often useful in focussing the patient's awareness on this area. Unsatisfactory or distorted relationships with a husband, fiancé or boyfriend may be discussed with both parties to divert attention away from the 'red herring' of food refusal onto the real, often sexual, fears and inadequacies. Psychotherapy is seldom successful unless the patient has reached 85% of her ideal weight (Dally and Gomez, 1979) and drugs (chlorpromazine or imipramine) may be used during the initial stage of weight gain.

Outcome

The majority of girls with primary anorexia nervosa recover completely to lead normal, contented lives, and may marry, have children and make good mothers. The youngest patients (11–14 years of age) are most likely to recover rapidly and have no recurrences.

About 10% of patients progress to chronic anorexia nervosa (lasting seven years or more).

It is likely that many milder forms are dealt with successfully by family and friends, perhaps with the support of the general practitioner, and thus never require psychiatric intervention in a formal setting.

Obesity

Obesity may be defined as 'a state in which there is excessive accumulation of fat' (Davidson et al, 1975). Fat accumulation may be considered as 'excessive' when it is at least 10% above normal, or desirable, weight for the patient's height and frame (Craddock, 1978).

Most people would unhesitatingly identify the severely emaciated anorexic girl as being ill, but to be fat may evoke entirely different responses. The fat lady is the butt of comedians' jokes and has been cruelly caricatured in generations of seaside post-cards. The anorexic girl may excite pity and concern but the fat person is likely to be contemptuously dismissed as a glutton.

The anorexic girl who pursues her quest for thinness to extremes is almost certain to occasion psychiatric referral and treatment, but the obese individual may continue to accumulate fat uninterrupted, save for occasional appeals from family, friends, conscience or general practitioner.

Obesity need not reflect underlying psychological conflict of the type found in anorexia nervosa, but many fat people are far from being the 'jolly' and contented individuals they are conventionally thought to be. The nurse may encounter the obese individual in the psychiatric hospital and, in many cases, the obesity may be either cause or effect of mental disorder.

Obese individuals will often attempt to rationalize their weight by blaming it on their 'glands', and, while there are a few endocrine disturbances which will lead to rapid weight increase, they tend to cause unmistakeable associated physical symptoms of the underlying illness which rapidly necessitate medical treatment.

The simple truth of the matter is that obesity is caused, in the vast majority of cases, by simple over-eating. If calories in excess of the body's requirements are consumed, the balance will be promptly stored as fat.

Overeating need not take the form of gluttonous gorging. Habitual consumption of a small excess of calories will steadily lead to obesity.

Emotional factors may be as prominent in overeating as in undereating. Overeating is common when people are under stress, and it has been suggested that neurotic traits and symptoms are to be found in obese people to a greater extent than in the non-obese (Sainsbury, 1980).

Withdrawal, or threatened withdrawal of affection, may cause regression to an earlier level of gratification where self-reward by eating may be used to create a feeling of security. The rapid increase in weight of those who give up smoking has also been explained on this basis (Sim 1974).

Overeating patterns may develop in childhood if an unhappy child substitutes the pleasures of food for the missing pleasure of love from his parents.

In adulthood, escape may also be sought from loneliness, anxiety or depression in the solace of food, which may become the only reliable pleasure in an otherwise bleak existence.

Treatment of obesity

In simple obesity, uncomplicated by underlying psychological conflict, the most effective treatment is still reduction of calorie intake by dieting, particularly if combined with exercise. The obese should be warned of the dangers of suddenly embarking upon strenuous exercise regimes however.

Massage will only serve to reduce the weight of the masseur, and patent nostrums like cider vinegar and other herbal concoctions claimed to 'dissolve fat' will most certainly reduce the bank balance but not the weight.

Vibrating electrical belts and other 'slimming machines' which allegedly 'break down fat' will certainly break down the composure of any unfortunate spectator but will have no effect upon adipose tissue.

The aspiring slimmer should also beware of relaxing with a drink in an attempt to take her mind off food. A single glass of whisky or sherry is the calorific equivalent of two eggs, a glass of milk, a helping of potatoes or a slice of bread and butter.

Commercially advertised slimming biscuits and cubes do nothing to retrain taste and eating habits permanently, and provide so little residue that intractable constipation is liable to develop.

The obese individual who expends considerable energy at work should be warned of the dangers of embarking upon 'crash' diets. Total starvation can only be undertaken under the most careful medical supervision in hospital and, even at that, there have been a few sudden deaths from heart failure.

Self-help groups are often effective as they provide an atmosphere of support and encouragement.

Draconian measures like 'apronectomy'—removal of fat from the abdominal 'apron' which may develop—may initially appear to have been satisfactory but prominent nodules, or lumps, of fat may develop post-operatively, leaving the patient in a worse condition than before surgery.

Wiring the teeth together, for five months or more, results in improvement in about 10% of cases, as there is a risk of bouts of compulsive overeating occurring in response to stress after the wiring is removed (Dally and Gomez, 1980).

In obesity complicated by underlying mental disorder, the problem may or may not resolve if the mental disorder is treated successfully. Faulty eating habits may have become firmly established by the time mental health improves, and may be difficult to eradicate.

Behavioural treatment of overeating may eradicate faulty eating habits and may be easily administered by the psychiatric nurse.

The programme is easily understood by patients and may be very effective in simple obesity or in residual overeating difficulties left after resolution of a neurotic disorder.

It has been demonstrated that obese persons are far more readily influenced by environmental factors than are the non-obese. 'External' factors such as palatability, time of day and availability of food are more likely to lead to impulsive eating than 'internal' factors such as hunger and interval of time since the last meal (Schachter, 1968).

Behavioural approaches aim at establishing control over environmental factors linked with overeating and are usually coupled with dietary advice and identification of the unwanted effects of overeating. The desired outcome is hopefully the development of the necessary self-control required to lose weight and maintain weight loss.

The programme is most widely used with outpatients, though the underlying principles may be usefully employed in weight reduction programmes for the in-patient.

Environmental control of eating

The patient is given dietary advice, and a suitable low calorie diet is constructed using the food-exchange principle. This involves compiling a varied list of foods of comparable calorific value from which the patient is thereafter free to select from the list as she wishes, so long as the daily total does not exceed her stipulated maximum. The unwanted effects of overeating are then discussed with the patient and general dietary advice is given, including the identification of foods of a high calorific value. The following programme of environmental control is then advocated:

1 Always eat at the same time and in the same place.
2 Remove foods from all places in the house other than the kitchen.
3 Only use foods that require preparation—avoid 'convenience' foods.
4 Make eating a 'pure experience'; that is, do *not* pair eating with other activities such as reading, watching television, listening to the radio or records, or talking on the telephone.
5 Chew food slowly and pause between mouthfuls.
6 Pause for 2–3 minutes before commencing a meal and pause for a similar period midway through the meal.

Drinking a pint of water before commencing a meal will give a feeling of 'fullness', as will the addition of natural bran to meals. Both of these measures may help to reduce food craving between meals.

Reduction of eating activities may be compensated for by the introduction of other activities incompatible with eating (for example, telephoning a friend or going for a walk).

Weight should be monitored and weight loss reinforced by the nurse making her approval apparent. The patient may also provide self-reinforcement by arranging visits to the theatre, buying new clothes or any other self-identified reinforcers, all made contingent on reaching target weights.

Key Concepts

1 Anorexia nervosa is a disorder characterized by food refusal, which may lead to debilitation or death.
2 It is commonest in adolescent girls but may occasionally affect males.
3 It is characterized by aversion to eating and a fanatical pursuit of thinness.
4 The patient does not suffer from true anorexia but, rather, learns to master her feelings of hunger.
5 Control of hunger may occasionally weaken, and the result may be episodes of compulsive overeating (bulimia).
6 Eating 'binges' may be followed by self-induced vomiting or abuse of purgatives.
7 Despite her reduced state, the patient nearly always shows both energy and alertness.

8 Physical signs and symptoms may be prominent and often include amenorrhoea, hypotension, lanugo and carotenaemia.
9 The patient does not regard her anorexia as a problem but, rather, tends to see it as the guiding principle of her life.
10 Theories abound as to the causes, but a central feature is often rejection of the female role.
11 The disorder is often precipitated by a stressful situation.
12 A secondary form affects older females and is often characterized by fatigue and genuine loss of appetite.
13 The secondary form involves a pursuit of thinness, not for its own sake, but rather for the effect it will have on others.
14 The secondary form is usually precipitated by relationship difficulties or unsatisfactory sexual experiences.
15 Primary anorexia nervosa may be treated conservatively (supervised diet and drugs) or by the use of behaviour therapy.
16 In behaviour therapy of anorexia nervosa, social privileges are removed and gradually returned, contingent on weight gain.

References

Barcai, A. (1971) Family therapy of anorexia nervosa. *American Journal of Psychiatry*, **128**: 286–290.

Bruch, H. (1970) Changing approaches to anorexia nervosa. *International Psychiatric Clinics*, **7**: 3–24.

Craddock, D. (1978) *Obesity and its Management*. Essex: Longman.

Dally, P. & Gomez, J. (1979) *Anorexia Nervosa*. London: Heinemann Medical Books.

Dally, P. & Gomez, J. (1980) *Obesity and Anorexia Nervosa*. London: Faber & Faber.

Davidson, S. et al (1975) *Human Nutrition and Dietetics*. London: Churchill Livingstone.

Evans, J. (1982) *Adolescent and Pre-Adolescent Psychiatry*. London: Academic Press.

Halmi, K., Powers, P. & Cunningham, S. (1975) Treatment of anorexia nervosa with behaviour modification—effectiveness of formula feeding and isolation. *Archives of General Psychiatry*, **32**(1): 93–96.

Sainsbury, M. J. (1980) *Key to Psychiatry*. Australia: Australia & New Zealand Book Co.

Schachter, S. (1968) Obesity and eating. *Science*, **161**: 751–756.

Sim, M. (1974) *Guide to Psychiatry*. London: Churchill Livingstone.

Slater, E. & Roth, M. (1969) *Clinical Psychiatry*. London: Baillière Tindall.

29

Suicide and Parasuicide

> 'Death hath a thousand doors to let out life:
> I shall find one.'
>
> *Philip Massinger*

The word suicide is usually taken to mean a fatal act of self-injury undertaken with *conscious* self-destructive intent, thus excluding self-destructive behaviours in which conscious intent is not apparent (speeding, drinking and driving, heavy cigarette smoking, anorexia nervosa, alcohol and drug abuse).

The term parasuicide refers to a deliberate act of self-harm which does not have a fatal outcome. Parasuicide is still sometimes described as 'attempted suicide', which is unsatisfactory as many persons so designated are *not* trying to kill themselves. Non-fatal acts of self-injury may be due to a combination of at least two tendencies, one of which may be the urge to self-damage, and possibly to self-destruction, the other of which may be the urge to elicit concern and love from other people. Parasuicide may thus be viewed as an extreme form of non-verbal communication, intolerable distress and inability to cope being announced by the act. Parasuicide is increasing steadily in frequency to the extent that, in many parts of Britain, deliberate self-poisoning has become the most common reason why women are admitted as emergencies to general hospitals and the second most common reason (after ischaemic heart disease) for similar admissions of men (Hawton and Catalan, 1982).

Suicidal behaviour tends to arouse strong emotional responses in most people, the act of suicide perhaps being regarded as 'self-murder' and thus tainted with sin or guilt. Despite the fact that neither the Old nor the New Testament directly forbids suicide, the Judeo-Christian ethic has tended to oppose it vehemently (in 693 the Council of Toledo proclaimed that a person who attempted suicide was to be excommunicated, and St Augustine described suicide as 'a greater sin that anyone might avoid by committing it').

The medieval church ferociously condemned suicide and insisted that the soul of a suicide was condemned to an eternity of hell. Dante (1265–1321) described the souls of suicides as being entangled in withered thorny trees where they were fed upon by monsters, inflicting wounds from which issued cries of lamentation and pain.

In the Middle Ages the corpses of suicides were degraded by being dragged through the streets followed by burial in non-consecrated ground, often at a crossroads with a stake driven through the heart and a stone over the face, preventing the spirit from returning to haunt the living (such a practice continued in London until 1823) (Morgan, 1979).

As late as 1961, attempted suicide was still a crime in England, where the law made provision for the hanging of the individual if he or she survived. Although explicit moral condemnation of suicidal behaviour is now rare there may often be moral residues implicit in the societal response to self-damaging behaviour, such patients often displaying awareness of stigma by describing their actions as a sign of 'weakness' or 'failure' and suffering debilitating (and quite unnecessary) loss of self-esteem.

Who Is Most at Risk?

Given that any person may be at risk if stress persistently overwhelms capacity to cope, it is possible to identify factors positively related to self-damaging behaviour. Emile Durkheim (1858–1917), one of the founding fathers of sociology, offered broad sociological explanations, insisting that suicide was always a social act. He distinguished three principal types of suicide:

1 *anomic* (under conditions of normlessness, the person being socially 'adrift' or 'uprooted').
2 *egoistic* (lack of ties with the community) and
3 *altruistic* (self-sacrifice for the good of society, as in the case of Japanese suicide pilots—kamikaze).

Durkheim's observations are broad generalizations, subject to some criticism by later sociologists. Perhaps the commonest generalization made is that the 'typical' suicide is male and elderly, while the 'typical' parasuicide is female and young.

Factors positively related to suicide:
1 Male sex
2 Increasing age
3 Widowhood
4 Single or divorced
5 Childlessness
6 Urban residence (especially in the 'zone of transition', e.g. 'bedsitland')
7 High standard of living
8 Economic crisis
9 Unemployment
10 Moderate to high alcohol consumption
11 Use of illicit drugs
12 Broken home in childhood
13 Mental disorder or chronic physical illness

Factors negatively related to suicide (reducing risk):
1 Female sex
2 Low density of population
3 Rural occupation
4 Religious affiliation or membership of any large well-integrated group with which the individual can identify and from which he can obtain support
5 The married state
6 Large number of children
7 Membership of the lower socioeconomic classes
8 War—there is an inverse relationship between suicide and homicide rates

Seasonal variations in rate have been reported. Peaks have been demonstrated in spring and in autumn. In Edinburgh, April and November have suicide rates which account for a quarter of the annual total (McCulloch and Philip, 1972).

Occupation may be associated with increased risk. Doctors, nurses and police officers are over-represented in the statistics, and occupational stress coupled with increased awareness of suicide methods are thought to be partially responsible.

Immigrants may suffer high levels of anomie and most immigrant groups in the United States have been found to have higher suicide rates than either native Americans or their fellow countrymen at home (Sainsbury, 1969).

Unemployment has been shown to bear a marked relationship to risk of self-harm. One study revealed that unemployed males were nineteen times more likely to harm themselves deliberately than those in employment (Platt, 1983). Risk of self-harm increases steadily as the period of unemployment lengthens.

Mental disorder

It has been found that on average one-third of persons committing suicide have been suffering from a neurosis or psychosis or a severe personality disorder. Suicide seems rare in the mentally handicapped (Stengel, 1970). This, however, reveals that two-thirds of persons who harm themselves do *not* suffer from mental disorder. 'Distress drives people to self-poisoning acts and distress is not the exclusive province of the mentally ill.' (Kessel, 1965) A common reaction to suicide is to insist that *anyone* who attempts suicide must be mentally disordered, at least at the time of the act. This may divert attention away from the situational and social causes of stress.

Jack London, in his classic study of the London poor (1903), writes vehemently of the frequency of the verdict 'temporary insanity' at coroners' inquests into suicides.

'Temporary insanity! Oh, these cursed phrases, these lies of language, under which people with meat in their bellies and whole shirts on their backs shelter themselves, and evade the responsibility of their brothers and sisters, empty of belly and without whole shirts on their backs.'

Birtchnell (1982) writes 'Probably, it is not that the suicide is caused by the depression, but that it arises out of the predicament which incidentally causes the person to be depressed'.

Despite the dangers of glib and complacent explanations of suicide which ignore situational stress, it would be equally inappropriate to minimize the increased risk associated with some forms of established mental disorder. Depressive disorders carry the highest suicidal risk, particularly those with prominent feelings of futility, pessimism, guilt and self-reproach. 'Invariably depressed patients want to die and many, though not all of them, commit or attempt suicide.' (Stengel, 1970) Chapter 13 discusses the assessment of suicidal risk in the depressed person.

Severe personality disorder may be characterized by powerful aggressive impulses, which are sometimes directed against self to find expression in either parasuicidal or suicidal behaviour. In schizophrenia there are occasional examples of suicidal behaviour in which the patient impulsively responds to delusional ideas or hallucinatory instructions. The grossly hallucinated, delusional or withdrawn patient should always be regarded as carrying an increased suicidal risk.

Marital problems

These were found to be the most common contributory factor in one study affecting 68% of females studied and 83% of males (Bancroft, 1979). More than two-thirds of married subjects had marital problems, and half of the men had been involved in extramarital relationships during the preceding year, as had a small minority of the women.

Problems with children

It has been found that parents who abuse or neglect their children and those regarded as at special risk of doing so have very high parasuicide rates (Roberts and Hawton, 1980).

Alcohol

In Edinburgh 48% of men who had committed parasuicide were found to have problems with alcohol (Holding et al, 1977) and another study revealed that alcohol had been taken within 6 hours preceding the event by 55% of men and by 25% of women, and often in amounts greater than usual (Morgan, 1979).

In all of the situations discussed, certain factors tend to repeatedly emerge: the person is subject to intolerable stress, and believes that life has become futile, and that others are powerless to help.

How Common Is Suicidal Behaviour?

This is difficult to ascertain. Many parasuicidal acts may be concealed because of stigma or fear of involuntary psychiatric hospitalization. Coroners' verdicts may be extremely unreliable as coroners in Roman Catholic and Moslem countries may return verdicts of accidental death to spare relatives' stigma. Stengel (1970) comments that 'this is why the very low suicide rates of the Republic of Ireland and Egypt are suspect'.

It has been estimated that in the world, every year, the equivalent of the population of Edinburgh kills itself, while the equivalent of the population of London indulges in an act of deliberate, non-fatal self-harm (parasuicide) (McCulloch and Philip, 1972). It has been estimated that these are gross underestimates and that actual rates are from two to ten times as high as official statistics suggest (Meyer and Salmon, 1984). Overall it has been estimated that about three times as many women as men commit parasuicidal acts, but three times as many men actually kill themselves (Marsella, 1980).

Methods Used

In England, drug overdoses account for about two-thirds of suicides among women and about a third of those among men (Morgan, 1979); in Japan, barbiturate overdose is the commonest method (Meyer and Salmon, 1984). Increase in the prescription rates of psychotropic drugs has created a situation whereby a wide range of lethal substances has been placed in the hands of those persons most likely to commit acts of self-poisoning. Tricyclic antidepressants are extremely cardiotoxic.

Men tend to use more violent methods than women (hanging, shooting, drowning, precipitation from a height), though it should be emphasized that the person intent on suicide will find the means in almost any environment. A broken window or light bulb will provide razor sharp fragments and psychiatric in-patients may clandestinely accumulate tablets.

Manipulative Versus Genuine Attempts

The term 'manipulative suicide attempt' tends to be widely used and has unfortunate implications. It would be a grave error of judgement to dismiss non-fatal acts of deliberate self-harm as 'attention-seeking' or 'manipulative' and to conclude that the person concerned has 'no intention' of 'genuinely' attempting suicide. Deliberate self-harm should never be regarded lightly as many parasuicides go on to complete the act at a later date. Among patients who have been involved in acts of deliberate self-harm, the suicide rate in the subsequent 12 months is about 100 times greater than in the general population (Gelder et al, 1983). The patient admitted to the accident and emergency department after an act of deliberate self-harm may encounter attitudes of hostility from nursing and junior medical staff, especially if the act is perceived as being of low lethality. Self-induced disorder is likely to be seen as an unwelcome addition to the workload, though persons surviving acts of high lethality are likely to be viewed as 'genuine' and thus tend to receive sympathy (Morgan, 1979).

Antipathy towards survivors of deliberate self-harm is described by London (1903) who recounts the attitude of a magistrate towards a young woman who attempted to drown herself in a canal: 'If you wanted to do it, why didn't you do it and get it done with? Why did you not get under the water and make an end of it, instead of giving us all this trouble and bother?'

Unsympathetic or hostile attitudes will add to feelings of despair and helplessness and may dramatically increase the likelihood of a repeat act, this time of high lethality. Remember that many lay people genuinely believe that 10 aspirins are a fatal overdose or that wrist slashing will cause almost immediate death from exsanguination. The nurse should try to see past the method used to assess the seriousness of the underlying suicidal intent.

It is true that there is a small percentage of individuals who regularly make suicidal gestures without any intention of causing self-harm. The poet and novelist, Laurie Lee, recalls one of his uncles thus:

'he committed suicide more than any other man I know but always in the most reasonable manner. If he drowned himself, then the canal was dry: if he jumped down a well, so was that: and when he drank disinfectant there was always an antidote ready, clearly marked to save everybody trouble'.

One day his uncle was sacked and vanished into the mist-shrouded woods to make an end of it. A search party of children eventually found him 'hanging' by his braces from an oak tree, his toes touching the ground. 'We approached the contorted figure with dread; we saw his baleful eye fixed on us. Our Uncle Sid was in a terrible temper. "You've been a bloody long time!" he said.' (Lee, 1959).

Most casualty departments have a small number of regular 'repeaters' of the Uncle Sid type, who tend to be discussed with a blend of despair and affection by the staff. It would be an error to regard all chronic repeaters as unlikely to commit serious acts of self-harm however. Repetition of acts of deliberate self-harm increases the chances that an individual will subsequently die from suicide (Hawton and Catalan, 1982). Chronic repeaters of the Uncle Sid type are relatively rare.

Child Suicide

Suicide is extremely rare in children under 14 years of age, though there is a dramatic rise in incidence at puberty and throughout adolescence (De Cantanzaro, 1981). Each year in Australia, the UK and the USA there are only one or two child suicides per million of the population, though acts of deliberate self-harm are distressingly common (Kosky, 1983). One study revealed that 72% of children in an in-patient unit had entertained the idea of suicide (Pfeffer et al, 1979). Suicidal behaviour is commonest in male children and is associated with personal experiences of loss, academic under-achievement, marital disintegration and past intrafamilial violence, including physical abuse of the index child. Suicidal children tend not to have a past history of antisocial behaviour, and classroom behaviour is unremarkable (Kosky, 1983).

Amongst children who do commit suicide almost half had made threats before (Gelder et al, 1983), so in children, as in adults, threats should be investigated with care.

Rational Suicide

It has been commented that 'there can be no doubt that suicide is occasionally the rational act of a mentally healthy person' (Gelder et al, 1983) and the ancient Greeks and Romans made a practice of rational suicide, such suicides falling into Durkheim's category of 'altruistic suicide' (suicide in response to a social ethic which permitted or dictated suicide under appropriate conditions).

The Roman philosopher, Seneca, commented: 'Just as I shall select my ship when I am about to go on a voyage or my house when I propose to take a residence, so shall I choose my death when I am ready to depart from life' (Seneca, AD 55). Rational suicide seems commonest in persons suffering from chronic, painful and incurable illnesses, and suicide notes tend to reflect concern with practical arrangements to be made after death, as opposed to the accusatory or emotive notes often left behind by the psychologically disturbed.

Suicide—Facts and Fiction

Many false beliefs persist about suicide including the following:

Fiction: suicide happens without warning.
Fact: suicidal individuals give many clues; 80% have to some degree discussed with others their intent to commit suicide (Meyer and Salmon, 1984). Suicidal feelings should never be regarded lightly.

Fiction: once people become suicidal they remain so.
Fact: suicidal persons remain so for limited periods, hence the value of intervention.

Fiction: suicidal behaviour is evidence of mental disorder.
Fact: as already noted, this is not so. Suicidal impulses usually arise from situational stress.

Fiction: suicidal tendencies are inherited.
Fact: there is no direct evidence of a genetic factor (Meyer and Salmon, 1984).

Fiction: once a person starts to come out of a deep depression, the risk of suicide reduces.
Fact: the risk of suicide is highest during the downswing into depression and during the upswing from the depth of a depression.

Fiction: once the depressed person commences antidepressant medication, suicide risk reduces.
Fact: psychomotor retardation lifts before mood in response to most antidepressants, creating a brief period of increased suicide risk (10–21 days after commencing treatment with tricyclics). Once mood starts to lift, the risk reduces.

Fiction: talking about suicidal feelings is morbid and should be discouraged.
Fact: the opposite is the case; patients should be encouraged to discuss troublesome feelings of this sort, thus reducing feelings of isolation and despair.

Fiction: persons with a history of several acts of deliberate self-harm have no intention of ever killing themselves.
Fact: they have a suicide risk that is 100 times that of the general population.

Fiction: patients with a history of deliberate self-harm are simply 'attention seekers' and should be treated unsympathetically and disapprovingly as this will discourage them from any repetition of this behaviour in the future.
Fact: harsh or unsympathetic treatment creates a gulf between staff and patient, is unethical, prevents effective communication (essential at a time of crisis) and increases the likelihood that the humiliated patient will 'really show them' that he/she means it the next time.

Nursing Care

By the time the psychiatric nurse meets the patient who has indulged in an act of deliberate self-harm, the patient will usually have spent some days in the general hospital. Gastric lavage will often have been carried out after self-poisoning, and slashed wrists sutured, the patient who has overdosed on cardiotoxic antidepressants will have spent 2–3 days on a cardiac monitor. The patient is likely to be traumatized physically and emotionally. Self-esteem may be low and feelings of despair high.

Nursing care is based to a large extent on the principles of crisis intervention, which are uncomplicated . . . 'the inexperienced therapist often feels that he lacks knowledge of sophisticated treatment techniques. He need not feel this, for crisis intervention is mostly a matter of common sense' (Hawton and Catalan, 1982).

Assessment of current situational stress, which precipitated the act of deliberate self-harm, is essential. Usually patients do not need a psychoanalyst but the services of a social worker. Current life difficulties must be identified and attempts made to reduce them (housing, financial, domestic difficulties). The psychiatrist will assess the patient's mental state and treatment will be commenced as appropriate. Coping resources and supportive relationships should also be assessed.

Planning supportive psychotherapy will help to restore lost self-esteem and self-confidence and will encourage resolution of personal problems. If there is overt depression and/or anxiety, then nursing care is planned accordingly. If low stress thresholds have been identified at assessment, then instruction in stress-proofing techniques (relaxation, breathing exercises, meditation and dietary modification) will be beneficial.

Implementation emphasizes the development of self-sufficiency. The nurse helps to establish goals and may suggest ways of attaining them, but the emphasis remains on the patient's striving for increased personal growth, independence and increased self-awareness. The nurse should try to avoid slipping into the role of Critical Parent, and interactions should focus firmly on the patient's Adult ego state.

If the patient's life difficulties centre on relationship difficulties with a partner or family member(s), it is helpful if these people are involved in counselling sessions.

Throughout the delivery of care the nurse should express unconditional positive regard, warmth and concern, without encouraging unhealthy dependence on the patient's part. The patient's self-esteem can be strengthened by reminding him of positive achievements and by warmly noting and reinforcing any gains made. Passive reliance on medication should be discouraged, as one study comments: 'Problems in personal relationships are unlikely to be altered directly by medication' (Hawton and Catalan, 1982).

Evaluation should (as always) be continuous and the care plan should be flexible enough to allow for steady movement as goals are realized and care moves on to fresh goals. Monitoring of mood and suicidal intent should be continuous, and observation should not be relaxed at the first signs of lifting of mood.

Planning for discharge should ensure that adequate follow-up is planned. The community psychiatric nurse and the social worker should be contacted at the earliest stages of discharge planning. Referral to other agencies may be helpful (social services, self-help groups, 'Gingerbread' groups for single parents, psychosexual problems clinics, marriage guidance clinics) and such referral must be made before discharge. An out-patient department appointment is usually made to enable ongoing psychiatric assessment.

Prevention

Prevention may be aimed at the social level or at the individual level. Social responses of an organized nature date back to 1906 when the Salvation Army established an anti-suicide department, the scope of which was limited to referrals from a few public agencies.

The Samaritans was founded by a clergyman in 1935 and is an organization based on the belief that the majority of suicides present not medical but social and spiritual problems. If medical difficulties are apparent the client is referred to a doctor.

The help offered by the Samaritans consists of 'befriending', that is the offer of 'friendship, neighbourly care, concern and love by people who are lay both medically and ecclesiastically' (Stengel, 1970). One quarter of the Samaritans are ex-clients.

Evidence of the efficacy of the Samaritans is contradictory. Some studies suggested a fall in suicide rate in cities with a Samaritan branch when compared to matched cities without Samaritan branches, though replications of the study failed to show any difference (Hawton and Catalan, 1982). Studies have also found that there are many differences between parasuicidal individuals and Samaritan clients. For example, the Samaritan clients showed a greater percentage of men and were more socially isolated (Kreitman and Chowdhury, 1973).

Despite the difficulties in evaluating the success of the Samaritans in preventing suicide, there can be little doubt that they use sound fundamental principles in helping those in despair. Initial telephone contact is often followed up by personal contact to make intervention at a time of crisis and, thereafter, support may be provided over a considerable period of time. The philosophy of the Samaritans is perhaps best summarized in this excerpt from an address given by an eminent suicide researcher to the Samaritans:

> 'They (the Samaritans) are trying to tell these people (suicidal individuals) "See, you can have friendship and love without risking your life" . . . the person threatened by suicide is like someone suffering from a deficiency disease and you are trying to make good that deficiency . . . by offering love and friendship, the stuff of life which they lack' (Stengel, 1970).

In the USA there are at least 200 organizations wholly or partly concerned with the prevention of suicide, the most notable of which are the suicide prevention centres which are staffed by psychiatrists, psychologists and social workers. These centres function as emergency clinics and offer 24-hour coverage.

The first American branch of the Samaritans opened in 1973 and, at present, the Samaritans are active in nine countries. Prevention programmes aimed at the individual level are largely exercises in primary prevention whereby vulnerable groups are identified and resistance increased. Suicide rates may be reduced if individuals are educated about stress and its effects at an early age. It is encouraging to note that many schools are now teaching children about stress, its causes and effects and its management. A large British insurance company has produced an excellent stress management teaching pack, aimed primarily at school children, and which is available (free) on request to all interested persons (Crusader Insurance Co., 1984). Education about the harmful effects of drug and alcohol abuse will also play a part in reducing suicidal morbidity, and these programmes should again be aimed at primary school children. The proliferation of voluntary agencies, the growth of community resources, increased education—all of these can only have a positive effect, but rising unemployment and social deprivation can only have a negative effect on overall rates of deliberate self-harm.

Though prevention rightly addresses itself to the question of social precipitants of self-harm, there will always be a pressing need for the identification of and assistance of the psychologically vulnerable. Suicide occurs in almost all societies and cultures, including primitive cultures, and tends to occur proportionately in all economic levels of society.

'The inner self is the part of us that is most vulnerable . . . the course of civilisation has shown us that, although we have mastered techniques for sealing off the mind by educating children to be stupid, people safely sealed off from dangerous ideas may still be exceedingly vulnerable to attacks on the self from within' (Henry, 1973).

Key Concepts

1 The term suicide refers to a deliberate and fatal act of self-harm.
2 The term parasuicide refers to a deliberate and non-fatal act of self-harm.
3 Non-fatal acts of self-harm frequently do not involve a desire to end life; they may be signals of intolerable distress—a cry for help.
4 Non-fatal acts of self-harm should never be regarded lightly, even if they occur on a repeater

basis. These individuals have a suicide risk that is 100 times that of the general population.
5 Only a third of persons exhibiting suicidal behaviour are suffering from mental disorder; the rest are usually experiencing intolerable situational stress which has exceeded capacity to cope.
6 Mental disorders, in particular the depressive disorders, carry an increased risk of suicide.
7 Suicide is commonest in males, while parasuicide is commonest in females.
8 Suicide rarely occurs without warning.
9 Suicidal impulses tend to remain intense for limited periods, hence the value of crisis intervention.
10 Nursing care involves careful observation and the building of a therapeutic nurse/patient relationship that will supply the friendship, concern, warmth and hope in which the patient is so often lacking.

References

Bancroft, J. (1979) Crisis intervention. In Bloch, (Ed) *An Introduction to the Psychotherapies*. Oxford: Oxford University Press.

Birtchnell, J. (1982) The life histories of some suicidal patients—pointers to the aetiology of suicidal behaviour. *British Journal of Clinical and Social Psychiatry*, 2(1): 1–7.

Crusader Insurance Co. (1984) Stress management teaching pack.

De Cantanzaro, D. (1981) *Suicide and Self-Damaging Behaviour*. London: Academic Press.

Gelder, M., Gath, D. & Mayou, R. (1983) Suicide and deliberate self-harm. In Henderson, Sir D. K. & Gillespie, R. D. (Eds) *Oxford Textbook of Psychiatry*. Oxford: Oxford University Press.

Hawton, K. & Catalan, J. (1982) *Attempted Suicide*. Oxford: Oxford University Press.

Henry, J. (1973) *On Sham, Vulnerability and Other Forms of Self-Destruction*. Australia: Allen Lane.

Holding, T., Buglass, D., Duffy, J. & Kreitman, N. (1977) Parasuicide in Edinburgh—a seven year review 1968–74. *British Journal of Psychiatry*, 130: 534–543.

Kessel, N. (1965) self-poisoning. *British Medical Journal*, 2: 1265–1336.

Kosky, R. (1983) Childhood suicidal behaviour. *Journal of Child Psychology and Psychiatry*, 24(3): 457–468.

Kreitman, N. & Chowdhury, N. (1973) Distress behaviour: a study of selected Samaritan clients and parasuicides (attempted suicide patients). *British Journal of Psychiatry*, 123: 1–8.

Lee, L. (1959) *Cider with Rosie*, p. 181. Harmondsworth: Penguin Books.

London, J. (1903) Suicide. In *People of the Abyss*. London: Journeyman Press.

Marsella, A. (1980) Depressive experience and disorder across cultures. In Triandis & Draguns (Eds) *Handbook of Cross-Cultural Psychology*. Herts: Allyn & Bacon.

McCulloch, J. & Philip, A. (1972) *Suicidal Behaviour*. Oxford: Pergamon Press.

Meyer, R. & Salmon, P. (1984) *Abnormal Psychology*. Herts: Allyn & Bacon.

Morgan, H. (1979) *Death Wishes—The Understanding and Management of Deliberate Self-Harm*. Chichester: John Wiley & Sons.

Platt, S. (1983) Unemployment and parasuicide in Edinburgh, 1968–82. *Unemployment Unit Bulletin*, **10**: 4–5.

Pfeffer, C. et al (1979) Suicidal behaviour in latency children. *Journal of the American Academy of Child Psychiatry*, **18**: 679–692.

Roberts, J. & Hawton, K. (1980) Child abuse and attempted suicide. *British Journal of Psychiatry*, **137**: 319–323.

Sainsbury, P. (1969) Social and community psychiatry. *American Journal of Psychiatry*, **125**: 105–112.

Stengel, E. (1970) *Suicide and Attempted Suicide*. Harmondsworth: Penguin Books.

VIII

MENTAL DISORDERS
AT THE EXTREMES OF LIFE

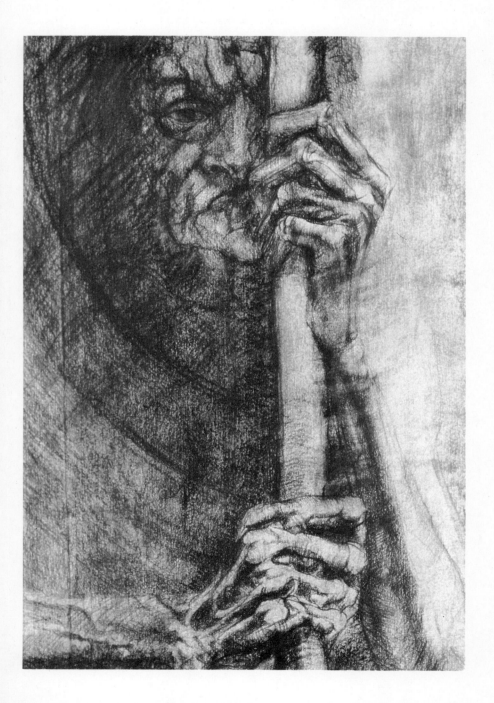

30

Mental Disorders of Childhood and Adolescence

'Who are *you*?' said the Caterpillar. Alice replied, rather shyly, 'I hardly know, sir, just at present—at least I know who I *was* when I got up this morning, but I think I must have been changed several times since then.'

Lewis Carroll: Alice's Adventures in Wonderland

The human infant is helpless, vulnerable and dependent for a longer time than the young of any other mammalian species. This dependency continues for a number of years and early experiences provided during this period play a critical part in shaping personality, and in determining the child's perceptions of adult roles and responsibilities. Developmental psychology is discussed in Chapter 5 and most of the models discussed suggest that there are critical periods in development when the child is most plastic and ready to acquire those behaviours necessary for optimal adjustment in later life. For example, Erikson (1963) has suggested that basic trust in others is a characteristic acquired during the first year of life through warmth and affection received from parenting figures. If this hypothesis is true, the lack of early affectionate care will result in the child growing up to be mistrustful of others and inadequate in social relationships.

The concepts of *maturation* and *learning* are basic to any considerations of development. Maturation refers to inherent aspects of growth which are largely independent of the environment and which proceed at their own rate, though an essential minimum of stimulation and support is needed. Learning refers to the acquisition of behaviours in response to *external* factors (e.g. reward, punishment, modelling). Most behaviour depends upon both maturation *and* learning; for example, a child learns to talk only when he has grown old enough to learn (maturation) but the language he learns is the one he hears (learning).

The importance of learning in the acquisition of behaviour was emphasized (some would say over-emphasized) in the writings of early behaviourist psychologists who saw the child as a tabula rasa (blank tablet) to be written upon by the experiences provided by the environment. A well-known example is the assertion of the behaviourist J. B. Watson that, given a child from birth, he could transform him into a criminal or a university professor, irrespective of his race or antecedents (Watson, 1914).

The learning theory viewpoint contends that children display maladaptive behaviour either because they have been reinforced (albeit inadvertently) for so behaving or because patterns of reinforcement have not been consistent (adaptive behaviour has not been consistently reinforced and maladaptive behaviour has not been punished or has not been associated with the absence of rewards). This viewpoint does not see maladaptive behaviour as the result of internal tensions or imbalance (e.g. impaired Ego boundaries or Super-Ego hypertrophy) in distinction to the psychoanalytical viewpoint which emphasizes early experiences as determinants of adult well-being.

Freud saw development in terms of conflict between the eternal antagonists of psychic life: biological drives (the Id) versus awareness of practical necessity (the Ego) versus perceptions of others' expectations of self (the Super-Ego). Unhealthy fixation at early developmental stages leads to self-defeating or anti-social behaviour later in life, as unresolved conflicts warp interpersonal relationships, according to this viewpoint.

One area of common ground between learning theory and psychoanalytical models of development consists of emphasis on the importance of coherent and stable patterns of relationships with parenting figures at early malleable developmental periods. The *socialization process* whereby children learn to fit in with, adapt to, and comfortably operate within the society into which they are born, is partially *active* (learning from parents and parental figures) and partially *passive* (absorbing almost by osmosis the values and attitudes of the peer group, though active modelling also plays a part here).

Parental approaches to socialization have been found to play a critical part in determining adjustment and well-being. Parents who use physical punishment frequently produce children with a high incidence of feeding problems (Sears et al, 1957) and also provide an aggressive model for their children to imitate (Bandura and Walters, 1963). Physical punishment has also been found to produce children who are low in self-esteem (Coopersmith, 1967) and unfriendly (Eron et al, 1963). Children who are physically punished by parents tend to inhibit aggression in the home but show increased aggression in other situations, such as school (Bandura and Walters, 1963). Parents who use *love-orientated* techniques in regulating behaviour (praise as reward, and withdrawal of love as punishment) have been found to produce children who have fewer feeding problems and who effectively develop a sense of conscience that effectively internalizes control (Sears et al, 1957).

Children do not imitate indiscriminately however; many persons' actions and attitudes are observed but are not copied. The child needs to see some similarity between himself and the model in order for him to take over some of the behaviour of the model. There is a tendency for girls to imitate their mothers and for boys to imitate their fathers (Danziger, 1971) and both adaptive and maladaptive behaviours may be so acquired. It seems that it is only the actions of *successful* models that are imitated. The child who witnesses another child receiving rewards (peer group approval, increased group status) for behaving aggressively is thereafter more likely to emulate the aggressive behaviour, whereas the child who observes aggressive behaviour to be unrewarding or unsuccessful is less likely to emulate the aggressive behaviour (Bandura and Walters, 1963).

Vicarious learning also applies to positive behaviour insofar as the child who observes another child being rewarded for adaptive behaviour is more likely to emulate that behaviour. Thus the process of becoming social, though largely unconscious, is by no means automatic. The microclimate of the family and the macroclimate of the greater society both provide stimuli to acquire new behaviours and provide opportunities to test newly acquired responses.

Adolescence is accompanied by a surge of activity in the socialization process as the physical changes of puberty herald the onset of the move away from dependence on the family and towards the peer group as a major source of social status and security.

Emerging needs for independence may lead to conflict with parents and parental figures and self-esteem is often both fragile and highly dependent on the judgement of others. Studies reveal that there is a relationship between parental interest and adolescents' self-esteem. Parental interest was found to be associated with high self-esteem and lack of parental interest with low self-esteem (Rosenburg, 1965).

Authoritarian parents and parental figures who simply tell adolescents *what* to do without explaining *why*, and without considering the wishes of the adolescent, do not eliminate dissent: they simply suppress it. Many children of authoritarian parents emerge from adolescence lacking in self-confidence, self-esteem and independence (Conger, 1979).

Above all, adolescence is a time of rapid-change—physical, sexual, intellectual, emotional and social. The speed of change may contribute to difficulties in establishing a coherent sense of identity. Erikson (1968) comments that 'Before the adolescent can successfully abandon the security of childhood dependence on others he must have some idea of who he is, where he is going and what the possibilities are of getting there'. Failure to achieve a sense of identity (the rather clichéd concept of the 'adolescent identity crisis') may arise where sound adult role models are lacking. Unfortunately, a common response to what Erikson calls '*identity confusion*' is development of a *negative*, deviant identity based on defiance and rebellion for their own sake.

Identity confusion is often associated with low self-esteem, and Coopersmith (1967) suggests that there are four major sources of self-esteem:

1 A feeling of *significance* based upon acceptance, attention and the affection of other people
2 An awareness of personal *competence* based on past and present achievements
3 A sense of *power* rooted in the ability to influence other people
4 A sense of *virtue* derived from adherence to one's own moral and ethical standards.

Adolescent boys in Coopersmith's study who were low in self-esteem reported that they found it harder to make friends, that they were more frequently 'listeners' than 'talkers' in groups, that they were more self-conscious in public, that they were too concerned with inner problems to be worried about broader social problems, that they were relatively sensitive to criticism and that they were likely to conform to group pressures. This study suggests both signs of low self-esteem and sources of self-esteem which may be developed.

Faulty social learning may lead to a variety of deeply engrained maladaptive behaviours which must be assessed carefully and objectively before intervention is attempted.

Assessing the Disturbed Child or Adolescent

The incautious use of traditional medical language and classification in assessing children and adolescents is not helpful. Hobbs (1975) outlines the reasons:

1 The failure of most diagnostic systems to adhere to consistent principles
2 Failure to base diagnostic categories on meaningful and observable behaviour
3 The questionable reliability and validity of the diagnostic categories currently in use
4 The reluctance of clinicians to stigmatize children with labels that may follow them throughout life

Psychiatric labels are easy to affix and notoriously difficult to remove, and once affixed, may prejudice life chances indefinitely. Their use becomes even more questionable when one considers the debate about their validity. Wells (1981) comments that 'diagnostic labels, particularly those used for children, have traditionally provided very little information relevant to selection of the most appropriate treatment procedures, course of treatment or treatment outcome'.

It is more helpful to examine the behavioural characteristics or presenting problems of children or adolescents referred for treatment. Treatment is best offered on the basis of out-patient referral either at a clinic or day centre. Admission to an in-patient facility has many disadvantages: it is stressful for child and parents, it is stigmatizing, it may lead to institutionalization and passive adoption of the 'sick role' and it makes accurate assessment difficult as separation from the family may lead to the development of a range of new deviant behaviours (secondary deviance)—'a child may become enuretic or encopretic once hospitalized' (Matson and Beck, 1981). A particularly undesirable state of affairs consists of the admission of a young adolescent to an adult psychiatric ward. Given the disadvantages of

in-patient treatment it may nevertheless be necessary under certain circumstances, for example suicidal or extremely aggressive behaviour or extreme withdrawal (Matson and Beck, 1981). Parental stress may have reached crisis point and in-patient treatment may then also be necessary.

Rutter (1975) comments that 'hospital care is very rarely adequate in itself and the co-ordination between in-patient and out-patient care is an essential element in the treatment programme'.

Wherever the treatment setting it is important that assessment involves use of clear and objective language that accurately describes the behaviours being examined. The deficits of diagnostic language as a vehicle for describing behaviour become particularly apparent at assessment.

> 'The serious pitfall of using diagnostic labels is the illusory impression it gives the user of having explained the behaviour. What it usually represents is a *re-naming* process. Particular villains are words like "minimal brain damage", "hyperactivity", "psychopathy", "disruptive"' (Herbert, 1981).

It is not helpful to use vague or casual observations (for example, 'John was aggressive all morning'). Where? How? With whom? What happened beforehand? When and how did he calm down? And with whom? Does 'all morning' mean the entire morning?

Vague reference to 'tantrums', 'withdrawal' or 'acting out' are equally unhelpful and convey little useful information to others. What one person means by 'aggression' or 'withdrawal' may be very different from someone else's opinion. It is possible for a child to be labelled hyperactive simply because the observer is particularly intolerant of high levels of activity. A better description would simply focus objectively on observable behaviour. For example, at 10 a.m. AB (staff member) and children were building a house with building blocks, watched by John who refused to participate when invited by AB. On the invitation being repeated, John walked from the room and sat in a corner in the quiet room where he covered his face with his arm and ignored the two other children present (Paul and Mary). He remained so until 10.15 a.m. when Paul approached him in a friendly manner and invited him to play at skittles with them. John responded by jumping to his feet and kicking and scratching Paul, whereafter he ran from the room and hid under the kitchen table, crying bitterly. He did not reply when approached by AB and offered no explanation for his behaviour.

Problematic behaviours must be described clearly if appropriate intervention is to be made.

Even with cautious and objective use of descriptive language it may be difficult to obtain consistent agreement among various adults as to the nature of the young person's disordered responses or behaviour, and even more difficult to reliably ascribe meaning to them. Parental reports of behaviour are often biased in one direction or another (Hetherington and Martin, 1979) and children do not necessarily agree with the way in which parents (and presumably other adults) evaluate their behaviour (Herjavic and Reich, 1982). Psychologist, physician, teacher, parent and nurse may have differing perceptions of a child's behaviour and may thus suggest differing solutions. The multidisciplinary approach to assessment is most appropriate and, if based upon objective factors, is most likely to lead to effective consensus and thus to effective intervention. Rutter (1975) comments that

'for the most part, child psychiatric disorders do not constitute diseases or illnesses' and 'as labels can bring about self-fulfilling predictions, and because most children with psychiatric disorders recover, this (labelling) should be avoided'.

Though incautious or casual use of diagnostic language is to be deprecated, careful approaches to classification have elicited representative disorders of childhood based on *patterns* of behaviour. Such representative disorders have often been arrived at by observing which behaviours *intercorrelate* or 'go together' (for example, children who steal are often also likely to play truant). Recognizable patterns of behaviour may constitute categories but this approach does not deny the uniqueness and individuality of each child—an individuality which will be quickly lost if the child is incautiously assigned to a category as the qualities thought to be associated with that category may distort observers' perceptions of the child. Diagnostic categories may become like moulds and there is a risk that the child's behaviour will be distorted by observational bias until it satisfactorily fits the mould.

Some pervasive developmental disorders have long been recognized and include two rare disorders often regarded as the primary forms of childhood psychosis: infantile autism and childhood schizophrenia.

Infantile autism

This was first described by Leo Kanner in 1943 and is therefore sometimes referred to as a *Kannerian psychosis*. Childhood autism is one of the greatest enigmas known to psychiatry wherein four distinctive characteristics are present:

1 An inability, since birth, to relate to other people
2 Failure to develop communicative language skills
3 An apparent obsession with maintaining regularity in the environment, and
4 The manifestation of isolated intellectual abilities—islets of performance (e.g. high artistic or musical abilities)—which distinguish autistic children from those who are mentally handicapped (Kanner, 1971).

When speech does develop (and in nearly half of the children it never does) it tends to be stereotyped and full of echoed phrases and reversal of personal pronouns (Rutter, 1975). Autistic children have good memories and appear to understand speech because when not watched too carefully they will often whisper well-formed, clearly enunciated sentences (Ney and Mulvihill, 1985). Additional features not present in mental handicap include wider variations on IQ tests, a greater likelihood of seizures, persisting delays in language development and more focal cognitive deficits (Rutter, 1978).

Other manifestations not crucial for diagnosis include *gaze avoidance* (Bhoyrub and Morton, 1983) (the child does not look other children or adults straight in the eye), repetitive motor patterns (e.g. constant whirling or hand flapping) and attempts at self-stimulation, which may include harmful behaviours such as head-banging or pinching or biting of self.

Autism is commoner in boys, and in about three-quarters of cases, there is a degree of associated mental retardation (Rutter, 1975). The causes of this fortunately rare condition remain obscure. Kanner noted that parents of autistic children were often highly intelligent but rigid and compulsive and this led him to propose that autism was the result of sustained contact with unfeeling *'refrigerator parents'* who were unable to relate to the child emotionally (Eisenburg and Kanner, 1956), though recent studies show that the incidence of psychological problems among parents of autistic children is no greater than average (Quay, 1979). Most researchers agree that language difficulty lies at the heart of the problem and neurological deficits have been suggested as causative factors. Autistic children show indications of right cerebral hemisphere dominance including distinct preferences for non-verbal stimuli, such as music (Blackstock, 1978). Auditory hypersensitivity causing withdrawal from the environment has also been suggested (Ney and Mulvihill, 1985). Debate about aetiology continues but does not detract from the fact that the nurse may continue to make a nursing diagnosis of withdrawal and severe communication difficulties.

Prognosis is often rather bleak as very few children recover fully. Of those with normal intelligence, about half will improve sufficently to make a reasonable social adjustment and hold a job, though scarcely any marry (Rutter, 1975). The sophistication of language usage by age five appears to be highly predictive of the severity of autistic symptoms in adolescence and early adulthood (Knopf, 1979). Many adults show evidence of their autistic childhood, often being 'rather quirky in their personal relationships and showing oddities of behaviour of one sort or another' (Bhoyrub and Morton, 1983).

Childhood schizophrenia

Unlike autism childhood schizophrenia does not begin until later childhood (between ages 2–11 years) and is usually preceded by a seemingly normal period of development. Cases before the age of seven years are rare (Rutter, 1975) and late childhood or early adolescence is the commonest period of onset. Schizophrenia in childhood does not differ essentially from schizophrenic reactions in adulthood (withdrawal, blunting or incongruity of affect, impaired relationships, thought disorder and bizarre or stereotyped behaviours). Regressive behaviours and deteriorating schoolwork are common and delusions and hallucinations may be present.

Prognosis tends to be better than in autism, and response to conservative treatment is often good. In nursing terms the problems presented usually do not differ significantly from those presented by autism (withdrawal, communication difficulties, social skills deficit).

Anxiety

Fears and phobias are especially common in early childhood (Rutter, 1975) and free-floating (non-

specific) anxiety is not uncommon. *School refusal*, formerly called 'school phobia', is an important manifestation of anxiety. This disorder is clearly more complex than a simple phobia (Kahn et al, 1980) and is most common in children just beginning school, though it remains a problem throughout the school years. This condition is thought to involve an unwillingness of the child to separate from the parent (and vice versa) rather than a specific fear of school, and most treatment approaches emphasize helping parents and child to develop consistently positive attitudes towards school attendance. One important study suggests that fear reduction through systematic desensitization or traditional psychotherapy resulted in only marginally greater improvement than no treatment at all (Miller et al, 1972).

Children may 'somatize' anxiety, that is transform it into a physical complaint (e.g. headache, nausea, abdominal pain) or express it behaviourally (e.g. tantrums, aggression).

If sources of fear are identified they may be approached gradually (e.g. animal fears) or adaptive approaches to the stimulus object may be modelled by the nurse. Social situations which evoke fear may be approached by *play therapy*, the nurse using puppets to explore and defuse the stimulus situation. The prognosis for childhood fears is good; most dissipate without specific treatment and a follow-up evaluation of a series of phobic children revealed that only 7% of the subjects were still phobic several months later (Miller et al, 1972).

Depression

This seems much less common in childhood than in adulthood. Child suicide is rare (see Chapter 29) and follow-up studies indicate that pre-pubertal children with emotional disorders do not often develop into adults with depression (Rutter, 1975). Depression in childhood does not always present as clearly as the equivalent state in adults and again may be somatized or acted out.

Enuresis

Enuresis or urinary incontinence occurring after bladder control has been established is a troublesome behaviour which is very common in childhood. Its most common form consists of bed-wetting (nocturnal enuresis) and affects up to 20% of all children by age seven (Quay and Werry, 1979). Important aetiological factors suggested have included expression of anger or hostility towards parents for some perceived wrong (Masling, 1982), simple inability to learn bladder control (Herbert, 1981), abnormalities of bladder and urinary tract (Bhoyrub and Morton, 1983) or regression associated with sibling rivalry or feelings of rejection.

Enuresis frequently runs in families, and the association between enuresis and emotional difficulties is more marked in girls and is also marked in those who wet during the day as well as at night (Rutter, 1975). Treatments have included classical conditioning methods, for example the 'bell and pad' method in which bed wetting completes an electrical circuit in a pad placed under the bottom sheet activating a bell which awakens the child who (hopefully) goes to the toilet. This method is moderately effective but relapse rates are high (Doleys, 1977). Operant conditioning techniques include 'dry bed' training which involves encouraging copious oral fluids, waking the child at hourly intervals and praising successful trips to the toilet, and providing aversive consequences for failure (e.g. sheet changing or practice of correct toilet responses). The results of this approach have been fairly encouraging (Azrin et al, 1974).

Family or situational stresses which have caused or contributed to enuresis will require exploration with a view to resolution.

Encopresis (Faecal Soiling)

This may consist of the passage of full motions into underpants or nightwear or may consist of faecal staining. In contrast to enuresis, encopresis usually occurs during the day. Encopresis is much rarer than wetting and is more likely to be indicative of significant psychological problems. The majority of children with encopresis have a disturbed relationship with one or both parents (Bhoyrub and Morton, 1983) but physical causes must be excluded. This problem behaviour may be an aggressive act directed against strict and over-fussy parents who over-emphasize cleanliness and toilet training. It may also arise out of a failure to adequately learn appropriate eliminatory patterns. In

every case psychosis and mental handicap must be excluded as these are commonly associated with encopresis.

Operant conditioning techniques have been used successfully in the treatment of encopresis and employ toilet training with rewards for appropriate eliminatory behaviour.

Abuse of drugs, solvents and alcohol increases in frequency in adolescents, and early adolescence is the peak incidence time for anorexia nervosa. For further discussion of these problems the reader is referred to the appropriate earlier chapters of this text.

A study of first time referrals to a child guidance clinic in London found that 47% presented problems of uncontrollable or unmanageable behaviour (tantrums, aggressiveness, non-compliance, overactivity), 14% displayed anxiety, fearfulness, specific fears and night terrors, 12% displayed habit disorders (enuresis, encopresis or head banging) and the remainder displayed speech and other miscellaneous disorders (Wolff, 1967).

So far we have discussed how the objective specification of behaviours is helpful in assessing young people and we have mentioned how related behaviours give rise to recognizable patterns which may be regarded as representative disorders of childhood. The behavioural approach is an effective antithesis to vague and inappropriate medical terminology but, if taken to extremes, can itself become unhelpful. Over-use of the behavioural approach can lead to a rigid and mechanistic approach (how does the rigid behaviourist respond towards the enuretic child between visits to the toilet?). Remember the emotions behind the behaviours. Rothenberg (1960) has written of children 'seething with greed from so much deprivation, with hate from so little love, with rage from needing and not getting, with love hidden deep and yet right on the surface'. Effective nursing intervention is based upon accurate behavioural assessment but the nurse also acts as a parental substitute in many cases, providing interpersonal stability, security, consistency and warmth, building self-confidence and self-esteem, providing positive learning experiences, providing a positive role model, providing social skills training, and being both source of feedback and careful listener.

As consideration of psychiatric disorders of childhood starts with behaviour and considers the organization of behaviour into patterns, so consideration of treatment interventions returns to behaviour.

Planning

Morgan (1984) identifies three learning tasks commonly undertaken in the behavioural approach to disturbed behaviour of childhood or adolescence:

1 The *learning* of a *desired* behaviour in which the child is deficient (e.g. bladder control, fluent speech, reading skills)

2 The *unlearning* of an *undesired* response (e.g. phobic anxiety, smearing of faeces, facial tics)

3 The *exchange* of one response for another (e.g. self-assertion in place of tearful withdrawal).

These learning tasks may be served by one (or any combination) or three primary types of learning:

1 *Conditioning.* This may be classical (learning by association) (for example, desensitization in which the feared object or situation comes to be associated with relaxation rather than anxiety, or treating enuresis with pad and bell so that 'holding on' and waking is associated with a full bladder instead of wetting). Operant conditioning (learning through consequences) may also be used (for example, increasing the frequency of desired responses by ensuring that these are followed by rewarding consequences such as reinforcement with praise, attention, privileges, tokens or sweets—remember the Premack Principle). Undesirable responses may be reduced in frequency by ensuring that they are not followed by rewarding consequences.

2 *Observational learning.* This is sometimes called 'vicarious learning', in which behaviours are learned by observing or imitating the actions of others (models). Modelling is particularly effective if opportunities are given for reinforced practice of what is learned. Practising the target behaviour alongside the model (participant modelling) is extremely useful in increasing the acquisition of desirable behaviours. Modelling will be effective if the subject is allowed to watch alternative ways of behaving which 'pay off' or are patently successful.

3 *Cognitive learning (learning through thinking).* This method, in which cause and effect relationships are explained and alternative behaviours are decided upon, is also useful. Teaching children to identify problem situations (e.g. aggressive behaviour) and to consider alternative approaches to these situations is an example.

These three primary types of learning may be compared to the three primary colours. In any one painting (as in any one treatment plan) the three primaries may be distinguished, though in any one given approach one may predominate. Pervading and providing a background to all three should be the presence of warmly humanistic nursing attitudes which recognize and respond to the individuality of each child.

Ney and Mulvihill (1985) in a comprehensive and imaginative guide to working with disturbed young people suggest three levels of intervention graded according to (a) the risk to the child, and (b) the skill and training necessary for the staff involved.

First level techniques (low risk) could be implemented by any member of regular staff and do not involve risk to the child, even if the techniques are administered incompetently or incompletely.

Second level techniques (moderate risk) require some specific supervised instruction if they are to be used safely and effectively.

Third level techniques (high risk) involve potential risk to the child and thus require a high level of instruction. This category also includes techniques that require a very high level of expertise.

Examples of techniques assigned to the categories suggested by Ney and Mulvihill are as follows:

First level techniques (low risk)

Play therapy (observation)

In children, play may be a more normal mode of expression than speech. When children play freely they express their thinking, including conflicts, fears, anxieties, imagination and intelligence. Careful observation and recording of a child's pattern of play can reveal a great deal that the child may not yet have put into words. Many children's games involve imaginary companions or elements of ritualistic behaviour and this may be regarded as normal. Play may not only be revealing—it can also be therapeutic: 'Play is of central importance in enabling young children to come to terms with stressful situations' (Bhoyrub and Morton, 1983).

Play may involve modelling clay, paints, sand, water, string, blocks and coloured pieces of fabric. Bendable human figures are particularly useful as they enable the child to model stressful scenarios from the home situation and generally allow projective representation (the child's feelings being projected into the scenes created). Mechanical one-purpose toys are not useful, and toys should generally stimulate the imagination and creative faculties and allow free expression.

In observational play the child is not directed or interacted with but is allowed to play freely, alone, or with another child. The child should be told that it's OK to do almost anything except break toys, harm himself or you. A brief narrative account of play patterns should be recorded.

Compliance training

This is a technique which assists a child in carrying out adult requests where there is a history of inappropriate or unnecessary disobedience. The child is presented with a hierarchy of requests with increasing probability of compliance. Each request is made once only and if the child begins to respond within 5 seconds, it is recorded as a compliance. Compliance is reinforced (sweet, token, gold star on chart, and always verbal praise and approval). Requests are made increasingly difficult but the child should succeed at 70–80% before more difficult tasks are requested (Ney and Mulvihill, 1985).

Self-esteem building

This first level technique is suited to depressed, anorectic or obsessive-compulsive children who have a negative or unrealistically critical view of self. The approach consists of obtaining a baseline measurement of positive self-statements and explaining to child and family the importance of self-esteem and how to obtain it. Self-praise is then modelled to the child ('I think I did a good job on that', 'Well, I'm pleased with the way that turned out'). Elicit self-praise with questions like: 'Do you thing you did that well?' and confirm self-praise: 'Yes, I think you did that well'. Encourage the child to monitor success rather than failure and, later in the programme, focus on more global personal qualities: 'I think I'm not so bad after all, in fact I think I'm all right'. The nurse should emphasize that:

> Liking yourself is OK
> Making mistakes is OK
> Taking pride in achievements is OK

Delayed gratification

This technique is suitable for demanding, impatient, anxious or immature children and consists of teaching children to wait realistically until their needs or desires are met. Baselines are again obtained and the object of the procedure explained to child and parents. Intervals should be increased as tolerated and should depend on the age of the child (e.g. 2 × the child's age). A 3-minute wait is a good starting point but the nurse should use her own judgement to decide whether any given request may be reasonably delayed. 'Nurse, I want to go to the toilet' is a very different category of request from 'Nurse, I want my milk now'. Gains should be reinforced and charted.

Second level techniques

Assertiveness training

This is a suitable approach for children who have internalized aggression or who have a passive-aggressive pattern of behaviour, and will also benefit timid or depressed children. Further indications include the anxiously over-pleasing child, the anorectic, encopretic, enuretic, battered, obese or phobic child (Ney and Mulvihill, 1985). Lack of assertiveness may lead to inappropriate reliance on adults and constant seeking for approval. The timid, dependent child is also likely to be viewed as 'wet' by the peer groups and may be rejected, abused or exploited. Assertiveness may be encouraged by placing young people in a position where they have to make demands, and then reinforcing positive responses. The unassertive child should also be encouraged to associate with peers rather than constantly seeking approval from adults.

Assertive behaviour has been defined as 'behaviour which enables a person to act in his own interests, to stand up for himself without undue anxiety, and to express his rights without denying the rights of others' (Alberti and Emmons, 1974). Lazarus (1973) suggests four categories of assertive behaviour:

1 The ability to say 'no'
2 The ability to make requests
3 The ability to express feelings
4 The ability to initiate, continue and terminate general conversation

Wilkinson (1983) comments that 'the aim of management of very insecure young people is that they become integrated and valued and able to make demands on others and be assertive'. Simple assertiveness training procedures involve explaining the rationale to child and parents and obtaining baseline measurements (at home or school or for the first two days of attendance at the day centre/unit). Demonstrate desirable assertive responses (modelling) using another staff member or child. Construct a hierarchy of situations to which the child responds with anxiety (for example, being called 'stupid' or being asked to read aloud in class). Rehearse self-affirming statements. For example: 'I'm not stupid; there are lots of things I'm good at'. Encourage use of these in role-play, reinforcing self-affirmative responses, until the child develops fluency. Work your way up the hierarchy, becoming more demanding of the appropriate social skills, and finish with 'homework assignments' (i.e. practice in real life). Observe and record progress.

Ney and Mulvihill (1985) point out that 'It is important for the child who cannot interpret social situations correctly to learn only those assertive responses that are unlikely to get him into trouble when used indiscriminately'. Assertiveness training will cause difficulties if it is misinterpreted or used over-enthusiastically by the child, culminating in abusive approaches or a tendency to habitually 'put down' other children.

Play therapy (corrective)

Structured use of play provides opportunities to model adaptive responses and discourage maladaptive responses. Target behaviours should be selected carefully and toys or play situations may be used to generate situations involving these behaviours. Structured play may be used to correct obsessional behaviours, teach social skills and build confidence.

Relaxation techniques

Standard relaxation exercises (see Chapter 17) may be effectively taught to children, and biofeedback equipment will prove useful and will help to capture the child's interest. Relaxation is a useful coping skill to teach and can be used effectively when the child becomes frustrated, agitated or angered (Herbert, 1981).

Self-control (the 'Turtle technique')

Self-control techniques may be usefully taught to impulsive or hyperactive children and involve teaching children to question their first responses

and restrain them appropriately. Schneider and Robin (1976) suggest the 'Turtle technique' for aiding self-control. This begins with a story to tell young children about a boy called Little Turtle who disliked school and used to get angry and tear up his papers in class. One day when he was feeling especially bad he met a talking tortoise who gave him advice:

> 'Hey there, I'll tell you a secret. Don't you realize you are carrying the answer to your problem around with you?' Little Turtle didn't know what he was talking about. 'Your shell, your shell', the tortoise said in his loud voice. 'That's why you have a shell. You can hide in your shell whenever you get that feeling inside of you that tells you you are angry. When you are in your shell you can have a moment to rest and figure out what to do about it. So next time you get angry, just go into your shell'.

The story continues with an account of how the boy remembered this advice the next time he got upset, so he pulled his arms in close to his body, put his head down so that his chin rested against his chest (demonstrate) and rested for a while until he knew what to do.

Turtle technique may be combined with relaxation therapy and teaching of social skills. Impulsive children may also be taught to inhibit impulsive reactions by counting to 10, turning in circles four times or muttering aloud for 30 seconds (Ney and Mulvihill, 1985).

Shaping techniques

This approach uses operant conditioning (learning through consequences) so that children learn that adaptive behaviours are rewarded (and rewarding) and that maladaptive behaviours are not. Nursing staff and parents may inadvertently reinforce the wrong behaviours by paying attention to those behaviours which irritate them most. Attention is a powerful reinforcer and will often maintain behaviour for a longer period than will tangible rewards.

Target behaviours are identified, baseline measurements of their incidence taken, the behaviour is modelled (it may be necessary to 'chain' it or break the behaviour down into small, easily managed steps) and successful responses are reinforced.

The Premack Principle may be used to select effective reinforcers (use a high intensity behaviour—something the child likes to do a lot of—to selectively return as a reward for increases in low intensity behaviour—something the child does not do a lot of). See Chapter 10 for fuller discussion of behaviour modification programmes. Parents must be aware of the programme and must continue it at home.

Third level techniques

Play therapy (interpretive)

'In the child play may be regarded as the speech of the unconscious. He may use the imaginary characters of his play to express his own disturbed feelings' (Kolb and Brodie, 1982). Interpretive play therapy differs from observational (first level) and corrective (second level) play therapy insofar as the observer attempts to interpret the themes emerging in play in an attempt to gain greater understanding of the emotional life of the child in general, and of unconscious conflicts in particular. Interpretations may be offered to the child for discussion: 'I see that you don't like the Mummy doll'. 'Why are you afraid of the Daddy doll leaving the house?'

Supervision and instruction are necessary if this approach is not to lead to transference neurosis in the child.

Empathy training

'Children are born self-centred, not necessarily selfish. They become selfish if they never have an opportunity to care for others.' (Ney and Mulvihill, 1985) Empathy involves the child's capacity to control behaviour by considering its effects on others. It represents 'a rather advanced state in the development of self-control and moral behaviour' (Herbert, 1981).

Some children may be poor at reading the emotions of others, and simple sensitivity training exercises will help to develop this skill. Group exercises in which each child takes turns in non-verbally expressing an emotional states (whispered by the nurse) will help. Suitable emotional states include anger, fear, pleasure, surprise, suspicion, perplexity and boredom.

As sensitivity to emotional states increases, children tend to become more careful of how they interact with others. The child may use a mirror to practise expressing his own emotional states non-verbally. Light-hearted role-play will help the child to gauge the effects of his behaviour on others. Stop

at intervals and ask: 'How do you think that would make someone feel?' And give feedback. The child should be taught to make empathetic statements: 'You look really sad'. 'Has that annoyed you?' You don't like it when I behave like this, do you?' 'You were pleased by that, weren't you?'

Older children and adolescents may benefit from group discussion of topics reflecting emotional states (e.g. 'being angry', 'feeling unhappy', 'good feelings about myself').

Evaluation of interventions should be ongoing and the approach may have to be modified if it becomes apparent that objectives have been met and that treatment may consequently move on to other areas. It may become apparent that the approach selected is not yielding the results, in which case reassessment may be necessary. No approach should be doggedly persisted with 'for its own sake'— compromise and improvisation will be necessary to meet the unique pattern of needs of any given child.

Discharge from treatment should not be unnecessarily delayed. 'It is not necessary or possible to "cure" all defects but young people should be able to survive and continue developing outside the hospital environment.' (Wilkinson, 1983) The goal of treatment is not to produce a meek, acquiescent 'robot' but a healthy young individual who now shows a decreased incidence of problem behaviours and an increased level of coping skills— without any loss of individuality.

Child Sexual Abuse

This is distressingly common. Statistics are uncertain and tend to be conservative but, nevertheless, estimate that 4–25% of females and 10% of males are sexually assaulted before the age of 18 years (Tucker, 1985). A survey of 1072 children who had been sexually assaulted revealed that 60% were over the age of 11 years, 27% were aged 6–10 years and 13% were under the age of 6 years. The youngest was a nine-month-old girl (Mrazek et al, 1981).

Short-term effects include anger, depression and confusion. Long-term effects (over which there is some dispute) may include promiscuity (often associated with alcohol and drug abuse), sexual coldness and relationship difficulties, an increased likelihood of adult depression, low self-esteem and disturbed parenting behaviours, including the likelihood that victims will physically or sexually abuse their own children (Porter, 1984).

Indicators that child sexual abuse has taken place or may be taking place include injuries (bruises, scratches) to the genital area, sexually transmitted infections, pain on micturition, recurrent urinary tract infections, torn or bloody underclothing, preoccupation with, or precocious knowledge of, adult sexual behaviour, regressive behaviour, lack of trust in familiar adults (or marked fear of men), nightmares (especially with sexual content) and marked reluctance to participate in physical activity or to change clothes for physical education, games, swimming or medical examination (Porter, 1984).

About three-quarters of all child sexual abuse emanates from someone the child already knows and trusts, and at least one in four child molesters are members of the same family as the child itself (Tucker, 1985). Family characteristics have long included the stereotype of the authoritarian father and the weak, dependent mother who is unable to protect her child. This may often be the case, but the opposite of this stereotype has also been described (Porter, 1984). Parental unemployment, alcohol abuse and financial problems have been found to be positively associated (Porter, 1984) but child sexual abuse transcends all socioeconomic groupings (Giarreto, 1981). Sexual abuse occurs in secret and may be kept a secret by the family, thus denying aid to both molester and victim.

Incest is a particular form of child sexual abuse which violates taboos and is likely to be kept secret. Father/daughter incest accounts for about three-quarters of cases and mother/son, father/son, mother/daughter and brother/sister incest account for the remaining one quarter (Kempe and Kempe, 1978). Most of the fathers concerned are introverted, socially isolated and family orientated and many are given the extra 'push' by a wife who arranges situations that allow privacy between father and daughter (Kempe and Kempe, 1978). Many fathers have atrophied sexual relationships with their spouses and some fear or hate women and have generally violent and destructive attitudes towards sexuality (Trowell, 1985).

Psychological tests reveal that incest victims see themselves as defenceless, worthless, guilty and threatened from all sides, particularly by the father and mother who would be expected to be their protectors (Kempe and Kempe, 1978). Favourable outcomes are associated with forgiving the parents, increased self-confidence and self-esteem and positive revisions of self-image.

Non-Accidental Injury to Children

Children have been physically abused for centuries, and a sixteenth century physician wrote a clear account of child abuse (Evans, 1985). Mitchell (1984) identifies factors which indicate increased risk of violence:

1 Family history of violence
2 History of failure to resolve potentially violent episodes leading to a belief that a violent outcome is to be expected and is almost inevitable
3 Poor self-esteem and associated loss of confidence in family members
4 Inability to put feelings into words leading to 'acting out' rather than 'talking out'
5 An abiding sense of loss, deprivation, hopelessness and worthlessness with no clear role or status in the family

Kempe and Kempe (1978) add the following factors:
   Parental experience of multiple stress (marital discord, divorce, debt, frequent moves, significant losses)
   Rigid, unrealistic expectations of the child's behaviour, impaired bonding, parental perceptions of the child as being difficult and provocative (whether or not the child is)

These researchers showed that abusive parents can be predicted with 76% accuracy (Kempe and Kempe, 1978). Signs of abuse include:

1 Doubtful or inconsistent explanations of fractures, cuts, bruises, scalds, burns and lacerations
2 Damage around the mouth and ears
3 Bites showing as crescent-shaped marks of a size incompatible with bites inflicted by other children
4 Cigarette burns
5 Bruising in areas unlikely to be affected by falls during play (e.g. centre of back, abdomen)
6 Bruising on upper arm, often indicating that the child has been tightly gripped and possibly shaken
7 Evidence of consumption of toxic substances. Repeated admissions for 'accidental' overdoses are highly suspicious. Some parents even continue to administer drugs after the child's admission to hospital (Evans, 1985).

8 Failure to thrive emotionally or physically, often with loss of weight, lethargy and fatigue

9 Undue fear of adults with apprehensive, withdrawn or aggressive behaviour

10 Attention-seeking behaviour directed against adults, with excessive attempts to please

11 Delayed speech development and regressive behaviour

If child abuse is suspected, the nurse should report her suspicions to her immediate superior. Accurate and detailed documentation is essential as records may be produced during court proceedings. It is usual to order X-rays and photographs, and the medical photography department should be clearly informed that the photographs may be required for legal purposes. Social worker and physician must be notified immediately.

Many children referred to child psychiatry facilities will come from disturbed family units and there will be increased risk of sexual or physical abuse. Awareness of indicators of abuse is essential: 'it is up to us, the health professionals, to be aware of the problem, to recognize abused children, to protect them and their brothers and sisters from further harm' (Evans, 1985).

Ney and Mulvihill (1985) suggest a *Rebonding for Battered Children* technique (third level) which aims to reduce aversive responses in both parent and child:

> 'Being beaten produces a situation whereby anything from the parents is seen as painful. This increases the child's resistance to the parents' direction which increases the parents' annoyance towards the child and results in more battering and pain'.

Bonding and aversive conditioning are explained to parent and child: 'We don't want you to be afraid of each other', and both are taught relaxation. Staff model responses of tolerance and the giving and receiving of positive verbal and physical strokes (cuddling, holding hands, warm, friendly verbal responses). This approach may be augmented by encouraging parent and child to note and discuss positive aspects of one another and by encouraging the child to discuss his/her feelings with the parent.

Family Therapy

Family therapy refers to those psychotherapeutic approaches based on the involvement of most, if not all, family members and is often based on systems' theory, which regards the family as a system and the persons constituting that family as components of the system. The family therapist looks at the problems presented by the 'index patient' or 'identified patient' as but one aspect of the functioning of the family system. If a football team is playing badly, it makes sense to consider the way the whole team plays together rather than to select one player and ignore the rest.

Walrond-Skinner (1981) comments that 'it is the system, not the individual, that must be the target of the family therapist's intervention, whatever his orientation'. The structure of the family is assessed and processes occurring within the family are identified. The aim is 'altering the family's "homeostasis" or fixed patterns of functioning, preferably in a way that will promote growth' (Barker, 1979). The approach may be analytical, behavioural or humanistic, and use is often made of role-play, modelling and contractual agreements between family members and between them and the therapist.

The outcomes hoped for include greater awareness of self and others within the family, increase in empathy and effective communication, and the acquisition of adaptive skills and approaches to be used in resolving conflict within the family. Above all, it is hoped that family therapy will produce greater awareness of the family as a system, of potentially harmful effects generated by the system, and of family members who may be casualties of the system.

The Use of Drugs in Child Psychiatry

Clearly this is a contentious area. There are obvious hazards associated with administering psychotropic drugs to children. Public concern is rising at the routine use of these drugs with adults, let alone children; benzodiazepine dependence, residual tardive dyskinesia caused by phenothiazines, and major side-effects (e.g. extrapyramidal symptoms) are increasingly being regarded with alarm. Drugs often simply suppress troublesome behaviour and, to that extent, may become a method of control rather than a means of treatment. Given these reservations, it is sometimes necessary to use medication (benzodiazepines, phenothiazines and antidepressants) as a temporary measure to make children more amenable to those non-physical treatments to which the majority of childhood difficulties satisfactorily respond.

The Role of the Nurse

Nursing young people can make great demands of the nurse. The nurse is companion, parental figure, friend, arbiter of quarrels, teacher, protector, confidante and authority figure. Nurses are 'adults who care enough to stay around and take whatever is hurled at them: whether it be chairs, love, abuse or jokes' (Wilkinson, 1983). The nurse teaches self-help skills, encourages and develops areas of interpersonal strength and helps make sense of what is often perceived as a confusing or threatening world.

Involvement is helpful to the development of therapeutic relationships. To understand children it is often necessary to partially enter their world, if the necessary empathy is to be built. Rigid routines are not helpful: children can behave like interpersonal quicksilver and slip through the framework of the most carefully constructed approaches. Flexibility, adaptability and the ability to improvise are helpful. Attitudes of warmth, understanding and calm consistency are helpful, and a sense of humour is absolutely essential. Tantrums, hyperactivity and acting out behaviour (in which emotional conflicts are expressed behaviourally) may tax the patience of the nurse to the extreme and create the risk of Critical Parent transactions dominating the nurse's interpersonal style.

Wilkinson (1983) describes the emotional reactions nurses may develop towards young people:

Anger that young people become psychiatrically disturbed, with parents for causing their child's problems, with the children for being násty to parents and themselves, with society and the institution for not providing just what the children need.

Despair that easy 'cures' are not available, at the perceived inadequacy of the nurse's interventions ('I am not good enough').

Sadness (and anger) when the children's sentiments match personal difficulties, past and present.

Elation when quite a small amount of change is observed.

Love for a special child and *guilt* because it is 'unprofessional'.

Resigned humour when it is recognized that all the other feelings will not go away.

There is always a risk of the child developing transference feelings towards the nurse, as feelings and emotions appropriate to parents are transferred onto the nurse who may find herself cast in the role of good or bad parent. Counter transference feelings may arise in the nurse as negative or positive feelings, based on unresolved areas in her own life, are generated towards the young person, often being aroused by transference feelings on the child's part.

The nurse will find herself working with other professionals (teacher, social worker, psychiatrist, clinical psychologist, educational psychologist, play therapist and occupational therapist) and the need for balanced, integrated teamwork is particularly apparent in the children's unit.

The nurse who comes to the care of young people for the first time may find it difficult to adapt to the often startling emotional immediacy and behavioural extremes of young people, and may find it hard to make the necessary adjustments in interpersonal style, perhaps on the basis of fears that it wouldn't be 'professional'. Rigid adherence to 'professionalism' often results in a cramped and inelastic interpersonal style which militates against understanding of and helpful involvement with children.

Children may demand a lot but they can give a lot in return.

Key Concepts

1 Human infants are born helpless and vulnerable and have a long period of dependence on parents during which critical moulding of personality takes place.

2 Parental approaches to *socialization* have been found to play a critical part in determining adjustment and well-being.

3 Punishment-orientated approaches to child-rearing may have negative consequences for the child's well-being, but love-orientated approaches are likely to have positive consequences.

4 Much childhood learning takes place as a result of *modelling* (*vicarious learning* in which the child learns by observing the behaviour of others and by noting its consequences).

5 Adolescence is marked by a surge, not just in physical growth, but in the socialization process.

6 Adolescence is marked by a search for *personal identity* and a move away from dependence on the family group towards dependence on the peer group.

7 *Identity confusion* in adolescence is often associated with low self-esteem, and low parental interest contributes to loss of self-esteem.

8 Assessment of young people should avoid unnecessary or inappropriate use of diagnostic medical terms and, instead, should focus on behaviour.

9 Patterns of intercorrelating behaviours (behaviours which tend to 'go together') constitute recognizable categories of behavioural problems.

10 *Infantile autism* is a rare but troublesome constellation of related difficulties—inability to relate to others, failure to develop communicative language skills, apparent obsession with environmental regularity and the associated presence of islets of performance.

11 *Childhood schizophrenia* together with autism constitutes the second developmental problem of a psychotic nature.

12 Fears and *anxiety* are common childhood difficulties and many children *somatize* anxiety (convert it into a physical complaint).

13 Depression is less common and child suicide is rare.

14 Habit disorders (*enuresis, encopresis*) and conduct disorders (*tantrums, hyperactivity, withdrawal*) are common reasons for referral.

15 Planning usually involves aiming to reduce undesired responses, to promote learning of desired responses or to exchange one type of response for another (e.g. assertion in place of withdrawal).

16 Conditioning (classical or operant), cognitive learning and observational learning (modelling) are three widely used categories of intervention.

17 Nursing interventions may be at first level (low risk), second level (moderate risk) or third level (high risk).

18 Examples of first level intervention are play therapy (observational), compliance training, self-esteem building and delayed gratification.

19 Second level techniques include assertiveness training, play therapy (corrective), relaxation techniques, self-control (e.g. Turtle technique) and shaping techniques.

20 Third level techniques include play therapy (interpretive) and empathy training.

21 Evaluation should be both objective and ongoing and should not seek unrealistically 'ideal' sets of responses.

22 Child sexual abuse (including incest) is common and has distressing psychological effects on the child to which the nurse should be alert.

23 Non-accidental injury to children is also common and, like child sexual abuse, is more likely to occur within disturbed family units.

24 The role of the nurse includes awareness of appropriate behavioural techniques, but technique alone is not enough—warm, flexible attitudes and the ability to improvise are needed.

25 The nurse should consider her own emotional responses to children and should be able to recognize *transference* and *counter transference* reactions.

26 Treatments used are diverse (e.g. behaviour therapy, family therapy and chemotherapy) and the nurse will operate within the framework of the multidisciplinary team.

References

Azrin, N., Sneed, T. & Fox, R. (1974) Dry bed training: rapid elimination of childhood enuresis. *Behaviour Research and Therapy*, **12**: 147–156.

Alberti, R. & Emmons, M. (1974) *Your Perfect Right: a Guide to Assertive Behaviour*. California (San Luis Obispo): Impact Press.

Bandura, A. & Walters, R. (1963) *Social Learning and Personality Development*. New York: Holt, Rinehart & Winston.

Barker, P. (1979) *Basic Child Psychiatry, 3rd edn*. London: Granada.

Bhoyrub, J. & Morton, H. (1983) *Psychiatric Problems in Childhood—a Guide for Nurses*. London: Pitman Books.

Blackstock, E. (1978) Cerebral asymmetry and the development of early infantile autism. *Journal of Autism and Childhood Schizophrenia*, **8**: 339–353.

Conger, J. (1979) *Adolescence*. London: Harper & Row.

Coopersmith, S. (1967) *The Antecedents of Self-Esteem*. San Francisco. W. H. Freeman.

Danziger, K. (1971) *Socialization*. Harmondsworth: Penguin Books.

Doleys, D. (1977) Behavioural treatment for nocturnal enuresis in children: a review of the literature. *Psychological Bulletin*, **84**: 30–43.

Eisenberg, L. & Kanner, L. (1956) Childhood schizophrenia. *American Journal of Orthopsychiatry*, **26**: 556–564.

Erikson, E. (1963) *Childhood and Society*, 2nd edn. New York: W. W. Norton.

Erikson, E. (1968) *Identity: Youth and Crisis*. New York. W. W. Norton.

Eron, L., Walder, L., Togio, R. & Lefkowitz, M. (1963) Social class, parental punishment for aggression and child aggression. *Child Development*, **34**: 849–867.

Evans, R. (1985) The silent victims. *Nursing Times*, November 27th, 59–60.

Giarreto, H. (1981) A comprehensive child sexual abuse treatment programme. In Mrazek, P. & Kempe, C. (Eds) *Sexually Abused Children and their Families*. Oxford: Pergamon Press.

Herbert, M. (1981) *Behavioural Treatment of Problem Children*. London: Grune & Stratton.

Herjavic, B. & Reich, W. (1982) Development of a structured psychiatric interview for children. *Journal of Abnormal Child Psychology*, **10**(3): 307–324.

Hetherington, E. & Martin, B. (1979) Family interaction. In Quay, H. & Werry, J. (Eds) *Psychopathological Disorders of Childhood*, 2nd edn. New York: John Wiley.

Hobbs, N. (1975) *The Futures of Children: Categories, Labels and their Consequences*. San Francisco: Jossey-Bass.

Kahn, J., Nursten, J. & Carroll, C. (1980). *Unwillingly to school: school phobia or school refusal? 3rd edn.* New York: Pergamon Press.

Kanner, L. (1971) Follow-up of eleven autistic children originally reported in 1943. *Journal of Autism and Childhood Schizophrenia*, **1**: 14–19.

Kempe, R. & Kempe, C. (1978) *Child Abuse*. London: Fontana.

Knopf, I. (1979) *Childhood psychopathology*. New Jersey: Prentice-Hall.

Kolb, L. & Brodie, H. (1982) *Modern Clinical Psychiatry*, 10th edn. Philadelphia: W. B. Saunders.

Lazarus, A. (1973) On assertive behaviour—a brief note. *Behaviour Therapy*, **4**: 697–699.

Masling, J. (1982) *Empirical Studies of Psychoanalytic Theories*. New Jersey: Erlbaum.

Matson, J. & Beck, S. (1981) Assessment of children in inpatient settings. In Hersen, M. & Bellack, A. (Eds) *Behavioural Assessment*. New York: Pergamon Press.

Miller, L. et al (1972) Comparison of reciprocal inhibition, psychotherapy and waiting list control for phobic children. *Journal of Abnormal Psychology*, **79**: 269–275.

Mitchell, A. (1984) Violence in the family—a programme for management. *Maternal and Child Health*, November, 342–348.

Morgan, R. (1984) *Behavioural Treatments with Children*. London: William Heinemann Medical Books.

Mrazek, P., Lynch, M. & Bentovim, A. (1981) Recognition of child sexual abuse in the United Kingdom. In Mrazek, P. & Kempe, C. (Eds) *Sexually Abused Children and their Families*. Oxford: Pergamon Press.

Ney, P. & Mulvihill, D. (1985) *Child Psychiatric Treatment. A Practical Guide*. Kent: Croom Helm.

Porter, R. (Ed.) (1984) *Child Sexual Abuse Within the Family*. London: Ciba Foundation.

Quay, H. (1979) Classification. In Quay, H. & Werry, J. (Eds) *Psychopathological Disorders of Childhood*, 2nd edn. New York: John Wiley.

Rosenberg, M. (1965) *Society and the Adolescent Self-Image*. Guildford: Princeton University Press.

Rothenberg, M. (1960) *Children with Emerald Eyes—Working with Deeply Disturbed Boys and Girls*. London: Souvenir Press (Educational & Academic).

Rutter, M. (1975) *Helping Troubled Children*. Harmondsworth: Penguin Books.

Rutter, M. (1978) In Rutter, M. & Schopler, E. (Eds) *Autism—a Reappraisal of Concepts and Treatment*. New York: Plenum Press.

Schneider, M. & Robin, A. (1976) The Turtle Technique: a method for the self control of impulsive behaviour. In Krumboltz, J. & Thoreson, C. (Eds) *Counselling Methods*. New York: Holt, Rinehart & Winston.

Sears, R., Maccoby, E. & Levin, H. (1957) *Patterns of Child Rearing*. Illinois: Evanston.

Trowell, J. (1985) Working with families where incest is actual or feared. *Health Visitor*, **58**: 189–191.

Tucker, N. (1985) A panic over child abuse. *New Society*, 18th October, 96–98.

Walrond-Skinner, S. (1981) In Walrond-Skinner, S. (Ed.) *Developments in Family Therapy—Theories and Applications since 1948*. London: Routledge & Kegan Paul.

Watson, J. B. (1914) *Behaviour: An Introduction to Comparative Psychology*. New York: Holt, Rinehart & Winston.

Wells, K. (1981) Assessment of children in outpatient settings. In Hersen, M. & Bellack, A. (Eds) *Behavioural Assessment*. New York: Pergamon Press.

Wilkinson, T. (1983) *Child and Adolescent Psychiatric Nursing*. Oxford: Blackwell Scientific Publications.

Wolff, S. (1967) Behavioural characteristics of primary school-children referred to a psychiatric department. *British Journal of Psychiatry*, **113**: 885–893.

31

Mental Disorders of Old Age (Functional)

> Her own mother lived the latter years of her life in the horrible suspicion that electricity was dripping invisibly all over the house.
>
> *James Thurber*

Old age is the last major segment of the life cycle and is often unnecessarily regarded in a negative fashion. Development does not stop with the arrival of old age but continues as this period of life brings its own developmental challenges and satisfactions. Negative stereotypes of old age are often reflected in '*ageist*' attitudes which see the elderly as being beset by failing physical, psychological and social abilities which render them ineffectual and relegate them to the background of the social landscape until they 'die of old age'. No-one ever died of 'old age'. People die of cardiovascular or neoplastic disease and ageing is a process, not a problem, a developmental period, not a difficulty.

Erikson (1963) suggests that old age brings the psychosocial crisis of integrity versus despair and a favourable outcome of this crisis consists of developing a sense of fulfilment and satisfaction with one's life, associated with willingness to face death.

Disengagement, the process whereby the ageing individual withdraws from those obligations and expectations governing active working life, may be characterized by satisfaction or frustration. Cultures which emphasize individualism and which view success or failure as the individual's responsibility tend to foster negative disengagement: 'it is here that old people feel useless, dread feeling dependent and play empty roles' (Cowgill and Holmes, 1972). Western industrial societies with a strong work ethic are thought to be more likely to bring about abrupt and often negative disengagement. In many African societies disengagement is balanced by re-engagement as people assume the role of elders, and societies which emphasize collective life (Russia, Samoa, Ireland, the Israeli kibbutz) provide greater security and satisfaction for their elderly members (Cowgill and Holmes, 1972).

Social trends analysis (1986) revealed that only 40% of people over the age of 65 years described themselves as 'healthy and independent', despite the fact that the purchasing power of the state pension has risen (pensioners in 1986 received 15% of the total national disposable income compared with 7% in 1951).

Retirement, death of spouse, social isolation, loss of occupational satisfaction, and failing physical abilities are all factors which may have lasting adverse effects on the psychosocial well-being of the individual. Retirement may have a particularly adverse effect on persons who have had tendencies to occupy themselves in their work to the exclusion of other interests. Work and life may become so interconnected that the loss of a job can demolish self-esteem and induce depression. Marriages may also suffer after retirement as unfulfilled areas of a marriage may be masked by being busy and going out to work. After retirement these problem areas may be impossible to evade, and research by the Marriage Guidance Council has shown that many of the problems faced by older couples are connected with changes in lifestyle brought about by retirement (Whitehouse, 1985). Retirement need not adversely affect relationships, though the demands it makes may make a radical revision of relationships necessary.

Most of the troublesome mental disorders of old age are those associated with declining integrity of the central nervous system (see Chapter 33) but a wide range of functional disorders may also necessitate intervention. The affective disorders (disorders of mood) are extremely common in the elderly and are probably even more common than brain failure (Gray and Isaacs, 1979). Depression (endogenous or exogenous) and bipolar or unipolar affective disorder may affect the elderly, and depressive states are by far the commonest functional disorder in the aged (Butler and Lewis, 1982). Suicide rates for the elderly are more than double those of people under 35 years of age (see Table 100) (Ross and Kreitman, 1975).

Table 100 Suicide.
Average annual suicide rates per million of population, England and Wales, 1969–71 by age and sex (Ross and Kreitman, 1975).

Age	Annual suicide rate	
	Men	Women
15–24	56	24
25–34	96	44
35–44	120	64
45–54	140	100
55–64	180	124
65–74	220	140
75–84	240	120

Depression in the elderly may follow the death of a spouse or other loved one and may also be associated with an increase in dependency. Physical diseases, especially those causing pain or incapacity, may also be associated with depression. Many drugs may induce depression in the elderly (e.g. methyldopa, digitalis, beta blockers, procainamide, barbiturates and tranquillizers (Davison, 1978).

The course of depressive disorders in the elderly has been studied and the conclusion is that the intensity lessens with age and the tendency to somatize the depression increases with age (Butler and Lewis, 1982). The elderly person who has somatized his or her depression may complain of vague unpleasant feelings, especially in the abdomen, without expressing firm convictions about a specific physical disease. Complaints may be reiterated endlessly to anyone who will listen and the patience of family and friends may be greatly strained. It has been suggested that the 'unlikeable' elderly patient should always be suspected of being depressed (Post, 1982) and should be assessed accordingly.

Treatment does not differ from that offered to younger patients, though the side-effects of anti-depressants may be more severe.

Bipolar affective disorder usually occurs before 30 years of age and may persist into old age, though this is uncommon. Unipolar disorders (manic or depressed type) may be present but mania in the elderly tends to be accompanied by aggression or paranoia rather than elation.

Paraphrenia is a form of schizophrenic disorder arising in old age in which the person develops persecutory delusions, though personality remains relatively intact. Paraphrenia is commonest in females and is often associated with social isolation and hearing impairment. Neighbours are often identified as sources of persecution, and delusions may be shared by husband and wife (folie à deux). Prognosis is variable and treatment is usually required for the remainder of life.

Hypochondriasis is common in the elderly and consists of preoccupation with bodily health, often with a belief in illness despite medical evidence to the contrary. Medical advice is sought at the least provocation, real or imaginary, and the patient may accumulate a large collection of patent medicines and remedies. It has been suggested that hypochondriasis serves the following functions (in persons of *any* age):

1 To symbolize and make concrete one's sense of defectiveness or deterioration
2 To serve as a ticket to interaction with care givers (or punishers) (e.g. doctors and nurses)
3 To displace anxiety from areas of greater concern
4 To serve as part of identification with a deceased loved one through similar symptoms
5 To serve as punishment for guilt
6 To avoid or inhibit unwanted behaviour or interactions
7 To punish others
8 To regulate (usually reduce) interpersonal intimacy (Busse, 1954)

Hypochondriasis is commonly associated with depressive feelings but may stand alone. It should not be dismissed but should be recognized as both a communication and an expression of a need to escape into the sick role. Anxiety (free-floating or phobic) may occur in the elderly, and conversion disorders may also arise.

Alcohol Dependence

The elderly are particularly vulnerable to alcohol problems, though the detection of elderly alcoholism may be difficult. One survey revealed that 9% of problem drinkers were over the age of 65 years (Hyatt, 1985) and it seems that female problem drinkers outnumber the males in this age group (Glatt, 1982). Elderly problem drinkers fall into two groups:

1 Those who have a lengthy history of problem drinking and have survived into old age, and
2 Those who have begun to drink to excess in old age, precipitating factors often including bereavement, loneliness, insomnia or chronic illness.

Moderate use of alcohol by the elderly is not harmful but safe limits may be half those applying to young adults (Age Concern Scotland). Alcohol (in excess) has particularly harmful effects on the elderly:

1 It worsens confusion by impairing memory.

2 It may lead to malnutrition as it interferes with vitamin absorption.

3 It will increase the likelihood of incontinence developing.

4 It is excreted less effectively than in young people and there is thus an increased risk of brain or liver complications.

5 It is expensive, and spending money on alcohol will worsen any existing financial problems.

6 It will tend to predispose to neglect of personal hygiene.

7 It increases risk of accidents.

Signs of alcohol abuse in the elderly include confusion, falls and decreased ability to cope, though accurate diagnosis is essential. It would be wrong to assume that the deteriorating elderly person has a drink problem simply because he/she visits the pub. There may be undiagnosed brain failure, diabetes or Parkinson's disease.

Tell-tale empty bottles may be concealed about the house but many elderly persons (especially females) go to elaborate lengths to discreetly dispose of incriminating empties. Elderly females had culturally restricted access to alcohol for many years; it was too stigmatizing for an elderly lady to visit the local pub regularly and equally shameful for her to be observed regularly making her way home clutching a clinking carrier bag bearing the logo of an off-licence. Supermarket shopping now gives easy access to cheap alcohol (e.g. sherry and other fortified wines) and a bottle may be discreetly transported home with the groceries.

Excessive alcohol consumption also increases heat loss (by causing vasodilation) and thus increases the risk of hypothermia, particularly when the risk of falls is also considered. The elderly person who is drinking excessively and who lives alone is at great risk, and remember that the term 'excessive drinking' refers to levels which would not be hazardous in a younger person.

Involutional Melancholia

This is a term used to describe depression arising in women who have reached or passed the menopause (the climacteric or involutional period). It was thought that physiological disturbances associated with the menopause contributed to these depressions but this now seems improbable. Research has failed to uncover any evidence that the onset of depression in women correlates with the menopause or that depression occurring in the involutional period is distinct from depression occurring at other stages of life (Weissman and Klerman, 1977; Weissman, 1979). The term is still unfortunately used, however, and is mentioned reluctantly.

Psychotherapy with the Elderly

Psychotherapy tends to be infrequently offered to elderly clients despite the major stresses often emerging at this developmental period. This may be partially due to the mistaken belief that elderly persons have a reduced capacity to cope with adversity, though these ageist stereotypes are increasingly being offset by recognition of the fact that older people are often beset by increased stresses and pressures. The problems of the elderly are increasingly being located in the environment, not the person.

Butler and Lewis (1982) identify some common themes in psychotherapy with older persons:

1 *New starts and second chances*. Retirement brings the opportunity to restructure social life in general and relationships in particular.

2 *Death in disguise*. Fears of death may be disguised or converted into anxiety, and suppression of troublesome thoughts and feelings about death will heighten anxiety.

3 *Keen awareness of time*. Remaining days may be running short and therapy may help develop a sense of immediacy, of the here and now, which will aid in the development of a sense of enjoyment and tranquillity.

4 *Grief and restitution*. Therapy must deal with grief, with losses of loved ones and with bodily dysfunction. One of the important goals of therapy is helping the older person to find a secure confidant, either in his family or in his circle of friends and acquaintances.

5 *Guilt and atonement*. Therapy in old age is a therapy of atonement and restitution. Facing genuine guilt as well as the attrition of the person's physical and emotional world is what makes therapy with the aged an intellectually and emotionally powerful experience.

6 *Need for assertion*. Helplessness may be reduced and self-esteem strengthened by recognizing the dignity and individuality of the elderly.

Reminiscence therapy involves recalling or reminiscing about the past with the aim of assigning new meanings and values to past experiences. It is best suited to a group of eight or nine elderly persons.

In essence this approach consists of a journey through or a summation of the participant's life and involves efforts to integrate experiences by mentally reliving them. The group leader starts by introducing topics that prompt a flow of reminiscences, and aids (music, poetry, scents, spices or photographs) may be used. Unfinished psychological 'business' may be completed in such a group and conflicts and ambiguities resolved.

Any approach to psychotherapy with the elderly should take account of the altered psychosocial perspectives of the elderly. Jung (1970) indicated the complexities of later life and the importance of an understanding of them. Thus:

'We cannot live in the afternoon of life according to the programme of life's morning, for what was great in the morning will be little at evening, and what in the morning was true, will at evening have become a lie. I have given psychological treatment to too many people of advancing years, and have looked too often into the secret chambers of their souls, not to be moved by this fundamental truth.'

Key Concepts

1 The years of later life are often unnecessarily viewed in a negative fashion. Ageing is a developmental stage, not a difficulty.
2 The later years tend to be associated with increases in stress rather than reduced capacity to cope.
3 Critical events of the later years often include retirement, death of a spouse and failing physical health.
4 Depression is common in old age and suicide rate increases with age.

5 *Hypochondriasis* is common in old age and is often a form of communication.
6 The elderly are particularly at risk of the effects of excessive alcohol use and safe limits may be half those applying in younger years.
7 Psychotherapy (individual or group) may help resolve the stresses associated with the life crises of later years.
8 *Reminiscence therapy* involves recalling and recounting life history in an attempt to resolve tensions, guilt and anxiety.

References

Age Concern Scotland (November, 1985) *Older People and Alcohol*. Edinburgh.

Busse, E. (1954) The treatment of hypochondriasis. *Tristate Medical Journal*, **2**: 7–12.

Butler, R. & Lewis, M. (1982) *Ageing and Mental Health 3rd edn*. London: C. V. Mosby.

Cowgill, D. & Holmes. L. (1972) *Aging and Modernisation*. New York: Appleton-Century-Crofts.

Davison, W. (1978) The hazards of drug treatment in old age. In Brocklehurst, J. (Ed) *Textbook of Geriatric Medicine, 2nd edn*. Edinburgh: Churchill Livingstone.

Erikson, E. (1963) *Childhood and Society, 2nd edn*. New York: W. W. Norton.

Glatt, M. (1982) *Alcoholism*. Kent: Hodder & Stoughton.

Gray, B. & Isaacs, B. (1979) *Care of the Elderly Mentally Infirm*. London: Tavistock Publications.

Hyatt, R. (1985) How to spot the elderly alcoholic. *Geriatric Medicine*, **15**(12): 20–24.

Jung, C. (1970) *Modern Man in Search of a Soul*. London: Routledge & Kegal Paul.

Post, F. (1982) Affective disorders in old age. In Paykel, E. (Ed) *Handbook of Affective Disorders*. Edinburgh: Churchill Livingstone.

Ross, D. & Kreitman, N. (1975) A further investigation of differences in the suicide rates of England, Wales and Scotland. *British Journal of Psychiatry*, **127**: 572–582.

Social Trends (1986) London: HMSO.

Weissman, M. (1979) Environmental factors in affective disorders. *Hospital Practice*, **14**(4): 103–109.

Weissman, M. & Klerman, G. (1977) Sex differences and the epidemiology of depression. *Archives of General Psychiatry*, **34**: 98–110.

Whitehouse, A. (1985) Changing relationships. In Greengroce, S. (Ed) *Ageing—An Adventure in Living*. London: Souvenir Press.

IX
PERSONALITY DISORDER

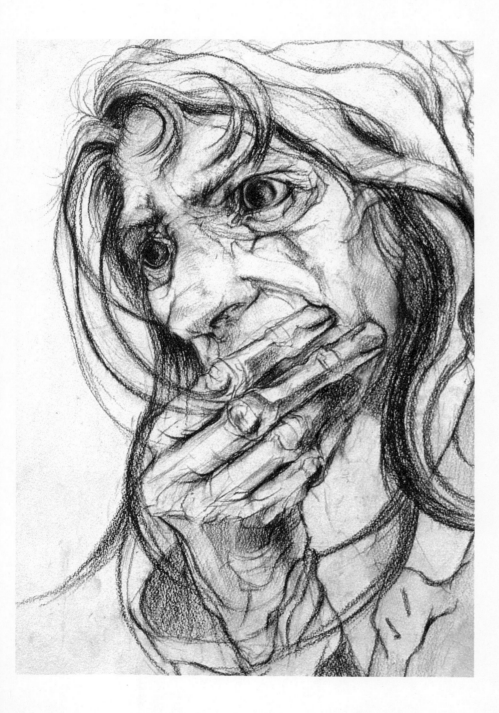

32

Personality Disorder

> '. . . to have stronger and more vehement passions for anything, than is ordinarily seen in others, is that which men call Madnesse . . .'
>
> *Thomas Hobbes: Leviathan (1651).*

The term *personality disorder* is used to describe psychiatric disorders characterized by seeming inability to conform with or accept the code of behaviour of the society in which the affected individual lives. Social adaptation tends to be faulty, interpersonal relationships tend to be erratic, and there may be a picture of extreme personality characteristics which are reflected in deeply ingrained maladaptive patterns of behaviour.

The presenting disorder is one of *character*, rather than mood or thought, and this led the Victorians to distastefully describe this group of disorders as 'moral deficiency'. The terms '*character neurosis*' or '*abnormal personality*' are now sometimes used to describe this controversial group of disorders.

Character may be defined as 'the acquired pattern of habits, attitudes and ideals which render a person's actions stable and predictable' (Walton, 1978). There is considerable transcultural variation regarding the criteria of 'stability' (see Chapter 3), and considerations of social deviance underline the risk that the 'bad' may be confused with the 'mad' as society uses psychiatry as a mechanism to expel dissidents, non-conformists and eccentrics (see Chapter 1).

An organized social response of intolerance to moral deviation became apparent during the seventeenth century when

> 'there was a regrouping of those whom society wished to expel and exorcise. It paid regard chiefly to the moral aspect of conduct. . . . All the conditions which the seventeenth and eighteenth centuries shut away had, in contemporary eyes, some moral fault to be punished and cleansed away . . .' (Lewis, 1967).

In 1676 Louis XIII decreed the establishment of an hôpital général in every city, in which were confined 'the debauched, spendthrift fathers, prodigal sons, blasphemers and libertines' (Szasz, 1973).

In 1835 J. C. Prichard, an English physician, coined the concept of 'moral insanity' in which

> 'the moral and active principles of the mind are strongly perverted or depraved, the power of self-government is lost or greatly impaired and the individual is found to be incapable . . . of conducting himself with decency and propriety in the business of life' (Sim, 1974).

Foolish Clothes and Strange Beards

This stern tone of moral censure is still apparent in some contemporary Russian psychiatric examinations. Wing (1978) summarizes the case history of a 'schizophrenic' Russian girl whose psychiatrist did not uncover any disorder of thought or perception but recorded that his patient was 'stubborn and rude to parents, often out late with boys, smoking and drinking. Began sexual intercourse at 16 . . . became interested in hippies "in foolish clothes and strange beards"'.

European classifications of personality disorder have included 'eccentrics, vagabonds, liars, swindlers, homosexuals, misanthropes, fanatics, the excitable and the insensitive' (Sim, 1974).

Lemert (1951) has pointed out that early sociological writings were permeated by strong elements of social values that were reflected in value-laden assumptions about the nature of deviance. What was implicit in much sociological writing was adherence to an ethic of 'residential stability, property ownership, sobriety, thrift, habituation to work, small business enterprise, sexual discretion, family solidarity, neighbourliness, and disciplines of the will'. Wing (1978) has described these values as 'the ideals of small-town America'.

Criticisms of the concept of personality disorder

abound, particularly in studies of deviance theory, and the newcomer to this field may be tempted to dismiss the concept as a tool of a repressive and intolerant society. Such an extreme stance would be unfortunate as the inescapable fact remains that the nurse will encounter patients who experience personal suffering as a result of personality quirks and will also encounter those from whose 'abnormality' society suffers. The controversy surrounding this area should, however, make the nurse aware of the dangers associated with describing behaviour that we find incomprehensible or offensive as 'abnormal'.

Classification of Personality Disorders

The term personality disorder is used in two different ways. Firstly to describe the individual who has neurotic personality traits but does not suffer from a fully blown neurosis (*neurotic personality disorder*). Such a person may complain continually of anxiety or depression, and their emotional instability may create havoc in the area of interpersonal relationships, causing much unhappiness and disruption to others. More commonly the term is synonymous with *psychopathic disorder*, the 1983 Amendment of the Mental Health Act, 1959, defining the psychopath as one suffering from 'a persistent disorder or disability (whether or not including significant impairment of intelligence) which results in abnormally aggressive or seriously irresponsible conduct on the part of the person concerned'.

In psychopathy there is a gross disparity between behaviour and prevailing social norms which tends to repeatedly bring the individual into conflict with society as a result of disregard both for social obligations and the feelings of others. The American term *sociopath* is finding more widespread use in the description of this type of personality disorder as it emphasizes the predominantly social nature of the deviance and may be less stigmatizing than the term 'psychopath' which tends to have rather lurid connotations to most lay people, these being contributed to in no small measure by the media's persistent misuse of the term.

In many cases there is no clear-cut distinction between sociopathic and neurotic disorder, and in any one patient there may be considerable overlapping.

Aetiology

The aetiology of personality disorders remains controversial and, to some extent, obscure. Studies have considered the relative effects of genetics and environment (nature and nurture) and it is probable that there is considerable overlapping between both areas.

It is probable that some important aspects of personality are substantially determined genetically (see Chapter 2) and constitutional factors in personality disorder have received some attention, though reliable evidence in the majority of cases is still lacking (Sim, 1974).

The possibility exists that the sociopath may be deficient in those bodily responses that give rise to the emotional experiences of anxiety, pity and guilt; in short, the development of a 'conscience' may be defective. Eysenck (1972) renders the layman's concept of 'conscience' more scientific by describing it as 'the sum of conditioned anxiety reactions to doing things labelled "wrong" or "naughty" in childhood and adolescence'. The failure of the emotionally unstable extrovert to develop quick and strong conditioned responses makes the development of a 'conscience' in him more difficult, and may explain the traits of impulsiveness and restlessness often associated with this personality type.

Extroverts habituate (or become used to) painful or unpleasant stimuli more readily than do introverts and show less anxiety when such a stimulus is impending (Hare, 1973) and these tendencies seem to be present in exaggerated amounts in many sociopaths, who show a tendency to fail to profit or learn from past experience, and who are often contemptuous of punishment.

The sociopath is often restless and stimulus-seeking. This may be due to low levels of cortical arousal or 'cortical immaturity', and studies of the EEG patterns of aggressive sociopaths revealed similarities to the EEG pattern of early childhood in a high percentage of cases (Sim, 1974). It now seems that there is no real connection between epilepsy and aggressive patterns of sociopathic behaviour, as was once thought to be the case (Sim, 1974), though marked personality disorder may develop after brain damage, the resultant disturbance being referred to as *pseudopsychopathy*.

The finding of an extra Y chromosome in many delinquent males led to the suggestion that the abnormal sex chromosome complement may predispose the individual towards delinquency—the so-called 'XYY man' hypothesis. Consistent correlations between chromosomal abnormality and delinquency have not emerged and it now seems that only in the presence of mental handicap *in males* is there a high correlation between the abnormal sex chromosome and crime (Sim, 1974).

Psychodynamic explanations include the suggestion by Bowlby (1944) that early maternal deprivation produced the '*affectionless personality*', characterized by lack of trust and inability to develop close personal relationships in adulthood. This personality type was thought to have a high correlation with the development of sociopathy in adulthood, the premise being that the sociopath had never had adequate opportunity to learn how to love, trust and develop appropriate emotional responses, having been reared in a loveless environment.

This viewpoint has been considerably amended by Bowlby (1958), and later studies bear out the suggestion that the critical factor is not separation from the mother in itself but rather the quality of relationships before, during and after separation (see Chapter 3).

The maternal deprivation theory is related to the psychoanalytical view that the Super-Ego is essentially the internalized voice of parental control, being the nearest psychoanalytical equivalent of the layman's concept of 'conscience'—'The institution of conscience was at bottom an embodiment first of parental criticism and subsequently that of society' (Freud, 1913). If parental criticism and guidance is lacking, then Super-Ego formation will be deficient and the adult will be lacking in this source of behaviour modifying feelings of guilt, anxiety, shame and remorse.

It seems probable that, although personality type is determined substantially by genetic influences, the development of sociopathic disorder is more likely to be the outcome of environmental influences, and research into causal factors continues.

Primary Sociopathy

Those sociopaths who show lack of anxiety, and from whose behaviour society suffers, have been called 'primary sociopaths' (or psychopaths) in distinction to the secondary group of personality disorders in which there are deeply ingrained neurotic features often including anxiety. The latter group tend to suffer as a result of their own personality, though they too may cause much distress to others.

Primary sociopathy is a disorder characterized by a cold lack of feeling for others, coupled with disregard for social obligations. There is a noticeable failure to learn from experience and a tendency to revert to immature and pleasure-seeking behaviour, regardless of the consequences, even if these include punishment. Tolerance to frustration is low and behaviour may be seriously irresponsible or impetuously violent, callous unconcern being displayed towards the consequences.

Ability to control impulses or to delay gratification may be poor, and plausible rationalizations or pathological lying may be used in an attempt to explain egocentric and thrill-seeking behaviour.

Social ineptitude may be persistent, leading the sociopath to be chronically in trouble. He thrives on excitement and may engineer 'exciting' events, often at the expense of others. There is a deep-seated inability to perceive adequately how his impulses harm others, coupled with an inability to comprehend accurately the feelings of other people. The consequences of his own actions may be lightly dismissed while he may sullenly exaggerate the restraining behaviour of others.

Major failures repeatedly occur in his marriage, work and social relationships, and anxiety responses to these may be noticeably lacking.

Rejection of authority, discipline and convention may be marked and unreliability is high, though expansive and insincere promises are readily made.

Emotions of love and affection may be readily expressed but tend to be felt in a shallow and insincere way. The sociopath may appear to be likeable and charming in a superficial way and may be adroit at manipulating and misleading others. He may lie to you, cheat you and deceive you but will come back time and time again expecting to be believed.

The disorder tends to reduce in intensity with age and a well-known psychiatric maxim is that 'there are no psychopaths over the age of forty'.

Drugs or alcohol may be misused so that secondary addictions are common, as are sexual deviations.

Classifications of primary sociopathic disorders vary but two types emerge repeatedly in the literature: the aggressive sociopath and the inadequate sociopath.

The *aggressive sociopath* displays general social destructiveness and hostility which may result in violence, theft, frauds, deception and swindling. These tendencies may lead to frequent brushes with the law, culminating in imprisonment.

The *inadequate sociopath* is chronically inept, passive and dependent, and may be placid and responsive or cold, withdrawn and apathetic. Many are aimless drifters, existing on the fringes of society and displaying a parasitic dependence on others.

Henderson (1939) suggested a third category, the *creative sociopath*, the individual in this instance often being gifted but erratic, with a history of chaotic interpersonal and social relationships. He suggested that Lawrence of Arabia and Joan of Arc may be examples of this category and later writers suggested that the world of show business may provide many well-known examples. This category has caused considerable debate and is now rarely used, perhaps because its use may have indicated moral and social prejudice rather than scientific objectivity on the part of the observer.

The Life History of the Sociopath

It is difficult to establish a clear picture of the life history of the sociopath as many live on the fringes of society and only become statistics when they fall foul of the law or are referred for treatment. In the latter case the sociopath tends to be low on cooperation and will often only complete treatment if detained in hospital. Various sources do, however, give some indication as to common life events.

Individuals with severe personality disorder may account for between a third and a half of all cases of suicide and parasuicide (Morgan, 1979), and this may reflect progressive worsening of situational stress with a background of recurrent quarrels, social disintegration, multiple imprisonment, and severe alienation from those around them. Many sociopaths become drug addicts, and British male heroin addicts have a suicide rate which is more than 50 times greater than that of the general population (James, 1967).

Studies of alcoholics presenting for treatment reveal that between 36% and 44% of them were diagnosed as suffering from personality disorder (Soloman, 1982).

Primary sociopathy is less common in females, but studies suggest that the risk of non-accidental injury to children is much increased in the case of mothers with personality disorder (Brockington and Kumar, 1982). Marital disharmony is predictably high, and relationships involving the sociopath may disintegrate against a background of violence, deceit or casual infidelity.

Acts of criminality, including theft, deception, violence, prostitution and drug offences are also predictably high, and imprisonment is common.

It has already been remarked that the severity of sociopathy seems to diminish with age ('no psychopaths over the age of forty') and, while some personality disorders seem to 'burn out' with age, the apparent decrease in circulating numbers in the older age groups may be partially explained by many serving lengthy prison sentences or receiving long-term treatment in hospitals for the criminally insane. Many may also die by their own hands or at the hands of others in one of the violent acts that punctuate the history of some sociopaths. The complications of drug and alcohol abuse may also further thin the ranks of the sociopaths.

Secondary Personality Disorders

These are sometimes referred to as *neurotic personality disorders* and should not be confused with true neurosis. Neurosis is a *reaction*, consisting of inappropriate responses to stress, and may be acute or prolonged. Neurotic personality disorder is a long-term effect of faulty development and constitution, and consists of maladaptive traits or tendencies which will be carried into every situation and which may colour all interactions. In considering these the reader should remember that the traits described are present, to a greater or lesser extent, in all of us, and should only be regarded as constituting a disorder when they create persistent disruption and unhappiness to self, others or both. Casual or ill-considered use of the following terms should be avoided, and the nurse should resist any temptation to use them as convenient explanations of behaviour which she finds incomprehensible or of which she disapproves.

Paranoid personality disorder

This disorder is marked by conspicuous and persistent *self-reference*, that is the tendency to misinterpret the words and actions of others as having special significance for, and being directed against, self. Such persons may be excessively jealous, quarrelsome and litigious (inclined to engage in law suits) and may go to extreme lengths to avenge imagined injustices. Suspicion of others may be marked, and real or imagined grievances may be nursed and magnified for inordinate periods of time. Self-importance may be excessive and aggression is not uncommon. Feuds may be enthusiastically embarked upon with neighbours or colleagues at work.

Affective personality disorder

In this disorder there is life-long predominance of a pronounced mood, which may be depressive or elated or alternately one and then the other. Such people may be gentle and likeable, although the whole approach to life is tinged with gloom or sadness, or they may be hostile, morose and spiteful.

Schizoid personality disorder

This disorder is marked by a tendency to withdrawal, with associated aloofness, cold indifference and a preference for fantasy and introspective reserve. Competitive situations may be avoided and behaviour may be mildly eccentric. There is often a childhood history of sensitivity, shyness and a preference for solitary pursuits, with the introversion becoming marked with adolescence. In adulthood, seclusiveness and unsociability may prevail.

Anankastic personality disorder

Typified by excessive conscientiousness, stubbornness, caution and rigidity. There is perfectionism and meticulous accuracy and a need to check excessively to ensure this. Inability to relax and chronic tension is often coupled with insecurity and self-consciousness. Sexual drives may cause considerable conflict, and self-doubt and self-criticism may lead to frequent feelings of shame or failure.

Explosive personality disorder

This disorder is marked by instability of mood with a tendency to intemperate outbursts of anger, hate or affection—the so-called 'short-circuit reactions'. The outbursts cannot be readily controlled by the affected person, who is not otherwise prone to anti-social behaviour. Relationships may be excellent between outbursts, though minor frustrations may suddenly precipitate an outburst. Intoxication increases the likelihood of outbursts occurring and impulsive suicidal attempts may be made.

Hysterical personality disorder

Behaviour is histrionic (theatrical or 'stagy') and there is emotional lability, excitability and dependency. There may be a craving for appreciation and attention, coupled with sexual immaturity (e.g. frigidity and over-responsiveness to stimuli). Emotional responses are shallow, and although superficial relationships may be excellent, there is great difficulty in sustaining long-term relationships or marriage. Flirtatious behaviour is common in the early stages of relationships, but rejection and frigidity are common once relationships become intense. The individual may 'love being in love' and a shallow and fickle emotionality may pervade relationships.

Suggestibility is high and hypochondriasis is common, and the individual may self-medicate with analgesics for a host of aches and pains and minor ailments. Dependence upon analgesics may develop and a hysterical neurosis may develop in response to stress.

Hysterical personality disorder is commoner in females and may be an equivalent of male primary sociopathy (Trethowan and Sims, 1983).

Asthenic personality disorder

This is marked by a weak, compliant inadequacy and lack of vigour, coupled with little capacity for enjoyment. There may be excessive dependence on others and the layman is likely to regard the overall picture as one of 'weakness of character'.

Treatment of Personality Disorder

Group psychotherapy and social skills training may be useful in the secondary forms, and treatment does not attempt to alter personality but promotes more adaptive responses and the formulation of positive interpersonal strategies. Reinforcement of gains may be incorporated into the treatment programme and significant others from the patient's background should be involved where possible. The asthenic may benefit from assertive training and the anankastic from desensitization or flooding. The tense, excited, affective type may profit from training in muscular relaxation and associated techniques (e.g. thought control).

Treatment in primary sociopathy unfortunately carries a poorer prognosis. The Report of the Committee on Mentally Abnormal Offenders (the 'Butler Report', 1975) gloomily concluded that 'The great weight of evidence presented to us tends to support the conclusion that psychopaths are not, in general, treatable, at least in medical terms'. Failure to learn constructively from past experience, coupled with hostility and poor self-regulation, together present a formidable obstacle to treatment.

Almost every conceivable approach has been tried, including some courageous and imaginative attempts to create specialist treatment centres, some of which have, in fact, claimed considerable success.

The Henderson hospital is perhaps the best known of these centres and uses a therapeutic community approach, with an emphasis on peer pressure and the restoration of normal social controls. Patients are held accountable for their own behaviour and the climate is permissive, with the staff avoiding the role of repressive authority figure. Some individual psychotherapy is given, though the group approach is the principal therapeutic tool, the emphasis being placed on the individual learning to accept responsibility for his own actions and learning to consider the effects of his actions on others, using social pressures derived from the group to create the appropriate climate.

Broadmoor, the famous prison hospital for the 'criminally insane', has used a behaviour modification approach with some degree of success. Adaptive behaviours were reinforced, while maladaptive responses led to withdrawal of privileges or the imposition of sanctions. Group approaches are not favoured as it was argued that 'some patients preferred to do nine months solitary rather than spend time arguing about why they had hit someone' (Sim, 1974).

Nursing Care

Assessment of the sociopathic patient should be made in clearly identifiable behavioural terms, and subjective value judgements should be avoided. Self-identification of problems by the patient should be made, but this is liable to reveal the patient's opinion that he is the innocent victim of an intolerant society. This exercise may nevertheless reveal areas of conflict and social difficulty for the patient, as well as a host of often petty grievances.

Significant others should be consulted and it not infrequently happens that this reveals a picture of widespread social deviance which differs radically from the patient's plausible rationalization about his presenting difficulties. Caution should be exercised in obtaining information from others who share the values of the patient's deviant subculture as they may simply regard this as an opportunity to indignantly confirm the injustice of the patient's circumstances and treatment.

The sociopathic patient will frequently have had sustained contact with social work services, and if the social worker can be contacted, this will help to provide a more dispassionate and broader picture of the patient's functioning.

The psychiatrist will assess the patient's type of disorder and will also identify key areas of maladaptive behaviour. Tranquillizers may be prescribed to control disturbed behaviour following admission and the psychiatrist may arrange individual psychotherapy sessions, often involving the psychology department. The psychology department may also administer psychometric tests to establish a clearer picture of the dimensions of the patient's personality disorder.

Planning of nursing activities will centre around the selection of strategies which may be realistically directed towards promoting a decrease in the incidence of maladaptive behaviour, with a corresponding increase in the level of adaptive behaviours. The behavioural approach may be coupled with group approaches aimed at discussing the patient's approaches to life and encouraging him to review his behaviour in an atmosphere of support and constructive criticism from fellow patients. Target behaviours may be established, for the patient and all staff who come into contact with the patient must be made aware of treatment goals in order that selective reinforcement may be used effectively.

The psychiatrist or psychologist may have established a programme of specific behavioural techniques for the secondary type of disorder, and the nurse should be involved in planning and implementation in this case. If the patient is simply whisked off to the psychology department at intervals for poorly specified or unspecified treatment, any resultant gains may be undone by a ward staff unaware of treatment goals.

Implementing the care plan should involve a firm but gentle approach and consistency and equanimity on the part of the nursing staff is vital.

The sociopath may feel animosity and resentment towards the nursing staff as they may be symbols of an authority and a social order he despises. These feelings may give rise to episodes of verbal or physical aggression, and contingency plans should be made for these.

The sociopath may also appear plausible and charming and the inexperienced nurse may become persuaded that he is indeed a likeable and innocent victim of a bigoted and unfair system. Should the patient suspect that the nurse feels like this he will rapidly, and often effectively, reinforce these feelings. The sociopath's capacity for manipulation may be immense and he may be a practised and polished liar. Vulnerable patients must be protected against possible exploitation by this type of patient, and vigilance is important. Violence may not only be directed against staff but against self or fellow patients. The risk of parasuicidal behaviour is often high and this underlines the need for discreet but careful observation.

Nurse/patient relationships in sociopathy are fraught with potential pitfalls. The patient will often be young and friendly and will often profess admiration or emotional attraction to the nurse. It may be very flattering for the nurse to be befriended by a young and attractive person, particularly one who presents himself as an oppressed and misunderstood underdog. He will rapidly use the nurse's Christian name and make it his business to familiarize himself with her interests and background. It may seem remarkably easy to relate to him, and the incautious nurse may find herself dropping her professional guard of objectivity and spending more time with him at the expense of other patients.

For this reason the approach should be a team approach and the content and pattern of interactions should be discussed with all other members of the team. This will reduce the likelihood of the patient successfully playing off one staff member against another, which is a real risk if the approach is unstructured.

Progress may be slow and setbacks frequent, but tenacity is essential if any progress is to be made. Do not expect dramatic breakthroughs. It has been ruefully said that 'If there is any group of patients who bring home to the nurse or therapist the fact that he is not the Almighty, but a weak instrument, it is this group of patients' (Sainsbury, 1980).

Key Concepts

1 Personality disorder is a category of disorder that is quite distinct from psychosis, neurosis and mental handicap.

2 The presenting disorder is one of *character*, rather than mood or thought.

3 This group of disorders is a controversial one, and much attention has been drawn to the fact that it may simply be used as a 'dustbin' for society's rejects, as the 'bad' become confused with the 'mad'.

4 Despite the controversies of deviance theory, clinical evidence does repeatedly suggest an identifiable group who suffer as a result of their own personality, or from whose personality society suffers. The term 'personality disorder' should nevertheless be used cautiously.

5 Personality disorders are considered to fall into two main groups. *Primary sociopathy* (or psychopathy) refers to that group from whose personality society suffers, as behaviour is predominantly antisocial. The secondary group consists of those who suffer as a result of their own personalities—the neurotic personality disorders.

6 Neurotic personality disorders differ from neurosis in that neurosis is a *reaction* to stress, whereas personality disorder reflects faulty development and socialization.

7 The aetiology of personality disorder is controversial, though much research suggests defective acquisition of adaptive interpersonal and social roles.

8 Primary personality disorder (sociopathy or psychopathy) is marked by absence of anxiety, guilt and remorse. Impulsive and egocentric patterns of immature behaviour may predominate, causing conflict with society.

9 *Secondary (neurotic) forms* consist of exaggeration of traits found in most people, and assume a variety of types.

10 Sociopathy is notoriously resistant to treatment but some specialist units have had some success using principles of therapeutic community or behaviour modification.

11 The nursing approach must be equable and consistent and a balance must be struck between sterile suspicion and incautious subjectivity.

References

Brockington, I. & Kumar, R. (1982) *Motherhood and Mental Illness*. London: Academic Press.

Eysenck, H. J. (1972) *Psychology is about People*. Australia: Allen Lane.

Freud, S. (1913) *Totem and Taboo*. (Translated by J. Strachey, 1960) Routledge & Kegan Paul.

Hare, R. D. (1973) Autonomic activity and conditioning in psychopaths. In Maher (Ed) *Abnormal Psychology*. Harmondsworth: Penguin Books.

James, I. P. (1967) Suicide and mortality among heroin addicts in Britain. *British Journal of Addictions*, **62**: 391–398.

Lemert, E. M. (1951) *Social Pathology*. New York: McGraw-Hill.

Lewis, A. (1967) Review of madness and civilization. In *The State of Psychiatry*. London: Routledge & Kegan Paul.

Morgan, H. G. (1979) *Death Wishes? The Understanding and Management of Deliberate Self Harm*. Chichester: John Wiley.

Report of the Committee on Mentally Abnormal Offenders (1975) the 'Butler Report', p. 90, London: HMSO.

Sainsbury, M. J. (1980) *Key to Psychiatry, 3rd edn*. Australia: Australia & New Zealand Book Co.

Sim, M. (1974) *Guide to Psychiatry, 3rd edn*. Edinburgh: Churchill Livingstone.

Solomon, J. (1982) *Alcoholism and Clinical Psychiatry*. New York: Plenum Books.

Szasz, T. (1973) *The Manufacture of Madness*. London: Paladin.

Trethowan, W. & Sims, A. (1983) *Psychiatry, 5th edn*. London: Baillière Tindall.

Walton, H. J. (1978) In Forrest, Affleck & Zealey (Eds) *Companion to Psychiatric Studies, 2nd edn*. Edinburgh: Churchill Livingstone.

Wing, J. K. (1978) *Reasoning about Madness*. Oxford: Oxford University Press.

X

ORGANIC STATES

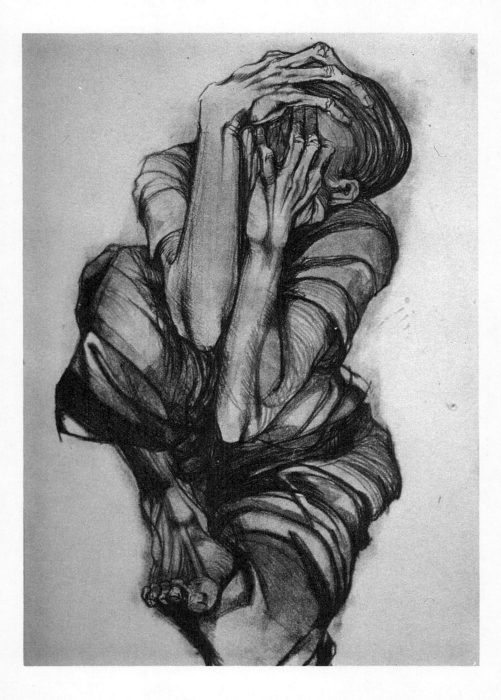

33

Organic States

Organic states are those resulting from some physical change in the brain substance, that is there is discernible cerebral pathology. These conditions are essentially neurological conditions but the clinical features often include psychosocial disorganization of a degree severe enough to warrant admission to the psychiatric hospital.

The brain is a fragile and sensitive organ which rapidly responds to any changes in its physiological equilibrium. It is a centre of high metabolic activity and requires a high continuous supply of blood to sustain this activity. An adult brain weighs about 1.5 kg and blood supply to the brain is about 800 ml/minute (16% of the cardiac output at rest). Blood flow to the brain is therefore 55 ml of blood per 100 g of brain tissue per minute compared with 2 ml per minute for skeletal muscle at rest and 40 ml per minute in exercise. This high rate of blood flow transports the large amounts of glucose and oxygen used by the brain as its basic fuels.

The principal fuel of the brain is *glucose*: in man during a fast of 2–3 days duration, about 180 g of glucose are produced in 24 hours (by glycogenolysis); of this, the brain and spinal cord use 140 g. Hypoglycaemia rapidly leads to confusion, progressing to stupor and unconsciousness; irreparable brain damage may ensue if glucose is not given promptly. Once brain cells die they will not be replaced.

Brain tissue also extracts a higher than average amount of *oxygen* from each 100 ml of blood. Each 100 ml of blood arrives carrying 19 ml of oxygen and leaves with only 13 ml; this constitutes an arteriovenous difference of 6, compared with a difference of 5 for the rest of the body. Cerebral anoxia of more than 2–3 minutes will lead to irreparable death of brain cells.

This high continuous supply of oxygen and glucose-rich blood reaches the brain by the internal carotid and vertebral arteries, which subdivide to form the cerebral arteries and arterioles. These culminate in capillary networks embracing the microscopic network of cells forming this delicate and sensitive organ. Interruption of blood supply may lead to areas of the brain becoming wastelands—areas of irreparable cellular death which will have marked effects on personality, behaviour and mood.

Cerebral blood vessels are very sensitive to metabolites and, in particular, to carbon dioxide and pH changes. A fall in pH (acidosis) dilates cerebral blood vessels, while a rise in pH (alkalosis) constricts the vessels (cotton wool soaked in sodium bicarbonate solution is used by neurosurgeons to stem bleeding from cerebral vessels). Changes in brain pH are frequently the result of changes in blood and cerebrospinal fluid carbon dioxide levels. Breathing a gas mixture containing 6% carbon dioxide will increase the cerebral blood flow by about 75%.

Overventilation, which leads to an eventual fall in alveolar and blood carbon dioxide, constricts the cerebral blood flow; the subject then becomes dizzy and light-headed and vision is affected. This sensitivity to carbon dioxide accounts for the *autoregulation* of cerebral blood flow; as carbon dioxide is a metabolite of the brain, any tendency for blood flow to fall will be opposed by the vasodilation which results from the accumulation of carbon dioxide. In cerebral arteriosclerosis of old age, the autoregulation mechanism may be lost so that a fall in blood pressure will reduce cerebral blood flow, causing confusion.

In the main, mental state seems to be more related to the brain's oxygen consumption than to its blood flow; thus, the coma of diabetic ketoacidosis is associated with a reduced cerebral oxygen uptake but no reduction in cerebral blood flow.

The brain is not only physiologically vulnerable but has anatomical vulnerabilities. This gelatinous, wrinkled organ is easily damaged by trauma and its protective casing of bone will lead to difficulties should intracranial pressure rise. There is little room for expansion inside the skull and space-occupying lesions will rapidly exert destructive pressure on the soft tissues of the brain. Neoplasms or haemorrhage will cause such a destructive rise in pressure, with resultant compression and displacement of delicate cerebral structures.

The oxygen and glucose-rich environment of the brain also provides a fertile breeding ground for microorganisms, and the result of cerebral infections may include residual disorder of personality. Trauma, neoplasm, infection, metabolic disturbance, disorders of blood supply or oxygen content—the possible causes of cerebral lesions are multitudinous.

Brain Mythologies

The belief that disordered thoughts, feelings or behaviour are caused by physical disturbances of the brain is an ancient one. Neolithic man used flint knives to remove large discs of bone from the skull, exposing the brain (an operation known as trepanning), possibly to allow the exit of 'evil spirits' occupying the skull of the mentally disordered. Surprisingly, many 'patients' survived as trepanned skulls often show signs of the regrowth of bone.

In medieval times the mentally disordered were sometimes 'treated' by the application of hot irons to the skull to relieve congestion of 'humours' of the brain. Victorian times saw the emergence of 'phrenology'—the 'science' of 'reading personality' by examining the bumps on the subject's skull.

Theodore Meynert, one of Freud's university teachers, confidently informed him that 'mental diseases are brain diseases' (Szasz, 1973). This belief that mental disorder was caused by physical disturbance of the brain gained impetus around the turn of the century when it was discovered that General Paresis of the Insane was caused by the organism of syphilis, Kraepelin asserting in 1917 that 'the diseases caused by syphilis are an object lesson. It is logical to assume that we shall succeed in uncovering the causes of many other types of insanity'. The development of psychosurgery added weight to the belief that mental disturbances were invariably related to disturbances of cerebral structure or function.

The resultant 'brain mythologies' may be dead but are far from being buried. Clare (1976) writes of 'the tendency amongst some psychiatrists to ground

mental phenomena, normal and abnormal, on a physical foundation, namely on a foundation of cerebral anatomy, physiology, biochemistry and pathology' and suggests that the growth of neurophysiological research contributed to the growth of 'the naive belief that psychic disease is brain disease'.

In functional psychosis, neurosis and personality disorder, there is no discernible cerebral pathology; although the 'programmes' transmitted by the patient may be regarded as faulty, there is no structural fault in the transmitter. In organic states the ability to transmit 'programmes' effectively is impaired, due to transmitter damage due to disease.

The consequences of neurological damage may or may not include variable degrees of psychic disturbance (temporary or permanent) but there is debate as to whether or not conditions like cerebral atrophy or arteriosclerosis may legitimately be viewed as 'psychiatric disorders'. They are perhaps best viewed as physical disorders which may be associated with psychiatric disturbance.

Classification of Organic States

Organic states are divided into two main types which vary in their duration, their onset and manifestations. These are acute and chronic states.

Acute Organic States

The *acute organic state* is sometimes also called *acute brain failure*, *acute brain syndrome*, *toxic-confusional state* or *acute delirious reaction*. These states tend to have an abrupt onset and a florid course, and most resolve rapidly without residual damage. States of acute brain failure are commonest in the very young and the very old and may have many causes. For example:

1 Infection (e.g. septicaemia, pneumonia, meningitis and encephalitis), though any acute systemic infection may cause one.
2 Intoxication (e.g. with alcohol, amphetamines, hypnotics, lead and industrial chemicals).
3 Metabolic disorder (e.g. hepatic and renal failure, hypo- or hyperglycaemia, malnutrition or electrolyte disturbance).
4 Cerebral catastrophe (e.g. head injury, subdural

haematoma, cerebrovascular accident, neoplasm, raised intracranial pressure and demyelinating disorders).

5 Cardiovascular disorders (e.g. cardiac failure, severe anaemia, anoxia, blood dyscrasias and hypercapnia).

6 Post-operative and post-anaesthetic complications

7 Epilepsy

8 Profound physical exhaustion

The cardinal feature is clouding of consciousness with confusion, restlessness and apprehension; hallucinations may occur and the patient will be prone to illusional misperception.

Delirium tremens is the classical example of the acute organic state, though concussion may also lead to a florid acute reaction. Most acute reactions subside and disappear without residual damage, though some may progress to a chronic organic state in which damage is permanent.

Chronic Organic States

This category consists of various forms of brain disorder which, as a general rule, give rise to *progressive* and *irreversible* deterioration of the mental faculties. These states of chronic brain failure are sometimes still collectively referred to as *dementia*, an unfortunate and stigmatizing term for which many alternatives are now being used (chronic brain failure, chronic brain syndrome, organic psychosyndrome).

The concept of brain failure (acute or chronic) is perhaps the most useful one and 'is used in a deliberate analogy with cardiac, renal or respiratory failure. It implies an inability of the organ system in question to carry out its functions in a normal way' (Anderson et al, 1982).

Anderson et al (1982) defend the use of the concept of brain failure:

> 'it avoids the use of emotive terms such as confusion and dementia. These may prejudice an attempt to find out the cause of the mental disturbance, which may well be reversible. (The second is that) it draws attention to the possibility of a very common occurrence, that of acute-on-chronic brain failure, in which both forms of disorder are present simultaneously'.

The use of the terms 'dementia' and 'senility' may constitute a potent recipe for therapeutic inertia. Isaacs (1974) says of the term 'senility':

> 'it offends the geriatrician; it requires an effort of will even to write it. In my mind's eye I see the word garbed in a cloak of black, with the blood of ill old people dripping from its lanky fingers. A melodramatic image perhaps; but how often has the attachment of this label to an ill old patient spelt the end of diagnostic and therapeutic endeavour, and condemned him to a slow death by stewing in his own urine?—Senility is not a diagnosis; it spells relegation for the patient and abdication by the doctor. I look forward to the day when the word 'senility' will have disappeared from acceptable medical terminology, as the word 'insanity' has done'.

Acute brain failure is often due to causes *outside* of the brain (congestive cardiac failure, systemic hypotension or infection, uraemia, dehydration, vitamin deficiency, drug toxicity, hypoglycaemia) and these non-cerebral factors will also worsen chronic brain failure by imposing an episode of acute failure on a brain which is already labouring to discharge its functions. Many of these factors are easily reversible and a diagnosis of brain failure should be a therapeutic beginning, not an end.

Chronic brain failure involves structural damage to the brain (which is irreversible), but abrupt intensification of confusion in chronic brain failure is often not due to a worsening of cerebral pathology but to simple non-cerebral causes which will respond rapidly to nursing intervention (faecal impaction, retention of urine, dehydration, pyrexia due to systemic infection).

The patient with brain failure exists in a state of fragile physiological equilibrium which necessitates high levels of awareness and observation on the part of nursing staff. Common causes of chronic brain failure include:

1 Infection—encephalitis, syphilis, trypanosomiasis, Jakob–Creutzfeld disease (slow virus)

2 Exogenous intoxications—chronic alcoholism, poisoning by lead, mercury or other heavy metals

3 Cerebral disasters—trauma, cerebrovascular accidents, multiple cerebral infarcts, neoplasms, anoxic damage, normal pressure hydrocephalus

4 Demyelinating disorders—chronic brain failure may occur in the advanced stages of multiple sclerosis and Schilder's disease

5 Heredofamilial and degenerative disorders—

Huntington's chorea, Pick's disease, Alzheimer's disease

The vast majority of patients suffering from chronic brain failure are elderly. *Cerebrosyphilis* is now rare and is unlikely to be encountered as antibiotics and effective screening practices have largely eliminated the complication of syphilis once known as 'general paralysis of the insane' which arose as the causal organism-ravaged cerebral and non-cerebral structures alike.

Improved safety practices in industry and higher safety standards for domestic products have reduced the incidence of cerebral damage arising from poisoning by mercury and lead (until recently a common component of household paint). The greatest health care problems arise from the growing numbers of elderly persons requiring in-patient care as a result of chronic brain failure, though it must be emphasized that brain failure is a *complication* of ageing, not an inevitable part of the ageing process.

The convention still tends to persist of dividing states of chronic brain failure into two groups: senile (occurring in old age, after 65 years) and pre-senile (states of chronic brain failure resembling those of old age but occurring before 65 years of age, often in middle life).

This arbitrary division is unsatisfactory for two reasons: (a) the dubious and unhelpful associations attached to the term senile, and (b) the fact that the clinical features of chronic brain failure in the aged differ in no essential respect from those encountered in the young (Trethowan et al, 1983).

Chronic brain failure in the elderly tends to be of two main types: multi-infarct and degenerative.

Multi-infarct type

This was formerly known as arteriosclerotic dementia and was once thought to be due to sclerosis and narrowing of the cerebral arteries and now recognized to be due to small areas of softening of the brain (infarcts) caused by repeated emboli which have broken away from atheromatous vessels in the neck. The history is often as follows:
1 One or more strokes
2 Hypertension
3 Symptomatic epilepsy
4 A stepwise course with plateaux of preservation, and
5 Relatively good preservation of personality and

effective response up to a late stage of the disorder (Bergman, 1978).

Onset is usually sudden following a small 'stroke', and relatives report that the patient was quite well until a brief episode during which he had difficulty in speaking. When these symptoms cleared up after a few hours, the first signs of mental impairment were noted. Thereafter, deterioration tends to progress in a stepwise manner if further small strokes occur. Relatives tend to report that the patient has 'good days' and 'bad days' and effective nursing care extends the 'good days' and minimizes the 'bad days'.

Tragically, many patients of this type retain a substantial awareness of their failing mental capacity and may experience associated depression. On 'good days' the elderly lady with this condition may suddenly revert to the person she always was—a calm, affectionate and caring mother who will apologize to her family for the 'trouble' she has caused, and efficiently resume her former domestic and social roles, only to slip into confusion and disorientation again without warning. It need hardly be said that the experience of caring for a person like this in the home situation is a harrowing and demanding one which will impose great stress on family members.

Degenerative type

This was formerly known as senile dementia, and in this type the underlying cerebral pathology is quite different. Brain cells undergo premature degeneration and death, and the brain undergoes a process of shrinkage and atrophy. Progress is progressive and inexorable and early features may include dyspraxia (inability to make skilled movements with accuracy) and dysphasia (speech disorder).

Unlike the sudden onset of the multi-infarct type, the degenerative type has an insidious onset. Initially, relatives tend to ascribe symptoms like emotional lability, memory loss and eccentric behaviour to ageing and are not unduly alarmed: 'it's just her age—what can you expect?'

Referral is made as the patient becomes progressively incapable of managing everyday living and causes concern by repeatedly wandering off, occasioning nocturnal searches of the streets by distressed relatives.

In the early stages, the patient is distressingly aware of failing intellect, and the resultant depression may require separate treatment. Physical health may be good and the special senses may be intact at this stage. As the disorder progresses, the patient becomes more and more perplexed and exhausted by the demands of everyday living. The patient shows progressive disorientation and may repeatedly get lost as she can't remember where she lives. Sphere of interest narrows and the patient eventually ceases to take interest in daily events. Memory loss is initially for recent events, though distant memory will also decay as the disorder progresses. Women may be unable to remember the names of their children, may forget that their husband died some years ago or may regress to the years of their youth. Eventually dyspraxia becomes marked and the patient may have difficulty in dressing and undressing. Personal hygiene is also likely to be neglected. Dysphasia is likely to become more marked until sentences become shorter and shorter; eventually scarcely two or three consecutive words can be produced.

Incontinence is likely in the later stages and confusion becomes so marked that it becomes inadvisable to leave the patient unattended, even for short periods, as behaviour may now be hazardous to self or others; for example, turning on the gas jet but forgetting to light it, wandering into the night street in mid-winter in night attire. Residential care is now necessary.

Alzheimer's disease is a condition resulting in chronic brain failure in middle life, one of the so-called pre-senile dementias. By the time 65 years of age is reached, Alzheimer's disease is said to affect one person in six (Trethowan and Sims, 1983), and this may be the commonest organic state leading to admission to the psycho-geriatric unit.

This disorder is characterized by generalized cerebral atrophy, and histological examination reveals the presence of cellular debris where healthy nerve cells had once existed. This debris includes neurofibrillary tangles (Alzheimer tangles)—twisted and tangled knots composed of the remnants of nerve cells and plaques of tissue degeneration. The condition is relentlessly progressive and commences after a phase of vague symptoms: headache, irritability and insomnia. Memory disturbance soon begins to arouse concern as forgetfulness leads to social disorganization. Severe disorientation usually follows at a relatively early stage and dyspraxia becomes evident.

Despite this background of progressive disability, the patient's behaviour may seem superficially normal for a long period.

Pick's disease is also a condition giving rise to chronic brain failure before the onset of old age. The pathological changes differ somewhat from those found in Alzheimer's disease insofar as atrophy affects the frontal and temporal lobes (in Alzheimer's disease the parietal lobes are markedly affected). The clinical features do not differ significantly from those of Alzheimer's disease, and accurate differential diagnosis may only be possible at autopsy.

Pick's disease is rarer than Alzheimer's disease but affects twice as many (if not more) women than men. In Alzheimer's disease the sex incidence appears to be about equal (Trethowan and Sims, 1983).

Huntington's chorea is a rare form of hereditary mental disorder giving rise to eventual chronic brain failure and confined to certain families. Because the condition is due to a non-sex-linked dominant gene, approximately 50% of the children of an affected parent are themselves liable to be affected. Cerebral degeneration begins in middle life and is preceded by the appearance of involuntary jerking movements (*choroid movements*) affecting the face and limbs. Involuntary writhing movements (*athetoid movements*) also tend to appear early in the course of the disorder and, eventually, a combination of choroid and athetoid movements (*choreoathetoid movements*) involves the face and upper limbs, spreading in due course to involve the whole body. Once choreoathetoid movements are firmly established, the patient suffers from explosive articulation, ataxia and continuous movements of the body and limbs while awake.

Mental symptoms initially consist of irritability, emotional lability and depression. Slowly, progressive intellectual deterioration ensues and the course of the disorder tends to be lengthy (10–20 years).

The tragedy of this condition is that the first symptoms do not appear until the fourth decade of life, by which time many patients have reproduced, passing the disease on to a further generation. No means of identifying the gene carriers has yet been found, though promising research continues.

Jakob–Creutzfeld disease is a rare degenerative brain disease having its onset in the fourth decade of life or later. It runs a rapid course and is usually fatal in the course of a year or so. The causative agent is thought to be a slow virus.

Normal pressure hydrocephalus is a condition in which the lateral ventricles can be seen to be grossly dilated when a brain scan is carried out, but in which the pressure of the cerebrospinal fluid is found to be normal (unlike the hydrocephalus of childhood in which cerebrospinal fluid pressure is so high that the sutures of the skull are forced apart).

Patients present with slowly progressive chronic brain failure, but the clinical picture is highly unusual insofar as incontinence of urine, ataxia and repeated falls may be pronounced, while intellectual impairment is still minimal. Early recognition of this condition is vital as it can be reversed if detected. Surgical intervention consists of a simple shunt which allows cerebrospinal fluid to drain off into the jugular vein. Nursing and medical staff should therefore be alert to the need for *early* investigation of any patient who presents with normal neurological findings, minimal intellectual impairment, incontinence and unsteady gait. Delay in diagnosis could be disastrous.

Wernicke's encephalopathy and *Korsakoff's psychosis* are organic complications of alcohol abuse and are therefore discussed in Chapter 24.

Frontal lobe syndrome is a condition that may arise due to head injury, cerebral neoplasm, psychosurgery or the residual lesions of infection. There is no gross deterioration of intellect but rather a disturbance of behaviour marked by lack of judgement, euphoria, tactlessness and fatuity. Behaviour may resemble that of the hypomanic patient. There is loss of finer feelings and deterioration of personal habits and hygiene.

Epilepsy is a symptom rather than a disease and the vast majority of sufferers do not experience any disorder of intellect or personality. Repeated attacks of status epilepticus may create the risk of residual brain damage however (this is true of epilepsy proper and of the epileptiform seizures sometimes arising in drug or alcohol withdrawal).

Clinical Features of Chronic Brain Failure

Despite the debates about the aetiology, classification and nomenclature of organic states, one can satisfactorily generalize about the clinical features and the resultant care problems liable to be commonly encountered by the nurse. Troublesome features include:

1 *Intellectual impairment.* This manifests itself in *impaired judgement.* The patient makes rash, foolish or inappropriate decisions which are quite out of keeping with previous patterns. Behaviour may become childishly impulsive and erratic and the patient becomes progressively impervious to appeals to reason. Intellectual impairment also manifests itself in difficulty in grasping new ideas and accepting new situations. Patterns of thinking become regressive and rigid.

2 *Memory impairment.* This is often severe and initially consists of loss of memory for recent events (anterograde amnesia). In the early stages distant events may be recalled with great clarity, though memory loss will become more pronounced until it extends to distant events. The patient may speak of persons long dead as though they were still alive.

3 *Confusion and disorientation.* These tend to worsen steadily, though they will fluctuate with overall physical condition. In advanced cases orientation for time, place and person are lost and the patient wears an expression of querulous perplexity. Disorientation for time may lead the patient to misidentify not only the month of the year but to misidentify the year by several decades. The patient may turn night into day and will often proceed to get dressed in the middle of the night, announcing when asked that he/she is going to work/going shopping/ going to take the children to school.

4 *Emotional lability.* Loss of emotional stability is often apparent before intellectual impairment becomes apparent. Emotional incontinence may occur, the patient is easily moved to anger or tears, and emotional outbursts (catastrophic reactions) may occur for very trivial reasons (e.g. difficulty in fastening a button). Catastrophic reactions tend to vanish as quickly as they appear and the patient seems to forget them in seconds. There may be enduring moods of depression or excitability or the patient may become self-centred and indifferent to the feelings of others.

5 *Habit deterioration.* The person suffering from chronic brain failure tends to be *disinhibited* and this may manifest itself in aggressive or promiscuous behaviour. Brain failure has not *caused* this behaviour but has *released* primitive behavioural patterns which are no longer inhibited, due to cortical damage. Habits, moral standards and personal hygiene inevitably deteriorate. Obscene language may be freely used and sexual advances made randomly, if feebly. Clothing will tend to become food stained and the patient will carry out excretory functions in a random and careless way, often

urinating in corners. Personality and behaviour may become a travesty of their former selves.

The overall picture of deterioration is harrowing in the extreme for relatives and they will need all the support and understanding that nursing staff can provide.

Treatment almost invariably requires admission for assessment. Accurate assessment must precede treatment intervention as many brain-failed patients are presenting with a crisis occurring 'below the neck', not above it (for example, a systemic infection, malnutrition or anaemia, which has precipitated an overlay of acute brain failure).

Many patients with early chronic brain failure can be returned to their families once infections have been treated, cardiovascular irregularities stabilized or malnutrition corrected. The provision of the maximum support from community agencies will be required. Advanced chronic brain failure will require in-patient care, and treatment will be palliative (directed against troublesome symptoms, not the underlying cause which is irreversible).

Skilled nursing care, more than any other factor, will help the patient to enjoy the life that is left with dignity, comfort and minimal distress.

Key Concepts

1 Organic states are those resulting from some *physical change* in the substance of the brain.
2 The brain is a sensitive and fragile organ, highly sensitive to changes in its physiological environment.
3 Acute organic states (toxic, delirious states) present with an episode of *acute brain failure*, which is usually florid but transient.
4 A small percentage of patients presenting with acute brain failure will present with residual *chronic brain failure* once the acute episode has subsided.
5 Chronic brain failure is irreversible and tends to be progressive.

6 Not all chronic failures are residues of acute failures, the commonest forms consist of *degenerative* and *multi-infarct* conditions affecting the elderly.
7 Brain failure is not a normal part of the ageing process but a complication of it.
8 Multi-infarct failure has a sudden onset, stepwise progression and relatively good preservation of the personality.
9 Degenerative failure has an insidious onset and inexorable progress.
10 *Pick's* disease and *Alzheimer's* disease are examples of degenerative states that tend to arise before the period of old age.
11 *Huntington's chorea* is an hereditary degenerative state, which will be transmitted to 50% of the offspring.
12 However caused, brain failure causes impairment of intellect, memory, mood, orientation and habits.
13 Treatment is palliative and in-patient care will be required in the later stages.
14 Relatives will require much support as caring for a brain-failed patient will impose great stresses on the family.

References

Anderson, Sir W. F., Caird, F., Kennedy, R. & Schwartz, D. (1982) *Gerontology and Geriatric Nursing*. Kent: Hodder & Stoughton.

Bergman, K. (1978) Psychogeriatrics. In Carver, V. & Liddiard, P. (Eds) *An Ageing Population*. Kent: Hodder & Stoughton.

Clare, A. (1976) *Psychiatry in Dissent*. London: Tavistock Publications.

Isaacs, B. (1974) Treatment of the 'irremediable' elderly patient. In Ware (Ed.) *Medicine in Old Age*. London: BMA.

Kraepelin, E. (1917) *One Hundred Years of Psychiatry* (translated by Wade Baskin, 1962) New York: Philosophical Library.

Szasz, T. (1973) *The Manufacture of Madness*. London: Paladin.

Trethowan, Sir W. & Sims, A. (1983) *Psychiatry, 5th edn*. London: Baillière Tindall.

34

Nursing Care of the Patient Suffering from Organic Mental Disorder

The nursing problems arising from the brain-failed patient are likely to be encountered in a variety of clinical settings. The nurse working in the paediatric unit may encounter states of acute brain failure in the toxic, delirious infant. General surgical wards will also occasionally produce cases of post-operative acute brain failure and the nurse working in the accident and emergency unit may encounter episodes of acute brain failure following head injury or drug or alcohol withdrawal. It has been estimated that 20% of beds in general medical wards are filled with confused elderly patients (Church, 1985).

The form of acute brain failure most likely to be encountered by the psychiatric nurse is the delirium tremens of alcohol withdrawal and similar toxic delirious states associated with drug withdrawal (especially barbiturates). Nursing care of acute brain failure is described in the section on nursing care of the alcohol-dependent patient, and this chapter will focus on the provision of care for the patient with chronic brain failure.

Most brain-failed patients encountered by the nurse will be elderly. Assuming that the population forecasts for 1992 are accurate, it has been predicted that 73.5% of all beds currently available for men and 93.7% of non-maternity beds currently available for women could be filled by the elderly (Bergman, 1978). Surveys of the population at age 65 years reveal that 10% have chronic brain failure and this figure rises with age to over 20% at age 80 onwards (Stafford-Clark and Smith, 1983). The younger patient with chronic brain failure will present similar problems to those encountered in the brain-failed elderly and the approach to nursing care is based on the same foundation.

In considering nursing care for the brain-failed

elderly it should be emphasized that the stresses experienced by elderly people are the result of complex interactions of *physical disorder*, *social deprivation*, *emotional disturbance* and the *mental impairment* caused by chronic brain failure. Negative approaches to care (as reflected in the use of labels like 'senile' or 'demented') are not helpful in the psychogeriatric unit. Opportunities for effective nursing intervention abound and skilled and perceptive nursing care, based on simple principles, will do much to restore and maintain a level of physical, psychological and social integrity often unnecessarily denied to the elderly.

Nursing intervention aims to promote maximal well-being in a client group characterized by diminishing awareness of the world around them and increasing difficulty in coping with the demands of daily living, a client group in whom diminishing physical efficiency often interacts with and compounds psychosocial difficulties. The broad aims of nursing care consist of measures aimed at the preservation of maximal *physical*, *psychological* and *social integrity*, commensurate with degree of disability, and the provision of effective care is dependent upon a high level of awareness of the effects of ageing in general and brain failure in particular.

The Ageing Process

Physical ageing

Before discussing assessment of physical state in the elderly we may briefly consider some of the physical changes associated with the ageing process.

The overall picture is one of declining organ efficiency, which reflects changes occurring at the cellular level with a gradual loss in the number of cells. An older person may have 30% fewer cells than the younger adult (Eliopoulos, 1979) and there is a redistribution of major body components. There is a decrease in the proportions of bone, intracellular water and skeletal muscle. Fat increases (from 15% at age 25 years to 30% at age 75 years) (Goldman, 1970) and extracellular water remains constant. Despite the proportionate increase in body fat, there is patchy atrophy of fat in some areas as age increases. There is deepening of the hollows of the intercostal and supraclavicular spaces, orbits and axillae, giving a bony appearance to the body contours. Life-long use and abuse of the body through accidents, athletic injuries, cigarette smoking, high alcohol intake and imbalanced diet are responsible for changes through wear and tear. Many of the excesses of youth will not come home to roost until old age. Organ systems are affected by the ageing process, as follows:

Cardiovascular system

Vessels lose their elasticity, and blood pressure increases to compensate for increased peripheral resistance. Cardiac output decreases by up to 40% between ages 25 and 45 years, stroke volume decreases and heart rate slows. The valves of the heart sclerose, becoming thicker and rigid, and arteries in the head, neck and extremities become more prominent. Sudden stress is not managed well by the aged heart as tachycardia responses are feebler and the heart takes longer to return to its baseline rate. Calcium lost from bone is deposited in the lumen of blood vessels.

Respiratory system

Alveoli and bronchioles are reduced in number, and vital capacity is reduced. Respiratory muscles become weaker and the aged individual has a less effective cough response, thus increasing the risk of respiratory problems. Oxygen utilization becomes less efficient.

Gastrointestinal system

The gastrointestinal system handles the changes of ageing better than most body systems but there are significant changes. Taste sensations decrease with age, and sweet and salt taste discernment tends to be lost before bitter and sour which may explain the fact that many elderly people tend to add excessive amounts of sugar and salt to beverages and food-stuffs. Mastication remains efficient (providing dental health is maintained or dentures, if worn, fit properly). The tendency to place the elderly on soft, pureed diets, lacking in taste, texture or visual appeal, is quite unnecessary. Decreased peristalsis, oesophageal dilation and relaxation of the cardiac sphincter slow oesophageal emptying. Many older people take longer over meals, not because they are being obtuse, but for sound physiological reasons.

Aging brings a decrease in gastric motility, acidity and emptying time, with an attendant loss of tolerance for bulky meals. The gastric contractions which signal hunger become feebler, increasing the risk of dietary neglect. Meals should be *lower in quantity but higher in quality* in view of gastrointestinal changes, and there may be marked intolerance of fatty foods associated with loss of lipase activity.

The large and small intestines show loss of absorbing cells, slower peristalsis and reduced blood flow. Research indicates that there is no evidence in support of the frequent claims that people get constipated as they get older (Brocklehurst, 1978). The elderly may complain of constipation as non-specific evidence of malaise or they may be 'bowel conscious' due to myths about autointoxication from the colon. Much 'constipation' in the elderly is probably due to nursing regimes founded on myths (unnecessary bed rest and needlessly 'soft' diets, low in residue). Excessive use of contact laxatives will eventually promote spasticity of the colon and will simply exacerbate constipation. Mobility, adequate fluid intake (2.5–3 litres daily) and a moderate residue diet, coupled with reassurance about bowel habits, should ensure healthy eliminatory patterns. Loss of external anal sphincter reflexes may lead to incontinence, and the elderly often have difficulty in distinguishing between flatus and faeces in the colon.

Genito-urinary system

Loss of nephrons occurs, and renal blood flow and glomerular filtration rate decrease. Bladder capacity decreases sharply so that a small volume of urine (of which a young person would be unaware) will cause feelings of 'desperation' in the elderly person (see Figure 16). Renal mass decreases with age; this may be due to atrophy caused by atherosclerosis. Filtration becomes less efficient and traces of protein in the urine are of no diagnostic significance (Eliopoulos, 1979). Most elderly men will show a degree of prostatic enlargement which, in combination with decreased bladder capacity and weakened bladder muscles, may create continence difficulties.

Musculoskeletal system

There is usually slight *kyphosis* (an increase in the posterior curvature of the spine), resulting in a slightly 'hump-backed' appearance. Height is reduced by approximately 2 inches between the ages of 20 and 70 years (Rossman, 1971). There is a decrease in bone mass, and bones become more porous and brittle, with an associated increase in the potential for fractures (especially of hip, ribs and vertebrae). A degree of *osteoporosis* (loss of density of bone) is common. Muscles fibres atrophy and there is a process of gradual replacement of muscle fibres with fibrous tissue, though aged persons who exercise regularly do not lose as much bone and muscle mass or tone as those who remain sedentary or inactive (Ebersole and Hess, 1981).

There is a tendency for the aged to tire more easily; exercise tolerance decreases, and the aged become less able to grip objects firmly. There may be muscle tremors, even in the resting state, and many elderly persons who are physically ill feel weak and shaky when standing and become terrified of falls.

Integumentary system (the skin)

Skin becomes less elastic and becomes thinner and more delicate, increasing the risk of pressure sores associated with bed rest. Finger nails become brittle and there is an increase in skin pigmentation and a decrease in the number of sweat glands.

Endocrine system

There is a reduction in the activity of the thyroid, adrenal and pituitary glands and the pancreas fails to release sufficient insulin in response to raised blood glucose levels. Decreased ability to metabolize glucose may lead to the elevation of blood glucose levels, presenting the geriatrician with a difficult task in deciding whether or not to consider the elderly person as diabetic or not. Reduction in thyroid activity leads to slowing of the basal metabolic rate and will impair oxygen consumption. Diminished hormone levels will lead to atrophy of the ovaries, uterus and vaginal tissues in elderly women, though libido remains present in both sexes.

Special senses

There is some diminution of sight, smell, sound, taste and touch. Diminished taste has already been mentioned and smell may diminish proportionately.

Sensation of pain may be sharply reduced and elderly persons may not feel pressure on bony prominences. Thus they may not respond to body messages to change position. This factor (combined with increased skin vulnerability and loss of subcutaneous fat) greatly increases the risk of pressure sores developing. Another condition that has been missed because of the lack of expected pain responses is appendicitis (Anderson, 1976), and transmission of hot and cold impulses may be delayed long enough for the elderly person to sustain serious tissue damage. Radiators and steam pipes should therefore be carefully guarded and the use of hot water bottles (often popular with the elderly) is not advised.

Decline in visual acuity is inevitable and all elderly persons eventually experience a degree of *presbyopia* or decreased ability of the eye to accommodate to close and detailed work. Individuals who are in their sixties need about twice as much light to see things as they did in their twenties (Ebersole and Hess, 1981). To aid failing vision it is best to increase the intensity of light on the object being studied; for example, it would be more helpful to focus a reading lamp on a newspaper than to increase the lighting intensity in the entire room. Night vision becomes poorer and the risk of falls at night is consequently increased. Secretion of tears diminishes and the need for eye care consequently increases.

The commonest type of hearing difficulty in the elderly is *presbycusis*, a progressive hearing loss in which high frequency sounds are lost first. As telephones, radios and television sets largely emit high frequency sound, this largely explains the tendency of many elderly persons to turn up volume controls to levels experienced as deafening by younger people. If the radio or television has tone controls, it will help to turn up the bass and turn down the treble (thus decreasing the percentage of high frequency sound).

Presbycusis also leads to difficulty in handling speech frequencies. Speech sounds distorted. Shouting *increases* the percentage of high frequency sound, so the voice should be low in pitch and only moderately loud.

Conductive hearing loss may be due to obstruction by ear wax (cerumen), and one study found that in one-third of elderly persons who complained of deafness, wax in the external auditory canal contributed to or even caused it (Green, 1970). Cerumen production increases with age.

The nervous system

There is a generalized delay in response and reaction time, and conduction velocity decreases with age.

Most of the neurophysiological deficits observed by the nurse are not due to the ageing process but are complications of it. Some specific deficits which may be encountered in the brain-failed patient are as follows:

Aphasia/dysphasia. Difficulty in the use of language which may take one of the following forms:

Nominal aphasia—the person can recognize objects but has difficulty in naming them appropriately (for example, the patient searching for the word 'slipper' may say 'thing for putting foot in').

Receptive dysphasia—speech may be normal but the person has difficulty in understanding what is being said to him.

Expressive dysphasia—an impairment in the production of speech which may range from mild word-finding problems through incomplete sentences to complete loss of speech.

It should be emphasized that dysphasia is not always indicative of brain failure. The patient recovering from a cerebrovascular accident will usually exhibit a variable degree of dysphasia which does *not* indicate intellectual deterioration and is often transient.

Apraxia/dyspraxia. This is loss of ability to carry out voluntary and purposeful movements. It commonly takes two forms:

Dressing apraxia—difficulty in dressing due to loss of the purposeful movements involved, e.g. in fastening buttons or tying shoelaces.

Constructional apraxia—difficulty in putting together parts to make a whole, e.g. assembling a jigsaw or making a simple drawing.

Agnosia. This is impaired ability to recognize things.

Visual agnosia—the patient may not only be unable to name a once familiar object but will be unable to recognize it for what it is.

Spatial agnosia—the patient is unable to find his way around once familiar surroundings.

Anosagnosia—another difficulty with spatial problems. The patient neglects part of his visual field or body; for example, a patient may eat half of his meal only and leave half untouched. The staff may compensate for this by turning the plate around and repeatedly reminding the patient of the neglected area (Church, 1985).

Dyslexia (difficulty with reading), *dysgraphia* (difficulty with writing) and *acalculia* (difficulty with simple arithmetic) may be the result of focal lesions (e.g. in multi-infarct brain failure).

In summarizing the physical effects of ageing, it should be emphasized that the overall picture is one of failing reserves. The elderly person may live in a state of fragile physiological equilibrium. Minor systemic infections which would be of mere nuisance value to a younger person may tax already labouring cardiovascular and respiratory systems to the point of failure.

Psychosocial well-being becomes intimately associated with physical well-being, and episodes of acute brain failure may be readily precipitated. The nurse's observational skills will never be more in demand than in caring for the brain-failed elderly. Their vulnerability and helplessness calls for nursing skills of the highest order.

Psychological changes

Although the ageing body may become slower and less flexible, this is less so of the mind. The elderly person in good health tends to do well on tests of *crystallized intelligence*—abilities that depend on knowledge and experience—until they die. Aspects of crystallized intelligence include vocabulary, the ability to see similarities between objects and situations and general information. *Fluid intelligence*—the capacity for abstract reasoning—seems to decline with age. Aspects of fluid intelligence include the ability to solve puzzles and the ability to modify problem-solving strategies. Shortly before dying, people often suffer a severe drop in intellectual abilities, a phenomenon called *death drop*.

Older people have difficulty in responding and performing quickly, and their performance is more adversely affected by time pressures than that of younger people.

Personality does not change dramatically with old age; 'in most of us, by the age of thirty, the character has set like plaster and will never soften again' (James, 1890). The calm and gentle elderly person was probably that way when younger, and the irascible elderly person was probably not noted for mildness in earlier years. Memory for recent events becomes poorer, though distant events may be recalled vividly.

Social changes

Evidence from a few studies suggests that the total amount of social participation increases during adolescence and early adult life and then remains fairly constant until towards the end of the normal working life, when it decreases sharply (Bromley, 1966). Retirement is a critical life event and brings more than loss of income—it may bring loss of self-esteem and loss of social contacts.

Psychosocial theories of ageing include *disengagement theory*, which views ageing as a process whereby society and the ageing individual gradually disengage, or withdraw from one another, to the benefit of both, as the aged can rest after a lifetime of labour, and power can be transferred to those who are younger and more able. Uncritical supporters of this viewpoint tend to assume that the years of retirement are spent in a mellow glow of achievement in which the elderly person contentedly rests and reflects on past accomplishments. To live in the real world we must accept that this is not always the case. People are living longer and a quarter of a century is a long time to spend feeding pigeons in the park. While some elderly persons may wish to disengage from society, others may experience disengagement as frustrating and depressing.

The opposite viewpoint is that of *activity theory*, which suggests that the elderly person should continue to maintain active involvement in the community and that society should apply the same norms to old age as it does to middle age, instead of engendering diminishing activity, interest and involvement as its members grow old.

The philosophy of encouraging an active lifestyle has obvious merits as inactivity tends to breed psychological and social inertia, whereas activity facilitates physical, psychological and social well-being—a philosophy which has obvious implications for nursing care.

Assessment of the Brain-Failed Patient

Careful and meticulous assessment is particularly important in the case of the brain-failed patient. As many patients will be unable to communicate effective descriptions of troublesome symptoms, the observational skills of the nurse are of paramount importance. Relatives are a source of vital information in respect of the patient's level of self-help skills, social skills, general activity pattern and likes and dislikes. Remember that hospitalization can be a stressful experience for the brain-failed patient as familiar cues and reminders which may have helped combat confusion and disorientation are now gone. Transient worsening of confusion and disorientation may occur until the patient becomes orientated to the hospital environment as a result of active nursing intervention.

There are a variety of assessment instruments which may be of use in assessing the capabilities of the brain-failed elderly. One such instrument is the Clifton Assessment Procedures for the Elderly (CAPE), which is useful in making initial broad assessment (see Appendix 3).

The associated problems of disorientation and confusion are often reflections of irreversible cerebral pathology but should nevertheless generate positive nursing responses as both may often be reduced in severity by simple *reality orientation* approaches and by carefully modifying the nursing approach to meet the needs of individual patients, so that failing abilities are not unduly taxed and relatively untouched areas are developed.

Reality Orientation

Reality orientation (RO) is a technique used to rehabilitate persons with memory loss, episodes of confusion and time–person–place disorientation. RO may be informal or formal. Informal RO continues for 24 hours a day, being a component of all nurse/patient interactions, and consists of reminders as to time, place and person, offered in a natural and consistent way, while activities of daily living are performed. A relaxed, friendly and reassuring manner is essential and inappropriate responses are gently corrected, while appropriate responses are reinforced verbally (praise) and non-verbally (a smile, handshake or squeeze of the arm or hand).

Repetition will be necessary and the pace should be unhurried. The nurse should remember that presbycusis will affect communication, so the approach should be tailored accordingly. Presbycusis primarily affects ability to hear high-pitched sounds, and sibilant consonants ('s', 'sh' and 'ch') may be difficult for the patient to differentiate in conversation.

Vowels (which have a low pitch) are more easily heard. Without consonants, high frequency pitched language becomes disjointed and difficult to comprehend. For example, the simple sentence 'How are you today?' may sound like: 'hOw ArE yOU tOdAy?' (-O, -A-E, -OU, -O-A?) to the individual with presbycusis (Hess and Day, 1977). Rapid speech should be avoided and background noise reduced to a minimum. Above all, patience is essential if communication is to be effective. RO is unlikely to be effective if it does not take account of hearing difficulties identified at assessment.

Addressing the confused person by his/her appropriate name or title will help to restore awareness and self-esteem. Avoid the unfortunately common practice of 'talking down' to elderly patients and avoid demeaning terms like 'Pops' or 'Gran'. Remember that staff do not have the right to unthinkingly use patients' Christian names on immediate acquaintance. Use of Christian names should be reserved until the common sense and good judgement of the nurse indicates that it is appropriate.

Responsiveness to the patients' non-verbal communications is an essential part of communication. Even in advanced brain-failure, many patients communicate eloquently by using body language. Is the patient restless and fidgety? Tense and withdrawn? Relaxed and smiling? Brain-failed patients are often surprisingly sensitive to body language (Lay and Woods, 1983), and poor memory often leaves them having 'first impressions' again and again. It is therefore helpful for the nurse to adopt a friendly and relaxed manner, make full use of non-verbal cues (e.g. smiles, touch) in order to reassure the patient, and underline verbal statements. Keep sentences short, slow, simple and heavily augmented by appropriate non-verbal communications.

At all costs, avoid reinforcing inappropriate ideas and responses for the purposes of expediency or to 'humour' the patient. Such reinforcement will worsen confusion and disorientation and will heighten associated distress. Should a confused patient get out of bed at 3 a.m. and announce that he is going to work, he should be reassuringly reorientated by simple reminders of place and time. For example: 'It's three o'clock in the morning, John. You are still in hospital. It is dark and raining. Let me help you back into bed'. Repeat these reminders as often as is necessary. Failing memory will be aided by information given by clocks, calendars, newspapers, notice boards and prominent labelling of doors.

The patient should be encouraged to personalize his/her bed space by placing familiar objects (photographs, ornaments, souvenirs) there, and personal clothing should be worn. It is often helpful to ask relatives to bring in a counterpane familiar to the patient (ensuring that it is not of a flammable material which would contravene fire safety regulations). Talk to relatives and patients to ascertain likes and dislikes (does he/she read a daily newspaper? If so, which one? Has he/she any dietary likes/dislikes? Are there any recreational activities/hobbies enjoyed by the patient? What does he/she enjoy talking about?).

Hospitalization should not mean an end to familiar and valued social activities and the nurse should be aware that it is dangerously easy for the brain-failed patient to lose individuality in the anonymity of the hospital ward.

Open visiting policies promote and maintain links with reality, and relatives should be encouraged to take the patient out for the day or weekend as often as is practicable. Relatives should also be made aware of the principles of informal reality orientation to ensure continuity of approach. Remember that seemingly trivial possessions and practices may be essential parts of a diminishing 'personal identity kit'.

Remember that visual spatial defects (e.g. neglect of one half of the visual field) may lead to inappropriate responses which may be wrongly ascribed to confusion alone. In the case of the patient who repeatedly returns to the wrong bed because of visual field deficit, it often happens that the simple expedient of moving the bed to the opposite side of the room will help (Holden and Woods, 1982).

Formal RO aims to enhance learning in a small group setting. It is a supplement to informal RO and is no substitute for it. 'Classes' meet daily (or at least five times a week) for 30–60 minute sessions which aim to reinforce members' orientation to time, place and person by relearning, restimulation and resocialization.

Kempton (1984) offers simple guidelines for therapists involved in formal RO classes:
1 Always call the person by name and encourage him to call others by their names.
2 Review basic information of time, place and person by the use of RO boards and cards, if necessary going through each letter individually to form the words.

3 Reinforce appropriate responses with verbal praise and touch.
4 If inappropriate responses are given, effort should be acknowledged and further clues given: ('that's close, Bill, but as yesterday was Sunday, today will be Monday').
5 Minimize frustration by asking questions that can be answered. If possible, encourage repetition of a simple fact after you state it.
6 Observe, and work with, non-verbal communications such as eye contact or facial expression in those who are least responsive.
7 Use activities that are simple but have meaning for the individual—identifying familiar objects, recognizing pictures—and so on.
8 Once the group is aware of basic time, place and person, then the names of former home towns, family, former occupations and so on can be discussed.
9 Encourage interest in current events by the use of newspapers, TV and radio.
10 Never set goals too high; establish attainable goals.
11 Use praise, small rewards or special favours to increase relearning.

Remember that RO will only be effective if underlying sensory or speech deficits are taken into account and, where possible, corrected.

Behavioural rehearsal may be used to augment RO and consists of prompting patients to learn by rehearsing actions. There is growing evidence that there may be some aspects of short-term memory that are spared even when there is considerable brain damage (Church, 1985) and one study showed that ward orientation involving behavioural rehearsal was considerably more effective than RO in improving the ability of patients to find specific ward areas, such as the toilet (Hanley et al, 1981).

Validation therapy is a companion to reality orientation and consists of accepting the disorientated person's feelings in whatever time or location is real to them, even though this does not correspond to our 'here and now' reality. This approach aims to *resolve* unfinished conflicts, to *restimulate* sensory memories, to *relive* past pleasures and to relieve boredom and stress by *retreating* from painful feelings of uselessness and loneliness. These are sometimes referred to as the 'four Rs' of validation therapy (Jones, 1985).

Validation therapy encourages reminiscences but does *not* reinforce delusional or inappropriate beliefs: 'At no time does the worker agree with false or questionable facts stated by the older person' (Jones, 1985). This approach acknowledges the reality of *feelings* associated with memories (positive or negative), and encourages their expression in order to finish unfinished business and resolve distress.

Consider a simple example: Bill gets out of bed at 3 a.m. on a cold winter's morning, is visibly agitated and announces that he has to get ready for work in the shipyard from which he retired 20 years ago. He does not respond to reminders of present reality. A validation therapy approach would accept his feelings of distress and urgency and would explore them by initiating a dialogue: 'Why are you in such a hurry?' 'Because they might lay me off if I'm late.' 'You seem very worried about that.' 'We haven't much money and there isn't any food in the house.' 'You seem to feel angry and helpless about that.' 'I do; it's my fault—I should be a better provider.' 'Can I do anything to make you feel better right now?'

Reminiscences will allow discharge of buried tensions and often have a visibly relaxing effect if steered towards resolution.

Validation therapy is thought to be most suited to clients who exhibit confusion and disorientation and who:

Have denied severe crises throughout life

Cling rigidly to familiar, and now inappropriate, roles

Tend to retreat from painful reality (consciously or unconsciously) and who tend to seek sanctuary in the past

This approach does not involve intense psychotherapeutic dialogue and can be used easily in many common situations. For example, 'Nurse, I want to go home.' 'What do you miss about home?' 'What do you want to do at home?' 'Does this place remind you at all of home?' Or, 'Nurse, I have to go and make the children's dinner.' 'You're thinking a lot about your children; did you like being a mother?'

In summary we may identify differing approaches to common problems arising from disorientation. Let us return to Bill as an example. He has announced that he has to go to work in the shipyard (at 3 a.m.). Nursing responses may be any of the following three types:

1 'The foreman 'phoned to say you have a day off.' I mention this type of response reluctantly and only because it is unfortunately common. This response simply reinforces Bill's mistaken belief and ensures further episodes of disturbed or distressed behaviour (disorientation therapy).

2 'It is three o'clock in the morning. You are still in hospital. You stopped work a long time ago. Relax and go back to bed (reality orientation).

3 'You talk about work a lot—did you enjoy working in the shipyard?' (validation therapy).

Promoting Sensory Stimulation

Sensory deprivation is a common problem among elderly clients and is often an integral part of rigid, task-orientated approaches which deny individuality and dignity. 'In many primitive societies the soul is imagined to leave the body at death or just prior to it; on the other hand society drives out the remnants of the soul of the institutionalized old person while it struggles to keep the body alive' (Henry, 1963).

Research suggests that problems associated with sensory deprivation include boredom, incoherent thinking, regression, emotional lability and inability to concentrate (Chodil and Williams, 1970). Impersonal and inflexible regimes may thus lead to further impairment of cognitive functioning. All too often measures adopted to provide sensory stimulation are inappropriate or are cursory cosmetic exercises. The author vividly recalls visiting a rehabilitation/assessment unit for the brain-failed elderly. A group of elderly ladies had been assembled in a circle and were mutinously singing: 'I'm hap-hap-hap-hap-happy' (wearing expressions ranging from depression through desperation to homicidal anger), the whole bizarre spectacle being proudly supervised by a beaming nursing assistant. There is also the seemingly widely held belief that elderly persons inevitably develop an insatiable craving for Scottish country dance music or the type of monotonous and sickly string orchestral music commonly heard in hotel foyers and elevators. Remember that the population in any hospital ward or residential centre for the elderly will include a rich mix of beliefs, attitudes, temperaments and preferences. Careful assessment will reveal preferences and tastes and it is not difficult to cater for most of these.

Repetition of stimuli is useful up to a point but there is a limit to the effectiveness of repetition. After a period of time, change is perceived more readily than continued repetition (Chodil and Williams, 1970) so that music of the same type, played at the same volume, may cease to penetrate consciousness at all—patients may become completely unaware of it.

Physical exercise, within the limitations of the patient, produces a variety of benefits and may stimulate cognitive functioning. One study compared the effects of exercise therapy with those of social therapy and found that after a 12-week period the group that had participated in exercise therapy showed significant improvement in cognitive functioning (Powell, 1974).

Many hospitals and residential homes have extensive grounds or gardens which provide suitable settings for gentle walks. Many patients will enjoy a little light gardening and others will enjoy the activities of indoor gardening provided by a collection of pot plants.

Institutions often have their own distinctive smells—an amalgam of disinfectant, urine, floor polish and cooking odours. Flowers and different soaps, perfumes and deodorants can be used to stimulate the sense of smell and provide welcome alternative odours.

The tendency to serve elderly persons with unnecessarily bland foods has already been mentioned and a variety of colours, tastes and textures should be aimed at. It is helpful to ascertain dietary likes and dislikes. If someone has successfully avoided carrots for 80 years, they are unlikely to suddenly develop a taste for them after hospitalization.

Some hospitals now permit alcoholic beverages to be served at certain events. One study revealed that persons served beer during a group session did not become more sociable than those who were given soda to drink, though everyone became more sociable during group interactions (Burril et al, 1974). Another study indicated that socialization was significantly increased when whisky, gin, vodka and wine were available during a social hour (Carroll, 1978). Intermittent claudication (exercise cramps in the legs due to ischaemia), which is common in the elderly, will benefit from alcohol ingestion . . . 'alcohol has a marked therapeutic effect in the condition' (Judge, 1978). It need hardly be said that alcohol should not be given to elderly patients without discussion with medical staff as alcohol may interact adversely with many drugs, and impaired liver or kidney function may contraindicate use of alcohol. Given these precautions it will not be often that elderly patients will be found unsuitable for occasional consumption of small amounts of alcoholic beverages.

A peculiar workhouse mentality pervades some geriatric homes and hospitals and manifests itself in segregation of the sexes and an absolute ban on alcohol. These parochial attitudes seem to emanate from a belief that growing old is a very serious business indeed and from the associated belief that social disengagement should be ensured with grim efficiency.

While sensory stimulation is important, it is equally important to ensure that sensory overload does not occur. Time span of attention will shorten with age and excessive demands on the patient's attention will lead to fatigue and anxiety. Ongoing evaluation of nursing intervention should ensure that sensory or social overload does not occur.

Assistance with Activities of Daily Living

Common problems and suggested nursing interventions may be summarized as follows:

1 *Maintaining a safe environment*

Falls are a common form of accident and the causes may be *extrinsic* or *intrinsic*.

Extrinsic causes arise from hazards in the environment. These include poor lighting, highly polished or wet floors, trailing dressing gowns or pyjama cords, badly fitting shoes or slippers, small pieces of occasional furniture (coffee tables, etc.) which may be stumbled over, trailing electrical cables, and light and easily overbalanced chairs. Carpet edges should be secured with metal strips and small rugs should not be used.

Falls in the lavatory or bathroom may be particularly serious, so careful observation is required in these areas. Non-slip bathmats and grab-rails reduce the likelihood of accidents in the bathroom, and confused patients should never be left alone in the bath due to the risk of drowning or scalding accidents.

Intrinsic causes of falls include drops in blood pressure associated with rising from a sitting or lying position. Sudden rising may cause a 60 mm drop in blood pressure (Eliopoulos, 1979), with resultant dizziness or fainting. *Drop attacks* are a common manifestation of *vertebrobasilar artery disease*. The two vertebral arteries pass through the foramina in the transverse processes of the cervical vertebrae and unite to form the basilar artery which enters the foramen magnum to feed the posterior area of the circle of Willis. Turning or extension of the neck may kink sclerosed vertebral arteries, causing momentary failure of blood supply. Sudden rotation of the head (as in looking over the shoulder) or flexion of the neck (as in looking up at a high shelf) may precipitate a drop attack. These attacks particularly affect elderly females and occur without warning, the patient suddenly falling on to her flexed knees and hands. Consciousness is either retained or only momentarily lost and the patient is normally able to rise to her feet immediately. The drop attack usually comes as a surprise to the patient: 'my legs just gave way and down I went'. Patients who are known or suspected to have vertebrobasilar artery insufficiency should not be involved in activities which involve sudden flexion of the neck or rotation of the head and should not be allowed to reach for objects on high shelves.

Fracture of the neck of the femur can occur with great ease in the elderly (even after a trivial fall) and careful examination should follow all falls. The unsteady old person may benefit from a walking aid (a Zimmer frame or walking tripod) and shoes and slippers must fit well and provide adequate support.

Confused 'wandering behaviour' increases the risk of accidents, and the limited living space available in hospital may promote restless wandering. One study revealed that an abrupt change from a person's home and routine to the new environment and routines of hospital may generate stress which many persons seek to release through methods developed earlier in life to reduce tension, such as taking a brisk walk or a long stroll. These behaviours arose from a stress-generated need for activity (Snyder et al, 1978). Provision of substitute activities and

Table 101 Risk of accidents.

Problem	Objective	Action
Risk of accidents due to confusion/sensory deficit/unsteadiness	To reduce risk of accidents	Render environment safe; provide appropriate aids

allowing escorted walks in the grounds will reduce tension and the likelihood of haphazard wandering in the ward.

2 Communication

Confusion and disorientation will result in inappropriate or disturbed communication patterns; the approach of choice is then reality orientation, with or without complementary validation therapy, as appropriate.

It also seems likely that the appropriate use of behaviour modification (shaping, prompting, behavioural rehearsal and reinforcement) can be effective with the brain-failed elderly (Church, 1985) and differential reinforcement should help to ensure that inappropriate verbalizations decrease in frequency, while appropriate patterns of verbalization increase in frequency. At all costs, ensure that hearing deficits are identified and treated appropriately. Do not assume that the use of a hearing aid means that hearing problems are being satisfactorily compensated for. Remember that the elderly have a tendency to:

Lose the batteries
Let the batteries run down
Confuse new and used batteries
Have difficulty manipulating batteries and handling controls
Refuse to wear a hearing aid

Try to ensure that both the auditory canal and the earpiece of hearing aids are free of impacted cerumen.

3 Expressing sexuality

Disinhibited sexual behaviour should be contained as humanely as possible and should not evoke negative and hostile staff responses of the 'dirty old man' type. Young nurses who may not have yet fully come to terms with their own sexuality may be particularly upset by sexual approaches, and the young nurse who may be secretly flattered by overtly admiring glances from a handsome young registrar, may over-react negatively should she receive same from a frail 85-year-old male (who is less likely to constitute a sexual threat).

Disinhibited sexual behaviour (verbal or physical) should not be reinforced, and the patient may be quietly led to a side room and left alone for a period of time. Boredom and lack of activity will increase the likelihood of inappropriate sexual behaviour, and constructive activities will reduce this likelihood.

4 Working and playing

Goffman (1961) identifies the deleterious effects of institutional living as arising from the three activities of work, rest and play taking place under the same roof, and from the 'stripping process' whereby inmates are stripped of individuality, autonomy and initiative. Passive adoption of the 'sick role' will ensue if nursing staff overenthusiastically organize the patient's life and deny individuality and initiative. The patient becomes dependent, needing and expecting to be taken care of by

Table 102 Communication.

Problem	Objective	Action
Reduced ability to communicate	To maximize remaining communication ability	Reality orientation; validation therapy
Inappropriate communication patterns		Behaviour modification
Sensory deficit		Provision of effective hearing aids

Table 103 Expressing sexuality.

Problem	Objective	Action
Inappropriate sexual behaviour	To reduce same	Behaviour modification; prevent boredom

Table 104 Working and playing.

Problem	Objective	Action
Risk of inactivity causing apathy/institutionalization/depression	To promote healthy and satisfying patterns of activity commensurate with patients' abilities	Provide structured and varied programme of activities centred around patients' needs and preferences

stronger, more 'adequate' persons. This process is likely to be marked in the case of the brain-failed elderly: 'We value youth and fear old age, which in our society confers no dignity but only losses' (Slater, 1964).

Many 'losses' ensuing after hospitalization are interpersonal losses and are as unnecessary as they are damaging. Simple programmes of activity militate against apathy and depression and restore texture and interest to daily living.

The first step should be careful assessment of the patients' likes/dislikes, recreational/social preferences and preferred patterns of activity which obtained until hospitalization. Assessment of the patients' capabilities is also essential to ensure that frail patients are not overtaxed. The possibilities are endless—outings, concerts, sing-songs, board games, discussion groups, indoor and outdoor gardening, ward pets (even if only a budgie or fish tank, though a cat or dog has been successfully introduced in many cases), visits by voluntary groups to organize concerts, carol singing, parties; celebrities are often most helpful about paying hospital visits. The patients should be allowed to practise religious worship of choice, and if visits to church are not practicable, padres can visit the ward. Encourage letter-writing and phone calls, keep a register of birthdays (of the patients and the next of kin) and celebrate these. A little imagination and energy will usually pay great dividends.

5 Sleeping

It is not uncommon for the elderly to have difficulty in falling asleep (remember that the elderly need more rest but less sleep) and, unfortunately, nursing care often resorts to the use of hypnotics to induce sleep. Hypnotics/sedatives do not induce natural sleep, often cause a 'hangover' the next morning and rapidly lose efficacy anyway. The 'hangover' effect may be marked due to the prolonged half-life of medications in the elderly, and the effects of sedatives may extend well into the daytime, causing confusion and sluggishness. Sedatives also decrease body movements during sleep and predispose the elderly to the many complications of reduced mobility.

Daytime activity will predispose to healthy sleep, particularly gentle exercise in the fresh air, and a warm bath before bedtime will promote relaxation. Ensure that the sleeping area is free of distracting background noise and that the room is well-ventilated. A night light will often reduce nocturnal restlessness as it enables recognition of familiar visual cues. Try to assess sleep requirements; an elderly person who requires less sleep cannot reasonably be expected to sleep from 8 p.m. until 8 a.m.

6 Eating and drinking

The elderly require a lower quantity and a higher quality of food. There is usually no need for bland institutional diets, and food should reflect the patient's preferences and be varied and interesting. Food intolerance (due to decreased gastric motility and slower emptying time) is common, and fried or fatty foods should be avoided in this case. Small amounts of alcohol (e.g. sherry) will stimulate the

Table 105 Sleeping.

Problem	Objective	Action
Insomnia	To promote healthy sleep patterns	Daytime activity
Nocturnal restlessness		Ensure that environment is conducive to sleep

Table 106 Eating and drinking.

Problem	Objective	Action
Food intolerance; indigestion	To provide a balanced and acceptable diet	Assess patients' needs and modify diet accordingly
Dysphagia		Partially assist at meals (if necessary)

appetite, and attractive presentation will stimulate interest.

Taste receptors for sweet and salt become less effective, and the common tendency of many elderly people to use too much sugar and salt may be compensated for by using artificial sweeteners and salt substitutes.

Malnutrition and dehydration are potential problems, and the elderly person who appears obese can actually be suffering from malnutrition. Careful monitoring of food and fluid intake is essential. Dysphagia may be a difficulty with some patients, and in this case a soft diet may be necessary. Sitting the patient in a high upright position will facilitate swallowing and reduce food intolerance (this position increases the size of the abdominal and thoracic cavities). Remember that food may be a great pleasure to the elderly and a little thought can ensure that mealtimes are one of the high spots of the day.

7 Personal cleansing and dressing

Loss of self-help skills and resultant neglect of personal hygiene and dress is often accepted and shrugged off as being inevitable in the brain-failed elderly, being ascribed to 'confusion'. Specific neuropsychological deficits are often responsible and, if these are identified, remedial action may be taken. In *ideomotor apraxia* the ability to perform simple over-learned gestures may be lost (e.g. brushing teeth or combing hair). Rhythm has been used to help with particular ideomotor apraxias (e.g. when the patient is attempting to brush the teeth); instituting a rhythmic cue such as tapping out a beat or saying out loud 'up-down' may aid the patient's performance (Church, 1985).

Dressing apraxia (difficulty in dressing due to loss of ability to make purposeful movements) may cause difficulties in dressing which may be reduced if clothes are laid out in order on the bed: underwear, outer clothes, stockings and shoes. Some assistance and prompting may also be necessary. Where possible, clothing may be simplified—slip-on shoes, front fastenings, larger zip-pulls, velcro fastenings or fewer buttons.

There may be an associated component of visuo-spatial difficulty so that the patient cannot make the appropriate movement to place the item of clothing on the appropriate part of the body. One approach to this difficulty involved the use of a large mirror to provide visual feedback so that patients could ensure that clothing was appropriately arranged and that zips and buttons were fastened (Church, 1985).

8 Breathing

The lungs lose elasticity with age, alveoli decrease in number, and there is loss of strength and increased rigidity of the respiratory muscles. As a result, the elderly person has an increased susceptibility to respiratory infections. Deep breathing exercises should be encouraged several times through the day, with the emphasis on forced expiration and attempts at expectoration following the exercises. The patient inhales to the count of one and then exhales to the count of three. Unnecessary inactivity or bed rest will greatly increase the risk of respiratory infection.

9 Elimination

Urinary incontinence may be a frequent problem with the brain-failed elderly and the causes may be

Table 107 Personal cleansing and dressing.

Problem	Objective	Action
Dressing dyspraxia and ideomotor apraxia, resulting in loss of self-help skills	To promote optimum self-sufficiency	Prompting, guiding, providing feedback and reinforcing; modifying clothing where necessary

Table 108 Breathing.

Problem	Objective	Action
Decreased respiratory activity; increased risk of respiratory infections	To promote optimal respiratory function	Deep breathing exercises

Table 109 Elimination.

Problem	Objective	Action
Incontinence	To promote healthy eliminatory patterns	Continence training
Constipation		Dietary modification; encourage activity

physical, psychosocial or both. Physical causes include lesions in the brain or spinal cord (following cerebral infarct, degenerative disease or cerebrovascular accident). The nerve pathways that are normally involved in the regulation of micturition may be damaged, resulting in three types of *neurogenic bladder*:

1 The *spastic* bladder (increased bladder tone causing urgency and decrease in volume, leading to frequency)

2 The *atonic* bladder (decreased bladder tone resulting in a large residual volume with overflow incontinence)

3 The *automatic* bladder (spinal cord lesion results in a lower centre for control; the small hypertonic bladder acts independently and frequently).

Specific neurological lesions aside, the elderly bladder tends to lose tone and has reduced capacity, leading to frequency, urgency and, sometimes, retention. Incontinence also has psychosocial dimensions. Sutherland (1976) describes some of the psychological causes of incontinence:

1 *Regression*—with associated incontinence may become a coping mechanism for dealing with the stresses of increasing infirmity

2 *Dependency*—nursing staff may unwittingly foster child-like dependence by excessively adopting the role of Nurturing Parent

3 *Rebellion*—anger and resentment expressed in a primitive manner

4 *Insecurity*—the anxiety evoked by sudden changes in environment or routine may result in incontinence which may become chronic

5 *Disturbance of conditioned reflexes*—the usual cues for elimination may be missing (e.g. privacy, lack of

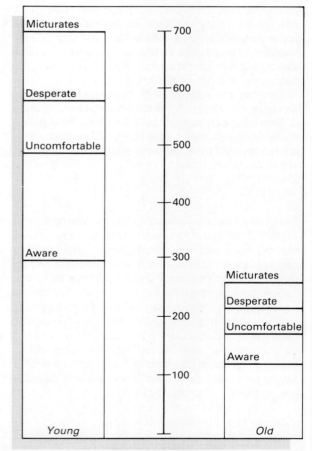

Bladder mechanism

Figure 16 A comparison of the bladder mechanism in the young and the old. (From Burns, E. et al with kind permission of the authors and the publisher, Heinemann.)

sufficient time, strange bathrooms and unusual receptacles)

6 *Sensory deprivation*—without adequate and appropriate stimulation, the individual loses the sense of being in a social relationship with the environment

To this list one may add depression which may lead to withdrawal and loss of interest, with associated incontinence and general decline of self-help behaviours.

If ageing of the genito-urinary system predisposes to incontinence, the precipitating factors are often psychosocial. Some simple principles will help to reduce the likelihood of incontinence:

1 Regularly ask patients whether they need to void and promptly answer calls for assistance. This will help to prevent episodes of incontinence (remember increased frequency and decreased bladder capacity). There is no point in asking elderly patients to 'wait for a few minutes'—they are often simply physically unable to do so).

2 Encourage oral fluids. Concentrated urine irritates the bladder and leads to incontinence.

3 Encourage an upright position while voiding.

4 Bladder retraining may be used and involves asking the patient to drink a glass of fluid and then make conscious efforts to retain urine. Two-hourly intervals are planned at first with steady increase as bladder capacity and control increase.

Routine 'toilet rounds', whereby every patient is offered a bedpan or urinal at routine intervals, are not helpful. Eliminatory patterns are highly individual and the likelihood of any given patient's need to void coinciding with the arrival of the toilet-round trolley is slight.

Urinary tract infections often cause associated incontinence, so the nurse should be alert to signs of these infections (pyrexia, urgency and scalding on micturition). If urinary tract infection is suspected, a urine specimen should be sent for bacteriological culture so that the causal organism may be identified and appropriate treatment commenced.

Occasionally, *retention with overflow* will develop. The bladder fills with a very large volume of urine which cannot be voided, although small amounts of urine escape through overtaxed sphincters to cause 'dribbling incontinence' wherein patients cannot use a bedpan or commode but frequently wet the bed with small amounts of urine. This situation is physically uncomfortable and psychologically distressing for the patient, and catheterization may be necessary.

Constipation may lead to *faecal impaction* in the elderly. A mass of faeces lying in the rectum or sigmoid colon will become progressively harder and drier if the patient suffers from chronic constipation. The faecal mass may eventually develop a consistency like plaster of Paris and will irritate the bowel wall. Irritation of the bowel wall will lead to production of large amounts of mucus which will combine with faecal material, liquefied by bacterial action to produce *spurious* (false) *diarrhoea*.

In spurious diarrhoea there is frequent leakage of small amounts of faecal liquid, causing spotting of bed linen or clothing. It would be disastrous if spurious diarrhoea were to be misidentified as true diarrhoea and treated with kaolin or similar solidifying agents, as this will worsen the impaction.

While taking a rectal temperature, the nurse may detect a resistance to the thermometer and find faeces on the thermometer when it is withdrawn. Gentle insertion of a lubricated finger will reveal the presence of a hard mass which is often also palpable through the abdominal wall. Once an impaction is detected, it should be softened (olive or arachis oil retention enema) and then removed (evacuant enema). Occasionally it will only be possible to remove an impaction manually, using a lubricated gloved finger. It must be emphasized that manual removal is not a routine nursing procedure and should only be undertaken by an experienced nurse after consultation with the medical staff. Impactions should never develop in the hospitalized patient and will not occur if the patient has adequate fluids, exercise within his/her capabilities, adequate fibre in the diet and treatment of minor constipation with aperients as necessary.

Faecal incontinence is much less common that urinary incontinence and will respond to similar measures, that is careful assessment and recording of individual eliminatory patterns, and ensuring prompt and easy access to the lavatory.

It is often helpful to have lavatory doors painted a different colour from all other ward doors so that the patient with failing eyesight or problems with orientation may find the appropriate door easily.

In the case of advanced and diffuse brain pathology, incontinence may not be responsive to nursing intervention and, in this case, incontinence aids may be used. These include incontinence garments (e.g. Kanga Pants), often incorporating an incontinence pad and penile sheaths permitting drainage into a collection bag. At their best, pads protect the bed rather than the patient and are likely to adhere to the skin causing maceration and breakdown of tissue. For this reason many hospitals do not use incontinence pads at all.

Catheterization is a last resort except in the case of terminally ill or unconscious patients as it creates a risk of urinary tract infections (which may ascend to the kidneys), leads to atrophy of the bladder muscles, and causes great loss of dignity. Before resorting to incontinence aids or catheters, the nurse should assume that *every* case of incontinence is remediable.

10 *Mobilizing*

Unnecessary and lengthy periods of immobility (in bed or out) are hazardous to the physical and psychological well-being of the brain-failed patient. The geriatric chair is to be particularly deprecated. These high-backed chairs with a locking table, which can be secured across the patient's lap, are still unfortunately used in many units, often as a means of restraint for confused elderly patients with a tendency to wander. Use of such a chair for lengthy periods will cause pressure sores, foster incontinence and cause lethargy and depression. It is suggested that the nurse tries sitting in one of these chairs (table in place) for an hour; the exquisite discomfort that will ensue will make this an experience most nurses will not hasten to repeat. Imagine the effects of spending most of the day in one.

Remember also that the elderly are more vulnerable to the effects of pressure (loss of subcutaneous fat, poor cutaneous blood supply, and thin, friable skin).

Table 113 Scoring system to determine vulnerability to pressure sores. (Norton et al 1962)

a *General physical condition*		b *Mental state*	
4	Good	4	Alert
3	Fair	3	Apathetic
2	Poor	2	Confused
1	Very bad	1	Stupor
c *Activity*		d *Mobility*	
4	Ambulant	4	Full
3	Walks with help	3	Slightly limited
2	Chairbound	2	Very limited
1	Bedfast	1	Immobile
e *Incontinence*		*Totals*	
4	Not		a = (1–4)
3	Occasional		b = (1–4)
2	Usually of urine		c = (1–4)
1	Doubly		d = (1–4)
			e = (1–4)
			Total = (5–20)

Each patient is scored daily (or several times daily if his condition changes).

Norton et al (1962) found that 75% of patients who developed pressure sores had a score of less than 15. 'Patients with a score of 14 or less are liable to develop pressure sores and when the score is lower than 12 the risk is very great indeed.'

Table 110 Mobilizing.

Problem	Objective	Action
Risk of problems associated with immobility (pressure sores, contractures, hypostatic pneumonia, thrombi, constipation, lethargy)	To promote healthy patterns of mobility compatible with patient's abilities	Encourage exercise; avoid unnecessary bed rest; teach joint exercises

Table 111 Controlling body temperature.

Problem	Objective	Action
Mechanisms for regulating body temperature often impaired	To ensure that the elderly person is protected against extremes of temperature	Assess resting temperature of individual; adjust environment as necessary
Body temperature lower in the elderly		Protect against hypothermia

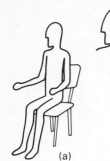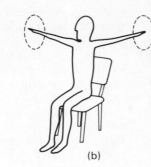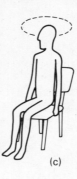

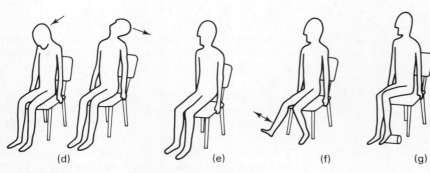

(a)   (b)   (c)

(d)   (e)   (f)   (g)

Figure 17 Exercises to do while sitting. From Eliopoulos (1979).

Norton et al (1962) have devised a scoring system to determine vulnerability to pressure sores (see Table 113), and careful assessment of risk will identify vulnerable patients. There is a wide range of exercises that can be carried out in or out of bed (see Figures 17 and 18) and which will reduce the risk of the complications of immobility. Morning exercises will loosen stiff joints and muscles and encourage activity, while bedtime exercises will promote relaxation and encourage sleep.

Physical exercise is beneficial in many ways but must be within the patient's capabilities, and exercise regimes should be discussed with the medical staff.

11 *Controlling body temperature*

Body temperature is lower in the elderly and may (normally) be as low as 35°C (95°F). The elderly person whose normal temperature is 35.5°C (96°F) may be febrile at 37.2°C (99°F), although this temperature falls within the normal range for the adult population. It is essential that baseline estimation of body temperature is established in the weeks after admission if pyrexia is to be correctly identified.

Thermoregulatory reflexes in the elderly often become defective. Studies revealed that cooling in the elderly was not followed by shivering, rise in metabolic rate or adequate vasoconstriction (Wollner and Spalding, 1978). As a result the elderly have an increased risk of *hypothermia*, which is a state in which 'deep body' or 'core' temperature falls below 35°C, measured either rectally or in freshly passed urine. Hypothermia may be caused by exogenous (exposure) or endogenous (internal) factors, and clinical disturbances which predispose to hypothermia include myxoedema, myocardial infarction, cerebrovascular accident, pneumonia, bronchitis and the effects of many drugs (including phenothiazines, barbiturates and alcohol). Clinical features of hypothermia include pallor (though the face may seem well perfused), apathy, disorientation, hallucinations, paranoid features, slurred speech, muscular rigidity and neck stiffness. The skin, particularly that of the abdomen, is ice cold but

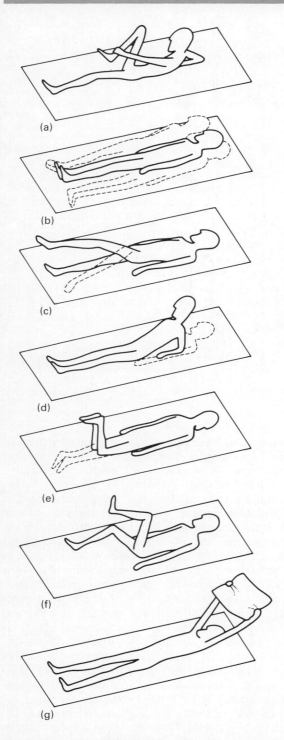

(a)

(b)

(c)

(d)

(e)

(f)

(g)

Figure 18 Exercises to do while lying down. From Eliopoulos (1979).

shivering is usually absent. A low-reading thermometer should be used to confirm the diagnosis.

Treatment consists of rewarming the patient slowly; this is best done by using blankets in a warm room, monitoring temperature (rectally) continuously and checking blood pressure every 30 minutes. If the blood pressure falls as the temperature rises, the patient is immediately re-cooled using fans, and rewarming commences when blood pressure is stable. (Wollner and Spalding, 1978).

Hypothermia is an acute emergency which accounts for many deaths in the community each winter. During the period between April 1983 and March 1984, which included a mild winter, over 36 000 more elderly people died in the winter months than in the summer months (the incidence of death from hypothermia is higher in Britain than in any other Western European country) (Burrows, 1985).

The elderly may also be susceptible to the effects of overheating in summer due to impaired thermoregulatory reflexes. It is likely that heat illness as a cause both of morbidity and mortality is much more common than is recognized and it may be a particular hazard when unclimatized elderly people go on holiday (Exton-Smith, 1969). Exposure to sun, even in Britain, should be carefully controlled and patients receiving phenothiazines are at additional risk of photosensitivity reactions.

12 Dying

It has been commented that 'for a long time nurses were more prepared to deal with the care of a dead body than with the dynamics involved with the dying process' (Eliopoulos, 1979). Dying is a complex and continually changing process that does not only affect the dying individual. Family, friends and care givers are also involved in the dynamics of the process.

Kubler-Ross (1969) suggests a five-stage model of reactions to impending death: *denial* ('It can't be true—there must be some mistake'), *anger* ('Why me?'), *bargaining* (attempts to negotiate a postponement of the inevitable), *depression* and *acceptance*. Relatives, friends and nursing staff often go through similar stages, and nurses may experience feelings of inadequacy—hospitals have an ethos of helping people to get better and the finality of impending death may lead to stasis of interpersonal nursing skills, physical symptoms being easier to attend to.

Table 112 Dying.

Problem	Objective	Action
Increased support needs associated with the dying process	To meet these needs in a systematic and patient-centred way	Assess physical, psychological and spiritual needs and adjust nursing care accordingly

Nursing measures should maintain independence, conserve energy, provide relief from pain and troublesome physical symptoms, promote trust, and ensure that the patient is listened to and treated as an individual until the end. The nurse should also be sensitive to the patient's spiritual needs and should ensure contact with and access by clergy as desired. Touching, comforting and being near the dying person are helpful nursing actions and the family will require support and assistance in dealing with feelings of anger, anxiety or guilt.

Community Care

Hospitalization need not be lengthy or final even for the brain-failed elderly patient. If adequate community support is arranged, many can be discharged once physical condition has been stabilized, and retraining has reduced the disruptive effects of psychosocial dysfunction. Persons over 65 years of age constitute 20% of all hospital discharges (Hunt, 1973), though severe behavioural disturbance may preclude discharge. Patients discharged from psycho-geriatric care are fewer in number than those discharged from geriatric care, but effective medical and nursing care will, nevertheless, make discharge feasible for many patients.

Careful assessment of home circumstances should precede discharge and this must include availability of support. Home-helps have a major part to play and are usually mature women employed by the local authority. The home-help will undertake cooking, shopping and laundry and will also provide friendship and emotional support. Meals on Wheels will also help to ensure adequate diet, though the service does not operate at weekends. Day hospital attendance will reduce strain on family and friends, allowing ongoing assessment, will provide valuable social stimulation for the elderly person. The community psychiatric nurse can monitor coping, both

of patient and family, and may continue retraining programmes commenced in hospital. The general practitioner and health visitor will assess physical well-being, and the social worker will also participate in multidisciplinary monitoring and will help to ensure access to community resources.

The tendency to view the confused elderly as being 'irremediable' is not helpful. Diffuse cerebral pathology may be inexorable, but skilled nursing and medical care can improve quality of life enormously. Isaacs (1974) says of one 69-year-old confused man:

'We did not "cure" him of his irremediable disease but we were privileged to watch the tide of his personality begin to flow again over the dry sand of his disability.'

Key Concepts

1 The vast majority of the brain-failed patients encountered by the nurse will be elderly, but the overall characteristics of brain failure in younger patients are the same.
2 Brain failure in the elderly is compounded by the physical effects of ageing (e.g. decreasing organ efficiency).
3 Neuropsychological deficits, which are commonly present, include *aphasia, apraxia, agnosia, anosagnosia, dyslexia, dysgraphia* and *acalculia*.
4 Communication difficulties may be compounded by *presbycusis* (high frequency deafness).
5 Assessment should be both careful and objective and the *Clifton Assessment Procedures* for the Elderly (CAPE) is an example of the type of rating scale that will prove useful.
6 *Reality orientation* (RO) will help to rehabilitate persons with memory loss and disorientation and may be informal or formal.

7 *Validation therapy* is a companion to RO and consists of accepting, and working with, feelings associated with disorientation.
8 *Sensory stimulation* should be promoted, and simple programmes are easily designed.
9 Much assistance with activities of daily living may be required but care plans should always respect the dignity and individuality of patients and should promote maximal psychosocial functioning commensurate with disability.
10 The risks of institutionalization, apathy and loneliness are always present in the psycho-geriatric unit and are reduced by individualization of patient care.

References

Anderson, Sir W. F. (1976) *Practical management of the elderly, 3rd edn.* Oxford: Blackwell Scientific Publications.

Bergman, K. (1978) Psychogeriatrics. In Carver, V. & Liddiard, P. (Eds) *An Ageing Population.* Kent: Hodder & Stoughton.

Brocklehurst, J. (1978) The large bowel. In Brocklehurst, J. (Ed) *Textbook of Geriatric Medicine and Gerontology.* Edinburgh: Churchill Livingstone.

Bromley, D. (1966) *The Psychology of Ageing.* Harmondsworth: Pelican.

Burril, R., McCourt, J. & Cutter, H. (1974) Beer: a social facilitator for FMI patients? *The Gerontologist,* **14**(5): 430.

Burrows, A. (1985) Hypothermia. *Journal of District Nursing,* **12**: 4–6.

Carroll, P. J. (1978) The social hour for geropsychiatric patients. *Journal of the American Geriatric Society,* **26**(1): 32–35.

Chodil, J. & Williams, B. (1970) The concept of sensory deprivation. *Nursing Clinics of North America,* **5**(3): 453.

Church, M. (1985) Forgotten something? *Nursing Times,* **81**(30): 22–24.

Ebersole, P. & Hess, P. (1981) *Towards Healthy Ageing—Human Needs and Nursing Response.* Oxford: C. V. Mosby.

Eliopoulos, C. (1979) *Geriatric Nursing.* London: Harper & Row.

Exton-Smith, A. (1969) Hazards of the elderly on holiday. *Community Health* (Bristol), **1**: 52–56.

Goffman, E. (1961) *Asylums.* Harmondsworth: Pelican.

Goldman, R. (1970) *Journal of the American Geriatrics Society,* **18**: 765.

Green, M. (1970) Incidence of deafness from wax. In Brocklehurst, J. (Ed) *Textbook of Geriatric Medicine and Gerontology.* Edinburgh: Churchill Livingstone.

Hanley, I., McGuire, R. & Boyd, W. (1981) Reality orientation and dementia: a controlled trial of two approaches. *British Journal of Psychiatry,* **138**: 10–14.

Henry, J. (1963) *Culture against Man.* New York: Random House.

Hess, P. & Day, C. (1977) *Understanding the Ageing Patient.* Bowie: R. J. Brady.

Holden, U. & Woods, R. (1982) *Reality Orientation: Psychological Approaches to the Confused Elderly.* Edinburgh: Churchill Livingstone.

Hunt, L. (1973) The elderly in hospital—recent trends in the use of medical resources. *British Medical Journal,* **4**: 83–85.

Isaacs, B. (1974) In Ware, M. (Ed) *Medicine in Old Age.* London: British Medical Association.

James, W. (1890) *The Principles of Psychology.* London: Macmillan.

Jones, G. (1985) Validation Therapy: a companion to reality orientation. *The Canadian Nurse,* **81**: 20–23.

Judge, T. (1978) Muscle. In Brocklehurst, J. (Ed) *Textbook of Geriatric Medicine and Gerontology.* Edinburgh: Churchill Livingstone.

Kempton, M. (1984) Keeping in touch (psychiatry forum). *Nursing Mirror,* **159**(18): 1–7.

Kubler-Ross, E. (1969) *On Death and Dying.* New York: Macmillan.

Lay, C. & Woods, R. (1983) *Caring for the Person with Dementia—a Guide for Families and Other Carers.* London: Alzheimer Disease Society Publication.

Norton, D., McLaren, R. & Exton-Smith, A. (1962) *An Investigation into Geriatric Nursing Problems in Hospital.* London: National Corporation for the Care of Old People.

Powell, R. (1974) Psychological effects of exercise therapy upon institutionalized geriatric mental patients. *Journal of Gerontology,* **29**: 157–161.

Rossman, I. (1971) *Clinical Geriatrics.* Philadelphia: J. B. Lippincott.

Slater, P. (1964) Cross-cultural views of the aged. In Kastenbaum, R. (Ed) *New Thoughts on Old Age.* New York: Springer.

Snyder, L., Rupprecht, P., Pyrek, J., Brekause, S. & Moss, T. (1978) Wandering. *The Gerontologist,* **18**: 272.

Stafford-Clark, D. & Smith, A. (1983) *Psychiatry for Students, 6th edn.* London: George Allen & Unwin.

Sutherland, S. (1976) The psychology of incontinence. In Wellington, F. (Ed) *Incontinence in the Elderly.* London: Academic Press.

Wollner, L. & Spalding, J. (1978) The autonomic nervous system. In Brocklehurst, J. (Ed) *Textbook of Geriatric Medicine and Gerontology.* Edinburgh: Churchill Livingstone.

XI

APPENDIXES AND INDEX

Appendix 1
General Relaxation Instructions

Begin by getting as comfortable as you can. Settle back comfortably. Just try to let go of all the tension in your body. Now take in a deep breath. Breathe right in and hold it (five-second pause). And now exhale. Just let the air out quite automatically and feel a calmer feeling beginning to develop. Now just carry on breathing normally and just concentrate on feeling heavy all over in a pleasant way. Study your own body heaviness. This should give you a calm and reassuring feeling all over (ten-second pause). Now let us work on tension and relaxation contrasts. Try to tense every muscle in your body. Every muscle: your jaws, tighten your eyes, your shoulder muscles, your arms, chest, back, stomach, legs, every part just tensing and tensing. Feel the tension all over your body—tighter and tighter—tensing everywhere, and now let it go, just stop tensing and relax. Try to feel this wave of calm that comes over you as you stop tensing like that—a definite wave of calm (ten-second pause).

Now I want you to notice the contrast between the slight tensions that are there when your eyes are open and the disappearance of these surface tensions as you close your eyes. So while relaxing the rest of your body just open your eyes and feel the surface tensions which will disappear when you close your eyes. Now close your eyes and feel the greater degree of relaxation with your eyes closed (ten-second pause). All right, let us get back to the breathing. Keep your eyes closed and take in a deep, deep breath and hold it. Now relax the rest of your body as well as you can and notice the tension from holding your breath. Study the tension. Now let out your breath and feel the deepening relaxation—just go with it beautifully relaxing now. Breathe normally and just feel the relaxation flowing into your forehead and scalp. Think of each part as I call it out—just relaxing—just letting go, easing up, eyes and nose, facial muscles. You might feel a tingling sensation as the relaxation flows in. You might have a warm sensation. Whatever you feel I want you to notice it and enjoy it to the full as the relaxation now spreads very beautifully into the face, into the lips, jaws, tongue, and mouth so that your lips are slightly parted as the jaw muscles relax further and further. As the throat and neck are relaxing (five-second pause), and the shoulders and upper back are relaxing, further and further, feel the relaxation flowing into your arms and to the very tips of your fingers (five-second pause). Feel the relaxation in your chest as you breathe regularly and easily. The relaxation spreads even under your armpits and down your sides, right into the stomach area. The relaxation becomes more and more obvious as you do nothing but just give way to the pleasant serene emotions which fill you as you let go more and more. Feel the relaxation—stomach and lower back, all the way through in a warm, penetrating, wavy, calm and down your hips, buttocks, and thighs to the very, very tips of your toes. The waves of relaxation just travel down your calves to your ankles and toes. Feel relaxed from head to toe. Each time you practise this you should find a deeper level of relaxation being achieved—a deeper serenity and calm, a good calm feeling.

Now to increase the feelings of relaxation at this point what I want you to do is just keep on relaxing and each time you exhale, each time you breathe out for the next minute, I want you to think the word *relax* to yourself. Just think the word *relax* as you breathe out. Now just do that for the next minute (one-minute pause). Okay, just feel that deeper relaxation and carry on relaxing. You should feel a deeper, deeper feeling of relaxation. To even further increase the benefits, I want you to feel the emotional calm, those tranquil and serene feelings which tend to cover you all over inside and out, a feeling of safe security, a calm indifference—these are the feelings which relaxation will enable you to capture more and more effectively each time you practise a relaxation sequence. Relaxation will let you arrive at feeling a quiet inner confidence—a good feeling about yourself (five-second pause). Now once more feel the heavy sensations that accompany relaxation as your muscles switch off so that you feel in good contact with your environment, nicely together, and the heavy good feeling of feeling yourself calm and secure and very, very tranquil and serene.

Now we can deepen the relaxation still further by just using some very special stimulus words. Let's use the words *calm* and *serene*. What I would like you to do is to think these words to yourself twenty times or so. Don't bother to count. Approximately twenty or thirty times just say to yourself *calm* and *serene* and then feel the deepening—ever, ever deepening—waves of relaxation as you feel so much more calm and serene. Now you just do that; take your time, think of the words and feel the sensations over and over (pause of about one minute). Good.

Now I am going to count backward from 10 to 1. At the count of 5 I would like you to open your eyes, and then by the time I reach 1, just kind of stretch and yawn and then you can switch off the recorder and just go back and relax on your own. Okay, now counting backward: 10, 9, 8, 7, 6, 5, open your eyes 4, 3, 2, and 1. Now just stretch and kind of yawn and then slowly get up and switch off the recorder and then you can go back and carry on relaxing as long as you wish.

Reprinted from *Behaviour Therapy and Beyond* (Lazarus, A.), 1971, with kind permission of the publisher, McGraw-Hill.

Appendix 2

The Nurse's Observation Scale for Inpatient Evaluation (NOSIE)

The NOSIE 30 is a flexible ward behaviour rating scale, produced by Honigfeld and Klett (1965). It takes the form of a simple questionnaire which asks the observer to consider certain aspects of the patient's behaviour, to produce an objective profile of patient functioning. In essence the questionnaire is a list of simple behavioural statements (e.g. Cries, Refuses to speak, Is sloppy) and the rater is asked to indicate whether each statement applies to the patient—Never, Sometimes, Often, Usually or Always—behaviour being observed over a three day period.

The scale elicits scores on six factors:

Social competence
Social interest
Personal neatness
Irritability
Manifest psychosis
and retardation (related to observable aspects of depressive symptomatology);

To produce scores for each of these six factors the ratings must be assigned numerical values. Note that NOSIE scores are based on the *sum* of two raters' evaluations and that, if one rater is used, the score *must be doubled*.

Scale items are scored as follows: Never—0, Sometimes—1, Often—2, Usually—3, Always—4 [these scores being transferred to the Hand Scoring Key, e.g. if in response to item 8 (Keeps his clothes neat) you had decided that 'Usually' was the appropriate category you would then enter a score of 3 against item 8 on the Hand Scoring Key].

Note that items marked * on the Hand Scoring Key receive *reflected* scores (0–4, 1–3, 2–2, 3–1, 4–0).

Positive factors (Competence, Interest, Neatness) are then added to yield a score for *total positive factors*.

Negative factors (Irritability, Manifest Psychosis, Retardation) are then added to yield a score for *total negative factors*.

You may now proceed to calculate *total patient assets* (*TOT*) which is arrived at in the following simple way—96 + *total positive factors* − *total negative factors*.

The profile sheet enables the rater(s) to plot the six factors by taking the score for each factor and marking it on the appropriate column with a dot or cross. Joining the dots will give an individual patient profile.

Use of the NOSIE will avoid or minimize observer bias and will enable effective baseline measurements to be taken. Thereafter progress (e.g. in a ward-based rehabilitation scheme or an individual behaviour modification programme) can be evaluated accurately and objectively —hopefully revealing an increase in positive factors and a decrease in negative factors (with a consequent increase in total patient assets.

The NOSIE scale is reproduced by kind permission of Dr Gilbert Honigfeld, for whose cooperation and assistance I am also grateful.

Copies of the NOSIE may be obtained from Dr Honigfeld, Sandoz Inc., 59 Route 10, East Hanover, New Jersey–079 36, USA.

More information may be found in the following articles:
Honigfeld, G. & Klett, C. (1965) The Nurses Observation Scale for Inpatient Evaluation. *Journal of Clinical Psychology*, 21: 65–71.
Honigfeld, G. Gillis, R. & Klett, C. (1966) NOSIE–30: A treatment sensitive ward behaviour scale. *Psychological Reports*, 19: 180–192.

NURSES OBSERVATION SCALE FOR INPATIENT EVALUATION (NOSIE-30)

Subject's name_____ Date_____

Rater's name_____ Title_____

DIRECTIONS

Please rate this patient's behaviour as you observed it *during the last three days only*. Indicate your choice by filling in one block for each item, using this key:

0 = Never   1 = Sometimes   2 = Often   3 = Usually   4 = Always

Use No. 2 pencil. Make your marks heavy and black. Erase mistakes completely.

0 === 1 === 2 === 3 === 4 ===   (1) Is sloppy.
0 === 1 === 2 === 3 === 4 ===   (2) Is impatient.
0 === 1 === 2 === 3 === 4 ===   (3) Cries.
0 === 1 === 2 === 3 === 4 ===   (4) Shows interest in activities around him.
0 === 1 === 2 === 3 === 4 ===   (5) Sits, unless directed into activity.
0 === 1 === 2 === 3 === 4 ===   (6) Gets angry or annoyed easily.
0 === 1 === 2 === 3 === 4 ===   (7) Hears things that are not there.
0 === 1 === 2 === 3 === 4 ===   (8) Keeps his clothes neat.
0 === 1 === 2 === 3 === 4 ===   (9) Tries to be friendly with others.
0 === 1 === 2 === 3 === 4 === (10) Becomes upset easily if something doesn't suit him.
0 === 1 === 2 === 3 === 4 === (11) Refuses to do the ordinary things expected of him.
0 === 1 === 2 === 3 === 4 === (12) Is irritable or grouchy.
0 === 1 === 2 === 3 === 4 === (13) Has trouble remembering.
0 === 1 === 2 === 3 === 4 === (14) Refuses to speak.
0 === 1 === 2 === 3 === 4 === (15) Laughs or smiles at funny comments or events.
0 === 1 === 2 === 3 === 4 === (16) Is messy in his eating habits.
0 === 1 === 2 === 3 === 4 === (17) Starts a conversation with others.
0 === 1 === 2 === 3 === 4 === (18) Says he feels blue or depressed.
0 === 1 === 2 === 3 === 4 === (19) Talks about his interests.
0 === 1 === 2 === 3 === 4 === (20) Sees things that are not there.
0 === 1 === 2 === 3 === 4 === (21) Has to be reminded what to do.
0 === 1 === 2 === 3 === 4 === (22) Sleeps, unless directed into activity.
0 === 1 === 2 === 3 === 4 === (23) Says that he is no good.
0 === 1 === 2 === 3 === 4 === (24) Has to be told to follow hospital routine.
0 === 1 === 2 === 3 === 4 === (25) Has difficulty completing simple tasks on his own.
0 === 1 === 2 === 3 === 4 === (26) Talks, mutters, or mumbles to himself.
0 === 1 === 2 === 3 === 4 === (27) Is slow-moving or sluggish.
0 === 1 === 2 === 3 === 4 === (28) Giggles or smiles to himself for no apparent reason.
0 === 1 === 2 === 3 === 4 === (29) Is quick to fly off the handle.
0 === 1 === 2 === 3 === 4 === (30) Keeps himself clean.

0 === 1 === 2 === 3 === 4 === 5 === 6 === 7 === 8 === 9 ===   Project Number
0 === 1 === 2 === 3 === 4 === 5 === 6 === 7 === 8 === 9 ===
0 === 1 === 2 === 3 === 4 === 5 === 6 === 7 === 8 === 9 ===
0 === 1 === 2 === 3 === 4 === 5 === 6 === 7 === 8 === 9 ===   Subject Code Number
0 === 1 === 2 === 3 === 4 === 5 === 6 === 7 === 8 === 9 ===
0 === 1 === 2 === 3 === 4 === 5 === 6 === 7 === 8 === 9 ===
0 === 1 === 2 === 3 === 4 === 5 === 6 === 7 === 8 === 9 ===   Treatment Group
0 === 1 === 2 === 3 === 4 === 5 === 6 === 7 === 8 === 9 ===   Rating Period
0 === 1 === 2 === 3 === 4 === 5 === 6 === 7 === 8 === 9 ===
0 === 1 === 2 === 3 === 4 === 5 === 6 === 7 === 8 === 9 ===   Rater

NOSIE-30   Hand Scoring Key

Subject_____ Code #_____ Date of Rating_____
Name of Rater 1_____ Position of Rater 1_____
Name of Rater 2_____ Position of Rater 2_____

> NOSIE factor scores are based on the sum of two raters' item responses. Therefore, if one rater is used, his *scores must be doubled.*

POSITIVE FACTORS

1 Social Competence (COM)

	Rater 1	Rater 2
11*	_____	_____
13*	_____	_____
21*	_____	_____
24*	_____	_____
25*	_____	_____
sum	_____ +	_____ =

2 Social Interest (INT)

	Rater 1	Rater 2
4	_____	_____
9	_____	_____
15	_____	_____
17	_____	_____
19	_____	_____
sum	_____ +	_____ =

3 Personal Neatness (NEA)

	Rater 1	Rater 2
1*	_____	_____
8	_____	_____
16*	_____	_____
30	_____	_____
sum	_____ +	_____ =

Total positive factors = sum COM + sum INT + sum NEA =

NEGATIVE FACTORS

4 Irritability (IRR)

	Rater 1	Rater 2
2	_____	_____
6	_____	_____
10	_____	_____
12	_____	_____
29	_____	_____
sum	_____ +	_____ =

5 Manifest Psychosis (PSY)

	Rater 1	Rater 2
7	_____	_____
20	_____	_____
26	_____	_____
28	_____	_____
sum	_____ +	_____ =

6 Retardation (RET)

	Rater 1	Rater 2
5	_____	_____
22	_____	_____
27	_____	_____
sum	_____ +	_____ =

Total negative factors = sum IRR + sum PSY + sum RET =

7. Total Patient Assets (TOT) =

96 + total positive factors [   ] − total negative factors [   ] = [   ]

*These items receive *reflected* scores:
0 = 4   1 = 3   2 = 2   3 = 1   4 = 0

Subject's name_____ No._____ Date_____

PROFILE SHEET – NOSIE-30

Normalized T-scores	Positive Factors — COM	Positive Factors — INT	Positive Factors — NEA	Negative Factors — IRR	Negative Factors — PSY	Negative Factors — RET	Total Patient Assets — TOT	Percentile values
	40	34–40	32	40	28–32	24	192–208	
							191	
80				37–39	25–27	23	190	99.9
				35–36		22	189	
					24	21	188	
75		32–33		34	23		187	99.4
		31					186	
				33		20	185	
	39	29–30		32			184	
				31	22	19	182–183	
70		28		29–30	21		180–181	97.7
		27		28	20		177–179	
				26–27	19	18	176	
		26		25			174–175	
		25		24	17–18	17	172–173	
65	38	24	31	22–23	16	16	171	93.3
		23		21	15		168–170	
		22		19–20			167	
		21		18	14	15	164–166	
	37	20	30		13		162–163	
60	36	19	29	16–17		14	159–161	84.1
	35	18		14–15	12	13	157–158	
	34	17	28	13	11	12	154–156	
	33	16			10		151–153	
		15	27	12	9	11	148–150	
55	32	14	26	10–11		10	146–147	69.1
	31	13			8		143–145	
	30	12	25	9	7	9	139–142	
			23–24	8			137–138	
		10–11	22		6		134–136	
50	29		21	7	5	8	132–133	50.0
	28	9	20	6			129–131	
	27	8	19	5		7	126–128	
	26	7	18	4	4	6	123–125	
		6	17				119–122	
45	24–25		15–16	3	3	5	115–118	30.9
	23	5	14				112–114	
	22	4	13	2	2	4	108–111	
	20–21		11–12				105–107	
	19		10				101–104	
40	18		9	1	1	3	98–100	15.9
	16–17	3	8			2	95–97	
	15	2	7				92–94	
	14		6	0			88–91	
	13				0		86–87	
35	12	1	5			1	84–85	6.7
	11						82–83	
	10	0	4				80–81	
	9		3			0	77–79	
			2				74–76	
30	8		1				72–73	2.3
							69–71	
	7						67–68	
							63–66	
	5–6						59–62	
25	4						58	.6
	3						57	
							50–56	
							45–49	
			0				42–44	
20	0–2						0–41	.1

Appendix 3

Clifton Assessment Procedures for the Elderly (CAPE)

The CAPE assessment procedure is a relatively brief method for assessing the cognitive (mental) and behavioural competence of the elderly and was produced by two psychologists (A. Pattie and C. Gilleard) working at the Clifton Hospital, York.

CAPE consists of two independent measures which can be used together to give an overall assessment of cognitive and behavioural disability or can be used separately, depending on the information required.

The *Cognitive Assessment Scale* (CAS) is a short psychological test which is most suited to evaluationg the existence and degree of impairment in mental functioning.

The *Behaviour Rating Scale* (BRS) is a rating scale which is completed by an observer familiar with the subject's behaviour and provides an overall measurement of the individual's behavioural disability level.

The information obtained from these two scales is recorded on a separate summary sheet, the CAPE report form, which allows individual scores to be compared to a five-point grading system, which indicates the level of dependency associated with each group.

The cognitive assessment scale (CAS)

The CAS consists of three sections.

1 *The information/orientation test*

This is made up of twelve questions designed to assess current information and orientation.

2 *The mental ability test*

This consists of four measures relating to well established skills involving counting, saying the alphabet, reading and writing.

3 *The psychomotor test*

This is the Gibson spiral maze which provides a measure of fine motor performance and hand–eye coordination.

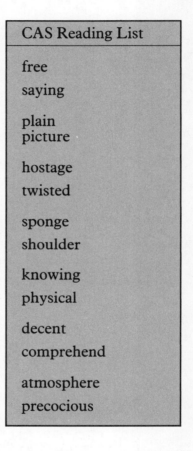

CAS Reading List

free

saying

plain
picture

hostage

twisted

sponge

shoulder

knowing

physical

decent

comprehend

atmosphere

precocious

Administering the CAS. A quiet, distraction-free room should be used and it should be ascertained whether or not the subject normally uses reading glasses. The test may be introduced as 'some questions I'd like to ask you' or 'some questions to see how your memory and concentration are at the moment'. The tester will need a stop-watch or a watch with a second hand, in addition to the test materials.

Questions may be re-phrased once or twice where necessary, no assistance or cues should be given and excessive repetition is not recommended.

CLIFTON ASSESSMENT PROCEDURES FOR THE ELDERLY (CAPE)
Cognitive Assessment Scale

Name: ....

Current address/placement: ....

....

Date of birth: .... **Occupation:** ....

Information/Orientation

Name:	Hospital/Address:	Colour of British Flag:
Age:	City:	Day:
D.o.B.:	P.M.:	Month:
Ward/Place:	U.S. President:	Year:

I/O Score...........................

Mental Ability

Count 1-20   *Time:* .... *Errors:*.........
    ≤ 10 secs – no errors   3
    ≤ 30 secs – no errors   2
    ≤ 30 secs – 1 error   1
                         0

Write name:
    Correct and legible   2
    Can write but not correctly 1
    Not able to   0

Alphabet   *Time:* .... *Errors:*..........
    ≤ 10 secs – no errors   3
    ≤ 30 secs – no errors   2
    ≤ 30 secs – 1 error   1
                         0

Reading: (See overleaf)
    10 words or more   3
    6-9 words   2
    1-5 words   1
    0 words   0

MAb Score ....

Psychomotor *Time:*.......................... *Errors:*..........................

Pm Score...

Scoring

Errors:	0-12	13-24	25-36	37-48	49-60	61-72	73-84	85-96	96+	N/C	N/A
Score:	10	9	8	7	6	5	4	3	2	1	0
Add Bonus 2 if 60 secs or under; 1 if 120 secs or under											

Assessed by: .... **Date:** ....

Directions and scoring criteria are as follows:

Information/orientation

Each correct response is given one point.

1 What is your name/full name?	First name and surname are both required.
2 How old are you?	Present age in years or predicted age next birthday, e.g. 79 next August.
3 What is your date of birth?	The date, month and year must all be correctly given.
4 What is this place/Where are you now?	The name of the hospital ward or recognition that it is a hospital ward is required for hospital patients; recognition that they are in their own home, social services accommodation or whatever for non-hospital subjects.
5 What is the name of this hospital/What is the address of this place?	Name of hospital is required, street address of the home, or, if in their own home, number and street name, as appropriate.
6 What is the name of this town/city?	The correct name of the town or city in which they are currently located.
7 Who is the Prime Minister?	Surname of the current PM is sufficient.
8 Who is the President of the United States of America?	Surname of the current president.
9 What are the colours of the British flag/Union Jack?	Red, white and blue.
10 What day is it?	The day of the week, not date, is required. (This can be explained once if the date is given).
11 What month is it?	Current month.
12 What year is it?	Current year.

Mental ability

Will you count up from 1 to 20 for me—as quickly as you can?	The prompt 1, 2, 3 may be given. Time in seconds and number of errors are recorded.
Now, can you say the alphabet—again as quickly as you can?	The prompt a, b, c may be given. Again the time taken and number of errors are recorded.
Will you read these words out loud for me?	A second test form is usually offered to the subject so that the examiner can mark the correctly read words on the test form being used.
Will/can you write your name here for me? Please write it clearly.	The name must include either first name and surname, correct and legible, or title (Mr, Miss, Dr) and surname. If there are errors, or the name is not clear, score 1, but if the person is unable to write out his name correctly or it is illegible, score 0.

Psychomotor

The Gibson spiral maze is a spiral design printed on a large card, with obstacles in the shape of the letter O along its pathway. A fresh card is used for each subject. The test is introduced to the subject as follows: 'This is like a maze—you start with your pencil at the little arrow here *(point)* and you go round and round. Try to keep on the white track and not touch these small black circles *(point)* or the thick black lines. Try to go as quickly as you can, until you come out at the end here *(point)*'. A maximum of *three* prompts are allowed, including only *one* repetition of

THE GIBSON SPIRAL MAZE

Copyright © H. B. Gibson 1961

T.....................................

E.....................................

Name..

Age..

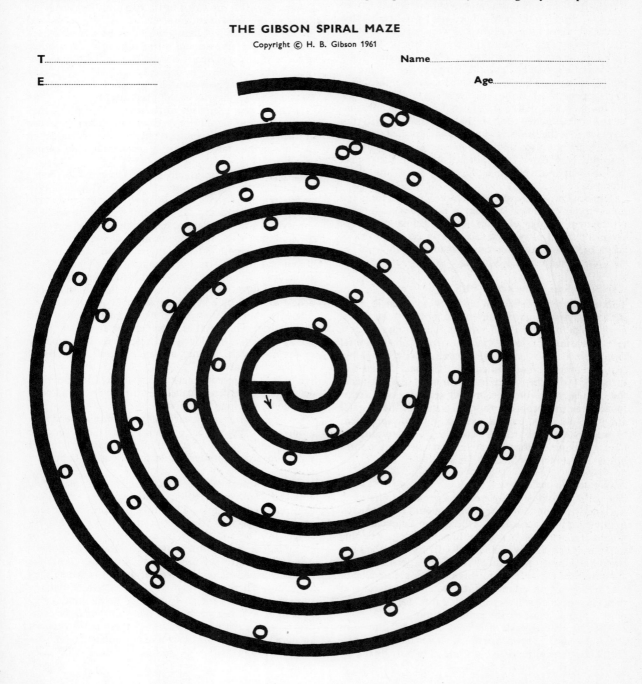

the instructions to avoid touching the black lines or circles.

As soon as the subject puts the pencil on the card to start, timing should begin.

Scoring. The time in seconds taken to complete the maze is recorded. The maximum amount of time allowed is four minutes, although the person need not be stopped at that point if it seems likely that he/she will shortly be able to complete it. (This, of course, is for the subject's morale only and the maze must still be scored as uncompleted.)

Errors are scored as 1 point if a circle or line is touched, but not penetrated by the pencil, and 2 points if the line or circle is penetrated. If the pencil remains on the black line for any length, 2 points are scored for each inch of continued contact/penetration. A maze is scored as N/C (not completed) if the subject completes at least the first circle of the maze but gives up before finishing, and after three prompts. It is scored N/A (not attempted) if the subject fails to complete even one circle of the maze, after three prompts.

Time and errors are recorded on the CAS test form and are then converted to a score out of 12. The score is based on the total number of errors, but additional points are given for speed of performance within certain levels of accuracy. This conversion can be made directly from the data provided on the CAS form.

The behaviour rating scale (BRS)

This is a shortened version of the Stockton geriatric rating scale which was originally developed for use in the assessment of elderly hospitalized patients. The rating scale provides measures of four principal areas of behavioural disability, namely 'physical disability' (Pd), 'apathy' (Ap), 'communication difficulties' (Cd) and 'social disturbance' (Sd). These are the same areas of disability as in the original scale, but the present scale excludes items found to be inappropriate to settings outside the hospital and items found to exhibit consistently poor agreement between raters (Gilleard and Pattie 1977). Two additional items covering sensory deficits are included in the form but do not contribute to the scale scores.

Administration and scoring
The scales should be completed by a person familiar with the elderly person to be rated. They should be instructed to rate each item according to the person's current functioning, i.e. what he *does* rather than what he may be able to do or at one time was able to do. In general, the rater should be advised to consider the elderly person's behaviour over the past week or fortnight. It is sometimes helpful, in cases of uncertainty by the rater, to suggest that they first consider whether the 0 or 2 rating applies and if neither applies to select the middle rating.

After the rating scale has been completed the form should be checked to ensure that no items have been missed. The scores of items 1–6 are added to provide the Pd score, 7–11 the Ap score, 12 and 13 the Cd score and items 14–18 the Sd score. The total score is simply the sum of all four sub-scales, which can range from 0 to 36.

The CAPE report form

The scores obtained on the CAS and BRS are entered on a separate report form which provides a useful way of summarizing the assessment information. All the scores are graded from A to E. These grades may be seen as representing levels of impairment in functioning. A description of the level of dependency is also given for each grade on the report form itself. The concept of dependency reflects the degree of support typically provided by society in association with given levels of disability.

Grade A represents no impairment in mental functioning and no significant behavioural disability. This characterizes the independent elderly, i.e. independence in daily living, making little or no demand on caring agencies.

Grade B indicates mild impairment in mental and behavioural functioning and is usually associated with elderly people requiring some support in the community. This level of low dependency can be found typically in warden-supervised accommodation, or among elderly people in the community receiving one or more services and a proportion of the more independent elderly in social services accommodation. Normally, hospital patients functioning at this level do not need long-term institutional care.

Grade C forms a moderate impairment/medium dependency group. People in this group are likely to need considerable support if they are to be maintained in the community. This level is more characteristic of social service homes for the elderly and hospitals, and is typically represented by the chronic, moderately disabled long-stay population in care.

Grade D represents marked impairment/high dependency. Such people are usually institutionalized and need considerable help in daily living.

Grade E, a severe impairment/maximum dependency group, are typical of psychogeriatric and geriatric patients, requiring a great deal of nursing attention and care, and are generally unable to look after their own needs.

The most reliable indices of dependency can usually be obtained from consideration of the two total scores, i.e. CAS total and BRS total. The sub-scale scores can be seen as offering a profile of disabilities which may be helpful in suggesting therapeutic or management strategies. For example, the report form allows identification of individuals whose degree of impairment is outside the range normally associated with the environment in which they are living. Where the level of disability is greater than the support offered by the environment, the individual may be seen to be at risk, and where there appears to be overprovision of environmental support there is both risk of encouraging unnecessary loss of independence and misuse of scarce resources.

CLIFTON ASSESSMENT PROCEDURES FOR THE ELDERLY (CAPE)
Behaviour Rating Scale

Name: ....Date of birth: ....

Current address/placement: ....

....

Please ring the appropriate number for each item

1 When bathing or dressing, he/she requires:
— no assistance ... 0
— some assistance ... 1
— maximum assistance ... 2

2 With regard to walking, he/she:
— shows no signs of weakness ... 0
— walks slowly without aid, or uses a stick ... 1
— is unable to walk, or if able to walk, needs frame, crutches or someone by his/her side ... 2

3 He/she is incontinent of urine and/or faeces (day or night):
— never ... 0
— sometimes (once or twice per week) ... 1
— frequently (3 times per week or more) ... 2

4 He/she is in bed during the day (bed does not include couch, settee, etc):
— never ... 0
— sometimes ... 1
— almost always ... 2

5 He/she is confused (unable to find way around, loses possessions, etc):
— almost never confused ... 0
— sometimes confused ... 1
— almost always confused ... 2

6 When left to his/her own devices, his/her appearance (clothes and/or hair) is:
— almost never disorderly ... 0
— sometimes disorderly ... 1
— almost always disorderly ... 2

7 If allowed outside, he/she would:
— never need supervision ... 0
— sometimes need supervision ... 1
— always need supervision ... 2

8 He/she helps out in the home/ward:
— often helps out ... 0
— sometimes helps out ... 1
— never helps out ... 2

9 He/she keeps him/herself occupied in a constructive or useful activity (works, reads, plays games, has hobbies, etc):
— almost always occupied ... 0
— sometimes occupied ... 1
— almost never occupied ... 2

10 He/she socializes with others:

— does establish a good relationship with others — 0
— has some difficulty establishing good relationships — 1
— has a great deal of difficulty establishing good relationships — 2

11 He/she is willing to do things suggested or asked of him/her:

— often goes along — 0
— sometimes goes along — 1
— almost never goes along — 2

12 He/she understands what you communicate to him/her (you may use speaking, writing, or gesturing):

— understands almost everything you communicate — 0
— understands some of what you communicate — 1
— understands almost nothing of what you communicate — 2

13 He/she communicates in any manner (by speaking, writing or gesturing):

— well enough to make him/herself easily understood at all times — 0
— can be understood sometimes or with some difficulty — 1
— can rarely or never be understood for whatever reason — 2

14 He/she is objectionable to others during the day (loud or constant talking, pilfering, soiling furniture, interfering with affairs of others):

— rarely or never — 0
— sometimes — 1
— frequently — 2

15 He/she is objectionable to others during the night (loud or constant talking, pilfering, soiling furniture, interfering in affairs of others, wandering about, etc.):

— rarely or never — 0
— sometimes — 1
— frequently — 2

16 He/she accuses others of doing him/her bodily harm or stealing his/her personal possessions — if you are sure the accusations are true, rate zero, otherwise rate one or two:

— never — 0
— sometimes — 1
— frequently — 2

17 He/she hoards apparently meaningless items (wads of paper, string, scraps of food, etc.):

— never — 0
— sometimes — 1
— frequently — 2

18 His/her sleep pattern at night is:

— almost never awake — 0
— sometimes awake — 1
— often awake — 2

Eyesight:
(tick which applies)

— can see (or can see with glasses)
— partially blind
— totally blind

Hearing:
(tick which applies)

— no hearing difficulties, without hearing aid
— no hearing difficulties, though requires hearing aid
— has hearing difficulties which interfere with communication
— is very deaf

Rated by: .... Date:...
        Staff/Relative

CLIFTON ASSESSMENT PROCEDURES FOR THE ELDERLY (CAPE)
Report Form

Name .... Age ....

Current address/placement ....

....

Date of birth .... Marital status ....

Relevant background information (rated sensory impairment, occupation, accommodation, etc.)

CAS Scores

Information/Orientation:................   Mental ability:................   Psychomotor:................

CAS Total

BRS Scores

Physical disability:................   Communication difficulties:................

Apathy:................   Social disturbance:................

BRS Total

Dependency Grade   Cognitive:................   Behavioural:................   Overall:

Recommendations

Assessed by: .... Date:..

Dependency grade

A—no impairment: independent elderly—comparable to those living without support in the community
B—mild impairment: low dependency—likely to include those needing some support in the community, warden-supervised accommodation and the better residents in residential accommodation
C—moderate impairment: medium dependency—people functioning at this level are likely to need residential care or considerable support and help if at home

D—marked impairment: high dependency—it is within this category that there is the greatest overlap between those in social services accommodation and those in hospital care
E—severe impairment: maximum dependency—this level is seen most often in psychogeriatric wards and the ones who remain in community homes/EMI hostels often present considerable problems to staff in terms of their demands on staff time

Grades	A	B	C	D	E
I/O	12,11	10,9	8,7,6	5,4,3	2,1,0
MAb	11	10,9,8	7,6	5,4	3,2,1,0
Pm	12,11,10	9,8,7	6,5,4	3,2	1,0
CAS total	35–30	29–24	23–16	15–9	8–0
BRS total	0–3	4–7	8–12	13–17	18+
Pd	0,1	2,3	4,5	6,7	8–12
Ap	0,1	2,3	4,5	6,7	8–10
Cd	0	0	0	1	2–4
Sd	0	1	2	3,4	5–10

From *Manual of the Clifton Assessment Procedures for the Elderly* (Pattie, A. & Gilleard, C.), 1979, with kind permission of the authors and the publisher, Hodder & Stoughton.
Copies of the test forms (and manual) are obtainable from P.O. Box 702, Dunton Green, Sevenoaks, Kent TN13 2YD.

Appendix 4

Notes on The Mental Health Act 1983 and The Mental Health (Scotland) Act 1984

In the course of the last 100 years, legislation has been in existence to protect people who, by virtue of their mental disorder, are deemed to be vulnerable to abuse from members of the public and from unscrupulous members of staff of the institutions in which they are being cared for.

At the end of the nineteenth century, the Lunacy Acts and the Mental Deficiency Acts were primarily designed to prevent compulsory detention in an 'asylum' of anyone who was not a danger to others or to him/herself as well as suffering from a mental disorder. Apart from the many sections of these Acts which regulated admission to institutions, discharge from, and care while in an institution, the Acts made provision for 'The Board of Control', a watchdog body with the duty to exercise protective functions on behalf of the mentally disordered.

The way the Lunacy Acts operated made it difficult, however, for people to obtain care and treatment unless they were in danger or a danger to others. In the 1930s, new legislation, the Mental Treatment Acts, made it possible to admit mentally disordered people, now referred to as 'patients', to institutions, renamed 'hospitals', on a voluntary basis. The protection against abuse which the Acts afforded applied also to voluntary patients.

To become a voluntary patient it was necessary to sign an application and patients had to give notice in writing of their intention to discharge themselves.

It was necessary to ensure the patients really understood what they were doing, and a medical officer had to ascertain that the patient was indeed 'volitional'. Many patients, though perfectly willing to be in hospital, were deemed not to be suitable for voluntary status because they were not regarded as volitional. Confused patients, severely depressed patients or schizophrenic patients who were very withdrawn, and severely mentally handicapped people had to be admitted under 'certificate' for this reason.

In the 1950s a Royal Commission recommended changes in legislation and in 1959 in England and Wales, 1960 in Scotland and 1961 in Northern Ireland, new legislation—'The Mental Health Acts'—came into operation. The main principles on which the Acts were based were:

1 That patients suffering from mental disorder should as far as possible be treated, in or outside hospital, on the same basis as patients suffering from any other disorder. They should be able to enter any hospital capable of offering treatment. They should enter hospital or leave hospital with no more formality or restrictions than any other patients.

2 That, outside hospital, provisions should be made for treatment and care comparable to those offered to people suffering from other disorders.

3 That hospitals which offered psychiatric treatment should be free to refuse admission if they felt unable to help the patient or for any other reason, just as other hospitals are.

4 That the provisions made for the fairly small number of patients who must be detained against their will should entail only a minimal amount of legal restriction.

5 In England and Wales, that special provisions for protection were no longer necessary.

In order to achieve these objectives, all previous legislation relating both to mental illness and what was formally known as mental deficiency was repealed. One Act replaced all former legislation and it covered disorders not formerly dealt with.

The term 'mental disorder' was used to cover all disorders dealt with under the Act. The definition in the Act of 'mental disorder' was: 'Mental illness, arrested or incomplete development, psychopathic disorder and any other disorder or disability of mind.' In Scotland the term 'psychopathic disorder' was not used.

There were four subdivisions of mental disorder recognized for the purposes of the compulsory provisions of the Act of 1959:

1 Mental illness
2 Severe subnormality
3 Subnormality
4 Psychopathic disorder

The Scottish Act did not define the categories. The term 'mental disorder' meant mental illness and mental defect. The latter term remained in use.

Admission without compulsion. Patients in all four of these categories could be admitted to any hospital without compulsion or application. It was not necessary that the patient should be capable of expressing a wish to be admitted. As long as he was not actively unwilling to enter hospital his admission could be informal.

Compulsory admission. In England and Wales and in Northern Ireland, for those patients who had to be admitted against their will, only the signatures of two specifically designated doctors were necessary. In Scotland, only emergency admissions were possible on the authority of medical officers. Within seven days an application to the Sheriff had to be made to obtain his authority for further compulsory detention.

In England and Wales and in Northern Ireland, no watchdog organization was appointed. When the Board of Control was dissolved in Scotland, the Mental Welfare Commission was appointed with the general brief of exercising protective functions. It had less power, however, than its predecessor, the Board of Control.

By the end of the 1970s it had become clear that the legislation of the 1960s had provided insufficient safeguards for patients. Following a review, a new Mental Health Act was passed in 1983 and a new Mental Health (Scotland) Act in 1984.

The Mental Health Act 1983

Application of the Act

The Act concerns 'the reception, care and treatment of mentally disordered patients, the management of their property and other related matters'. The definition of mental disorder is a mental illness, arrested or incomplete development of mind, psychopathic disorder or any other disorder or disability of mind. For most purposes of the Act it is not enough for a patient to be suffering from one of the four specific categories of mental disorder set out in the Act:
1 Mental illness
2 Mental impairment
3 Severe mental impairment
4 Psychopathic disorder

It is important to note that no person shall be treated as suffering from mental disorder by reason of promiscuity or other immoral conduct, sexual deviancy, or dependence on alcohol or drugs.

The Scottish Act does not define the categories. The words mental subnormality and mental deficiency cease to have effect.

Admission without compulsion

Informal admission should be the normal mode of admission to hospital whenever a patient is willing to be admitted and be treated without the use of compulsory powers. It is not necessary that the patient should be capable of expressing a wish to be admitted. As long as he is not actively unwilling to enter hospital the admission can be informal. The majority of patients enter hospital as informal admissions.

Compulsory admission: England and Wales

Some patients suffering from mental disorder may have to be compulsorily admitted to and detained in hospital or received into guardianship. There are a number of different powers under which a patient may be compulsorily detained in hospital; as follows:

The emergency admission

An application may be made by an approved social worker or by the nearest relative of the patient in exceptional circumstances. The applicant must state that it is of urgent necessity that the patient should be admitted and detained for assessment, and that compliance with the normal procedures would involve undesirable delay. Only one medical recommendation is required, but the practitioner concerned must have seen the patient within the previous 24 hours. The application is effective for 72 hours.

Admission for assessment

Admission to and detention in hospital for assessment may be authorized where a patient is (a) suffering from mental disorder of a nature of degree which warrants the detention of the patient in hospital for assessment (or for assessment followed by medical treatment) for at least a limited period, and (b) he ought to be so detained in the interests of his health or safety, or with a view to the protection of others. Detention is for up to 28 days. An application for admission must be made by either the patient's nearest relative or an approved social worker. An application for admission must be accompanied by written recommendations from two medical practitioners, one of whom must be approved as having special experience in the diagnosis and treatment of mental disorder.

Admission for treatment

The grounds for admission for treatment are first that the patient is suffering from one or more of the four forms of mental disorder as previously described. Secondly, the mental disorder must be of a nature or degree which makes it appropriate for the patient to receive medical treatment in hospital. Thirdly, for a patient suffering from psychopathic disorder or mental impairment there is an additional condition that medical treatment is likely to alleviate or prevent a deterioration in the patient's condition. Treatment need not be expected to cure the patient's disorder; medical treatment should enable the patient to cope more satisfactorily with his disorder or it should stop his condition from becoming worse. Fourthly, it must be necessary for the health or safety of the patient or for the protection of others that he should receive this treatment and it cannot be provided unless he is detained. Application for admission for treatment must be made by either an approved social worker or the patient's nearest relative. The person who is to be regarded as nearest relative is defined in the Act. This must be accompanied by written recommendations from two medical practitioners, one of whom must be approved as having special experience in diagnosis and treatment of mental disorder. Detention for treatment is for a maximum period of six months unless the order is renewed.

Patients already in hospital

A patient may be compulsorily detained for up to 72 hours if the doctor in charge of his treatment reports that an application for admission ought to be made. If the doctor is not obtainable, a first level nurse trained in nursing people suffering from mental illness or mental handicap may detain an informal patient on behalf of the managers for a period of up to six hours, while a doctor is found. It must appear to the nurse that (a) the patient is suffering from mental disorder to such a degree that it is necessary for his health or safety, or for the protection of others, for him to be immediately restrained from leaving hospital and (b) it is not practicable to secure the immediate attendance of a doctor for the purpose of furnishing a report. The nurse must record these facts in writing.

Safeguards for patients and staff

Patients who feel they are wrongfully detained may apply to a *Mental Health Review Tribunal* to have their case considered. The tribunal has the power to discharge a patient from hospital. Patients admitted for assessment may apply within the first 14 days of detention. Patients admitted for treatment may apply within the first six months of detention, and again within six months if the detention order is renewed. In addition, a *Mental Health Act Commission* will ensure that hospitals have adopted and are following proper procedures for using the powers of detention. The Commission will also assist in giving staff guidance on good practice, which will be included in a Code of Practice. The Mental Health Act Commission is a new body. It has evolved a structure in which it will operate in independent groups from several regional offices.

Patients' information

The hospital managers must provide certain information to detained patients and their nearest relatives. This is to ensure that the detained patient understands the nature of his detention and his right to apply to a Mental Health Review Tribunal. They must also inform the person with whom the patient had last been living.

Consent to treatment

Compulsory detention does not mean that the patient may be automatically compelled to accept treatment. There are safeguards to ensure that either a second opinion or consent to treatment or both are obtained in the case of certain forms of treatment.

Treatment requiring consent and a second opinion

This section of the Act applies to the following forms of treatment where outcome is irreversible.
1 Psychosurgery—any surgical operation for destroying brain tissues or the function of the brain.
2 Surgical implantation of hormones. The Mental Health Act Commission must be notified to consider the validity of the patient's consent. They will jointly issue a certificate but, before doing so, the medical member will consult with a nurse and one other professional who have been concerned with the patient's treatment.

Treatment requiring consent or a second opinion

This section of the Act applies to the following forms of treatment.
1 The administration of medicine if three months or more have elapsed since medicine was first administered during that period of detention.
2 Electroconvulsive therapy.

If the patient does not consent to a treatment, the Mental Health Act Commission must be consulted for a second opinion. In addition the medical member will consult with a nurse and one other professional and the responsible medical officer before giving a second opinion.

Urgent treatment

Special conditions are set out for treating patients in an emergency but they exclude those treatments mentioned above. Such treatments will be necessary to save the patient's life, to prevent serious deterioration of his condition, to alleviate serious suffering by the patient or to prevent the patient from behaving violently or being a danger to himself or to others. In cases where treatment is not immediately necessary or it is proposed to continue treatment after the initial urgent administration, it will be necessary to contact the Mental Health Act Commission.

Withdrawing consent

If a patient withdraws his consent to any treatment, the treatment must not be given or must cease to be given immediately.

Powers of the Courts and the Home Secretary

In certain circumstances patients may be admitted to and detained in hospital on the order of a Court, or may be transferred to hospital from penal institutions on the direction of the Home Secretary. The courts also have the powers to remand to hospital for a medical report, to remand to hospital for treatment, and to obtain interim hospital orders.

Patients' property may be protected by the 'Court of Protection'.

Application of the Mental Health (Scotland) Act 1984

Unlike the Mental Health Act Commission in England and Wales, *The Mental Welfare Commission* in Scotland is not new. Under the 1984 Act it has increased duties and increased power. It is concerned with exercising 'protective function in respect of mentally disordered persons who may be incapable of adequately protecting their persons or their interests', whether they are compulsorily detained or not, and wherever they are, whether in hospital or in the community. (The Mental Health Act Commission in England and Wales is concerned only with detained patients.)

In Scotland there is no Mental Health Review Tribunal. Detained patients may appeal for discharge either to the Sheriff or to the Mental Welfare Commission, which has the power to order the discharge of a patient against medical advice.

The Mental Welfare Commission has the duty to bring to the attention of the managers any matter which they consider appropriate to secure the welfare of any patient by:

1 Preventing ill treatment
2 Remedying any deficiency in care or treatment
3 Preventing or redressing loss or damage to his property

Curator bonis

The Mental Welfare Commission has the power to petition for the appointment of a *curator bonis* to administer a patient's property and affairs.

The duties of the Mental Welfare Commission to visit, interview and examine patients who are compulsorily detained and to visit patients on leave of absence, and the power to hold enquiries and require persons to give evidence, are laid down in the Act.

Compulsory detention of patients

Provisions for Emergency Admission are similar to those in England and Wales. The term 'short-term detention' is used for detention up to 28 days and 'long-term detention' for a period of detention beyond that. Short- and long-term detention must be authorized by the Sheriff.

Nurses have the power to detain a patient for only two hours.

The Mental Welfare Commission is informed at specified intervals of the movements in and out of hospital, of renewal of authority to detain a patient and of matters concerning guardianship.

Safeguards concerning consent to treatment are similar to those which apply in England and Wales.

Patients may be detained in hospital on the order of a court, under the Criminal Procedure (Scotland) Act 1975. The Secretary of State is empowered to make an order restricting discharge.

Reprinted from Psychiatric Nursing (Altschul & McGovern) by kind permission of Baillière Tindall.

Appendix 5
Some Useful Addresses

Addiction problems

Alcoholics Anonymous, UK General Services Office, PO Box 514, 11 Redcliffe Gardens, London SW10.

Al-Anon Family Groups UK, 61 Dover Street, London SE1 4YF.

Alcohol Concern (The National Agency of Alcohol Misuse), 3 Grosvenor Crescent, London SW1 6LD.

Accept Clinic (for heavy drinking problems and problems with tranquillizers), 200 Seagrave Road, London SW6.

Ash (Action on Smoking and Health), Margaret Pike House, 5–11 Mortimer Street, London W1.

Drink Watchers, 200 Seagrave Road, London SW6.

Medical Council on Alcoholism, 31 Bedford Square, London WC1.

Scottish Council on Alcoholism, 147 Blythswood Street, Glasgow G2 4EN.

Northern Ireland Council on Alcoholism, 36/40 Victoria Street, Belfast.

Release (drug problems), 1 Elgin Avenue, London W9.

APA (Association for the Prevention of Addiction), 11 Grosvenor Street, Cardiff CF5 1NH.

ISDD (Institute for the Study of Drug Dependence), 1–4 Hatton Place, Hatton Garden, London EC1N 8ND.

Narcotics Anonymous, PO Box 246, London SW10.

Tranquillizer Withdrawal Support, 160 Tosson Terrace, Heaton, Newcastle NE6 5EA.

Tranx Release, Jane Bristow, 106 Welstead Avenue, Aspley, Nottingham.

Families Anonymous (for the friends and relatives of those with a drug problem), 88 Caledonian Road, London N1.

Gamblers Anonymous, 17/23 Blantyre Street, Cheyne Walk, London SW10.

Bereavement and stillbirth/miscarriage

Miscarriage Association, 18 Stoneybrook Close, West Bretton, Wakefield, West Yorkshire, WF4 4TP.

Stillbirth and Neonatal Death Society, Argyle House, 29/31 Euston Road, London NW1.

Foundation for the Study of Infant Deaths (counsel bereaved and anxious parents and give information), 5th floor, 4 Grosvenor Place, London SW1X.

Compassionate Friends (helps people who have lost a child of any age) B. Trimmer, 2 Norden Road, Blandford, Dorset.

Cruse (support group and counselling service in bereavement and for the carers of widows and widowers), Cruse House, 126 Sheen Road, Richmond, Surrey TW9.

Counselling

British Association for Counselling, 37a Sheep Street, Rugby, Warwickshire CV21 3BX.

Scottish Association for Counselling, 14 Caiystane Hill, Edinburgh EH10 6SL.

Developmental problems

National Autistic Society, 276 Willesden Lane, London NW2.

National Council for Special Education, 1 Wood Street, Stratford on Avon.

Fears and phobias

The Phobics Society, Katherine Fisher, 4 Cheltenham Road, Chorlton-cum-Hardy, Manchester M21 1QN.

Phobias Confidential, 1 Clovelly Road, Ealing, London W5 5HF.

The Open Door Association (agoraphobia), Mona Woodford (National Organizer), 447 Pensby Road, Heswall, Wirral, Merseyside.

Depression

Depressives Associated, 19 Merley Ways, Wimborne Minster, Dorset BH21 12N.

(this organization was formerly known as Depressives Anonymous).

Anorexia nervosa

Anorexia Aid, The Priory Centre, 11 Priory Road, High Wycombe, Buckinghamshire.

Anorexic Family Aid (AFA), Sackville Place, 44–48 Magdalen Street, Norwich, Norfolk NR3 1JE.

Schizophrenia

Schizophrenia Association of Great Britain, International Schizophrenia Centre, Bryn Hyfryd, The Crescent, Bangor, Gwynedd LL57 2AG.

National Schizophrenia Fellowship, J. Meirion Thomas (General Sec.) 79 Victoria Road, Surbiton, Surrey.

Suicide/parasuicide

The Samaritans (Secretary's office), 17 Uxbridge Road, Slough SL1 1SN.

Sexual and relationship difficulties

National Marriage Guidance Council, Herbert Gray College, Little Church Street, Rugby, Warwickshire.

General

MIND (National Association for Mental Health), 22 Harley Street, London W1.

Scottish Association for Mental Health, 40 Shandwick Place, Edinburgh EH2 4RT.

Appendix 6
Patient Assessment Form

The patient assessment form provides basic background
information on one side with guidelines for assessors on
the reverse.

Hospital _____ Ward/Unit _____ Date of admission _____ Date of assessment _____

Surname _____ Forename(s) _____ Age _____ Date of birth _____

Male ☐   Single ☐   Prefers to be addressed as _____ Type of accommodation _____

Female ☐   Married ☐   Address _____

  Widowed ☐   Length of time at this address _____ Family/Others at this residence _____

  Divorced ☐   Next of kin – name _____ Relationship _____

  Separated ☐   Address_____ Tel. no._____

Significant others – relatives/dependants _____ Any others specified by patient _____

Occupation _____ Name and address of general practitioner _____

Religious beliefs _____ _____

Reason for admission/referral

Diagnosis _____ Past history _____ Significant life crises _____

Patient's Perception of Self – Describe actual or potential problems identified by patient (see over).	**Others' Perceptions of Patient** (spouse/relatives/ friends) – see over.
	SUMMARY – Identify problems – actual (A) or potential (P). **Physical** (Use appropriate ALs to identify problems).
Nursing Perception of Patient – Describe objectively any actual or potential problems apparent at assessment, including any activities of living (see over) with which patient requires assistance.	
	Psychological – Identify the problems of (a) thought (b) mood (c) behaviour.
Signature of assessors: (1) _____ (2) _____ Date:_____	**Social**

Guidelines for Assessors

1 Patient's perception of his own level of functioning – That is, what does he/she complain of? What does he/she feel unable to do? Has there been a discernible change in the level of psychosocial functioning of late? If so, how has it manifested itself? How are the patient's relationships with others – at home/at work/socially? Is he/she socially active or inactive? Have there been any recent crises or changes in life circumstances?

2 Nurse's perceptions of patient's functioning – Objective assessment is important and the modified AL model (given below) may prove useful here.

3 Others' perceptions of patient's functioning – How do 'significant others' (family, spouse, friends) feel about the patient's level of functioning? Is there social/domestic stress? Do they express anxieties or doubts about his functioning? What does he complain of to them? What changes have they noticed? Is he insightful about his difficulties? How has his behaviour affected the family unit?

Activities of Living (ALs)

Roper (1976) has identified twelve ALs in respect of which patients may have actual or potential health problems and with which they may therefore require assistance. The twelve ALs are as follows:

1 Maintaining a safe environment – Has the patient any sensory deficit (poor eyesight, poor hearing or any loss of sensation?) Are adjustments in the patient's environment necessary due to confusion or suicidal feelings?

2 Communication – Does the patient communicate freely or is he withdrawn and uncommunicative? Is the content of his speech coherent and rational or does it reflect underlying thought disorder? Is he anxious or suspicious? Does he maintain eye contact? Are his non-verbal communications congruent with his verbal communications? Can he read and write? Remember that communication can be affected by mood, level of intelligence, personality traits and current awareness of reality.

3 Expressing sexuality – Do the patient's attitudes reflect an appropriate level of psychosexual maturity? Does the patient express sexual fears or anxieties? Does the patient express disordered sexual thoughts or feelings?

4 Working and playing – What is the patient's occupation? Where does he work? Are there any indications of difficulties in the work situation? What are his hobbies and interests? Is he socially active or isolated? Are difficulties in interpersonal and social relationships apparent? Does he have many friends? Does he complain of loss of efficiency or drive?

5 Sleeping – Does the patient suffer from insomnia? Does he feel refreshed or unrefreshed on waking? Does he suffer from 'early morning waking'? Is his mood lower in the mornings? Does he take sleeping tablets? Does he waken during the night? At what time does he usually retire to bed? What factors increase or decrease his sleep? Does he suffer from nightmares?

6 Eating and drinking – Does the patient take an adequate diet? Is there any evidence of anorexia or food refusal? Does the patient express delusional beliefs about his food? Is there any indication of excessive alcohol consumption or loss of control over alcohol consumption? Is the patient well-nourished or undernourished? Does he eat alone or with others? Is the patient able to eat and drink independently?

7 Personal cleansing and dressing – Is there evidence of self-neglect or loss of interest in personal hygiene? Does the patient express an interest in his/her appearance? Does the patient require assistance with cleansing and dressing due to confusion? Is there any loss of self-help skills in relation to cleansing and dressing. Does the patient's clothing reflect financial hardship?

8 Breathing – Does the anxious patient complain of difficulty in breathing or 'tightness in the chest'? Does he have any pain or discomfort associated with breathing? Does the patient smoke? If so, how many a day? Is he smoking more or less lately? Does he have anxieties associated with smoking?

9 Elimination – Does the patient experience frequency of micturition? Does he have constipation associated with low food/low fluid intake? Does he express delusional beliefs about bowel function?

10 Mobilizing – Is the patient physically active/overactive/inactive? Does the patient with cerebral pathology have any paralysis/anaesthesia/muscular pain or discomfort?

11 Controlling body temperature – Is there any evidence of flushing, excessive perspiration, goose flesh or shivering? Is there any evidence of pyrexia or hypothermia in the confused patient who may not be able to express any associated feeling or discomfort? Does the drug addict or alcoholic who may have been 'living rough' have any evidence of infection, as evidenced by pyrexia?

12 Dying – Does the patient express fears of death unjustified by his physical condition? Does he express suicidal or homicidal feelings? Is the patient preoccupied by fears of death?

Index

From Baillière Tindall

The Essential Text For All Nursing Students ...
and Recommended Reading for Qualified Nurses ...

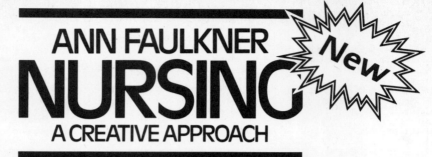

ANN FAULKNER
NURSING
A CREATIVE APPROACH

New

"The aim of the book is to teach nurses to identify patients' deficits and needs from the individual's perspective of his disease, so that creative and coherent care may be planned within the framework of the nursing process." Ann Faulkner (from the Preface)

For the first time we have an introduction to and review of nursing practice which captures the essence of the nursing process as an accepted basis for nursing care *but* goes much further in encouraging the nurse to consider the experience of illness from the patient's point of view.

In this comprehensive, psychology-based text the author has succeeded in combining considerable clinical detail with a constant awareness of the patient's feelings and requirements in a variety of hospital situations.

FEATURES OF THIS BOOK INCLUDE:

- **The Nursing Process,** as an implicit framework throughout the text. The philosophy and process of nursing are explained as they apply during the course of illness and the process is reinforced through headings and sub-headings in the text.

- **Emphasis on Patient Education** encourages the nurse to involve the patient, and to teach him to understand and respond positively to his illness and problems. There is also emphasis on general Health Education.

- **A Practical and Realistic Approach to Care** is described while the concept of the patient as an individual remains the main theme throughout.

- **Case Histories** are included to reinforce the theories of the holistic approach to nursing through *realistic* sketches of everyday nursing situations.

- **Potential Problems are Identified** and rational, caring solutions are suggested.

- **The Observation of the Physical and Psychological State of the Patient** is stressed with clear descriptions of signs to watch for and examples from case histories.

- **Practical Advice on Counselling and Communication** is given to ensure that the patient's individual problems are handled compassionately and continuously during his stay in hospital *and* after discharge.

- **A Wide Range of Illnesses** is covered and references to relevant nursing research are incorporated. Guidance is given to further study and personal reflection.

- **High Quality Illustrations** are included throughout the two-colour text emphasizing and complementing the message of the book.

ABOUT THE AUTHOR ...

Ann Faulkner PhD, MA, MLitt, SRN, RCNT, Dip. Ed., is Director of the Communication in Nursing Education Project at Manchester University; a former winner of the Baillière Prize for Nursing Studies, she is currently engaged in teaching and research related to communication in nursing practice and has a special interest in patients with cancer. In writing this book Ann Faulkner has drawn on her own nursing experience and wide clinical knowledge. This readable text reflects her caring attitude to patients and their problems. With rare clarity, she has been able, in this book, to pass on her insight into the complex relationships surrounding illness.

Prices, specifications and availability are subject to change without prior notification.
This book will be available through all leading booksellers.

BAILLIÈRE TINDALL   W.B.SAUNDERS

1, St Annes Road, Eastbourne, East Sussex BN21 3UN, UK

TABLE OF CONTENTS

This book is vital reading for all student nurses, and qualified nurses at all stages in their careers will appreciate this as a refreshing reappraisal of the many and varied needs of the patients in their care.

Paperback   464pp   225 ills   0 7020 1083 9   Baillière Tindall (UK)   August 1985